American Medical Association

Manual of Style

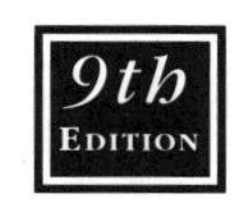

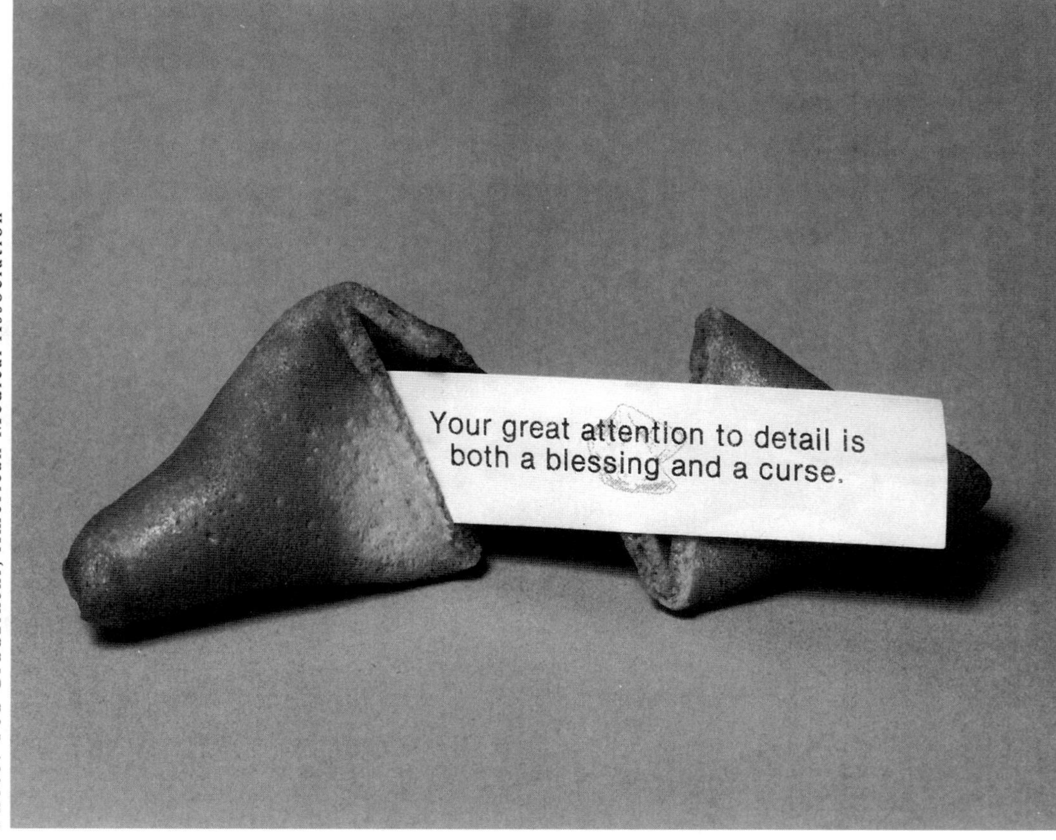

Photo: Ted Grudzinski, American Medical Association

American Medical Association
Manual of Style

A Guide for Authors and Editors

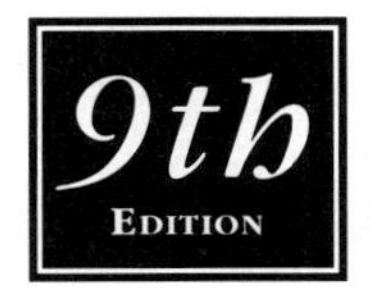

Cheryl Iverson, MA
(*Chair*)

Annette Flanagin, RN, MA

Phil B. Fontanarosa, MD

Richard M. Glass, MD

Paula Glitman

Jane C. Lantz, ELS

Harriet S. Meyer, MD

Jeanette M. Smith, MD

Margaret A. Winker, MD

Roxanne K. Young, ELS

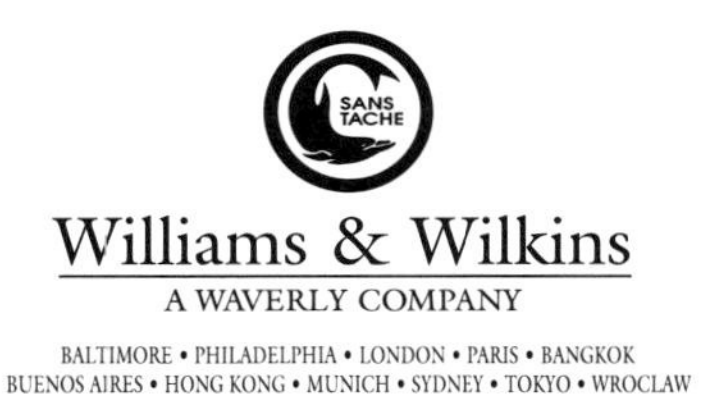
Williams & Wilkins
A WAVERLY COMPANY
BALTIMORE • PHILADELPHIA • LONDON • PARIS • BANGKOK
BUENOS AIRES • HONG KONG • MUNICH • SYDNEY • TOKYO • WROCLAW

Editor: Maureen Barlow Pugh
Marketing Manager: Elizabeth Haigh
Production Coordinator: Marette Magargle-Smith
Designer: Paul Fry
Cover Designer: Paul Fry
Typesetter: Bi-Comp, Inc.
Printer & Binder: RR Donnelley & Sons Co.

515 North State Street
Chicago, Illinois 60610 USA

351 West Camden Street
Baltimore, Maryland 21201-2436 USA

Rose Tree Corporate Center
1400 North Providence Road
Building II, Suite 5025
Media, Pennsylvania 19063-2043 USA

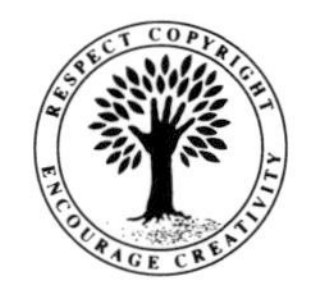

Printed in the United States of America

Library of Congress Cataloging-in-Publication Data

American Medical Association manual of style : a guide for authors and
editors.—9th ed. / Cheryl Iverson (chair) . . . [et al.]
p. cm.
Includes bibliographical references and index.
Other title: Guide for authors and editors.
ISBN 0-683-40206-4
1. Medical writing—Handbooks, manuals, etc. 2. Authorship—Style
manuals. I. Iverson, Cheryl. II. American Medical Association.
[DNLM: 1. Writing. WZ 345 A511 1997]
R119.A533 1997
808′.06661—dc21
DNLM/DLC
for Library of Congress 97-19246
CIP

The publishers have made every effort to trace the copyright holders for borrowed material. If they have inadvertently overlooked any, they will be pleased to make the necessary arrangements at the first opportunity.

To purchase additional copies of this book, call our customer service department at (800) 638-0672 or fax orders to (800) 447-8438. For other book services, including chapter reprints and large quantity sales, ask for the Special Sales department.

Canadian customers should call (800) 665-1148, or fax (800) 665-0103. For all other calls originating outside of the United States, please call (410) 528-4223 or fax us at (410) 528-8550.

***Visit Williams & Wilkins on the Internet:* http://www.wwilkins.com or contact our customer service department at custserv@wwilkins.com.** Williams & Wilkins customer service representatives are available from 8:30 am to 6:00 pm, EST. Monday through Friday, for telephone access.

98 99 00
3 4 5 6 7 8 9 10

Foreword

When Emily Flint died in the spring of 1996 at her home in Bedford, Mass, at the age of 85, her colleagues at the *Atlantic Monthly* paid her tribute in the July issue. When she was managing editor of the magazine during the 1950s and 1960s, not a word of those 2 decades ever escaped her eye, they wrote. And, although she never published a word in the magazine under her own name, her experience did find its way into some trenchant remarks that the *Atlantic*'s editors have now graciously passed on to today's generation of writers and editors. They are as applicable today as then: "The principles of good writing and good editing are the same," she said: "clarity, organization, and style."[1]

A generation and more earlier William Strunk, Jr, professor of English at Cornell University, had issued similar advice—imperatives, actually—to his students at Cornell, in the now-classic *The Elements of Style.* Only 43 pages long, it has since been known affectionately by Strunk's soubriquet, "the *little* book," even after E. B. White revised it (and almost doubled the number of pages) in 1959. If one could extract the essence of the message given by Flint, Strunk, and White, it would boil down to 2 words: Be clear.

This new edition of the *American Medical Association Manual of Style* has been prepared for just that purpose. It is a consensus of all that a group of *JAMA* and AMA *Archives* Journals editors believe is necessary to make a published manuscript clear and readable and, not least, reliable and authoritative. This new edition is designed, as were its more recent predecessors, not only for authors and editors, but for readers as well. If one may take a computer analogy, before a document sent from one terminal can be received by another and made intelligible to a human reader, it must conform to certain mutually agreed on standards and conventions. So it is with the publication of manuscripts in *JAMA* and the AMA *Archives* Journals. If the reader and the author are to be able to "shake hands," they must observe the same standards. Otherwise communication is impossible, or at best the data received are unclear or even misleading.

At one time *JAMA* and the AMA *Archives* Journals had no manual of style, or, more correctly, no manual of style that existed in written form. Copy editors, or manuscript editors as they are also known, carried everything in their heads. When an editor had a question about usage, nomenclature, punctuation, or some other matter in a manuscript, he or she simply asked another copy editor, who might either have the information or be able to supply a reference; sometimes an ad hoc group gathered and made a decision on the spot. If that was not sufficient, or if there were several equally good choices, or if perhaps an author objected, the "Chicago Style Manual," as it was known familiarly, served as referee.

Sometime during the mid-1960s, when the pace of everything, not least publishing, began accelerating, these decisions were collected and codified into a set of written rules. The result was the American Medical Association's first style manual for its scientific journals, a slim little volume of fewer than 70 pages with a green cardboard cover. It was helpful, except that soon things were moving even faster. Even as more papers were being written and submitted, and multiple authors, even multiple institutions, on a single manuscript were becoming the norm, the time to publication was being compressed. The acceleration of this change is reflected in the number and increasing size of the revised editions of the *AMA Manual of Style* that have been necessary since that first "in-house" edition: Eight.

This ninth, latest, and largest edition is compact nevertheless when one considers the amount and type of information provided to authors, editors, and readers. It should be remembered, too, that to produce a book such as this is, like the art of painting or the art of medicine, an ongoing process that adapts the past to the present to enable it to accommodate the future. It requires, for example, the patience and persistence of a Paul Cézanne as well as the brilliance and insight of a Claude Bernard. Every statement, every usage, every rule must be reexamined, rethought, and a consensus established as to which, among all the possibilities, is the best and clearest. And the choices that are made must cover not only the present, but a future that can only be guessed at.

The English of today has perhaps become a lingua franca, used not only in science and medicine across the world and in outer space, but even, as a *New York Times* editorial[2] noted, as the language of airports, the Internet, and rock music as well. Yet, at least in the language of medicine, one—whether reader, author, or editor—can move confidently, knowing that words mostly mean what they say, that sentences still have verbs and are marked by periods at the end, and that the same condition or disease will be both named and spelled the same regardless of who is writing about it. Moreover, when questions do arise—whether of which category is best suited to one's manuscript, which bibliographic particulars should be included in a reference and in what order they should be listed, how many authors can be named in a byline, what constitutes fraud or plagiarism, how to punctuate, how to refer to a virus or to an isotope, what "inclusive language" means, not to mention grammar and composition—there is a "little" book one can have recourse to that contains what Strunk and White called "the elements of style." Like their own *little* book, it is a rule book, but it is also more. It is a manual for the "dressing of thoughts," as Dickens so happily defined style on one occasion. There may be nothing, for example, quite so elegant as a comma, correctly placed. Yet if, like Will Strunk, the authors of the ninth edition of the *AMA Manual of Style* have deep sympathy for other authors, they have even deeper sympathy for readers. Hence, their final injunction to authors, again from Strunk and White: Be clear.

M. Therese Southgate, MD
Senior Contributing Editor, *JAMA*

REFERENCES

1. The Editors. 745 Boylston Street. *Atlantic Monthly.* July 1996:6.

2. How not to write English [editorial]. *New York Times.* March 14, 1996:A22.

PREFACE

The frontispiece is our whimsical allusion to something we take very seriously. We have added new sections, fresh examples, and revised policies—attempting to attend to the smallest detail with a minimum of cursing.

What's new in this edition?

- An expanded chapter on legal and ethical concerns in publishing, including copyright and intellectual property, authorship, and the rights and responsibilities of authors, editors, and reviewers
- An extensive chapter on statistics, featuring a section on study design and a large glossary of statistical terms, their definitions, and preferred presentation, including notes on common errors
- A completely updated chapter on nomenclature, including several new subsections
- New policies for eponyms and numbers style, with rationale and examples
- A larger references section, featuring new examples, including style recommendations for electronic references
- An expanded discussion of inclusive language and abbreviations
- A larger section on figures and tables, with a description of types of figures and their most appropriate use
- A new section on typography
- Current information on electronic publishing, including copyright issues and reference style, and a description of how rapid changes in the publishing environment have affected manuscript processing, from copyediting to printing
- End-of-chapter references (rather than end-of-book references) for greater ease of use; in chapters with many distinct subsections, we have included end-of-section references

What remains? Chapters that are at the heart of every editor's and author's concern, such as capitalization, grammar, correct usage, and punctuation, remain—all updated with new examples.

The work on the ninth edition proceeded much as that on the eighth. The committee divided the work, did independent research and writing, and critiqued chapters or sections at biweekly meetings. This cycle was repeated 2 or 3 times for most chapters and in some cases complete agreement was not reached: rather we agreed to disagree, and the majority opinion, even if not the opinion of every committee member, became the policy.

New to this edition is the attribution of "principal author" for each chapter or section. Because this was truly a group effort, we do not claim sole authorship but rather seek through this means to provide accountability.

After review by the committee, the draft of the manual (all or part) was reviewed by more than 70 in-house and external journal editors, managing editors, manuscript editors, and other critics. To these reviewers, we owe a tremendous debt. Their contributions were important in enhancing the substance of the manual, correcting errors, and polishing presentation. Any errors or omissions in the manual are solely the responsibility of the committee.

It is our hope that this book will be the basis for the development of digital versions to serve our users online as well as offline. We will take advantage of software and Internet technology to provide responsive, updated material in between printed editions of the *Manual of Style.* We welcome your comments regarding what would benefit you as a user. To comment or to note corrections, write to Cheryl Iverson, AMA, 515 N State St, Room 10240, Chicago, IL 60610 (e-mail: cheryl_iverson@ama-assn.org).

Cheryl Iverson, MA
Chair, AMA Style Manual Committee

Acknowledgments

The individuals listed below reviewed all or part of the manual in draft form. Their advice and comments were invaluable in adding clarity, polish, and additional substance to the manual. Any errors are solely the responsibility of the Style Manual Committee.

Janet Byron Anderson, PhD
Richard E. Appen, MD
Susan R. Benner, MLS
Marjorie A. Bowman, MD, MPA
Charlene Breedlove, MA
Carol Cadmus, ELS
Diane L. Cannon
Barbara J. Clark
Mary Coerver
Lois Ann Colaianni
Helene M. Cole, MD
Thomas B. Cole, MD, MPH
David S. Cooper, MD
Catherine D. DeAngelis, MD, MPH
Lois DeBakey, PhD
Judith Dickson, MS, ELS(D)
John H. Dirckx, MD
Faith T. Fitzgerald, MD
Susan Goeks
David Goldblatt, MD
Vickey Golden
Marsha F. Goldsmith
Rick Goodman, MD
Phil Gunby
Suzanne M. Hewitt, MPA
Wayne Hoppe, JD
Colleen M. Hubona
Robin Husayko
Edward Jyväskylä†
Laura King, MA
Elizabeth Knoll, PhD
Linda Knott
Carol L. Kornblith, PhD
Diane Berneath Lang
Thomas A. Lang, MA
Leonard A. Levin, MD, PhD
Stephen P. Lock, MD
Lorraine W. Loviglio
Faith McLellan, ELS
Peter M. Marzuk, MD
Carin M. Olson, MD
Karen Patrias
Roy M. Pitkin, MD
Charl Richey
Don Riesenberg, MD
Lee Ann Riesenberg, RN, MS
Povl Riis, MD, DHonC
Peggy Robinson, ELS
Jennifer Sperry, MA
Joan Stephenson, PhD
Marty Suter
Masaaki Terada, MD
Kate Whetzle, MA
Chris Zielinski

† Deceased.

In addition, 2 others must be singled out for special acknowledgment: George D. Lundberg, MD, Editor-in-Chief, Scientific Information and Multimedia, AMA, and Editor, *JAMA,* supported the research and writing of this new edition by members of his staff, and Nicole Netter, Lake Bluff, Ill, copyedited this edition.

CONTENTS

PREPARING AN ARTICLE FOR PUBLICATION

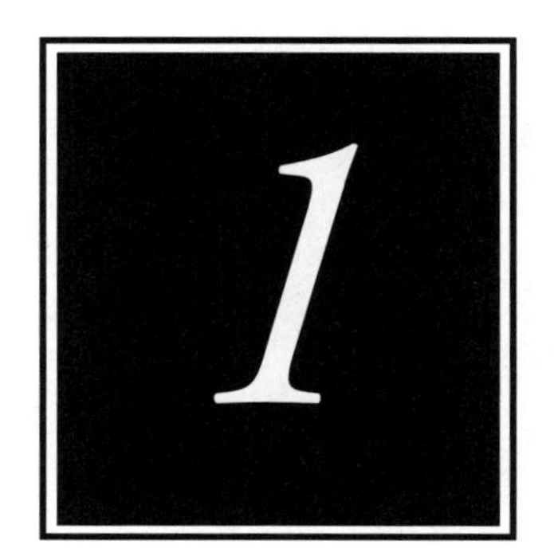

Chapter 1

1.0 Types of Articles

Effective written communication requires the author to consider the intended message and audience and use a form appropriate to both. Medical articles usually fit into one of the following main types.

1.1 ■ **REPORTS OF ORIGINAL DATA.**—Published reports of original research are the backbone of medical and scientific communications. Critical evaluation and replication of the findings of such reports are key aspects of quality control and progress in science and medicine; the clinical applications of original research are a major source of benefits for patients. Journals often categorize reports of original data as Original Articles, Original Contributions, or Original Reports—section headings that emphasize the new findings such articles intend to communicate. Short articles (in *JAMA,* those that occupy no more than 3 journal pages) that report new data may be called Brief Reports. Studies that address basic issues of physiology or pathology may be called Research Reports or Clinical Investigations. In *JAMA,* articles that report preliminary findings are called Preliminary Communications.

Articles that report original research results usually follow the traditional IMRAD (Introduction, Methods, Results, and Discussion) format. Changing the acronym to AIMRAD would give appropriate emphasis to the Abstract, which has become increasingly important in this era of information expansion and electronic databases. Structured abstracts, which provide summary information in one of several standard formats, have enhanced value and are now required by many medical journals for all reports of original data.[1] (See 2.5, Manuscript Preparation, Abstract, and 2.8, Manuscript Preparation, Parts of a Manuscript, Headings, Subheadings, and Side Headings, for guidance in preparing these sections.)

1.2 ■ **REVIEW ARTICLES.**—Review articles attempt to collate and summarize the available information on a particular topic, in contrast to reporting original data. Reviews carry great practical importance because clinicians often use them as guides for clinical decisions. This use highlights the importance of ensuring that reviews are systematic and not overly influenced by the opinions and biases of the authors. Systematic reviews specify the methods used to search for, select, and summarize the information to minimize bias and the chance of missing important data.[2] Some reviews use meta-analysis, a set of statistical techniques that combine quantitative results from independent studies. (See 17.2.7, Statistics, Meta-analysis.) All review articles should include a description of the methods used to perform the review. Structured abstracts for review articles provide authors a framework for the information that should be provided and enable readers to grasp quickly the methods and conclusions of a review.[3] (See 2.5.2, Manuscript Preparation, Structured Abstracts for Review Manuscripts [Including Meta-analyses].)

1.3 ■ **DESCRIPTIVE ARTICLES.**—Descriptions or observations that lack the systematic rigor of original research are often published as Case Reports (for patient descriptions), Clinical Observations, Special Articles, or Special Communications. To merit publication, such articles should make novel observations that can stimulate research or should provide useful delineations of topics of particular interest to a journal's readership. Because the scientific value of single case reports is often limited, many journals prefer to consider them Letters to the Editor and publish them only if they make a unique observation that merits systematic investigation.[4] Some medical journals publish case reports as educational tools. Grand Rounds presentations published in journals typically combine descriptive case material with a review of the major issues raised by the case. A standard format for descriptive articles does not exist. A short abstract may be helpful and usually is written in an unstructured narrative form.

1.4 ■ **CLINICAL PRACTICE GUIDELINES AND CONSENSUS STATEMENTS.**—Governmental and private organizations often develop recommendations for the diagnosis, treatment, and prevention of various disorders. These recommendations regarding appropriate clinical decisions usually are made by a group of experts after they assess the available evidence. Recommendations may be published as consensus statements developed at a conference or as clinical practice guidelines (sometimes called practice parameters) developed over time. In either case, publication of the recommendations should identify the sponsor and the participating experts, describe the evidence that supports the recommendations, and explain how the conclusions were reached. Structured abstracts can be helpful in summarizing this information.[5,6] (See 2.5.3, Manuscript Preparation, Structured Abstracts for Consensus Statements.)

1.5 ■ **ARTICLES OF OPINION.**—Editorials are short essays that usually express the views of the editor or the policies of the journal. They may be written by the editor, a member of the editorial staff or board, or an invited author. Editorials may comment on an article or articles in the same issue of the journal, providing additional context and opinion regarding implications, or they may deal with a separate topic of concern to the journal's readers. In the past, it was common for authors of journal editorials not to be identified, as is still the usual practice for newspaper editorials. This has become much less common as authorship responsibility has received increasing emphasis in medical publishing. (See 3.1.3, Ethical and Legal Considerations, Unsigned Editorials, Anonymous Articles, Pseudonymous Authors.) Journals infrequently publish unsolicited articles of opinion as editorials. Opinion pieces that represent only the views of the authors may be published in journal sections called Commentary, Sounding Board, Viewpoint, or Controversies.

1.6 ■ **CORRESPONDENCE.**—Recognizing that Letters to the Editor are an essential aspect of postpublication review, the International Committee of Medical Journal Editors has recommended that all biomedical journals "have a section carrying comments, questions, or criticisms about articles they have published and where the original authors can respond."[7] Published letters frequently comment on an article that was published in the same journal. Such letters and replies from the authors can provide lively and useful interchanges. Often 1 or 2 letters are chosen as representative of the responses to a particular article. Letters that do not pertain to a previous article may report original research data, describe a problem, report a case, or express an opinion. Journals usually have strict limitations on the number of words and references in published letters. Letters submitted for publication require statements of authorship responsibility, disclosure of conflicts of interest, and copyright transfer, and they may be subject to peer review and revision. Correspondents should always indicate whether letters sent to the editor are to be considered for publication.

1.7 ■ **REVIEWS OF BOOKS, JOURNALS, AND NEW MEDIA.**—Readers of such reviews seek both an overview of the product and an assessment of its quality relative to similar works. Thus, these reviews usually include description and opinion, both of which may extend to broader issues raised by the work. Individual style and expression can be included in these critiques, but supporting evidence for the reviewer's praise or criticism is essential.

1.8 ■ **OTHER TYPES OF ARTICLES.**—Journals publish other items and articles that do not fit into any of the major categories. Examples include the personal reflections in A Piece of My Mind in *JAMA,* news articles, reports on conferences, poetry, obituaries, and articles based on clinical photographs. Authors should examine several issues of a journal to ensure that a submission is appropriate and read the journal's instructions for authors to determine requirements regarding various types of articles.

ACKNOWLEDGMENT

Principal author: Richard M. Glass, MD

REFERENCES

1. Rennie D, Glass RM. Structuring abstracts to make them more informative. *JAMA.* 1991;266:116-117.

2. Cook DJ, Mulrow CD, Haynes RB. Systematic reviews: synthesis of best evidence for clinical decisions. *Ann Intern Med.* 1997;126:376-380.

3. Mulrow CD, Thacker SB, Pugh JA. A proposal for more informative abstracts of review articles. *Ann Intern Med.* 1988;108:613-615.

4. Riesenberg DE. Case reports in the medical literature. *JAMA.* 1986;255:2067.

5. Hayward RSA, Wilson MC, Tunis SR, Bass EB, Rubin HR, Haynes RB. More informative abstracts of articles describing clinical practice guidelines. *Ann Intern Med.* 1993;188:731-737.

6. Olson C. Consensus statements: applying structure. *JAMA.* 1995;273:72-73.

7. International Committee of Medical Journal Editors. Uniform requirements for manuscripts submitted to biomedical journals. *JAMA.* 1997;277:927-934.

Chapter 2

2.0 Manuscript Preparation

Preparation of a scholarly manuscript requires thoughtful consideration of the topic and anticipation of the reader's needs and questions. Certain elements either are standard parts of all manuscripts or are used so often as to merit special instruction. These elements are discussed in this section in the order in which they appear in the manuscript.

The preparation of any manuscript for publication should take the requirements of the intended journal into account; this may enhance the chances for acceptance and expedite publication. For the author, this requires familiarity with the journal to which the article is submitted. Most journals publish instructions for authors, which serve as useful guides; some publishers also publish style manuals, which provide in-depth instruction (see 22.1, Resources, Readings). For those journals that subscribe to the Uniform Requirements for Manuscripts Submitted to Biomedical Journals,[1] as the journals published by the AMA do, adherence to these guidelines will be acceptable, although the individual journal may make changes to suit its house style or require more items than the Uniform Requirements. Many journals also publish manuscript checklists (Table 1).

Some journal publishers may request submission of material on disk (Table 2), sent via e-mail, or as printed paper copies ("hard copy") suitable for electronic scanning (see 4.2, Editorial Assessment and Processing, Editorial Processing).

2.1 ■ TITLES AND SUBTITLES.

—Titles should be concise, specific, and informative, and should contain the key points of the work. Overly general titles are not desirable (see also 2.1.7, Names of Cities, States, and Countries).

Avoid: Cocaine Use and Homicide
Better: Cocaine and Homicide in Men in New York City, 1996

TABLE 1. MANUSCRIPT CHECKLIST

- Include original manuscript and 3 photocopies.
- Include statements—signed by each author—on (*a*) authorship criteria and responsibility, (*b*) financial disclosure, and (*c*) copyright transfer *or* federal employment.
- Include statement signed by corresponding author that written permission has been obtained from all persons named in the Acknowledgment.
- Include research or project support/funding in an acknowledgment.
- Double-space manuscript (text and references) and leave right margins unjustified (ragged).
- Check all references for accuracy and completeness. Put references in proper format in numerical order, making sure each is cited in the text.
- Send 4 sets of all illustrations. Black-and-white illustrations are nonreturnable. Four-color illustrations will be returned 3 months after publication.
- Provide and label an abstract.
- Include written permission from each individual identified as a source for personal communication.
- Include informed consent forms for identifiable patient descriptions, photographs, and pedigrees.
- Include written permission from publishers and authors to reproduce or adapt previously published illustrations and tables.
- On the title page, designate a corresponding author and provide a complete address, telephone and fax numbers, e-mail address, and word count.

TABLE 2. GUIDELINES FOR CREATING AN ELECTRONIC MANUSCRIPT*

- The lowercase letter *l* should not be substituted for the number 1 (one) and the capital letter *O* should not be substituted for zero, and vice versa.
- Words at the ends of lines should not be hyphenated unless the hyphen is normally part of the word.
- *After all revisions are made on the electronic copy of the manuscript,* print a paper copy ("hard copy"). Save the electronic file containing the manuscript as text only (ASCII [American Standard Code for Information Interchange]) without formatting codes and copy it onto a disk.
- Label the disk with the name and version number of the operating system and word-processing software, the corresponding author's name, the manuscript number (if the publisher has provided one), and the date.
- To prevent data from being erased from the disk, avoid attaching paper clips or any other metal or magnetic objects to it.
- Before mailing the disk, place it in a disk mailer or between 2 pieces of cardboard to protect it from being damaged.
- Always include 4 dated hard copies that match the disk copy exactly.

**The disk of an article should be provided only* after *final revision. This avoids potential confusion in processing different versions of the same article.*

Similarly, although the subtitle is frequently useful in expanding on the title, it should not contain key elements of the study as a supplement to an overly general title.

Avoid: Psychiatric Disorders: A Rural-Urban Comparison
Better: Rural-Urban Differences in the Prevalence of Psychiatric Disorders

Avoid: Multiple Sclerosis: Sexual Dysfunction and Response to Medications
Better: Sexual Dysfunction and Response to Medications in Multiple Sclerosis

Avoid: Hospitalization for Congestive Heart Failure: Explaining Racial Differences
Better: Racial Differences in Hospitalization Rates for Congestive Heart Failure

However, too much detail is also to be avoided. Subtitles should complement the title by providing supplementary information that will aid in information retrieval by computer or manual search. Examples of good title and subtitle combinations follow:

> *BRCA1* Testing in Families With Hereditary Breast-Ovarian Cancer: A Prospective Study of Patient Decision Making and Outcomes

> Prevention of Systemic Infections, Especially Meningitis, Caused by *Haemophilus influenzae* Type b: Impact on Public Health and Implications for Other Polysaccharide-Based Vaccines

Phrases such as "The Role of," "The Effects of," "The Treatment of," and "Report of a Case of" can usually be omitted from both titles and subtitles. Subtitles may be used to amplify the title; however, the main title should be able to stand alone (ie, the subtitle should not be a continuation of the title or a substitute for a succinct title):

> *Avoid:* An Unusual Type of Pemphigus: Combining Features of Lupus Erythematosus
> *Better:* Pemphigus With Features of Lupus Erythematosus

> *Avoid:* Von Hippel-Lindau Disease: Affecting 43 Members of a Single Kindred
> *Better:* Von Hippel-Lindau Disease in 43 Members of a Single Kindred

Declarative sentences are used frequently as titles of news stories and opinion pieces (eg, "Experts Set 1996 Influenza Vaccine and Plan for Unpredictable Pandemic," "Spate of Lawsuits May Finally Find Chink in Tobacco Industry's 'Impenetrable Armor' "). However, in scientific articles, they tend to overemphasize a conclusion, and AMA journals avoid them.

> *Avoid:* Fibromyalgia Is Common in a Postpoliomyelitis Clinic
> *Better:* Frequency of Fibromyalgia in Patients With Postpoliomyelitis Syndrome

> *Avoid:* Microdialysis Reduces Tissue Edema
> *Better:* Reduction of Tissue Edema by Microdialysis

Questions are more appropriate for editorials, commentaries, and opinion pieces (see examples below) than for original research articles.

> Translating Medical Science Into Medical Practice: Do We Need a National Medical Standards Board?

> Levothyroxine and Osteoporosis: An End to the Controversy?

> Toward Improved Glycemic Control in Diabetes: What's on the Horizon?

Randomized controlled trials should be identified in the title or subtitle because this information is helpful to researchers performing a meta-analysis:

> A Randomized Trial of Physical Rehabilitation for Frail Nursing Home Residents

> Influenza Vaccination in the Elderly: A Randomized, Double-blind, Placebo-Controlled Trial

Sometimes a subtitle will contain the name of the group responsible for the study, especially if the study is large and has been known by its group name or acronym (see also 11.9, Abbreviations, Collaborative Groups):

> Lowering Dietary Intake of Fat and Cholesterol in Children With Elevated Low-Density Lipoprotein Cholesterol Levels: The Dietary Intervention Study in Children (DISC)

Informed Consent in Emergency Research: Consensus Statement From the Coalition Conference of Acute Resuscitation and Critical Care Researchers

Prevention of Stroke by Antihypertensive Drug Treatment in Older Patients With Isolated Systolic Hypertension: Final Results of the Systolic Hypertension in the Elderly Program (SHEP)

2.1.1 ***Quotation Marks.***—If quotation marks are required in the title or subtitle, they should be *double,* not *single* (see 6.6.3, Punctuation, Quotation Marks, Titles).

Example: Above All "Do No Harm": How Shall We Avoid Errors in Medicine?

2.1.2 ***Numbers.***—Follow AMA style for numbers included in titles (see 16.0, Numbers and Percentages).

Examples: Educational Programs in US Medical Schools, 1994-1995

Quality of Care for Medicare Patients With Acute Myocardial Infarction: A 4-State Pilot Study From the Cooperative Cardiovascular Project

Randomized Trial of 3-Day Antimicrobial Regimen for Treatment of Acute Cystitis in Women

Laboratory Analysis of Blood Samples From 54 Patients With HIV-1 Infection

If numbers appear at the beginning of a title or subtitle, they—and any unit of measure associated with them—should be spelled out. Exceptions may be made for years (see also 16.2.1, Numbers and Percentages, Spelling Out Numbers, Beginning a Sentence, Title, Subtitle, or Heading).

Examples: Primary and Secondary Prevention Services in Clinical Practice: Twenty Years' Experience in Development, Implementation, and Evaluation

Seventy-five Years of the *Archives of Surgery:* 1920 to 1995

2.1.3 ***Drugs.***—If drug names appear in the title or subtitle, (1) use the approved generic or nonproprietary name, (2) omit the nonbase moiety unless it is required (see 12.4, Nomenclature, Drugs), and (3) avoid the use of proprietary names unless (*a*) several products are being compared, (*b*) the article is commenting on only 1 brand of the product in question, or (*c*) the number of ingredients is so large that the resulting title would be clumsy and a generic term, such as "multivitamin tablet," would not do.

2.1.4 ***Genus and Species.***—Genus and species should be expanded and italicized in the title or subtitle and an initial capital letter should be used for the genus but not the species name, just as in the text (see also 12.12, Nomenclature, Organisms).

2.1.5 ***Abbreviations.***—Avoid the use of abbreviations in the title and subtitle, unless space considerations require an exception (see also 11.0, Abbreviations).

2.1.6 ***Capitalization.***—Capitalize the first letter of each major word in titles and subtitles. Do not capitalize articles, prepositions of 3 or fewer letters, coordinating conjunctions (*and, or, for, nor, but*), or the *to* in infinitives. *Do* capitalize a 2-letter verb, such as *Is*. Exceptions are made for some expressions:

> Ethical Questions Surrounding In Vitro Fertilization
>
> Permanent Duplex Surveillance of In Situ Saphenous Vein Bypasses
>
> Universal Screening for Tuberculosis Infection: School's Out!

For capitalization of hyphenated compounds, see 8.4, Capitalization, Titles and Headings.

2.1.7 ***Names of Cities, States, and Countries.***—Include cities, states, or countries in titles only when essential (eg, unique to that site), with results that may not be generalizable to other locations.

> The Epidemic of Gang-Related Homicides in Los Angeles County From 1979 Through 1994

In other cases, include this information in the abstract and the text only (see also 11.5, Abbreviations, US States, Territories, and Possessions; Provinces; Countries).

> *Avoid:* Pertussis Infection in Adults With Persistent Cough in Nashville, Tenn
> *Better:* Pertussis Infection in Adults With Persistent Cough
>
> *Avoid:* Hospitalization Charges, Costs, and Income for Trauma-Related Injuries at the University of California, Davis, Medical Center in Sacramento
> *Better:* Hospitalization Charges, Costs, and Income for Trauma-Related Injuries at a University Trauma Center

2.2 ■ **BYLINES AND END-OF-TEXT SIGNATURES.**—In major articles, authorship is indicated by a byline, which appears immediately below the title or subtitle. The byline should contain each author's full name (unless initials are preferred to full names), including, for example, Jr, Sr, II, III, and middle initials, and highest academic degree(s). In letters, editorials, book reviews, and news stories, the authors' names appear as signatures at the end of the text, rather than as a byline on the first page. The authors' names and academic degrees are used, as in the byline. Further information given in the signature varies with the journal. The author should consult a recent issue for style and format. Authors should be consistent in the presentation of their names in all published works for ease of use by indexers, catalogers, and database searchers.

2.2.1 ***Authorship.***—All persons listed as authors should qualify for authorship (see 3.1, Ethical and Legal Considerations, Authorship Responsibility, and 3.1.2, Ethical and Legal Considerations, Guest and Ghost Authors). Order of authorship should be determined by the authors (see 3.1.5, Ethical and Legal Considerations, Order of Authorship). According to the International Committee of Medical Journal Editors,

> Each author should have participated sufficiently in the work to take public responsibility for the content. Authorship credit should be based only on substantial contributions to (1) conception and design, or analysis and interpretation of data; and to (2) drafting the article or revising it critically for important intellectual content; and on (3) final approval of the version to be published. Conditions (1), (2), and (3) must all be met.[1]

Editors may ask authors to describe what each author contributed, and this may be published at the editor's discretion.

Persons who made subsidiary contributions may be listed, with their permission, in the Acknowledgment section (see 2.10.2, Other Assistance, and 3.2, Ethical and Legal Considerations, Acknowledgments). *JAMA* requires justification to list more than 6 authors in the byline (see 3.1.4, Ethical and Legal Considerations, Number of Authors).

In rare cases, authors may request that their names be withheld from publication. In those cases, the author must meet the authorship criteria but the byline may reflect the author's desire for anonymity (see 3.1.3, Ethical and Legal Considerations, Unsigned Editorials, Anonymous Articles, Pseudonymous Authors):

George B. Smith, MD; Name Withheld on Request of Second Author

2.2.2 ***Degrees.***—Journals should establish their policies on inclusion of authors' degrees. AMA journal policy is as follows: If an author holds 2 doctoral degrees (eg, MD and PhD, or MD and JD), either or both may be used, in the order preferred by the author. If the author has a doctorate, degrees at the master's level usually are not included, although exceptions may be made when the master's degree represents a specialized field or a field different from that represented by the doctorate (eg, MD, MPH).

Academic degrees below the master's level usually are omitted unless these are the highest degrees held. Exceptions are made for specialized professional certifications, degrees, and licensure (eg, RN, RD, COT, PA) and for specialized bachelor's degrees (eg, BSN, BPharm) and combination degrees (eg, BS, M[ASCP]).

Generally, US fellowship designations (eg, FACP or FACS) and honorary degrees (eg, PhD[Hon]) are omitted. However, non-US designations such as the British FRCP or FRCS and the Canadian FRCPC are included. (See 11.1, Abbreviations, Academic Degrees and Honors.)

If an author is on active duty in the armed services, only the service designation should be used (see also 11.2, Abbreviations, US Military Services and Titles).

CPT James B. Dane, MC, USA; LTC Carl Seller, Jr, MC, USA

2.2.3 ***Multiple Authors, Group Authors.***—When the byline contains more than 1 name, use semicolons to separate the authors' names.

Melvin H. Freedman, MD, FRCPC; E. Fred Saunders, MD, FRCP; Louise Jones, MD, PhD; Kurt Grant, RN

John E. Ware, Jr, PhD; Martha S. Bayliss, MSc; William H. Rogers, PhD; Mark Kosinski, MA; Alvin R. Tarlov, MD

Thomas G. Delap, FRCS; Antonios Kaberos, MD; William E. Grant, FRCSI; Michael P. Stearns, FRCS

When a byline or signature contains the name of a group and 1 or more individuals' names, use *for* followed by the name of the group only if the individuals named qualify for authorship and are writing for the group.

William A. Tasman, MD; for the Laser ROP Study Group

Occasionally a specific subgroup of a larger group will be listed as the author:

Executive Committee for the Symptomatic Carotid Atherosclerotic Study

The Writing Group for the DISC Collaborative Research Group

If only a group or subgroup is listed as the author and no specific individual is named anywhere in the article, a person should be named as corresponding author (see also 2.3.8, Reprint or Correspondence Address).

Byline: The Diabetes Control and Complications Trial Research Group

Footnotes: Corresponding author: David M. Nathan, MD, Diabetes Unit, Massachusetts General Hospital, 32 Fruit St, Boston, MA 02114-2698.

Reprints: DCCT Research Group, Box NDIC/DCCT, Bethesda, MD 20892.

Use *and* followed by the name of the group if each member of the group as well as the individuals named in the byline or signature qualify for authorship. In this case, every member of the group must sign a statement that he or she meets the criteria for authorship (see 3.1.6, Ethical and Legal Considerations, Group and Collaborative Authorship, and 11.9, Abbreviations, Collaborative Groups).

Debra L. Hanson, MS; Susan Y. Chu, PhD; Karen M. Farizo, MD; John W. Ward, MD; and the Adult and Adolescent Spectrum of HIV Disease Project Group

If each member of the group qualifies for authorship, the group name may be listed in the byline or signature without naming any individuals (see 2.3.3, Author Affiliations, and 2.10.4, List of Participants in a Group Study).

Council on Scientific Affairs, American Medical Association

2.3 ■ FOOTNOTES TO TITLE PAGE.

2.3 ■ FOOTNOTES TO TITLE PAGE.—Footnotes should be avoided within the text. Such explanatory material usually can be incorporated into the text parenthetically. The footnotes discussed are those that may appear at the bottom of the first page of major articles.

2.3.1 ***Order of Footnotes.***—The preferred order of the footnotes at the bottom of the first page of an article in AMA publications is as follows. *Note:* Not all articles will include *all* of these.

JAMA

- Author affiliations
- Financial disclosure (see 3.5.1, Ethical and Legal Considerations, Author's Disclosure)
- Death of an author (death dagger [†]) (see 2.3.5, Death)
- Previous presentations (ie, "read before" or "presented at" notices)
- Disclaimer (if necessary to separate author's views of those of employers, funding agencies or organizations, or others)
- Corresponding author or reprint address

Byline: John A. Doe, MD; Myrtle S. Coe, MD†; Simon T. Foe, RN

Footnotes: From the Department of Pediatrics, Baylor College of Medicine, Houston, Tex.

Dr Doe is a consultant to Baxter Diagnostics Inc, Miami, Fla.

†Dr Coe died February 27, 1996.

Presented in part at the Society of General Internal Medicine annual meeting, April 30, 1994, Washington, DC.

The views herein are those of the authors and are not necessarily those of the Robert Wood Johnson Foundation.

Reprints: John A. Doe, MD, Department of Pediatrics, Baylor College of Medicine, 1 Baylor Plaza, Houston, TX 77030 (e-mail: jdoe@baylor.edu).

Archives Journals

- Author affiliations and financial disclosure
- Death of author

(In the *Archives* Journals, the additional material published on the first page of an article in *JAMA* is given in the Acknowledgments [see 2.10, Acknowledgments] and is preceded by the acceptance date.)

2.3.2 ***Acceptance Date.***—Some journals include the date of the manuscript's acceptance; others include the date of acceptance and the date revised and, when relevant, the date the revised version was received. Those AMA journals that include the acceptance date use the following form:

Accepted for publication May 15, 1996.

2.3.3 ***Author Affiliations.***—The institutions with which an author is professionally affiliated, including location, are given in a footnote. Title and academic rank are *not* included in this footnote. List the affiliations in the order of the authors' names as given in the byline, but, for ease of grouping, combine the listings of authors affiliated with the same institution (eg, if the byline includes authors A, B, and C and if authors A and C are at the same institution, list the institution of authors A and C first and then the institution of author B) and list authors in private practice at the end.

Byline: Gary T. Jeng, MS; James R. Scott, MD; Leon F. Burmeister, PhD
Affiliation: From the Department of Preventive Medicine, University of Iowa, Iowa City (Mr Jeng and Dr Burmeister); and the Department of Obstetrics and Gynecology, University of Utah, Salt Lake City (Dr Scott).

Byline: Daniel G. Deschler, MD; Robert Osorio, MD; Nancy L. Ascher, MD, PhD; Kelvin C. Lee, MD
Affiliation: From the Departments of Otolaryngology-Head and Neck Surgery (Drs Deschler and Lee) and General Surgery (Drs Osorio and Ascher), University of California, San Francisco.

Byline: Jeremiah Brown, Jr, MD; John H. Fingert; Chris M. Taylor; Max Lake, MD; Val C. Sheffield, MD, PhD; Edwin M. Stone, MD, PhD
Affiliation: From the Departments of Ophthalmology (Drs Brown and Stone, Mr Fingert, and Ms Taylor) and Pediatrics (Dr Sheffield), University of Iowa, Iowa City. Dr Lake is in private practice in Salina, Kan.

The affiliation listed, including departmental affiliation if appropriate, should reflect the author's institutional affiliation at the time the work was done. If the author has since moved, the current affiliation also should be provided.

From the Department of Health Policy and Management, The Johns Hopkins University School of Hygiene and Public Health, Baltimore, Md. Dr Lloyd is now with the Department of Emergency Medicine, St Luke's Hospital, Milwaukee, Wis.

If several authors are affiliated with different institutions or different departments at the same institution, this information should be indicated parenthetically.

From the Hematology Laboratory Service, Duke University Medical Center, Durham, NC (Dr Ioachim); and the Hematology Department, Ball Memorial Hospital, Muncie, Ind (Dr Hanson).

From the Departments of Pediatrics (Dr Nelson), Pathology (Dr Ellenberg), and Radiology (Dr Chan), Emory University School of Medicine, Atlanta, Ga.

From the Rocky Mountain Poison and Drug Center, Denver Department of Health and Hospitals (Dr Dart, Ms Stark, and Mr Fulton), and Colorado Emergency Medicine Research Center, University of Colorado Health Sciences Center (Drs Dart and Lowenstein and Ms Koziol-McLain), Denver, Colo.

If the byline includes names of Chinese, Japanese, or Vietnamese origin, or other names in which the family name is traditionally given *first,* the author should be asked to verify the surname when it is used parenthetically in the affiliation footnote.

For large groups, the name of the group may be given in the byline, and an affiliation footnote may refer the reader to the end of the article or to another publication for a complete listing of the participants (see also 2.2.3, Multiple Authors, Group Authors, and 2.10.4, List of Participants in a Group Study).

A complete list of the members of the Human Fetal Tissue Working Group appears at the end of this article.

A complete listing of the centers and selected committees that participated in this study was published previously (*Arch Ophthalmol.* 1994;112:482).

If the byline contains the names of several individuals and a group name, a combination of the forms mentioned should be used.

Byline: Sanjay Sharma, MD; Arif Naqvi, MD; Susan M. Sharma, MD; Alan F. Cruess, MD; Gary C. Brown, MD; for the Retinal Emboli of Cardiac Origin Group

Affiliation: From Queen's University, Kingston, Ontario. A complete list of the members of the Retinal Emboli of Cardiac Origin Group is given at the end of this article.

2.3.4 ***Financial Disclosure.***—AMA journals require each author to submit to the editor a statement that specifies whether the author has financial or proprietary interest in the subject matter or materials discussed in the manuscript, including (but not limited to) employment, consultancies, stock ownership, honoraria, and paid expert testimony. If the manuscript is accepted, the editor decides whether this information is published (see 3.5, Ethical and Legal Considerations, Conflicts of Interest). The financial disclosure statement is usually published with the affiliation footnote on the first page of the article. (*Note:* In *JAMA,* it is published as a separate footnote.)

Dr Healthy has received monetary compensation for speaking engagements from several pharmaceutical companies, including some that manufacture ACE inhibitors. [This is for an article on randomized trials of ACE (angiotensin-converting enzyme) inhibitors.]

Dr Healthy has testified as an expert witness in litigation matters involving resuscitation equipment. [This is for an article on cardiopulmonary resuscitation.]

Dr Healthy has a proprietary interest in patent 4 724 522 and other patents covering tangential refractory photokeratectomy. None of the other authors or contributors has proprietary or financial interest in the technology or devices used in this study.

Drs Healthy and Wise are consultants for Humphrey Instruments Inc, San Leandro, Calif.

Dr Healthy was paid by Wyeth-Ayerst for his role in analyzing the data and writing the manuscript. Dr Wise was employed by and owned stock in Wyeth-Ayerst while the study and analysis were being conducted.

Note: The financial disclosure may be a disclosure of *no* potential conflicts of interest. This is not obligatory, and the choice not to include such a statement should not be misinterpreted as an indication of a conflict. The absence of this statement is not self-incriminating.

The authors have no commercial, proprietary, or financial interest in the products or companies described in this article.

The authors have no commercial, proprietary, or financial interest (as consultant, reviewer, or evaluator) in fluorouracil.

2.3.5 ***Death.***—If an author of an article is deceased at the time of publication, a death dagger (†) should follow the author's name in the byline, and one of the following footnotes should be inserted after the affiliation footnote:

†Dr Parhad died June 26, 1996.

†Deceased.

2.3.6 ***Previous Presentations.***—The following forms are used for material that has been read or exhibited at a professional meeting. The original spelling and capitalization of the meeting name should be retained. Provide the exact date and location of the meeting.

Presented in part at the annual sessions of the Society of General Internal Medicine, Washington, DC, April 30, 1993, and San Diego, Calif, May 4, 1995.

Presented as a poster at the 46th Annual Scientific Assembly of the North Carolina Academy of Family Physicians, Greensboro, March 24-27, 1994.

2.3.7 ***Disclaimer.***—A footnote of disclaimer is used to separate the views of the authors from those of employers, funding agencies, organizations, or others. This notation precedes the reprint address. Editors should retain the author's phrasing.

The views expressed herein are those of the authors and do not necessarily reflect the views of the US Army or the US Department of Defense.

Use of trade names or names of commercial sources is for information only and does not imply endorsement by the US Public Health Service or the US Department of Health and Human Services.

Opinions in this article should not be interpreted as the official position of the International Committee of the Red Cross.

2.3.8 ***Reprint or Correspondence Address.***—A complete mailing address (street address, if possible, with ZIP or postal code, and e-mail address, if the author wishes) is provided in a footnote for readers who want reprints or for authors who do not intend to offer reprints but would like their addresses to be included for informal correspondence with interested readers. Even for a single author, the full name of the person to be addressed should be included. Follow the custom of individual countries regarding the placement of the ZIP or postal code.

Reprints: Daniel M. Barry, MD, Bridge Defense Foundation, 111 N First St, French Lick, IN 47432.

Reprints: Jeremy L. Freeman, MD, Mount Sinai Hospital, 600 University Ave, Room 401, Toronto, Ontario, Canada M5G 1X5.

Reprints: Andreas U. Monsch, PhD, Memory Clinic, Kantonsspital, Hebestrasse 10, 4031 Basel, Switzerland.

Reprints: Itsuzo Shigematsu, MD, MPH, FRCP, Radiation Effects Research Foundation, 5-2 Hijiyama Park, Minami-ku, Hiroshima 732, Japan.

Reprints: S. Goya Wannamethee, PhD, Department of Public Health, Royal Free Hospital School of Medicine, Rowland Hill Street, London NW3 2PF, England.

Corresponding author: Norbert E. Schindlbeck, MD, Medizinische Klinik, Klinikum Innerstadt der Universität, Ziemstrasse 1, 80336 Munich, Germany.

Corresponding author: Kenneth F. C. Fearon, MD, University Department of Surgery, Royal Infirmary, Lauriston Place, Edinburgh EH3 9YW, Scotland.

If the author does not intend to offer reprints, use the following footnote:

Reprints not available from the author.

If requests for reprints are to be sent to one author and a second author wants to receive correspondence about the article, list the corresponding author's name and address first and the address of the author to whom reprint requests are to be sent second.

Corresponding author: Paul R. Cieslak, MD, Oregon Health Division, 800 NE Oregon St, Suite 772, Portland, OR 97232 (e-mail: cieslak@state.or.us).

Reprints: Foodborne and Diarrheal Diseases Branch, Mail Stop A-38, Centers for Disease Control and Prevention, 1600 Clifton Rd, Atlanta, GA 30333.

Note: E-mail addresses may be included, *at the author's discretion,* either alone or in conjunction with a mailing address:

Reprints: J. Megginson Hollister, PhD, University of Pennsylvania, Neuropsychiatry Section, 10th Floor, Gates Building, Philadelphia, PA 19104-4283 (e-mail: meggin@hirisk.psych.upenn.edu).

Corresponding author: Mary T. Wright, Northwestern University Medical School, 45 E Grand Ave, Room 403, Chicago, IL 60610 (e-mail: mwright@nwu.edu).

Corresponding author: Patrick L. Twomey, MD (e-mail: patt@itsa.ucsf.edu).

2.4 ■ **RUNNING FOOT.**—Printed pages customarily carry the journal name or abbreviation, volume number, date of issue, and page number. They may also include a shortened version of the article title. When this information appears at the top of the page, it is called a *running head*; when it appears at the bottom of the page, as it does in AMA publications, it is called a *running foot.*

2.4.1 ***Name of the Publication.***—Use the accepted *Index Medicus* abbreviations of journal names (see 11.10, Abbreviations, Names of Journals) and the following forms, as applicable to the journal involved:

JAMA:	JAMA, July 17, 1996—Vol 276, No. 3
Archives Journals:	Arch Intern Med/Vol 155, Feb 27, 1995

Note that journals will differ in the amount of information included in their running feet and that the style for some abbreviations (eg, the month in the *Archives* example) may differ from that used elsewhere in the publication.

2.4.2 ***Title of the Article.***—The shortened version of the title should be kept short (approximately 45 characters and spaces in *JAMA*). If there are 2 authors, their surnames should be joined by an ampersand. If there are 3 or more authors, the surname of the first should be used, followed by "et al." No punctuation follows the running foot.

Title:	Taking Health Status Into Account When Setting Capitation Rates
Running Foot:	Adjusting Capitation Rates—Fowles et al
Title:	Decline in Hospital Utilization and Cost Inflation Under Managed Care in California
Running Foot:	Decline in Hospital Utilization and Costs—Robinson
Title:	Domestic Production vs International Immigration: Options for the US Physician Workforce
Running Foot:	Domestic vs International Physician Workforce—Kindig & Libby

In some instances, the article will be identified in the running head or foot by its editorial department rather than by its title and author, eg, Editorials, Commentary, Letters.

2.5 ■ **ABSTRACT.**—In this age of electronic data dissemination and retrieval, a well-written abstract has become increasingly important in directing readers to articles of potential clinical and research interest. The abstract of a research report summarizes the main points of an article: (1) the study objective or background, (2) the study design and methods, (3) primary results, and (4) principal conclusions. Empty narrative expressions, such as "X is described," "Y is discussed," "Z is also reviewed," do not add meaning and should be avoided. For reports of original data and for review articles, meta-analyses, and consensus statements, structured abstracts are recommended (see specific instructions [sections 2.5.1-2.5.3] from *JAMA*,[2] adapted from Haynes et al[3]).

2.5.1 ***Structured Abstracts for Reports of Original Data.***—Authors submitting manuscripts reporting original data should prepare an abstract of no more than 250 words under the following headings: Context, Objective, Design, Setting, Patients or Other Participants, Intervention, Main Outcome Measure(s), Results, and Conclusions. The content that follows each heading should be as follows:

1. Context.—The abstract should begin with a sentence or two summarizing the rationale for the study, providing the clinical (or other) reason for the study question.

2. Objective.—The precise objective or question addressed in the report should be stated. If more than 1 objective is addressed, the main objective should be indicated and only key secondary objectives stated. If an a priori hypothesis was tested, it should be stated.

3. Design.—The basic design of the study should be described. The duration of follow-up, if any, should be stated. As many of the following terms as apply should be used.

A. Intervention studies: randomized controlled trial; nonrandomized controlled trial; double-blind; placebo controlled; crossover trial; before-after trial.

B. For studies of screening and diagnostic tests: criterion standard (that is, a widely accepted standard with which a new or alternative test is being compared; this term is preferred to "gold standard"); blinded or masked comparison.

C. For studies of prognosis: inception cohort (subjects assembled at a similar and early time in the course of the disorder and followed thereafter); cohort (subjects observed forward in time, but not necessarily from a common starting point); validation cohort or validation sample if the study involves the modeling of clinical predictions.

D. For studies of causation: randomized controlled trial; cohort; case-control; survey (preferred to "cross-sectional study").

E. For descriptions of the clinical features of medical disorders: survey; case series.

F. For studies that include a formal economic evaluation: cost-effectiveness analysis; cost-utility analysis; cost-benefit analysis.

For new analyses of existing data sets, the data set should be named and the basic study design disclosed.

4. Setting.—To assist readers to determine the applicability of the report to their own clinical circumstances, the study setting(s) should be described. Of particular importance is whether the setting is the general community, a primary care or referral center, private or institutional practice, or ambulatory or hospitalized care.

5. Patients or Other Participants.—The clinical disorders, important eligibility criteria, and key sociodemographic features of patients should be stated. The numbers of participants and how they were selected should be provided, including the number of otherwise eligible subjects who were approached but refused. If matching is used for comparison groups, characteristics that are matched should be specified. In follow-up studies, the proportion of participants who completed the study must be indicated. In intervention studies, the number of patients withdrawn because of adverse effects should be given.

For selection procedures, these terms should be used, if appropriate: random sample (where "random" refers to a formal, randomized selection in which all eligible subjects have a fixed and usually equal chance of selection); population-based sample; referred sample; consecutive sample; volunteer sample; convenience sample. These terms assist the reader to determine an important element of the generalizability of the study. They also supplement (rather than duplicate) the terms used by professional indexers when articles are entered into computerized databases.

6. Intervention(s).—The essential features of any interventions should be described, including their method and duration of administration. The intervention should be named by its most common clinical name (for example, the generic term "chlorthalidone"). Common synonyms should be given as well to facilitate electronic text-word searching. This would include the brand name of a drug if a specific product was studied.

7. Main Outcome Measure(s).—The primary study outcome measurement(s) should be indicated as planned before data collection began. If the paper does not emphasize the main planned outcomes of a study, this fact should be stated and the reason indicated. If the hypothesis being reported was formulated during or after the data collection, this information should be clearly stated.

8. Results.—The main results of the study should be given. Measurements that require explanation for the expected audience of the manuscript should be defined. Important measurements not included in the presentation of results should be declared. As relevant, it should be indicated whether observers were blinded to patient groupings, particularly for subjective measurements. Because of the current limitations of retrieval from electronic databases, results must be given in narrative or point form rather than tabular form if the abstract is to appear in computerized literature services such as MEDLINE. The results should be accompanied by confidence intervals (for example, 95%) and the exact level of statistical significance. For comparative studies, confidence intervals should relate to the differences between groups. For nonsignificant differences for the major study outcome measure(s), the clinically important difference sought should be stated and the confidence interval for the difference between the groups should be given. When risk changes or effect sizes are given, absolute values should be indicated so that the reader can determine the absolute as well as the relative impact of the finding. Approaches such as "number needed to treat" to achieve a unit of benefit are encouraged when appropriate; reporting of relative differences alone is usually inappropriate. If appropriate, studies of screening and diagnostic tests should use the terms "sensitivity," "specificity," and "likelihood ratio." If predictive values or accuracy is given, prevalence or pretest likelihood should be given as well. No data should be reported in the abstract that do not appear in the rest of the manuscript.

9. Conclusions.—Only those conclusions of the study that are directly supported by the evidence reported should be given, along with their clinical application (avoiding speculation and overgeneralization), and indicating whether additional study is required before the information should be used in usual clinical settings. Equal emphasis must be given to positive and negative findings of equal scientific merit.

To permit quick and selective scanning, the headings outlined above should be included in the abstract. For brevity, parts of the abstract can be written in phrases rather than complete sentences. (For example: "3. *Design.* Double-blind randomized trial," rather than "3. *Design*. The study was conducted as a double-blind, randomized trial.") This technique may make reading less smooth but facilitates selection scanning and allows more information to be conveyed per unit of space.

2.5.2 ***Structured Abstracts for Review Manuscripts (Including Meta-analyses).***—Authors submitting review manuscripts and reports of the results of meta-analyses should prepare an abstract of no more than 250 words under the following headings: Objective, Data Sources, Study Selection, Data Extraction, Data Synthesis, and Conclusions. The manuscript should also include a section that addresses the methods used for data sources, study selection, data extraction, and data synthesis. Each heading should be followed by a brief description:

1. Objective.—The abstract should begin with a precise statement of the primary objective of the review. The focus of this statement should be guided by whether the review emphasizes such factors as cause, diagnosis, prognosis, therapy, or prevention. It should include information about the specific population, intervention, exposure, and test or outcome that is being reviewed.

2. Data Sources.—A succinct summary of data sources should be given, including any time restrictions. Potential sources include experts or research institutions active in the field, computerized databases and published indexes, registries, abstract booklets, conference proceedings, references identified from bibliographies of pertinent articles and books, and companies or manufacturers of tests or agents being reviewed. If a bibliographic database is used, the exact indexing terms used for article retrieval should be stated, including any constraints (for example, English language or human subjects) and the dates of the search.

3. Study Selection.—The abstract should describe the criteria used to select studies for detailed review from among studies identified as relevant to the topic. Details of selection should include particular populations, interventions, outcomes, or methodologic designs. The method used to apply these criteria should be specified (for example, blind review, consensus, multiple reviewers). The proportion of initially identified studies that met selection criteria should be stated.

4. Data Extraction.—Guidelines used for abstracting data and assessing data quality and validity (such as criteria for causal inference) should be described. The method by which the guidelines were applied should be stated (for example, independent extraction by multiple observers).

5. Data Synthesis.—The main results of the review, whether qualitative or quantitative, should be stated. Methods used to obtain these results should be outlined. Meta-analyses should state the major outcomes that were pooled and include odds ratios or effect sizes and, if possible, sensitivity analyses. Numerical results should be accompanied by confidence intervals, if applicable, and exact levels of statistical significance. Evaluations of screening and diagnostic tests should address issues of sensitivity, specificity, likelihood ratios, receiver operating characteristic curves, and predictive values. Assessments of prognosis should include summarizations of survival characteristics and related variables. Major identified sources of variation between studies should be stated, including differences in treatment protocols, cointerventions, confounders, outcome measures, length of follow-up, and dropout rates.

6. Conclusions.—The conclusions and their applications should be clearly stated, generalization limited to the domain of the review. The need for new studies may be suggested.

2.5.3 ***Structured Abstracts for Consensus Statements.***—Authors submitting manuscripts that report consensus statements should prepare an abstract of no more than 250 words under the following headings: Objective, Participants, Evidence, Consensus Process, and Conclusions. This format should also be used to report clinical practice guidelines that were developed by consensus. While the descriptions are summarized in the abstract, they should be expanded in the text. References supporting the text should be provided. The content under each heading is as follows:

1. Objective.—Describe the issue, purpose, and intended audience for the consensus statement. The issue may be framed as a series of key questions; as a targeted health problem with relevant patients and providers; or as practice options with health and economic outcomes. The purpose may be to guide clinical practice; to develop public policy; to determine whether insurance will cover innovative therapy; or to set norms for evaluating clinical performance. The audience may include primary care clinicians, specialist physicians, researchers, health planners, and/or the public.

2. Participants.—Explain how people became participants (eg, selection by staff members of the sponsoring agency, nomination by supporting associations, or self-designation). Explain whether meetings were open or closed. Describe the number of participants (particularly panel members or subgroups responsible for developing the statement) and their areas of expertise. Disclose the sponsor or funding source.

3. Evidence.—Describe data sources, selection, abstraction, and synthesis. (See section 2.5.2 for more information.) If a formal literature review was prepared, describe who wrote it and whether it was reviewed. Explain the use of unpublished data and the influence of expert opinion and comments from other participants.

4. Consensus Process.—Describe the basis for drawing conclusions (some techniques involve causal pathways, decision rules, or assigning values to alternative outcomes). Explain the process by which consensus was achieved, such as voting, the Delphi technique, group meetings, or the nominal group process. Explain who wrote the statement (a single person or a writing committee); whether it was drafted before it was presented to the group or after the group had expressed its opinions; and the time during which it was written. Describe who reviewed the statement and how suggestions for revision were incorporated.

5. Conclusions.—Summarize the consensus statement. Conclusions may include what benefits, harms, and costs are expected if the recommendations were implemented. Include important minority views.

2.5.4 ***Unstructured Abstracts.***—For other major manuscripts, a conventional unstructured abstract of no more than 150 words should be included. Abstracts are not required for opinion pieces and special features such as news articles. Consult the journal's instructions for authors for special requirements in individual publications.

2.5.5 ***General Guidelines.***—A few specific guidelines to consider in preparing either type of abstract follow:

- Do not begin the abstract by repeating the title.
- Do not cite references.
- Avoid abbreviations (see 11.0, Abbreviations).
- Provide results for main outcome measures with confidence intervals whenever possible (if not, *P* values) (see 17.1, Statistics, The Manuscript).
- Include major terms and describe databases and study groups (related to the subject under discussion) in the abstract, since the abstract can be text-searched in many retrieval systems.
- Include the stated hypothesis, if applicable.
- Include nothing in the abstract that is not in the article.
- Include the active moiety of a drug at first mention (see 12.4, Nomenclature, Drugs).
- Avoid proprietary names or manufacturers' names unless they are essential to the study (see 12.5, Nomenclature, Equipment, Devices, and Reagents).
- If an isotope is mentioned, spell out the name of the element when first used and provide the isotope number on the line (see 12.9, Nomenclature, Isotopes).

2.6 ■ KEY WORDS.

—Some medical journals publish a short list (3-5 terms, no more than 10) of key words at the end of the abstract. These descriptors are provided by the author and are the terms the author believes represent the key topics presented in the article. The AMA journals do not use key words. Articles in AMA journals are indexed by professional indexers by means of, for example, Medical Subject Headings (MeSH) for indexes such as *Index Medicus* and databases such as MEDLINE.

2.7 ■ EPIGRAPHS.

—On occasion an author will use an epigraph, a short quotation set at the beginning of the article, to suggest the theme of the article. In AMA journals, epigraphs are set in italics, beginning flush left, with the signature set in roman type, underneath the quotation, flush right with the longest line of the quotation. If the work cited appears in the reference list, a superscript number should indicate the source. Otherwise, the title of the work should be indicated.

The medical profession seems to have no place for its mistakes.... And if the medical profession has no room for doctors' mistakes, neither does society.

David Hilfiker[1]

2.8 ■ PARTS OF A MANUSCRIPT, HEADINGS, SUBHEADINGS, AND SIDE HEADINGS.

2.8 ■ PARTS OF A MANUSCRIPT, HEADINGS, SUBHEADINGS, AND SIDE HEADINGS.—Although not all articles will conform to a single pattern because format and section headings vary with the type of article (see 19.0, Typography), a consistent pattern of organization for all headings should be used for original research articles (see also 17.1, Statistics, The Manuscript).

Introduction: The introduction, which usually is *not* given a heading, should provide the objective of the study and state the hypothesis or research question (purpose statement), how and why the hypothesis was developed, and why it is important. It should convince the expert that you know what you are writing about and fill in the gaps for the novice.

Methods: This section should include, as appropriate, a description of (1) study design or type of analysis and period of study, (2) condition, factors, or disease studied, (3) details of sample (eg, study subjects and the setting from which they were drawn), (4) intervention(s), (5) outcome measures, and (6) statistical analysis. Enough information should be provided to enable an informed reader to replicate the study.

Results: The results given in the manuscript should be specific and relevant to the research hypothesis. Characteristics of the study subjects should be followed by presentation of results, from the broad to the specific. The "Results" section should not include implications or weaknesses of the study, but should include validation measures if conducted as part of the study. Results should not discuss the rationale for the statistical procedures used. Data in tables and figures should not be duplicated in the text (see 2.13, Tables, and 2.14, Figures).

Comment: AMA journals avoid the use of the heading "Discussion" here, as that heading is reserved for symposium proceedings, or articles in which a discussion follows the presentation of a paper. The "Comment" or "Discussion" should be a formal consideration and critical examination of the study. The research question or hypothesis should be addressed in this section and the results should be considered in the context of other studies. (*Note:* A lengthy reiteration of the results should be avoided.) The study's limitations and the generalizability of the results should be discussed, as well as mention of unexpected findings with suggested explanations. The type of future studies needed, if appropriate, should be mentioned. This section should end with a clear, concise conclusion that does not go beyond the merits of the study.

2.8.1 ***Levels of Headings.***—Regardless of the headings used, a consistent style or typeface should be used for each level throughout a manuscript so that the reader may graphically distinguish between primary and secondary headings.

The styles used for the various levels of headings will vary from publisher to publisher and, within publishing houses, from one category of article to another (see also 19.0, Typography).

2.8.2 ***Number of Headings.***—There is no requisite number of headings. However, because headings below the first level are meant to divide a primary part into secondary parts, there should usually be a minimum of 2 secondary headings.

Headings reflect the progression of logic or the flow of thought in an article and thereby guide the reader. In the online environment, use of the same major headings as in the structured abstract aids in hypertext links. Headings also help break up the copy, making the article more attractive and easier to read. Headings may be used even in material such as editorials and reviews, which usually do not follow the organization described above for research articles. (Other typographic and design elements, such as pullout quotations, bullets [■], enumerations, tabulations, figures, and tables, may also be used for these purposes [see also 19.0, Typography].)

2.8.3 ***Items to Avoid in Headings.***

- Avoid using a single abbreviation as a heading, even if the abbreviation has been expanded earlier in the text. If the abbreviation appears as the sole item in a heading, spell it out (see 11.11, Abbreviations, Clinical and Technical Terms).
- Avoid expanding abbreviations for the first time in a heading. Spell the abbreviation out in the heading if that is its first appearance and introduce the abbreviation, if appropriate, at the next appearance of the term.
- Avoid citing figures or tables in headings. Cite them in the appropriate place in the text that follows the heading.

2.9 **■ ADDENDA.**—The use of addenda is discouraged in AMA publications. If material is added after a manuscript has been accepted for publication (eg, an additional case report, longer follow-up, data or information on recent legislation, or studies that bear on the present article), this is best handled by incorporating the information in the text or by adding a final paragraph to the existing manuscript: "Since the manuscript was accepted for publication. . . ." If desired, this paragraph may be set off by extra space and/or a half-column-wide centered hairline rule. Any references cited for the first time in this final paragraph or addendum should follow the numbering of the existing reference list.

Note: If substantial material (eg, new figures, new tables, several additional cases) is added after acceptance of the manuscript or if the conclusions change after acceptance, the editor should be notified; additional peer review may be required.

If an article is part of a multipart article series, a sentence to that effect may be added as the last paragraph of the article. This usually is italicized and may also be set in reduced type.

This article is the first of a 3-part series. The second part will appear next month.

2.10 **■ ACKNOWLEDGMENTS.**—Acknowledgments are unnumbered endnotes that follow the body of the article and precede the references. These are considered to be a continuation of the text, so that abbreviations expanded in the text may stand without expansion here. (See also 2.3, Footnotes to Title Page, where some additional types of acknowledgment footnotes are discussed. Placement of these may vary among journals.) Examples of various types of acknowledgments follow.

2.10.1 ***Funding or Grant Support.***—Funding or grant support or provision of supplies used in the study should be acknowledged first. Grant or contract numbers should be included whenever possible. The complete name of the funding institution or agency should be given, along with the city and state or country in which it is located. Although funding or grant support is usually listed in the Acknowledgments, the context of the grant should be examined vis-à-vis the subject of the manuscript. A private grant may need to be treated as a financial disclosure (see 2.3.4, Financial Disclosure).

> This study was supported by research grants R01 EY03812 and R01 EY03454 from the National Eye Institute, Bethesda, Md.
>
> The fluorouracil used in this study was provided by Hoffmann-La Roche Inc, Nutley, NJ.

If individual authors were the recipients of funds, their names should be listed parenthetically.

> This study was supported in part by grant CA34988 from the National Institutes of Health, Bethesda, Md, and by a teaching and research scholarship from the American College of Physicians, Philadelphia, Pa (Dr Fischl).
>
> This study was supported by a 1993 Special Projects Award of the Ambulatory Pediatric Association, McLean, Va (Dr Rappley).
>
> This work was supported by research grant R01 MH45757 from the National Institute of Mental Health, Rockville, Md (Dr Klein).

If an author is a fellow or investigator doing research sponsored by an organization, that information may be included in the Acknowledgments.

> Dr Caskey is a Howard Hughes Medical Institute Investigator.
>
> Dr Blank is a fellow of the American Cancer Society.

2.10.2 ***Other Assistance.***—Acknowledgment of other forms of assistance (eg, statistical review, preparation of the report, performance of special tests or research, editorial or writing assistance, or clerical assistance) may also be included. When specific individuals are named, their given names and highest academic degrees (see 2.2.2, Degrees) should be included and their written permission to be named should be obtained by the author (see 3.2, Ethical and Legal Considerations, Acknowledgments).

> Robert C. Della Rocca, MD, performed the biopsy, contributed the orbital computed tomographic scan, and provided the exenteration specimen; Ramon Font, MD, confirmed our histopathologic diagnosis.
>
> We thank John Hewett, PhD, and Jane Johnson, MA, for statistical support.
>
> The photographs that constitute Figure 1 were provided by Hans-Peter M. Freihofer, MD, Department of Maxillofacial Surgery, University Hospital of Nijmegen, Nijmegen, the Netherlands.
>
> The Branch Retinal Vein Occlusion Study Group is grateful for the contributions of the many referring ophthalmologists, without whom this study could not have been carried out, and to the study patients, whose faithfulness to the study led to conclusions that promise hope for others with branch vein occlusion.

JAMA and the *Archives of Ophthalmology* require authors to disclose any substantial writing and editing assistance and to recognize those persons responsible for such assistance. This information should be included in the Acknowledgments, and permission to be identified should be obtained from all named individuals (see 3.2, Ethical and Legal Considerations, Acknowledgments). In such cases, institutional affiliations may be included:

> William Wise, PhD, Dynapharm Inc, Newark, NJ, contributed to the writing of this article; and Sarah Jewel, MA, Medical Writers Corp, Chicago, Ill, helped edit the initial manuscript.
>
> We thank Cheryl Christensen for manuscript preparation and Stephen Ordway for editorial assistance.

2.10.3 ***Miscellaneous Acknowledgments.***—Occasionally, other types of announcements are listed in the Acknowledgments.

> This is report 54 in a series on chronic disease in former college students.
>
> This article has been reviewed by the Publications Committee of the Collaborative Study of Depression and has its endorsement.
>
> This article is dedicated to the memory of my mentor, friend, and father, Clifford C. Lardinois, Sr, MD.

2.10.4 ***List of Participants in a Group Study.***—If the study was by a group of persons, the names of the participants may be listed in the Acknowledgments (see also 2.3.3, Author Affiliations). Alternatively, the list of participants may be placed in a box wherever it best fits in the layout or the reader can be referred to a previously published list of the group's members.

2.10.5 ***Reproduction of Figures and Tables.***—Credit for reproduction of a figure or a table, even if modified, should be given in the figure legend or the table footnote, not in the Acknowledgments (see 2.13, Tables, and 2.14, Figures).

2.10.6 ***National Auxiliary Publications Service (NAPS) or Availability of Material in Other Forms or Databases.***—If data related to a manuscript (1) are not presented in the manuscript but are available through NAPS, (2) are available from the author or other source, or (3) are available in digital format (from the author or other source [eg, floppy disks, CD-ROM]), or are online, information on how to obtain this material may be given in the Acknowledgments.

> See NAPS document 05144 for 24 pages of supplementary material. Order from NAPS, c/o Microfiche Publications, PO Box 3513, Grand Central Station, New York, NY 10163-3513. Remit in advance, in US funds only, $8.65 for photocopies and $4 for microfiche. There is a $15 invoicing charge on all orders filled before payment. Outside the United States and Canada, add postage of $4.50 for the first 20 pages and $1 for each 10 pages of material thereafter, or $1.50 for the first microfiche and $0.50 for each subsequent microfiche.
>
> A complete list of documents surveyed is available on request from the author.
>
> The original data set is available from the New York State Department of Health, Albany.
>
> These documents are also available via the Internet (http://www.library.ucsf.edu/tobacco).
>
> Additional studies are available from the UK Cochrane Centre, NHS R&D Programme, Summertown Pavillion, Middleway, Oxford OX2 7LG, England (e-mail: ichalmers@cochrane.co.uk).

2.11 ■ **APPENDIXES.**—AMA journals generally do not use appendixes. On rare occasions, however, they serve a useful purpose for data that cannot be presented easily as a table or a figure and are too central to the article to be deposited in NAPS or some other repository. In these cases, appendixes are cited in the text as a table or figure would be cited (eg, Appendix 1) and are usually placed at the end of the article, before the references. If the appendix cites references but contains no figures or tables, it should be placed before the reference list for the article, and the references should be sequential with those in the text. If the appendix contains figures or tables, but cites no references, the appendix should be placed after the text and text reference list, and the figures and tables should be numbered separately in the appendix and the text (eg, Appendix Table, Appendix Figure 1). If the appendix has figures or tables and references, the appendix should be placed after the text and text reference list, and both the figures and tables and the references should have new numbering (eg, Appendix Figure 1, Appendix Table 1, and a separate reference list beginning with reference 1).

2.12 ■ **REFERENCES.**—References serve 2 primary purposes—documentation and acknowledgment. Authors may cite a reference to support their arguments or lay the foundation for their theses; in this case, the emphasis is on documentation. They may also cite a reference as a source of information or credit other authors; in this case, the emphasis is on acknowledgment.

References are a critical element of a manuscript and, as such, the reference list demands close scrutiny by authors, editors, peer reviewers, copy editors, and proofreaders. Authors bear primary responsibility for all reference citations. Editors and peer reviewers should examine manuscripts for completeness, accuracy, and relevance of documentation and references. Copy editors and proofreaders are responsible for assessing the completeness of references and for ensuring that references are presented in proper style and format.

Much has been written about problems with bibliographic inaccuracies[4] (eg, the first author's name is misspelled, the journal name is incorrect, the year of publication or the volume or page numbers are incorrect). Such errors make it difficult for the interested reader to retrieve the documents cited. An even more serious problem is inappropriate citation (eg, a speculative commentary is cited in a way that implies proved causality; an article about an association between diet and heart disease in *men* is cited as if it represents data on the association in all adults). Not only is accuracy critical for the integrity of the individual document, but because authors may sometimes rely on secondary rather than primary sources, an inaccurate citation in a document's reference list may be replicated in subsequent articles whose authors do not consult the primary source. Authors should always consult the primary source and should never cite a reference that they themselves have not read[5-8] (see also 2.12.21, Abstracts and Other Material Taken From Another Source, and 2.12.48, Secondary Citations and Quotations [Including Press Releases]).

2.12.1 ***Reference Style and the Uniform Requirements.***—For greater uniformity in "technical requirements for manuscripts submitted to their journals," the International Committee of Medical Journal Editors, meeting in 1978 in Vancouver, British Columbia, developed the Uniform Requirements for Manuscripts Submitted to Biomedical Journals.[1] Suggested formats for bibliographic style, developed for uniformity by the US National Library of Medicine (NLM), are included in that document, which has been revised and updated several times. Editors of approximately 500 journals have agreed to receive manuscripts prepared in accordance with this uniform style. Although Uniform Requirements is intended to aid authors in the preparation of their manuscripts for publication, not to dictate publication style to journal editors, "many journals have drawn on them for elements of their publication style."[1] References that adhere exactly to the Uniform Requirements will be acceptable without challenge in manuscripts submitted for publication to AMA journals, and any necessary changes will be made by AMA copy editors.

The reference style followed by AMA journals is also based on recommendations of the NLM described in the *National Library of Medicine Recommended Formats for Bibliographic Citation.*[9] Both the Uniform Requirements and AMA style represent modifications of the NLM style but follow the general principles outlined in the NLM document. Whatever reference style is followed, consistency throughout the document and throughout the publication (journal, book) is critical.

Each reference is divided by periods into the following ***bibliographic groups*** (listed in order):

- Author(s)
- Title
- Edition
- Imprint group (place and name of publisher, date of publication, volume number, issue number, inclusive page numbers)
- Physical description (physical construction or form)
- Series statement
- Supplementary notes (identifiers of the uniqueness of the reference or material necessary for added clarity)

The period serves as a field delimiter, making each bibliographic group distinct and establishing a sequence of bibliographic elements in a reference. The items within a bibliographic group are referred to as ***bibliographic elements.*** Bibliographic elements may be separated by the following punctuation marks:

- A semicolon: if the elements are different or if there are multiple occurrences of logically related elements within a group; also, before volume identification data
- A comma: if the items are subelements of a bibliographic element or a set of closely related elements
- A colon: before the publisher's name, between the title and the subtitle, and after a connective phrase (eg, "In," "Taken from," "Located at," "Accompanied by," "Available from")

2.12.2 ***Reference List.***—Reference to information that is retrievable is appropriately made in the reference list. This includes but is not limited to (1) articles published or accepted for publication in scholarly or mass circulation print or electronic journals, magazines, or newspapers, (2) books that have been published or accepted for publication, (3) papers presented at professional meetings, (4) abstracts, (5) theses, (6) CD-ROMs, films, videotapes, (7) package inserts or a manufacturer's documentation, (8) monographs, (9) official reports, (10) databases, (11) legal cases, and (12) patents.

References should be listed in numerical order at the end of the manuscript (except as specified in 2.12.3, References Given in Text, and 2.12.5, Numbering). Each reference is a separate entry.

References to material not yet accepted for publication or to personal communications (oral, written, and electronic) are not acceptable as listed references and instead should be included parenthetically in the text (see 2.12.3, References Given in Text, 2.12.46, Electronic Citations, and 2.12.47, Unpublished Material).

2.12.3 ***References Given in Text.***—Parenthetical citation in the text of references that meet the criteria for inclusion in a reference list should be restricted to those features that do not use reference lists, such as news articles or obituaries. In the text (1) author(s) may not be named, (2) the title may not be given, (3) the name of the journal is abbreviated only when enclosed in parentheses, and (4) inclusive page numbers are given.

> The findings were reported by Kessler et al (*Arch Gen Psychiatry.* 1995;52:1048-1060).
>
> The results were reported by Kessler et al in the *Archives of General Psychiatry* (1995;52:1048-1060).
>
> The *JAMA* article (1995;274:1591-1598) on the frequent failure of physicians to heed dying patients' wishes was picked up by *Time* (December 4, 1995:76) and *Newsweek* (December 4, 1995:74-75) as well as many major newspapers (eg, *Chicago Tribune.* December 3, 1995;§1:19).

2.12.4 ***Minimum Acceptable Data for Print References.***—To be acceptable, a reference to print journals or books must include certain minimum data, as follows:

> *Journals:* Author(s). Article title. *Journal Name.* Year;volume:inclusive page numbers.
>
> *Books:* Author(s). *Book Title.* Place of publication: publisher; year:inclusive pages.

Enough information to identify and retrieve the material should be provided. More complete data (see 2.12.12, References to Journals, Complete Data, and 2.12.28, References to Books, Complete Data) should be used when available. (For detailed information on references to material available in electronic form and unpublished material, see 2.12.46, Electronic Citations, and 2.12.47, Unpublished Material.)

2.12.5 ***Numbering.***—References should be numbered consecutively by means of arabic numerals in the order in which they are cited in the text. Unnumbered references, in the form of a selected reading list, are rarely used in AMA journals. If they are, these references would appear alphabetically in a list separate from the specifically cited reference list.

2.12.6 ***Citation.***—Each reference should be cited in the text, tables, or figures in consecutive numerical order by means of superscript arabic numberals. A reference may be cited *only* in a table or a figure legend and not in the text if it is in sequence with references cited in the text (see Example F1). For example, if Table 2 contains reference 13, which does not appear in the text, this is acceptable as long as the last reference cited (for the first time) before text citation of Table 2 is reference 12. (See Example F1 for an illustration of this in a published article.)

Use arabic superscript numerals *outside* periods and commas, *inside* colons and semicolons. When *more than* 2 references are cited at a given place in the manuscript, use a hyphen to join the first and last numbers of a closed series; use commas without space to separate other parts of a multiple citation.

> As reported previously,[1,3-8,19]
>
> The derived data were as follows[3,4]:

cant difference between dorzolamide and acetazolamide was observed. The reason could be that the topical route cannot deliver the drug to all the sites where carbonic anhydrase is present and active. For whatever reason, dorzolamide suppressed flow by 17%, approximately half as much as acetazolamide did in the same subjects (30% suppression). The reduction of aqueous flow by dorzolamide is also less than that of other oculohypotensive drugs that have been studied by similar techniques, as illustrated in **Table 4**.

Could the limited suppression of flow have been the result of applying a submaximal dose? In the present study, 2% dorzolamide was administered topically for longer than 24 hours. In previous studies, the effect on intraocular pressure appeared quickly[23] and did not increase with continual dosing.[26] These studies also showed that administering concentrations greater than 2% did not increase its effect.[21] The flow was measured in this study during the time when the peak effect of dorzolamide should have occurred. For these reasons, it seems unlikely that a higher dose, a longer period of dosing, or a change in the timing of the measurements would have altered the outcome.

Dorzolamide is used to treat glaucoma. The effect that makes it useful is its ability to lower intraocular pressure. One might ask whether measurements of aqueous flow in normal persons, rather than intraocular pressure in persons with glaucoma, is of any value in predicting the efficacy of dorzolamide. To answer this question, one must keep in mind 3 facts. First, carbonic anhydrase inhibitors have not been shown to have any ocular hypotensive effect mediated by anything other than a reduction of flow. Second, patients with various kinds of glaucoma have been found to have normal aqueous humor production.[42-45] Third, studies of other aqueous-suppressing drugs on aqueous flow in healthy subjects have been predictive of effects of these drugs on intraocular pressure in glaucoma (Table 3). Thus, it seems that measurement of aqueous flow in healthy subjects would be a predictive surrogate of the intraocular pressure effects of one aqueous flow suppressant vs another in patients with glaucoma.

Table 2. Diurnal Effects of Aqueous Humor Flow for United States and Sweden Groups

	Mean±SD Aqueous Humor Flow, μL/min			
Treatment	8 AM-10 AM	10 AM-12 PM	12 PM-2 PM	2 PM-4 PM
Placebo	3.44±0.83	3.28±0.75	3.09±0.74	2.93±0.63
Dorzolamide hydrochloride	2.98±0.86	2.75±0.66	2.51±0.65	2.36±0.58
Acetazolamide	2.48±0.64	2.33±0.59	2.14±0.44	1.95±0.39
Both drugs	2.52±0.65	2.33±0.55	2.12±0.45	1.90±0.35

Table 4. Previous Studies of Aqueous Humor Flow

Drug	Inhibition of Aqueous Flow, %	Year Reported	Source
Acetazolamide	27	1982	Dailey et al[33]
	20	1985	Topper and Brubaker[34]
	21	1992	McCannel et al[35]
	30	1997	Present study
Aplonidine hydrochloride	35	1988	Gharagozloo et al[36]
Betaxolol hydrochloride	32	1983	Reiss and Brubaker[37]
Clonidine hydrochloride	21	1984	Lee et al[38]
Dorzolamide hydrochloride	17	1997	Present study
Levobunolol hydrochloride	32	1989	Gaul et al[39]
Timolol maleate	47	1978	Yablonski et al[40]
	35	1978	Coakes and Brubaker[41]
	33	1982	Dailey et al[33]
	30	1985	Topper and Brubaker[34]
	39	1992	McCannel et al[35]

EXAMPLE F1 The last reference cited *before* the Table 4 citation is reference 32. References 33 through 41 are cited *in* the table. The remaining references (references 42-45) are cited in the text that follows the citation of Table 4.

Avoid placing a superscript reference citation immediately after a number or an abbreviated unit of measure to avoid any confusion between the superscript reference citation and an exponent.

Avoid: The 2 largest studies to date included 26[2] and 18[3] patients.
Better: The 2 largest studies to date included 26 patients[2] and 18 patients.[3]

Avoid: The largest lesion found in the first study was 10 cm.[2]
Better: The largest lesion found in the first study[2] was 10 cm.

When a multiple citation involves more than 23 characters (including spaces and punctuation), use an asterisk in the text and give the citation in a footnote at the bottom of the page (see Example F2). Reference numerals in such a footnote are set full size and on the line rather than as superscripts. The spacing is different from that in superscript reference citations.

As reported previously,*

**References 3, 5, 7, 9, 11, 13, 21, 24-29, 31.*

If the author wants to cite different page numbers from a single reference source at different places in the text, the page numbers are included in the superscript citation and the source appears only once in the list of references. The superscript

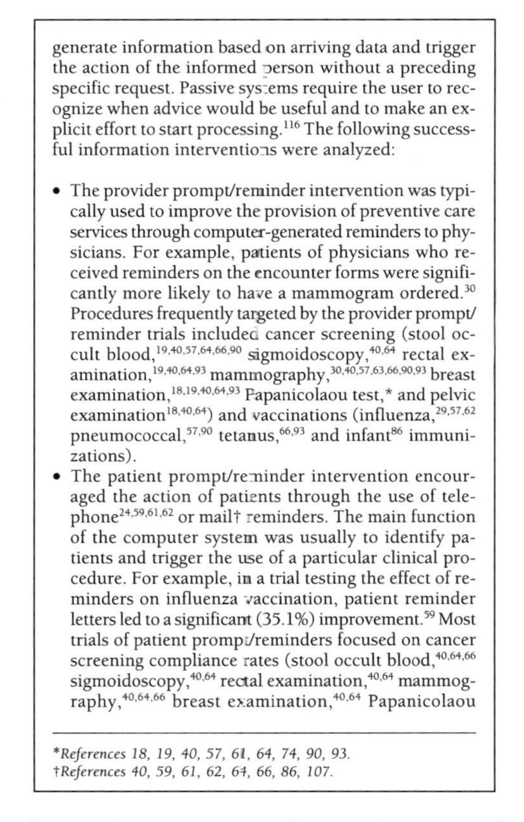

generate information based on arriving data and trigger the action of the informed person without a preceding specific request. Passive systems require the user to recognize when advice would be useful and to make an explicit effort to start processing.[116] The following successful information interventions were analyzed:

- The provider prompt/reminder intervention was typically used to improve the provision of preventive care services through computer-generated reminders to physicians. For example, patients of physicians who received reminders on the encounter forms were significantly more likely to have a mammogram ordered.[30] Procedures frequently targeted by the provider prompt/reminder trials included cancer screening (stool occult blood,[19,40,57,64,66,90] sigmoidoscopy,[40,64] rectal examination,[19,40,64,93] mammography,[30,40,57,63,66,90,93] breast examination,[18,19,40,64,93] Papanicolaou test,* and pelvic examination[18,40,64]) and vaccinations (influenza,[29,57,62] pneumococcal,[57,90] tetanus,[66,93] and infant[86] immunizations).
- The patient prompt/reminder intervention encouraged the action of patients through the use of telephone[24,59,61,62] or mail† reminders. The main function of the computer system was usually to identify patients and trigger the use of a particular clinical procedure. For example, in a trial testing the effect of reminders on influenza vaccination, patient reminder letters led to a significant (35.1%) improvement.[59] Most trials of patient prompt/reminders focused on cancer screening compliance rates (stool occult blood,[40,64,66] sigmoidoscopy,[40,64] rectal examination,[40,64] mammography,[40,64,66] breast examination,[40,64] Papanicolaou

*References 18, 19, 40, 57, 61, 64, 74, 90, 93.
†References 40, 59, 61, 62, 64, 66, 86, 107.

EXAMPLE F2 For references that occupy more than 23 characters and spaces, bottom-of-page footnotes are used. This example shows 2 such footnotes within a single column.

may include more than 1 page number, citation of more than 1 reference, or both, and all spaces are closed up.

> These patients showed no sign of protective sphincteric adduction.[3(p21),9]
>
> Westman[5(pp3,5),9] reported 8 cases in which vomiting occurred.

In listed references, do not use *ibid* or *op cit*.

2.12.7 ***Authors.***—Use the author's surname followed by initials without periods. In listed references, the names of all authors should be given unless there are more than 6, in which case the names of *the first 3 authors* are used, followed by "et al."

Note spacing and punctuation. Do not use *and* between names. Roman numerals and abbreviations for Junior (Jr) and Senior (Sr) *follow* author's initials.

The NLM guidelines recommend listing the first 10 authors and, if more than 10, the first 10 and "et al." For space considerations, and because "et al" means "and others" (ie, more than 1—a problem in citing an article with 11 authors and listing the first 10 followed by "et al"), we have elected to depart from the NLM guidelines on this point.

One author:	Doe JF.
Two authors:	Doe JF, Roe JP III.
Six authors:	Doe JF, Roe JP III, Coe RT Jr, Loe JT Sr, Poe EA, van Voe AE.

More than 6 authors:	Doe JF, Roe JP III, Coe RT Jr, et al.
One author for a group:	Doe JF, for the Laser ROP Study Group
One author and a group:	Doe JF, and the Laser ROP Study Group
More than 6 authors for a group:	Doe JF, Roe JP III, Coe RT Jr, et al, for the Laser ROP Study Group
More than 6 authors and a group:	Doe JF, Roe JP III, Coe RT Jr, et al, and the Laser ROP Study Group

When mentioned in the text, only surnames of authors are used. For a 2-author reference, list both surnames; for references with more than 2 authors or authors and a group, include the first author's surname followed by "et al," "and associates," "and coworkers," or "and colleagues."

Doe[7] reported on the survey.

Doe and Roe[8] reported on the survey.

Doe et al[9] reported on the survey.

Do not use the possessive form *et al's*; rephrase the sentence.

The data of Doe et al[9] support our findings.

2.12.8 ***Prefixes and Particles.***—Surnames that contain prefixes or particles (eg, von, de, La, van) are spelled and capitalized according to the preference of the persons named.

1. van Gylswyk NO, Roche CI.
2. Van Rosevelt RF, Bakker JC, Sinclair DM, Damen J, Van Mourik JA.
3. Al-Faquih SR.
4. Kang S, Kim KJ, Wong T-Y, et al.

2.12.9 ***Titles.***—In titles of articles, books, parts of books, and other material, retain the spelling, abbreviations, and style for numbers used in the original. However, *all* numbers are spelled out at the beginning of a title (although exceptions are made for years; see 2.1.2, Numbers). See below for capitalization and typeface style.

Articles and Parts of Books: In English-language titles, capitalize only (1) the first letter of the first word, (2) proper names, and (3) abbreviations that are ordinarily capitalized (eg, DNA, EEG, VDRL). Do not enclose article and book chapter titles in quotation marks. However, if a book, book chapter, or article title contains quotation marks in the original, retain them as double quotation marks (unless both double *and* single quotation marks are used).

Journals, Books, Government Bulletins, Documents, and Pamphlets: Capitalize the first letter of each major word in titles and subtitles. Do not capitalize articles, prepositions of 3 or fewer letters, coordinating conjunctions (*and, or, for, nor, but*), or the *to* in infinitives (see 2.1.6, Capitalization, for exceptions). *Do* capitalize a 2-letter verb, such as *Is*.

Capitalization: For journal article titles, follow the capitalization in *Index Medicus.* For books, pamphlets, reports, government documents, and parts of books, retain the capitalization used in the original or consult the author or publisher. *Note:* In non-English-language titles, capitalization does not necessarily follow the same rules. For example, in German titles (both articles and books), all nouns *and only nouns* are capitalized; in French, Spanish, and Italian book titles, capitalize only the first word, proper names, and abbreviations that are capitalized in English.

Names of Organisms: In all titles, follow AMA style for capitalization of scientific names of organisms and use of italics (see 8.1.7, Capitalization, Organisms, and 12.12, Nomenclature, Organisms). Use roman type for genus and species names in book titles.

2.12.10 ***Non–English-Language Titles.***—Non-English-language titles may be given as they originally appeared, without translation:

1. Hachulla E, Hatron PY, Robert Y, Devulder B. Artérite digitale, thrombose et syndrome hyperéosinophilique: une complication exceptionnelle. *Rev Med Interne.* 1995;16:434-436.
2. Aranete MRG, Mascola L, Eller A, et al. Transmissão de HIV atraves de inseminacão artificial de doador. *JAMA-GO.* 1995;3:1956-1972. Originally published, in English, in: *JAMA.* 1995;273:854-858.

If non-English-language titles are translated into English, bracketed indication of the original language should follow the title:

3. Salmon RJ, Vilcoq JR. Breast cancer after preventive subcutaneous mammectomy [in French]. *Presse Med.* 1995;24:1167-1168.

If both the non-English-language title and the translation are provided, both may be given, as shown, with the non-English-language title given first, followed by the English translation, in brackets:

4. Kolmos HJ. Antibiotika i almen praksis [Antibiotics in general practice]. *Ugeskr Laeger.* 1996;158:258-260.

Non-English-language titles should be verified from the original when possible. Consult a dictionary in the appropriate language for accent marks, spelling, and other particulars.

Reference to the primary source is always preferable, but if the non-English-language article is not readily available or not accessible, the translated version is acceptable. The citation should always be to the version consulted.

Such words as *tome* (volume), *fascicolo* (part), *Seite* (page), *Teil* (part), *Auflage* (edition), *Abteilung* (section or part), *Band* (volume), *Heft* (number), *Beiheft* (supplement), and *Lieferung* (part or number) should be translated into English.

2.12.11 ***Subtitles.***—Style for subtitles follows that for titles (see 2.12.9, Titles) with regard to spelling, abbreviations, numbers, capitalization, and use of italics, except that for *journal articles* the subtitle begins with a *lowercase* letter. A colon and space separate title and subtitle. If the subtitle is numbered, as is common when articles in a series have the same title but different—numbered—subtitles, use a comma after the title, followed by a roman numeral immediately preceding the colon.

1. Guyatt GH, Sackett DL, Sinclair JC, Hayward R, Cook DJ, Cook RJ, for the Evidence-Based Medicine Working Group. Users' guides to the medical literature, IX: a method for grading health care recommendations. *JAMA.* 1995;274:1800-1804.

References to Journals

2.12.12 ***Complete Data.***—A complete journal reference includes the following:

- Authors' surnames and initials
- Title of article and subtitle if any

- Abbreviated name of journal
- Year
- Volume number
- Part or supplement number, when pertinent, and issue month or number when pagination is not consecutive throughout a volume
- Inclusive page numbers

2.12.13 ***Names of Journals.***—Abbreviate and italicize names of journals. Use initial capital letters. Abbreviate according to the listing in the current *Index Medicus*[10] (see 11.10, Abbreviations, Names of Journals). Include parenthetical designation of a city if it is included in the abbreviations given in *List of Journals Indexed in Index Medicus*[10]; for example, *Acta Anat (Basel), J Physiol (Lond)*.

In journal titles listed in *Index Medicus,* information enclosed in brackets should be retained *without* brackets, eg, *J Comp Physiol A* for *J Comp Physiol [A]*.

If the name of a journal has changed since that used at the time the reference was published, retain the name used during the time of publication but use the currently recommended NLM abbreviations for the words involved. For example, the journal formerly called *Transactions of the Ophthalmological Societies of the United Kingdom* is now called *Eye*. If a citation was from the older-named journal, do not change the journal name to *Eye,* but do use the current style of abbreviating the former title: *Trans Ophthalmol Soc U K.*

2.12.14 ***Page Numbers and Dates.***—Do not omit digits from inclusive page numbers. The year, followed by a semicolon, the volume number, a colon, the initial page number, a hyphen, the final page number, and a period are set without spaces.

1. Davis JT, Allen HD, Powers JD, Cohen DM. Population requirements for capitation planning in pediatric cardiac surgery. *Arch Pediatr Adolesc Med.* 1996;150:257-259.

2.12.15 ***Discontinuous Pagination.***—For an article with discontinuous pagination, the cited parts of which appear in the same issue, follow this example:

1. Altman LK. Medical errors bring calls for change. *New York Times.* July 18, 1995:C1, C10.

2.12.16 ***Journals Without Volume Numbers.***—In references to journals that have no volume numbers or that have volume numbers but paginate each issue beginning with page 1, use one of the following styles:

1. Timmerman MG. Medical problems of adolescent female athletes. *Wis Med J.* June 1996:351-354.
2. Hardy AM. Incidence and impact of selected infectious diseases in childhood. *Vital Health Stat 10.* 1991;No. 180:5.
3. Hastings C. Differences in professional practice model outcomes: the impact of practice setting. *Crit Care Nurs Q.* November 1995;18:75-86.

2.12.17 ***Parts of an Issue.***—If an issue has 2 or more parts, the part cited should be indicated in accordance with the following example:

1. Newman KM, Johnson CL, Jean-Claude J, Li H, Ramey WG, Tilson MD. Cytokines which activate proteolysis are increased in abdominal aortic aneurysms. *Circulation.* 1994;90(pt 2):224-227.

2.12.18 ***Issue Number.***—Do not include the issue number or month except in the case of a special issue (see 2.12.19, Special or Theme Issue) or when pagination is not consecutive throughout the volume (ie, when each issue begins with page 1). In the latter case, the month or the date of the issue is preferable to the issue number.

1. Taulbee P. Maryland Quality Project puts new focus on processes of care. *Rep Med Guideline Outcomes Res.* June 1994;5:10-11.

2.12.19 ***Special or Theme Issue.***—The NLM *Recommended Formats*[9] defines a special or theme issue as follows: "Special issues are frequently published to present the papers from conferences. . . . They may also be published to commemorate a specific event or to bring together papers on a specific subject." AMA journals refer to these as theme issues. References to all or part of a special or theme issue of a journal should be cited as follows:

1. Marais AD, Firth JC, Batemon M, Jones J, Mountney J, Marten C. Atorvastatin is a powerful and safe agent for lowering plasma cholesterol concentrations in heterozygous familial hypercholesterolaemia. *Atherosclerosis.* 1994;109(special issue):316. Abstract 226.
2. Winker MA, Flanagin A, eds. Emerging and reemerging global microbial threats. *JAMA.* 1996;275(theme issue):163-256.

Special or theme issues may be published as supplements (see also 2.12.20, Supplements). In this case, the following form is used:

3. Warrell DA, Molyneux ME, Beales PF, eds. Severe and complicated malaria. *Trans R Soc Trop Med Hyg.* 1990;84(suppl 2):1-65. Theme issue.

2.12.20 ***Supplements.***—The following example illustrates the basic format:

1. Lagios MD. Evaluation of surrogate endpoint biomarkers for ductal carcinoma in situ. *J Cell Biochem.* 1994;19(suppl):186-188.

If pagination is not consecutive with that of the volume, use the following form; there may be several supplements to a volume, each referred to by month.

2. Novick LF, Glebatis DM, Striacof RL, MacCubbins PA, Lessner L, Berns DS. New York State HIV Seroprevalence Project, II: Newborn Seroprevalence Study: methods and results. *Am J Public Health.* May 1991;81(suppl):15-21.

If the supplement is numbered, use the following form; pagination in each supplement is independent of that in others.

3. Schmidt D. Behavioural abnormalities and retention rates of anti-epilepsy drugs during long-term treatment of epilepsy: a clinical perspective. *Acta Neurol Scand.* 1995;92(suppl 162):7-10.

When numbered supplements have several parts, each with independent pagination, use the following form:

4. Sofferman RA. The recovery potential of the optic nerve. *Laryngoscope.* 1995;105(suppl 72, pt 3):1-38.

The following example shows the pagination that may be found in a supplementary issue:

5. Ball P. Bacterial resistance to fluoroquinolones: lessons to be learned. *Infection.* 1994;22(suppl 2):S140-S147.

Other variations, akin to supplements, use a form similar to that for supplements. An example of a supplement (Recommendations and Reports) published June 17, 1994, is shown below; there is an issue of the *Morbidity and Mortality Weekly Report* (weekly) with that date as well.

6. Centers for Disease Control and Prevention. Compendium of animal rabies control, 1994. *MMWR Morb Mortal Wkly Rep.* 1994;43(RR-10):1-9.

2.12.21 ***Abstracts and Other Material Taken From Another Source.***—Several types of published abstracts may be cited: (1) an abstract of a complete article taken from another publication, as in the "Abstracts" section of *JAMA,* (2) a published abstract of a paper before presentation at a conference, and (3) a rewritten abstract of a published article with an appended commentary. (For examples of abstracts presented at meetings, published or unpublished, see 2.12.39, Serial Publications, and 2.12.47, Unpublished Material.)

Ideally, reference to any of these types of abstracts should be permitted only when the original article is not readily available (eg, non-English-language articles or papers presented at meetings but not yet published). If an abstract is published in the society proceedings section of a journal, the name of the society before which the paper was read need not be included.

- Abstract of a complete article taken from another publication:

1. Falco NA, Upton J. Infantile digital fibromas [abstract]. *J Hand Surg Am.* 1995;20:1014-1020. Taken from: *JAMA.* 1996;275:1462*b*.
2. Salmon RJ, Vilcoq JR. Breast cancer after preventive subcutaneous mammectomy [in French; English abstract]. *Presse Med.* 1995;24:1167-1168. Taken from: *JAMA.* 1996;274:1896*b*.

- Published abstract of a paper to be presented at a conference:

3. Schwartz RH, O'Donnell R, Mann L, Baugh J. Adolescents who smoke cigarettes: criteria for addiction, health concerns, and readiness to quit [abstract]. *AJDC.* 1993;147:417. Abstract 3.

If an abstract number is given, it appears in the final field.

- Rewritten abstract of a published article with an appended commentary:

4. Long-term clomiphene therapy may increase the risk of ovarian cancer [abstract]. *Arch J Club/Womens Health.* October 1995:43. Abstract of: Rossing MA, Daling JR, Weiss NS, Moore DE, Self SG. Ovarian tumors in a cohort of infertile women. *N Engl J Med.* 1994;331:771-776.

2.12.22 ***Special Department, Feature, or Column of a Journal.***—When reference is made to material from a special department, feature, or column of a journal, the department should be identified only in the following cases:

- The cited material has no byline or signature. (This is preferable to citing Anonymous, unless "Anonymous" or something similar was actually used [see 2.2, Bylines and End-of-Text Signatures].)

1. Health effects of sanctions on Iraq [editorial]. *Lancet.* 1995;346:1439-1440.
2. Case records of the Massachusetts General Hospital: weekly clinicopathological exercises. *N Engl J Med.* 1995;333:1625-1630. Case 38-1995.

- The column or department name (1) might help the reader identify the nature of the article and (2) is not apparent from the title itself. In these cases, the inclusion of the department or column name is optional and should be used as needed, at the editor's discretion.

3. Voelker R. Hypnosis for diagnosis [Quick Uptakes]. *JAMA.* 1996;275:272.
4. Seifer SD, Grumbach K. Migrating docs: studying physician practice location [letter]. *JAMA.* 1995;274:1914.

Identification of other special departments, features, or columns may not require additional notation (eg, book or journal reviews, cover stories) as their identity will be apparent from the citation itself:

5. Schreiner GE, reviewer. *Ann Intern Med.* 1995;123:975-976. Review of: Kissick WL. *Medicine's Dilemmas: Infinite Needs Versus Finite Resources.*
6. Bowden VM, Long MJ, reviewers. *JAMA.* 1995;273:1395. Review of: Cohen GD, ed. *American Journal of Geriatric Psychiatry.*
7. Southgate MT. The Cover (Felix Nussbaum, *Carnival Group*). *JAMA.* 1993;269:477.

2.12.23 ***Other Material Without Named Author(s).***—Reference may be made to material that has no named author or is prepared by a committee or other group. The following forms are used:

1. National Institute of Neurological Disorders and Stroke rt-PA Stroke Study Group. Tissue plasminogen activator for acute ischemic stroke. *N Engl J Med.* 1995;333:1581-1587.
2. NIH Consensus Development Panel on Cochlear Implants in Adults and Children. Cochlear implants in adults and children. *JAMA.* 1995;274:1955-1961.

2.12.24 ***Discussants.***—If reference citation in the text names a discussant specifically rather than the author(s), eg, "as noted by Allo,[1]" the following form is used (see also 2.12.48, Secondary Citations and Quotations [Including Press Releases]).

1. Allo MD. In discussion of: McKindley DS, Fabian TC, Boucher BA, Croce MA, Proctor KG. Antibiotic pharmacokinetics following fluid resuscitation from traumatic shock. *Arch Surg.* 1995;130:1321-1329.

2.12.25 ***Corrections.***—If the reference citation is to an article with a published correction, provide both the information about the article and the information about the published correction, if available, as follows:

1. Nelson HD, Nevitt MC, Scott JC, Stone KL, Cummings SR, for the Study of Osteoporotic Fractures Research Group. Smoking, alcohol, and neuromuscular and physical function of older women [published correction appears in *JAMA.* 1996;275:446]. *JAMA.* 1994;272:1825-1831.

2.12.26 ***Retractions.***—If the reference citation is to an article that has since been retracted, or to the retraction notice itself, use the appropriate example shown below, as adapted from Uniform Requirements.[1] Uniform Requirements notes, "Ideally, the first author should be the same in the retraction as in the article, although under certain circumstances the editor may accept retractions by other responsible people."[1] (See also 3.4.3, Ethical and Legal Considerations, Editorial Policy for Detecting and Handling Allegations of Scientific Misconduct.)

- Article containing retraction:

1. Garey CE, Schwarzman AL, Rise ML, Seyfried TN. Ceruloplasmin gene defect associated with epilepsy in EL mice [retraction of Garey CE, Schwarzman AL, Rise ML, Seyfried TN. In: *Nat Genet.* 1994;6:426-431]. *Nat Genet.* 1995;11:104.

- Article retracted:

    2. Liou GI, Wang M, Matragoon S. Precocious IRBP gene expression during mouse development [retracted in: *Invest Ophthalmol Vis Sci.* 1994;35:3127]. *Invest Ophthalmol Vis Sci.* 1994;35:1083-1088.

2.12.27 ***Duplicate Publication.***—The following form is suggested for citation of a notice of duplicate publication (see also 3.3, Ethical and Legal Considerations, Duplicate Publication).

1. Shadey IM. Notice of duplicate publication: Prevalence of measles in day-care centers [duplicate publication of Shadey IM. Measles in children attending day care: an epidemiological assessment. *J New Results.* 1994;32:150-154.]. *JAMA.* 1994;270:2004-2008.

References to Books

2.12.28 ***Complete Data.***—A complete reference to a book includes the following:

- Authors' surnames and first and middle initials
- Chapter title (when cited)
- Surname and first and middle initials of book authors or editors (or translator, if any)
- Title of book and subtitle, if any
- Volume number and volume title, when there is more than 1 volume
- Edition number (do not indicate first edition)
- Place of publication
- Name of publisher
- Year of copyright
- Page numbers, when specific pages are cited

2.12.29 ***Reference to an Entire Book.***—When referring to an entire book, rather than pages or a specific section, use the following form (see also 2.12.7, Authors).

1. Sherlock S, Dooley J. *Diseases of the Liver and Biliary System.* 9th ed. Oxford, England: Blackwell Scientific Publications; 1993.
2. LaFollette MC. *Stealing Into Print: Fraud, Plagiarism, and Misconduct in Scientific Publishing.* Berkeley: University of California Press; 1992.
3. Sutcliffe AJ, ed. *The New York Public Library Writer's Guide to Style and Usage.* New York, NY: HarperCollins Publishers Inc; 1994.

2.12.30 ***Reference to a Chapter in a Book.***—When citing a chapter of a book, capitalize as for a journal title (see 2.12.9, Titles); do *not* use quotation marks. Inclusive page numbers of the chapter should be given (see also 2.12.36, Page Numbers or Chapter Number).

1. Nahas GG, Goldfrank LR. Marijuana. In: Goldfrank LR, Flomenbaum NE, Lewin NA, Weisman RS, Howland MA, Hoffman RS, eds. *Goldfrank's Toxicologic Emergencies.* 5th ed. Norwalk, Conn: Appleton & Lange; 1994:889-898.
2. Cole BR. Cystinosis and cystinuria. In: Jacobson HR, Striker GE, Klahr S, eds. *The Principles and Practice of Nephrology.* Philadelphia, Pa: BC Decker Inc; 1991:396-403.
3. Huth EJ. Revising prose structure and style. In: *How to Write and Publish Papers in the Medical Sciences.* 2nd ed. Baltimore, Md: Williams & Wilkins; 1990:109-136.
4. Haddy FJ, Buckalew VM. Endogenous digitalis-like factors in hypertension. In: Laragh HJ, Brenner MB, eds. *Hypertension: Pathophysiology, Diagnosis, and Management.* New York, NY: Raven Press; 1995:1055-1067.

2.12.31 ***Editors and Translators.***—Names of editors, translators, translator-editors, or executive and section editors are given in accordance with the following forms:

1. Plato. *The Laws*. Taylor EA, trans-ed. London, England: JM Dent & Sons Ltd; 1934:104-105. [Plato is the author; Taylor is the translator-editor.]
2. Gwei-Djen L, Needham J. Diseases of antiquity in China. In: Kiple KF, ed; Graham RR, exec ed. *The Cambridge World History of Human Disease.* New York, NY: Cambridge University Press; 1993:345-354. [Gwei-Djen and Needham are the authors of a chapter in a book edited by Kiple, for which Graham was the executive editor.]
3. Bloom FE. Neurotransmission and the central nervous system. In: Gilman AG, consulting ed; Hardman JG, Limbird LE, eds-in-chief; Molinoff PB, Roddon RW, eds. *Gilman's The Pharmacological Basis of Therapeutics.* 9th ed. New York, NY: McGraw-Hill Book Co; 1996:267-293. [Bloom is the author of a chapter in a book edited by Molinoff and Roddon, for which Gilman was the consulting editor and Hardman and Limbird were the editors-in-chief.]
4. Jacobson MS, ed. *Pediatric Atherosclerosis Prevention: Identification and Treatment of the Child With High Cholesterol.* Chur, Switzerland: Harwood Academic Publishers; 1991. Lanzkowsky P, ed. Monographs in Clinical Pediatrics.
5. Goligorsky MS, ed. *Acute Renal Failure: New Concepts and Therapeutic Strategies.* New York, NY: Churchill Livingstone; 1995. Stein JH, ed. Contemporary Issues in Nephrology; No. 30.
6. Warner R, ed. *Alternatives to the Hospital for Acute Psychiatric Treatment.* Washington, DC: American Psychiatric Press; 1995. Clinical Practice Series; No. 32.

No authors are named in examples 4 through 6 above. Each book has an editor and is part of a series; in examples 4 and 5, the series also has an editor. *Note:* The name of the series, as well as the series editor, if any, is given in the final field. If the book has a number within the series, the number is also given in the final field.

2.12.32 ***Volume Number.***—Use arabic numerals for volume number if the work cited includes more than 1 volume.

If the volumes have no separate titles, merely numbers, the number should be given after the general title.

1. Bithell TC. Hereditary coagulation disorders. In: Lee GR, Bithell TC, Foerster J, Athens JW, Lukens JN, eds. *Wintrobe's Clinical Hematology.* Vol 2. 9th ed. Philadelphia, Pa: Lea & Febiger; 1993:1422-1472.
2. Widiger TA, Frances AJ, Pincus HA, Ross R, First MB, Davis WW. DSM-IV *Sourcebook.* Vol 2. Washington, DC: American Psychiatric Press; 1996.

If the volumes have separate titles, the title of the volume referred to should be given first, with the title of the overall series of which the volume is a part given in the final field, along with the name of the general editor and the volume number, if applicable.

3. Creager MA, ed. *Vascular Disease.* St Louis, Mo: Mosby; 1996. Braunwald E, ed. *Atlas of Heart Disease*; vol 7.

In the example shown, Creager is the editor of *Vascular Disease,* which is volume 7 in the series *Atlas of Heart Disease.* Braunwald is the editor of the entire series.

When a book title includes a volume number, use the title as it was published. Three examples are given below. *Note:* The volume number does not need to be repeated in its customary place after the title if it is included *in* the book's title.

4. Rous SN. *1995 Urology Annual Volume 9.* New York, NY: WW Norton & Co; 1995.
5. Lewin B. Gene numbers: repetition and redundancy. In: *Genes V.* New York, NY: Oxford University Press; 1994:703-731.
6. Hames BD, Higgins SJ, eds. *Gene Probes 1.* New York, NY: Oxford University Press; 1995. Rickwood D, Hames BD, eds. The Molecular Approach Series.

2.12.33 ***Edition Number.***—Use arabic numerals to indicate an edition, but do not indicate a first edition. If a subsequent edition is cited, the number should be given. Abbreviate "New revised edition" as "New rev ed"; "Revised edition" as "Rev ed"; "American edition" as "American ed"; and "British edition" as "British ed."

1. Frolich ED. Pathophysiology of systemic arterial hypertension. In: Schlant RC, Alexander RW, eds. *Hurst's The Heart: Arteries and Veins.* 8th ed. New York, NY: McGraw-Hill Book Co; 1994:1391-1401.
2. Baker PC, Keck CK, Mott FL, Quinlan SV. *NYLS Child Handbook: A Guide to the 1986-90 National Longitudinal Survey of Youth and Child Data.* Rev ed. Columbus: Ohio State University; 1993.

2.12.34 ***Place of Publication.***—Use the name of the city in which the publishing firm was located at the time of publication. Follow AMA style in the use of state names (see 11.5, Abbreviations, US States, Territories, and Possessions; Provinces; Countries). Do not list the state name if it is part of the publisher's name. If more than 1 location appears, use the one that appears first in the edition consulted. A colon separates the place of publication and the name of the publisher.

1. Perkins AC. *Nuclear Medicine: Science and Safety.* London, England: John Libbey; 1995.
2. Chalmers I, Altman DG. *Systematic Reviews.* London, England: BMJ Publishing Group; 1995.
3. Scioscia AL. Reproductive genetics. In: Moore TR, Reiter RC, Rebar RW, Baker VV, eds. *Gynecology & Obstetrics: A Longitudinal Approach.* New York, NY: Churchill Livingstone; 1993:55-77.
4. Dougherty CJ. *Back to Reform: Values, Markets, and the Health Care System.* New York, NY: Oxford University Press; 1996.
5. Parkes MB. *Pause and Effect: An Introduction to the History of Punctuation in the West.* Berkeley: University of California Press; 1993.

2.12.35 ***Publishers.***—The full name of the publisher (publisher's imprint, as shown on the title page) should be given, abbreviated in accordance with AMA style (see 11.7, Abbreviations, Business Firms) but *without* punctuation. Even if the name of a publishing firm has changed, use the name that was given on the published work.

Consult the latest edition of *Books in Print*[11] to verify names of publishers.

2.12.36 ***Page Numbers or Chapter Number.***—Use arabic numerals, unless the pages referred to use roman pagination (eg, the preliminary pages of a book).

1. Litt IE. Special health problems during adolescence. In: Nelson WE, senior ed; Behrman RE, Kliegman RM, Arvin AM, eds. *Nelson Textbook of Pediatrics.* 15th ed. Philadelphia, Pa: WB Saunders Co; 1996:541-560.
2. Grossman J. Preface. In: *The Chicago Manual of Style.* 14th ed. Chicago, Ill: University of Chicago Press; 1993:vii-xi.

If a book uses separate pagination within each chapter, follow the style used in the book.

3. Trunkel AR, Croul SE. Subacute and chronic meningitides. In: Bleck TP, ed. *Central Nervous System and Eye Infections*. Philadelphia, Pa: Current Medicine; 1995:2.1-2.27. Mandell GL, ed. *Atlas of Infectious Diseases*; vol 3.

Inclusive page numbers are preferred. The chapter number may be used instead if the author does not provide the inclusive page numbers.

4. Shils ME. Magnesium. In: Shils ME, Young VR, eds. *Modern Nutrition in Health and Disease.* 7th ed. Philadelphia, Pa: Lea & Febiger; 1988:chap 6.

Special Materials

2.12.37 ***Newspapers.***—References to newspapers should include the following, in the order indicated: (1) name of author (if given), (2) title of article, (3) name of newspaper, (4) date of newspaper, (5) section (if applicable), and (6) pages. Newspaper titles are *not* abbreviated.

1. Gianelli DM. AMA launching ethics institute for research, outreach projects. *American Medical News.* November 4, 1996:1, 75.
2. Steinmetz G. Kafka is a symbol of Prague today; also, he's a T-shirt. *Wall Street Journal.* October 10, 1996:A1, A6.
3. Auerbach S. Tomorrow's MDs unready for managed care? studies say that medical schools' training methods are behind the times. *Washington Post.* September 17, 1996;Health section:11.
4. Travis D. Advertising our dishonor: my industry should be ashamed of itself for pushing cigarettes on kids. *Washington Post.* September 8, 1996:C3.
5. Grady D. So, smoking causes cancer: this is news? *New York Times.* October 27, 1996;sect 4:3.

2.12.38 ***Government Bulletins.***—References to bulletins published by departments or agencies of the US government should include the following information, in the order indicated: (1) name of author (if given); (2) title of bulletin; (3) place of publication; (4) name of issuing bureau, agency, department, or other governmental division (in this position, *Department* should be abbreviated *Dept;* US Government Printing Office should be used only if the name of the issuing bureau, agency, or department cannot be obtained); (5) date of publication; (6) page numbers, if specified; (7) publication number, if any; and (8) series number, if given.

1. US Bureau of the Census. *Statistical Abstract of the United States: 1993.* 113th ed. Washington, DC: US Bureau of the Census; 1993.
2. US General Accounting Office. *Trauma Care: Life-saving Systems Threatened by Unreimbursed Costs and Other Factors.* Washington, DC: US General Accounting Office; 1991. Publication HRD 91-57.
3. *Clinical Practice Guideline Number 5: Depression in Primary Care, 2: Treatment of Major Depression.* Rockville, Md: Agency for Health Care Policy and Research, US Dept of Health and Human Services; 1993. AHCPR publication 93-0551.
4. Food and Drug Administration. *Jin Bu Huan Herbal Tablets.* Rockville, Md: National Press Office; April 15, 1994. Talk Paper T94-22.

2.12.39 ***Serial Publications.***—If a monograph or report is part of a series, include the name of the series and, if applicable, the number of the publication.

1. Steahr TE, Roberts T. *Microbial Foodborne Disease: Hospitalizations, Medical Costs and Potential Demand for Safer Food.* Storrs: Food Marketing Policy Center, University of Connecticut; 1993. Private Strategies, Public Policies and Food System Performance Working Paper Series, No. 32.

2. Hardy AM. *AIDS Knowledge and Attitudes for Oct-Dec 1990: Provisional Data From the National Health Interview Survey*. Hyattsville, Md: National Center for Health Statistics; 1991. Advance Data From Vital and Health Statistics, No. 204.
3. Miller JE, Korenman S. *Poverty, Nutritional Status, Growth and Cognitive Development of Children in the United States*. Princeton, NJ: Princeton University Office of Population Research; 1993. Working Paper 93-5.

2.12.40 ***Theses and Dissertations.***—Titles of theses and dissertations are given in italics. References to theses should include the location of the university (or other institution), its name, and year of completion of the thesis. If the thesis has been published, it should be treated as any other book reference (see 2.12.28, References to Books, Complete Data).

1. Knoll EG. *Mental Evolution and the Science of Language: Darwin, Müller, and Romanes on the Development of the Human Mind* [dissertation]. Chicago, Ill: Committee on the Conceptual Foundations of Science, University of Chicago; 1987.
2. King L. *Modern Literary Apparitions and Their Mind-Altering Effects* [master's thesis]. Evanston, Ill: Northwestern University; 1994.

2.12.41 ***Special Collections.***—References to material available only in special collections of a library take this form:

1. Hunter J. An account of the dissection of morbid bodies: a monograph or lecture. 1757;No. 32:30-32. Located at: Library of the Royal College of Surgeons, London, England.

2.12.42 ***Package Inserts.***—Package inserts may be cited as follows:

1. Lamasil [package insert]. East Hanover, NJ: Sandoz Pharmaceuticals Corp; 1993.

2.12.43 ***Patents.***—Patent citations take the following form:

1. Furukawa Y, Kishimoto S, Nishikawa K, inventors; Takeda Chemical Industries Ltd, assignee. Hypotensive imidazole derivatives. US patent 4 340 598. July 20, 1982.

2.12.44 ***Audiotapes, Videotapes.***—Occasionally, references may include citation of audiotapes or videotapes. The form for such references is as follows:

1. The Right to Die . . . *The Choice Is Yours* [videotape]. New York, NY: Society for the Right to Die; 1987.
2. *Obsessive-compulsive Disorder: Pharmacotherapy and Psychotherapy* [videotape]. Washington, DC: American Psychiatric Press; 1995. Alger I, ed; Treatment of Psychiatric Disorders Video Series.
3. Cohen LB, Basuk PM, Waye JD. *Video Guide to Flexible Sigmoidoscopy* [videotape]. New York, NY: Igaku-Shoin Medical Publishers; 1995.

2.12.45 ***Transcript of Television or Radio Broadcast.***—Citation of transcripts to television or radio broadcasts take the following form:

1. Lundberg GD. The medical profession in the 1990s [transcript]. American Medical Television. September 15, 1993.
2. An American dilemma [transcript]. "60 Minutes." CBS television. January 14, 1996.

2.12.46 ***Electronic Citations.***—The NLM *Recommended Formats*[9] document includes guidelines for many types of electronic citations, examples of which are given. As electronic forms of documents proliferate and the number of citations to them increases, additional guidelines likely will be required. Already, specific guidelines on these forms of citations are appearing.[12-14] The recommendations in this section combine those in NLM's *Recommended Formats*[9] and those at the Li/Crane Web site.[14] When citing an electronic document that also exists in print form, you should cite the version you consulted. Annotation of an additional version of the same publication might also be helpful.[15]

Software: To cite software, use the following form. When the computer program is mentioned only in passing and is not the subject of the report, the software used does not need to be added to the reference list. However, in these cases, the manufacturer of the software, and the manufacturer's location, should be included in parentheses in the text (see 12.5, Nomenclature, Equipment, Devices, and Reagents).

1. *Epi Info* [computer program]. Version 6. Atlanta, Ga: Centers for Disease Control and Prevention; 1994.

Software Manual: If it is not the software but the software manual or guide that is being cited, use the following form, which follows that for citation of a book (see 2.12.28, References to Books, Complete Data).

1. Dean AG, Dean JA, Coulombier D, et al. *Epi Info, Version 6: A Word-Processing, Database, and Statistics Program for Public Health on IBM-Compatible Microcomputers.* Atlanta, Ga: Centers for Disease Control and Prevention; 1994.
2. Dixon WJ, Brown MB, Engelman L, Jennirch RI, eds. *BMDP Statistical Software Manual.* Los Angeles: University of California Press; 1990.

Online Journals: References to articles cited in online journals may take 1 of the 2 following forms:

- Journals without volume and page information: For online journals that do not use the typical year, volume, and page format of print journal citations, a document number, preceded by a date of publication, may be used.

  1. Harrison CL, Schmidt PQ, Jones JD. Aspirin compared with acetaminophen for relief of headache. *Online J Curr Clin Trials* [serial online]. January 2, 1992;doc 1.

- Journals with volume and page information: Citations to online journals that do use year, volume, and page formats take a form similar to that of citations to print journals. The inclusion of date accessed (consulted) is appropriate and especially important when articles in online journals that allow changes to be made in the article after its publication are cited.

  1. Friedman SA. Preeclampsia: a review of the role of prostaglandins. *Obstet Gynecol* [serial online]. January 1988;71(1):22-37. Available from: BRS Information Technologies, McLean, Va. Accessed December 15, 1990.

CD-ROMs: When citing a book or monograph in a CD-ROM format, use the following form:

1. *The Oxford English Dictionary* [book on CD-ROM]. 2nd ed. New York, NY: Oxford University Press; 1992.
2. *The American Heritage Dictionary: Reference Tool for Windows* [book on CD-ROM]. Cambridge, Mass: SoftKey International Inc; 1995. Based on: *American Heritage Dictionary of the English Language, Third Edition.* Boston, Mass: Houghton Mifflin Co; 1992.
3. *AMA Drug Evaluations Annual 1993* [book on CD-ROM]. Jackson, Wyo: Teton Data Systems; 1993. Based on: Sugden R, ed. *AMA Drug Evaluations Annual*

1993. Chicago, Ill: American Medical Association; 1993. STAT!-Ref Medical Reference Library.

4. *Williams Obstetrics* [book on CD-ROM]. Jackson, Wyo: Teton Data Systems; 1993. Based on: Cunningham FG, MacDonald PC, Grant NF, Leveno KJ, Gilstrap LC III. *Williams Obstetrics.* 19th ed. East Norwalk, Conn: Appleton & Lange; 1993. STAT!-Ref Medical Reference Library.

Citation of a journal article on CD-ROM takes the following form:

5. Gershon ES. Antisocial behavior. *Arch Gen Psychiatry* [serial on CD-ROM]. 1995;52:900-901.

Databases: When citing a database, use the following form:

1. CANCERNET-PDQ [database online]. Bethesda, Md: National Cancer Institute; 1996. Updated March 29, 1996.

World Wide Web: Citations to material on a Web site take the following form:

1. Rosenthal S, Chen R, Hadler S. The safety of acellular pertussis vaccine vs whole-cell pertussis vaccine [abstract]. *Arch Pediatr Adolesc Med* [serial online]. 1996; 150:457-460. Available at: http://www.ama-assn.org/sci-pubs/journals/archive/ajdc/vol_150/no_5/abstract/htm. Accessed November 10, 1996.
2. Gostin LO. Drug use and HIV/AIDS [*JAMA* HIV/AIDS Web site]. June 1, 1996. Available at: http://www.ama-assn.org/special/hiv/ethics. Accessed June 26, 1997.
3. LaPorte RE, Marler E, Akazawa S, Sauer F, et al. The death of biomedical journals. *BMJ* [serial online]. 1995;310:1387-1390. Available at: http://www.bmj.com/bmj/archive/6991ed2.htm. Accessed June 26, 1997.
4. FDA/CFSAN resources page. Food and Drug Administration Web site. Available at: http://vm.cfsan.fda.gov/;aplrd/sodium.txt. Accessed June 23, 1997.
5. Health on the Net Foundation. Health on the Net Foundation code of conduct (HONcode) for medical and health web sites. Available at: http://www.hon.ch/Conduct.html. Accessed June 26, 1997.
6. Health Care Financing Administration. 1996 statistics at a glance. Available at: http://www.hcfa.gov/stats/stathili.htm. Accessed December 2, 1996.

E-mail: References to e-mail messages, as to other forms of personal communication (see also 2.12.47, Unpublished Material), should be listed parenthetically in the text and should include (1) the name of the person who sent the message, (2) the sender's e-mail address, and (3) the date the message was sent. An example of an e-mail citation, appearing in running text, appears below:

Unlike e-mail addresses, URLs [uniform resource locators] may be case-sensitive (J. M. Kramer, K. Kramer [jmkramer@umich.edu], e-mail, March 6, 1996).

2.12.47 ***Unpublished Material.***—References to unpublished material may include articles or abstracts that have been presented at a society meeting but not published and material accepted for publication but not published. If, during the course of the publication process, these materials *are* published or accepted for publication, and if the author is familiar with the later version, the most up-to-date bibliographic information should be included.

Items Presented at a Meeting but Not Published: These oral presentations take the following form:

1. Eisenberg J. Market forces and physician workforce reform: why they may not work. Paper presented at: Annual Meeting of the Association of American Medical Colleges; October 28, 1995; Washington, DC.

2. Jones JL, Hanson DL, Ward JW, Kaplan JE. Incidence and trends in AIDS-related opportunistic illnesses in injecting drug users and men who have sex with men. In: Program and abstracts of the XI International Conference on AIDS; July 7-12, 1996; Vancouver, British Columbia. Abstract We.C.3418.
3. Donegan J. Anesthesia for patients with ischemic cerebrovascular disease. Refresher course lectures presented at: American Society of Anesthesiologists; October 17-21, 1981; New Orleans, La.

Once these presentations do become published, they take the form of reference to a book, journal, or other medium in which they are ultimately published, as in the example shown (see 2.12.28, References to Books, Complete Data):

4. Slama K, ed. *Tobacco and Health: Proceedings of the Ninth World Conference on Tobacco and Health, Paris, France, 10-14 October 1994.* New York, NY: Plenum Press; 1995.

Material Accepted for Publication but Not Published: Formats suggested for both journal articles and books, accepted for publication but not yet published, are shown below:

5. Klassen TP, Watters LK, Feldman ME, Sutcliffe T, Rowe PC. The efficacy of nebulized budesonide in dexamethasone-treated outpatients with croup. *Pediatrics.* In press.
6. Akil H, Morano MI. The biology of stress: from periphery to brain. In: Watson SJ, ed. *Biology of Schizophrenia and Affective Disease.* Washington, DC: American Psychiatric Press. In press.
7. Mrak RE. Ultrastructural diagnosis of tumors of the nervous system. In: Garcia JH, ed. *Diagnostic Neuropathology.* Vol 4. New York, NY: Oxford University Press. In press.

Some publications require that authors demonstrate proof that acceptance for publication has been granted.[9,16] Some publishers also prefer the term *forthcoming* to *in press* because they feel that the latter is not appropriate for electronic citations,[9,16] in which case online designation would also be used, as shown in 2.12.46, Electronic Citations.

In the list of references, do not include material that has been submitted for publication but has not yet been accepted. This material, with its date, should be noted in the text as "unpublished data," as follows:

These findings have recently been corroborated (H. E. Marman, MD, unpublished data, January 1996).

Similar findings have been noted by Roberts[6] and H. E. Marman, MD (unpublished data, 1996).

Numerous studies[12-20] (also H. E. Marman, MD, unpublished data, 1996) have described similar findings.

If the unpublished data referred to are those of the author, indicate this as follows:

Other data (H.E.M., unpublished data, 1996). . . .

Do not include "personal communications" in the list of references. The following forms may be used in the text:

In a conversation with H. E. Marman, MD (August 1996). . . .

According to a letter from H. E. Marman, MD, in August 1996. . . .

Similar findings have been noted by Roberts[6] and by H. E. Marman, MD (written communication, August 1996).

According to the manufacturer (H. R. Smith, oral communication, May 1996), the drug became available in Japan in January 1995.

The author should give the date of the communication and indicate whether it was in an oral or written form. Highest academic degrees should also be given. On occasion, the affiliation of the person might also be included to better establish the relevance and authority of the citation.

See also 2.12.46, Electronic Citations, E-mail.

Some journals now require that the author obtain written permission from the person whose unpublished data or personal communication is thus cited.[1,16] (See 3.2.1, Ethical and Legal Considerations, Permission to Name Individuals.)

2.12.48 ***Secondary Citations and Quotations (Including Press Releases).***— Reference may be made to one author's citation of, or quotation from, another's work. Distinguish between citation and quotation (ie, between work mentioned and words actually quoted). In the text, the name of the original author, rather than the secondary source, should be mentioned (see also 2.12.24, Discussants). As with citation of an abstract of an article rather than citation of the original document (see 2.12.21, Abstracts and Other Material Taken From Another Source), citation of the original document is preferred unless it is not readily available. Only items actually consulted should be listed. The forms for listed references are as follows:

1. Gordis E. Relapse and craving: a commentary. *Alcohol Alert.* 1989;6:3. Cited by: Mason BJ, Kocsis JH, Ritvo EC, Cutler RB. A double-blind, placebo-controlled trial of desipramine for primary alcohol dependence stratified on the presence or absence of major depression. *JAMA.* 1996;275:761-767.

Occasionally, though rarely, a more complex citation "history" is required.

2. Wang YX, Jin X, Jiang HF, et al. Studies on the percutaneous absorption of four radioactive labeled pesticides. *Acta Acad Med Primae Shanghai.* 1981;8:370. Cited by: Bartelt N, Hubbell JP. *Percutaneous Absorption of Topically Applied 14C-Permethrin in Volunteers: Final Medical Report.* Research Triangle Park, NC: Burroughs Wellcome Co/Fairfield American Corp; 1989:378-410. Publication 86182. Cited by: *Permethrin (Permanone Tick Repellent): Risk Characterization Document (Revised).* Sacramento: Dept of Pesticide Regulation, California Environmental Protection Agency; 1994.
3. Leary WE. Quoted by: Smoking Control Advocacy Resource Center (SCARC) Action Alert. *Issue: Study Correlates Advertising With Increased Youth Consumption.* Washington, DC: Advocacy Institute; March 15, 1994.
4. Cigarette smoking among American teens rises again in 1995 [press release]. Ann Arbor: University of Michigan Survey Research Center; December 15, 1995.

2.12.49 ***Classical References.***—Classical references may deviate from the usual forms in some details. In many instances, the facts of publication are irrelevant and may be omitted. Date of publication should be given when available and pertinent.

1. Shakespeare W. *A Midsummer Night's Dream.* Act 2, scene 3, line 24.
2. Donne J. *Second Anniversary.* Verse 243.

For classical references, *The Chicago Manual of Style*[17] may be used as a guide.

3. Aristotle. *Metaphysics.* 3. 2.966b 5-8.

In biblical references, do not abbreviate the names of books. The version may be included parenthetically if the information is provided. References to the Bible are usually included in the text.

The story begins in Genesis 3:1.

Paul admonished against succumbing to temptation (I Corinthians 10:6-13).

Occasionally they may appear as listed references at the end of the article.

4. I Corinthians 10:6-13 (RSV).

2.12.50 ***Legal References.***—A specific style variation is used for references to legal citations. Because the system of citation used is complex, with numerous variations for different types of sources and among various jurisdictions, only a brief outline can be presented here. For more details, consult *The Bluebook: A Uniform System of Citation.*[18]

Method of Citation: A legal reference may be included in full in the text or in the reference list, or partially in the text and partially in the reference list.

In a leading decision on informed consent (*Cobbs v Grant,* 502 P2d 1 [Cal 1972]), the California Supreme Court stated. . . .

In a leading decision on informed consent,[1] the California Supreme Court stated. . . .

In the case of *Cobbs v Grant* (502 P2d 1 [Cal 1972]). . . .

In the case of *Cobbs v Grant*[1]. . . .

Citation of Cases: The citation of a case (ie, a court opinion) generally includes, in the following order:

- The name of the case in italics (only the names of the first party on each side are used, never with "et al," and only the last names of individuals)
- The volume number, name, and series number (if any) of the case reporter in which it is published
- The page in the volume on which the case begins and, if applicable, the specific page or pages on which is discussed the point for which the case is being cited
- In parentheses, the name of the court that rendered the opinion (unless the court is identified by the name of the reporter) and the year of the decision. If the opinion is published in more than 1 reporter, the citations to each reporter (known as parallel citations) are separated by commas. Note that *v*, 2d, and 3d are standard usage in legal citations.

1. *Canterbury v Spence,* 464 F2d 772,775 (DC Cir 1972).

This case is published in volume 464 of the *Federal Reporter,* second series. The case begins on page 772, and the specific point for which it was cited is on page 775. The case was decided by the US Court of Appeals, District of Columbia Circuit, in 1972.

The proper reporter to cite depends on the court that wrote the opinion. Table T.1 of *The Bluebook* contains a complete list of all current and former state and federal jurisdictions.

US SUPREME COURT. Cite to *US Reports* (abbreviated as US). If the case is too recent to be published there, cite to *Supreme Court Reporter* (SCt), *US Reports, Lawyer's Edition* (LEd), or *US Law Week* (USLW)—in that order. Do *not* include parallel citation.

US COURT OF APPEALS (FORMERLY KNOWN AS CIRCUIT COURTS OF APPEALS). Cite to *Federal Reporter,* original or second series (F or F2d). These intermediate appellate-level courts hear appeals from US district courts, federal administrative agencies, and other federal trial-level courts. Individual US Courts of Appeals, known as circuits, are referred to by number (1st Cir, 2d Cir, etc), except for the District of Columbia Circuit (DC Cir) and the Federal Circuit (Fed Cir), which hears appeals from the US Claims Court and from various customs and patent cases. Citations to the *Federal Reporter* must include the circuit designation in parentheses with the year of the decision.

2. *Wilcox v United States,* 387 F2d 60 (5th Cir 1967).

US DISTRICT COURT AND CLAIMS COURTS. Cite to *Federal Supplement* (F Supp). (There is only the original series so far.) These trial-level courts are not as prolific as the appellate courts; their function is to hear the original cases rather than review them. There are more than 100 of these courts, which are referred to by geographical designations that must be included in the citation (eg, the Northern District of Illinois [ND Ill], the Central District of California [CD Cal], *but* District of New Jersey [D NJ], as New Jersey has only 1 federal district).

3. *Sierra Club v Froehlke,* 359 F Supp 1289 (SD Tex 1973).

STATE COURTS. Cite to the appropriate official (ie, state-sanctioned and state-financed) reporter (if any) *and* the appropriate regional reporter. Most states have separate official reporters for their highest and intermediate appellate courts (eg, *Illinois Reports* and *Illinois Appellate Court Reports*), but the regional reporters include cases from both levels. Official reporters are always listed first, although an increasing number of states are no longer publishing them. The regional reporters are the *Atlantic Reporter* (A or A2d), *North Eastern Reporter* (NE or NE2d), *South Eastern Reporter* (SE or SE2d), *Southern Reporter* (So or So2d), *North Western Reporter* (NW or NW2d), *South Western Reporter* (SW or SW2d), and *Pacific Reporter* (P or P2d). If only the regional reporter citation is given, the name of the court must appear in parentheses with the year of the decision. If the opinion is from the highest court of a state (usually but not always known as the supreme court), the abbreviated state name is sufficient (except for Ohio St). The full name of the court is abbreviated (eg, Ill App, NJ Super Ct App Div, NY App Div). A third, also unofficial, reporter is published for a few states; citations solely to these reporters must include the court name (eg, *California Reporter* [Cal Rptr], *New York Supplement* [NYS or NYS2d]).

4. *People v Carpenter,* 28 Ill2d 116, 190 NE2d 738 (1963).
5. *Webb v Stone,* 445 SW2d 842 (Ky 1969).

When a case has been reviewed or otherwise dealt with by a higher court, the subsequent history of the case should be given in the citation. If the year is the same for both opinions, include it only at the end of the citation. The phrases indicating the subsequent history are set off by commas, italicized, and abbreviated (eg, *aff'd* [affirmed by the higher court], *rev'd* [reversed], *vacated* [made legally void, annulled], *appeal dismissed, cert denied* [application for a writ of certiorari, ie, a request that a court hear an appeal, has been denied]).

6. *Glazer v Glazer,* 374 F2d 390 (5th Cir), *cert denied,* 389 US 831 (1967).

This opinion was written by the US Court of Appeals for the Fifth Circuit in 1967. In the same year, the US Supreme Court was asked to review the case in an application for a writ of certiorari but denied the request. This particular subsequent history is important because it indicates that the case has been taken to the highest court available and thus strengthens the case's value as precedent for future legal decisions.

Citation of Statutes: Once a bill is enacted into law by the US Congress, it is integrated into the US Code (USC). Citations of statutes include the official name of the act, the title number (similar to a chapter number), the abbreviation of the code cited, the section number (designated by §), and the date of the code edition cited.

7. Comprehensive Environmental Response, Compensation, and Liability Act, 42 USC §9601-9675 (1988).

This example cites sections 9601-9675 of title 42 of the US Code.

If a federal statute has not yet been codified, cite to Statutes at Large (abbreviated Stat, preceded by a volume number, and followed by a page number), if available, and the Public Law number of the statute.

8. Pub L No. 93-627, 88 Stat 2126.

The name of the statute may be added if it provides clarification.

9. Labor Managment Relations (Taft-Hartley) Act §301(a), 29USC §185a (1988).

Citation forms for state statutes vary considerably. Table T.1 in *The Bluebook* lists examples for each state.

10. Ill Rev Stat ch 38, §2.

This is section 2 of chapter 38 of Illinois Revised Statutes.

11. Fla Stat §202.

This is section 202 of Florida Statutes.

12. Mich Comp Laws §145.

This is section 145 of Michigan Compiled Laws.

13. Wash Rev Code §45.

This is section 45 of Revised Code of Washington.

14. Cal Corp Code §300.

This is section 300 of California Corporations Code.

Citation of Federal Administrative Regulations: Federal regulations are published in the *Federal Register* and then codified in the Code of Federal Regulations.

15. 55 *Federal Register* 36612 (1990) (codified at 26 CFR §52).

If a rule or regulation is known by its name, the name should be given.

16. Medicare, Medicaid and CLIA programs: regulations implementing the Clinical Laboratory Improvement Amendments of 1988 (CLIA), 57 *Federal Register* 7002 (1992).

Regulations promulgated by the Internal Revenue Service retain their unique format. Temporary regulations must be denoted as such.

17. Treas Reg §1.72 (1963).
18. Temp Treas Reg §1.338 (1985).

Citation forms for state administrative regulations are especially diverse. Again, Table T.1 in *The Bluebook* lists the appropriate form for each state.

Citation of Congressional Hearings: Include the full title of the hearing, the subcommittee (if any) and committee names, the number and session of the Congress, the date, and a short description if desired.

19. *Hearings Before the Consumer Subcommittee of the Senate Committee on Commerce,* 90th Cong, 1st Sess (1965) (testimony of William Stewart, MD, surgeon general).
20. *Discrimination on the Basis of Pregnancy, 1977: Hearings on S995 Before the Subcommittee on Labor of the Senate Committee on Human Resources,* 95th Cong, 1st Sess (1977) (statement of Ethel Walsh, vice-chairman, EEOC).

Citations to Services: Many legal materials, including some reports of cases and some administrative materials, are published by commercial services (eg, Commerce Clearing House [CCH Inc]), often in looseleaf format. These services attempt to provide a comprehensive overview of rapidly changing areas of the law (eg, tax law, labor law, securities regulation) and are updated frequently, sometimes weekly. The citation should include the volume number of the service, its abbreviated title, the publisher's name (also abbreviated), the paragraph or section or page number, and the date.

21. 7 Sec Reg Guide (P-H) ¶2333 (1984).

This example cites volume 7, paragraph 2333, of the *Securities Regulation Guide,* published by Prentice-Hall in 1984.

22. 54 Ins L Rep (CCH) 137 (1979).

This is volume 54, page 137, of *Insurance Law Reports,* published by Commerce Clearing House in 1979.

23. 4 OSH Rep (BNA) 750 (1980).

This is volume 4, page 750, of the *Occupational Safety and Health Reporter,* published by the Bureau of National Affairs in 1980.

2.13 ■ **TABLES.**—By virtue of their capacity to present detailed information effectively and in ways that text alone cannot, tables are an essential component of many scientific articles. Tables can condense, summarize, organize, and display complex or detailed data and therefore are commonly used to present study results.

The purpose of a table is to present data or information and support statements in the text. Information in the table must be accurate and consistent with that in the text in context and style. However, a properly designed and constructed table should be able to stand independently, without the requirement of explanation from the text.

2.13.1 ***Tables vs Figures.***—Tables and figures (eg, graphs, charts, and maps; see 2.14, Figures) are used to express and demonstrate relationships among numerical data and other types of information (Table 3). A well-structured table is perhaps the most efficient way to convey a large amount of data in a scientific manuscript. As text, the same information may take considerably more space; if summarized as a figure, key details of exact data may be less apparent.

Text may be preferred if the information can be presented concisely (Example T1). For qualitative information, text should be used if the relationships among data are simple and data are few, whereas a figure (eg, a diagram) should be used if the relationships are complex.[19] For quantitative information, a table should be used when the display of exact values is important, whereas a figure (eg, a graph) should be used to demonstrate patterns or trends.[19] Tables also are preferable to graphics for many small data sets and also are preferred when data presentation

TABLE 3. GUIDELINES FOR USING TEXT VS TABLES VS FIGURES TO DISPLAY NUMERICAL DATA

Uses of text
- Present quantitative data that can be given concisely and clearly
- Describe simple relationships among qualitative data

Uses of tables
- Present more than a few precise numerical values
- Present large amounts of detailed quantitative information in a smaller space than would be required in the text
- Demonstrate detailed item-to-item comparisons
- Display many quantitative values simultaneously
- Display individual data values precisely
- Demonstrate complex relationships in qualitative data

Uses of figures
- Highlight patterns or trends in data
- Demonstrate changes or differences over time
- Display complex relationships among quantitative variables
- Clarify or explain methods
- Provide information to enhance understanding of complex concepts
- Provide visual data to illustrate findings (eg, graphics, photographs, x-ray films, maps)

requires many specific comparisons. Regardless of the tabular or graphical presentation, the same data should not be duplicated in a table and a figure or in the text.

Priorities in the creation and use of tables and figures are to emphasize important information efficiently and to ensure that each table and figure makes a clear point. In addition to presenting study results, tables and figures can be used to explain or amplify the methods or highlight other key points in the article. Like a paragraph, each table or figure should be cohesive and focused. To be most effective, tables and figures should present ideas and information in a logical sequence. The relationship of tables and figures to the text and to each other should be considered in manuscript preparation, editorial evaluation, peer review, article layout, and publication.

When used properly, tables and figures add variety to article layout and are visually compelling and distinct components of scientific manuscripts. However,

Table 1. Severity of Injury Among 142 Injured Patients

Injury Severity Score	Patients, No. (%)
0-4	30 (21)
5-10	69 (48)
11-20	42 (30)
>20	1 (1)

Of the 142 injured patients, 30 (21%) had an Injury Severity Score (ISS) of 0 to 4; 69 (48%) had an ISS of 5 to 10; 42 (30%) had an ISS of 11 to 20; and 1 (1%) had an ISS greater than 20.

EXAMPLE T1 Presentation of data as a table (top) and as text (bottom). The information can be presented as text concisely and completely. Text is preferred in this instance instead of the table.

The operative procedures performed among the patients with bowel obstruction included the following:

Procedure	No.
Bypass	
Enterocolostomy	15
Enteroenterostomy	13
Gastrojejunostomy	1
Cutaneous stomas	
Colostomy	11
Enterostomy	4
Lysis of adhesions	14
Bowel resection with anastomosis	3
Adjunctive procedures	20
Tube jejunostomy	3

One or more bypass procedures were the most common approach to relieve obstruction. Tube gastrostomy or tube jejunostomy was a frequent adjunctive procedure to vent the gastrointestinal tract in patients with prolonged postoperative ileus or persistent obstruction.

EXAMPLE T2 In-text tabulation. The information is presented concisely and helps add variety to break up running text. These data also could be presented in a small table.

authors and editors of scientific publications should avoid using tables and figures simply to break up text or primarily to impart visual interest. Considering the potential of tables and figures to convey information, authors and editors should strive to ensure the relevance and accuracy of these powerful tools.

2.13.2 ***Types of Tables.***—*Tabulation:* A tabulation is a brief, informal, in-text table that may be used to set material off from text.[20] Tabulations are part of the text and require the text to explain their meaning. Tabulations usually consist of 1 or 2 columns of data. A tabulation is set off from text by the use of space above and below and also may have boldface column headings. Titles, numbering, and rules are unnecessary. The tabulation should be centered within a single typeset column and may be set in reduced type (Example T2).

Formal Table: A formal table (as distinguished from a tabulation) displays information arranged in columns and rows (Example T3 and 2.13.4, Table Components) and is used most commonly to present numerical data. Each formal table has a title, is numbered consecutively as referred to in the text, and should be positioned as close as possible to its first mention in the text. Formal tables usually are set off from the text by horizontal rules, boxes, or white space.

Textual Tables: A textual or word table displays words, phrases, or sentences in list form. These formal tables are used to emphasize key points, to summarize information, and to reduce the narrative text (Example T4).

Matrix: A matrix is a tabular structure that uses numbers, short words (eg, no, yes), or symbols (eg, bullets, check marks) and provides a visual image in table form.[20] A matrix depicts mutual relationships among items in columns and rows and allows for comparisons among entries. Each entry in the matrix presents information about the combination of items represented by the cell (Example T5).

2.13.3 ***Organizing Information in Tables.***—For a table to have maximum effectiveness, the information it contains must be arranged logically and clearly so that the

Table number and title

Table 1. Risk Factors for Cardiac Arrest*

Characteristic	Patients With Cardiac Arrest (n = 225)	Controls (n = 234)
Age, mean (SD), y	54 (11)	55 (10)
Men	180 (80)	175 (75)
White	192 (85)	187 (90)
Medical history		
Diabetes	29 (13)	31 (13)
Hypertension	68 (30)	55 (24)
Previous CAD	49 (22)	21 (9)
Previous MI	32 (14)	16 (7)
Body mass index, mean (SD), kg/m^2	26 (4)	25 (3)
Total cholesterol, mean (SD), mmol/L [mg/dL]	6.23 (0.08) [241 (3.1)]	5.85 (0.06) [226.2 (2.5)]

* Values are number (percentage) unless otherwise indicated.
CAD indicates coronary artery disease; MI, myocardial infarction.

Column headings

Stubs (row headings)

Field with data cells

Footnotes

EXAMPLE T3 Components of a formal table.

reader can quickly understand the key point and find the specific data of interest. Information in tables should be organized into columns and rows by type and category, thereby simplifying access and display of data and information.

During the planning and creation of a table, the author should consider the primary comparisons of interest. Because readers usually make comparisons first horizontally (from left to right) and then vertically (from top to bottom), the primary comparisons should be shown horizontally across the table. Data that

Table 1. Common Elements of Problem Solving in Smoking Cessation Treatments

Component	Examples
Recognition of dangerous situations Identification of events, internal states, or activities that are thought to increase the risk of smoking or relapse	Being around other smokers Being under time pressure Getting into an argument Experiencing urges or negative moods Using alcohol
Development of coping skills Identification and practice of coping or problem-solving skills, which typically are intended to cope with dangerous situations	Learning to anticipate and avoid dangerous situations Learning cognitive strategies that will reduce negative moods Accomplishing lifestyle changes that will reduce stress, improve quality of life, or produce pleasure Learning cognitive and behavioral activities that distract attention from smoking urges
Provision of basic information The provision of basic information about smoking and successful quitting	Explaining the nature and time course of withdrawal Discussing the addictive nature of smoking Emphasizing that any smoking (even a single puff) increases the likelihood of full relapse

EXAMPLE T4 Text table. The arrangement of the stub headings and the indention of runover lines in the stub entries create an hierarchical order for the entries. The entries in the table categories use parallel construction to create consistency. Adapted from *JAMA.* 1996;275:1273.

Table 1. Objectives of Proposals to Reform Medical Education*

Objectives	Report Year															
	1910	1932	1940	1953	1959	1965	1966	1970	1972	1982	1983	1984	1989	1991	1992	1993
Serve changing public interest	X	X		X		X	X	X		X		X	X	X		X
Address physician workforce needs	X	X			X	X		X	X							
Cope with burgeoning knowledge	X	X	X		X	X	X	X	X	X	X	X			X	X
Foster generalism; decrease fragmentation		X		X			X		X	X		X	X	X	X	X
Apply new educational methods		X		X		X			X		X	X	X			
Address changing nature of illness burden						X		X				X		X	X	
Address changing nature of practice					X	X	X	X	X			X				
Increase quality and standards of education	X	X	X	X	X	X		X	X		X	X				

*The objectives are listed roughly in order of their overall centrality to reform proposals, in terms of the quantity and quality of the attention they are accorded within and across the reports. X denotes that the objective is present in the report year. No entry indicates objective not present.

EXAMPLE T5 Matrix. The letter "X" is used in the matrix entries to denote the presence of an objective for a given year. In this matrix with dichotomous entries (X = yes, no entry = no), the empty cells are acceptable, provided the lack of entry is explained. Adapted from *JAMA*. 1995;274:708.

depict cause-and-effect or before-and-after relationships should be arranged from left to right if space allows or, alternatively, from top to bottom. Similar data elements should be arranged vertically rather than horizontally. Information being compared (such as numerical data) should be juxtaposed within adjacent rows or adjacent columns to facilitate comparisons among items of interest.

Although tables frequently are used to present many quantitative values, authors should remember that tabulating all collected study data is unnecessary, and actually may distract and overwhelm the reader. Data presented in a table should be pertinent and meaningful.

2.13.4 ***Table Components.***—Formal tables in scientific articles conventionally contain 5 major elements: title, column headings, row headings (table stubs), body (data field) consisting of individual cells (data points), and footnotes (Example T3). Details pertaining to elements of style for table construction vary among publications; what follows is based on the general style of AMA journals.

Title: Each table should have a brief, specific, descriptive title, usually written as a phrase rather than as a sentence. The title should distinguish the table from other data displays in the article. The title should convey the topic of the table succinctly but should not provide detailed background information or summarize or interpret the results.

Tables should be numbered consecutively according to the order in which they are mentioned in the text. The word *Table* and the table number are part of the table title. If the article contains only 1 table, it is referred to in the text as "Table" and the title of the table does not include the designation "Table." For articles with more than 1 table, the tables are numbered consecutively, with the number of the table given after the word "Table" in the title and followed by a period. The capitalization style used in titles should be followed for table titles (see 2.1.6, Capitalization). The following are examples of table titles:

Table 1. Symptoms and Signs of Chronic Fatigue Syndrome

Table 5. Relationship of Blood Pressure and Intraocular Pressure in Patients With Open-angle Glaucoma

Column Headings: The main categories of information in the table should have their own columns. In tables for studies that have independent and dependent variables, the independent variables conventionally are displayed in the left-hand column and the dependent variables in the columns to the right. Each column should have a brief heading that identifies and applies to all items listed in that column. If necessary, the unit of measure should be indicated in the column heading (unless it is given in the table stub) and is preceded by a comma. Column headings are set in boldface type. If necessary, column subheadings may be used. For more complex headings, braces may be used or additional explanatory information may be provided in the footnotes (Example T6).

If all elements in a column are identical (eg, if all patients were men and a column indicated the patients' sex), this information could be provided in a footnote or in the table title rather than in a separate column.

In column headings, guidelines regarding numbers and abbreviations may be relaxed somewhat to save space, with abbreviations expanded in a footnote. However, when space allows spelled-out headings, expansions are preferable to abbreviations. The capitalization style used in titles should be followed (see 2.1.6, Capitalization).

Table 1. Outcome and Cost-effectiveness Results for Base-Case and Worst-Case Scenarios for 2 Extreme Demographic Categories*

	White Women Aged 60 y				White Men Aged ≥ 85 y			
	Base Case		Worst Case		Base Case		Worst Case	
Result	THA	No THA	THA	No THA	THA	No THA	THA	No THA
Expected years in ACR class I	13.27	0	4.79	0	3.36	0	1.34	0
Expected years in ACR class II	7.13	0	11.56	0	1.59	0	3.19	0
Expected years in ACR class III	1.38	14.88	3.52	18.10	0.09	4.47	0.34	4.76
Expected years in ACR class IV	0.60	7.73	1.98	4.51	0.02	0.63	0.12	0.34
Life expectancy, y	22.38	22.61	21.85	22.61	5.06	5.10	4.99	5.10
QALY†	13.70	6.82	7.63	6.43	4.16	2.16	3.13	2.61
Expected cost, $ ‡	47 649	165 440	68 478	38 499	30 580	21 432	48 265	7 338

*THA indicates total hip arthroplasty; ACR, American College of Rheumatology; and QALY, quality-adjusted life-year.
†QALY discounted at 5% for base case and 8% for worst case.
‡Expected costs discounted at 5% for base case and 8% for worst case.

EXAMPLE T6 Column headings and 2-level subheadings with use of braces to group data. Adapted from *JAMA.* 1996;275:862.

Table Stubs (Row Headings): The left-most column of a table contains the table stubs (or row headings), which are used to label the rows of the table and apply to all items in that row. If a unit of measure is necessary and is not included in the column heading, it should be included in the stub heading. Stub headings are capitalized according to style for sentences, not titles. Therefore, if a symbol (such as a percent sign), an arabic numeral, or a lowercase Greek letter begins the entry, the first word to follow should be capitalized.

Stub headings are left-justified, and indentions are used to depict hierarchical components of the stub headings. The first indentation is a 1-em indentation, and runover lines or secondary indentations use a 2-em indentation.

For a table that may be readily divided into parts to enhance clarity or for 2 closely related tables that would be better combined, cut-in headings are useful. The cut-in heading is placed above the table columns (below the column heads) and applies to all tabular material below. Cut-in headings are set boldface, are centered, and have a 1-point rule above but no rule below them (Example T7).

Field: The field or body of the table presents the data. Each data entry point is contained in a cell, which is the intersection of a column and a row. Table cells may contain numerals, text, or symbols. Data in the field should be arranged logically so the reader can find an individual data point in the table easily. For instance, time order should be used for data collected in sequence (Example T8). Similar types of data should be grouped. Numbers that are added or averaged should be placed in the same column. Different types of data or information should not be mixed within a single column.

Missing data and blank space in the table field (ie, an empty cell) may create ambiguity and should be avoided, unless an entry in a cell does not apply (eg, a column head does not apply to one of the items in the stub).[16]

In most cases, an indicator, rather than blank space, should be used for cells that lack data.[16] The numeral "0" should be used to indicate that the value of the data in the cell is 0. Ellipses (. . .) may be used to indicate that no data are available for a cell or that the category of data is not applicable for a cell. However, ellipses should not be used to denote different types of missing elements in the same table. Other designations, such as NA (for "not available" or "not applicable") or

Table 1. Selected Pregnancy Outcomes and Neonatal Measurements in the Zinc Supplement and Placebo Subgroups by Body Mass Index (BMI) Categories*

	BMI ≥26 kg/m^2			BMI <26 kg/m^2		
Characteristic	Zinc Supplement (n = 155)	Placebo (n = 145)	*P*	Zinc Supplement (n = 134)	Placebo (n = 134)	*P*
Maternal Characteristics						
Age, y	24.8	24.2	.32	22.9	21.2	.01
BMI, kg/m^2	33.4	33.0	.64	22.3	22.2	.57
Current smoker, %	7.7	5.5	.44	3.0	3.0	.98
Pregnancy Outcome						
Birth weight, g	3240	3241	.99	3190	2942	.005
Gestational age, wk	39.0	38.7	.47	38.6	37.9	.08
Preterm birth <32 wk, %	3.2	5.5	.33	3.0	6.8	.15
Birth weight <1500 g, %	3.9	3.5	.84	2.3	6.0	.12
Anthropometric Measurements						
Crown-heel length, cm	50.2	49.8	.41	50.3	49.7	.20
Head circumference, cm	34.3	34.0	.50	34.1	33.4	.005
Abdominal circumference, cm	33.3	33.1	.64	32.8	32.6	.58
Arm length, cm	9.9	9.7	.27	9.9	9.6	.03
Subscapular skinfold, mm	4.2	3.9	.05	3.9	3.6	.06
Neonatal Outcome						
Neonatal hospital stay, d	3.9	4.5	.47	3.1	4.9	.10
Neonatal sepsis, %	0.7	1.4	.52	0	2.2	.08

*Values are means unless otherwise indicated.

EXAMPLE T7 Use of cut-in headings. Adapted from *JAMA.* 1995;274:466.

Table 1. Women in US Medical Schools*

Academic Year	Women Applicants, No. (%)	Women in Entering Class, No. (%)	Total Women Enrolled, No. (%)	Graduates, No. (%)
1985-1986	11 562 (35.1)	5788 (34.2)	21 624 (32.5)	4930 (30.8)
1986-1987	11 267 (36.0)	5866 (35.0)	22 082 (33.4)	5092 (32.1)
1987-1988	10 411 (37.0)	6087 (36.5)	22 539 (34.3)	5356 (33.7)
1988-1989	10 264 (38.4)	6205 (37.0)	22 902 (35.1)	5225 (33.5)
1989-1990	10 546 (39.2)	6404 (38.2)	23 501 (36.1)	5197 (33.9)
1990-1991	11 785 (40.3)	6499 (38.7)	24 164 (37.2)	5593 (36.1)
1991-1992	13 700 (41.4)	6777 (39.8)	24 911 (38.0)	5483 (35.7)
1992-1993	15 619 (41.8)	7100 (41.8)	25 933 (39.3)	5924 (38.1)
1993-1994†	17 957 (42.0)	7213 (42.2)	26 737 (40.2)	5951 (38.2)
1994-1995	18 968 (41.8)	7191 (42.2)	27 497 (41.0)	6216 (39.1)
1995-1996	19 779 (42.5)	7351 (43.2)	27 976 (41.8)	6528 (40.7)‡

*Data are from *Medical School Admission Requirements,* Association of American Medical Colleges, Section for Student Services.

†Meharry Medical College, Nashville, Tenn, did not report for 1993-1994; 1992-1993 data were used.

‡Estimated in April 1996.

EXAMPLE T8 Time ordering of data to facilitate identification of data points by year. Adapted from *JAMA.* 1996;276:717.

Table 1. Health and Functional Status in Surviving Patients Who Had Suspected Gram-negative Sepsis

Measure*	Surviving Patients	US General Population	*P*†
SF-36			
Physical function	61.08	84.15	<.001
General health perceptions	60.93	71.95	.004
Emotional role	83.33	81.26	.008
Physical role	66.07	80.96	.02
Mental health	78.91	74.74	.18
Vitality	66.37	60.86	.16
Bodily pain	79.12	75.15	.33
Social function	81.14	83.28	.59
Change in health	35.71	NA	...
Barthel Performance Scale	85	NA	...

*Mean scores for the Medical Outcomes Survey 36-Item Short-Form Health Survey (SF-36), the Barthel Performance Scale. NA indicates not applicable.
†Ellipses indicate *P* value not computed.

EXAMPLE T9 Designation of missing data. Ellipses are used to show that values for those table cells were not computed, whereas "NA" is used to indicate data points that were "not applicable." Adapted from *JAMA*. 1995;274:344.

ND (for "not determined") may be used, provided their meaning is clear and unambiguous.[16] Tables in which ellipses or abbreviations are to denote missing data should include footnotes that explain these items (Example T9).

Totals: Totals and percentages in tables should correspond to values presented in the text and should be verified for accuracy. Any discrepancies (eg, because of rounding error) should be explained in a footnote.

Boldface type for true totals (ie, those that represent sums of values given in the table) should be used with discretion and careful consideration. Boldface should be used only if it adds clarity or emphasis, but should not be used routinely (eg, simply to designate subtotals within a table). When boldface type is used to designate true totals, the word *Total* and the numerical totals are set boldface. When the word *Total* is used in the table stub, it should be set flush left. For true totals, any additional words in the stub (eg, Total No. of Patients) should all be set boldface and should follow the capitalization style used in titles (see 2.1.6, Capitalization).

Alignment of Data: Horizontal alignment (across rows) must be considered in setting tables. If the table stubs contain lines of text that exceed the width of the stub column (runover lines in the table stub) and the cell entries in that row do not, the field entries should be aligned across the first or top line of the table stub entry. This "top-line alignment" of data applies to tables that have numbers, words, or both as cell entries. If some entries within the table cells contain information that cannot be contained on a single line in the cell (runover lines in the table field), the table entries in that row also should be aligned across on the first or top line of the stub entry (Example T10).

Vertical alignment within each column of a table is important for the visual presentation of data. Whenever possible, columns of data should be aligned on common elements, such as decimal points, plus or minus signs, hyphens (used in ranges), virgules, or parentheses (Example T11). If table entries consist of

Table 1. Application of Hill's Criteria for Causal Inference

Criterion	Outcome: Antral Gastritis	Outcome: Duodenal Ulcer	Outcome: Gastric Ulcer	Outcome: Recurrent Abdominal Pain
Experimental evidence in humans (eg, human challenge studies)	Yes	No	No	No
Temporal sequence (ie, does cause precede effect?)	Yes*	No	No	No
Strength of the association (ie, is the magnitude of the association strong?)	Yes	Yes	Equivocal	Equivocal
Consistency of the association (ie, has the association been replicated by others?)	Yes	Yes	Equivocal	Equivocal
Specificity of the association (ie, 1 cause, 1 effect)	Yes	Equivocal	No	No
Biological plausibility/coherence/analogy (ie, does the association make biological sense?)	Yes	Yes	Yes	No
Biological gradient (ie, is there a dose-response relationship?)	No	No	No	No

*Two adult challenge studies.

Table 2. Comparison of Diagnostic Techniques in the Identification of Pedal Osteomyelitis in Patients With Diabetes

Investigation	Sensitivity, %	Specificity, %	Positive Predictive Value, %
Probe to bone	66	85	89
Plain radiograph	28-93	50-92	74-87
Technetium Tc 99m bone scan	68-100	18-79	43-87
Indium 111 leukocyte scan	45-100	67-89	75-85
Magnetic resonance imaging	29-100	78-89	50-93

Table 3. Accuracy of the Clinical Examination for Detecting Mitral Regurgitation*

Finding	Reference Standard (No. of Patients)	Positive Likelihood Ratio (95% CI)†	Negative Likelihood Ratio (95% CI)†	Quality Grade
Murmur audible in mitral area	Echocardiogram: moderate to severe MR (394)	3.9 (3.0-5.1)	0.34 (0.23-0.47)	B
Murmur audible below mitral area	Cardiac catheterization: moderate to severe MR (35)	3.6 (1.9-7.7)	0.12 (0.02-0.50)	C
Late or holosystolic murmur	Echocardiogram: moderate to severe MR (80)	1.8 (1.2-2.5)	0.0 (0.0-0.8)	C
Any murmur during acute MI	Cardiac catheterization: moderate to severe MR (206)	4.7 (1.3-11.0)	0.66 (0.25-1.00)	C
With transient arterial occlusion, murmur increases in intensity	Cardiac catheterization: severity not stated (231)	7.5 (2.5-23.0)	0.28 (0.13-0.60)	B

*CI indicates confidence interval; MR, mitral regurgitation; and MI, myocardial infarction.
†The applicable likelihood ratio when the finding is present.

Example T10 Alignment of data on the basis of horizontal alignment with top line of overrun entry in stub headings. Text entries in table cells (Table 1) and numerical entries in table cells (Table 2) should be aligned with first line of the stub entry. In tables with overrun stub entries and mixed elements in the data fields (ie, some cells with words and other cells with numbers), each entry should be aligned with the top line of the stub entry to which it applies (Table 3). Adapted from *JAMA*. 1997;277:568, and *JAMA*. 1995;273:722.

Table 1. Geometric Mean Cotinine Levels in Non–Tobacco Users by Home and Work ETS Exposure: NHANES III, 1988-1991*

	Sample Size (Unweighted)	Geometric Mean Cotinine, ng/mL	95% Confidence Interval
No. of smokers in home			
0	5382	0.14	0.13-0.16
1	1349	0.73	0.62-0.86
>1	600	1.24	1.07-1.43
No. of hours exposed at work for ages ≥17 y			
0	3861	0.16	0.14-0.18
1-3	487	0.33	0.29-0.39
>3	538	0.46	0.39-0.55
Ages 4-11 y			
No home ETS exposure	1071	0.11	0.10-0.14
Home ETS exposure only	713	1.14	0.97-1.34
Ages 12-16 y			
No home ETS exposure	379	0.11	0.09-0.15
Home ETS exposure only	268	0.80	0.62-1.04
Ages ≥17 y			
No home or work ETS exposure	3154	0.12	0.11-0.13
Home ETS exposure only	722	0.70	0.58-0.83
Ages ≥17 y (workers only)			
No home or work ETS exposure	1332	0.13	0.11-0.14
Work ETS exposure only	779	0.31	0.28-0.35
Home ETS exposure only	315	0.65	0.52-0.81
Home and work ETS exposure	246	0.92	0.76-1.13

*ETS indicates environmental tobacco smoke; NHANES, National Health and Nutrition Examination Survey.

EXAMPLE T11 Vertical alignment of data elements in columns. Alignment is on the units digit in the column for Sample Size, on the decimal marker in the column for Geometric Mean, and on the hyphen in the column for the 95% Confidence Interval. Adapted from *JAMA*. 1996;275:1238.

lengthy text, the flush-left format should be used with a 1-em indent for runover lines. If entries in a column are mixed (ie, if no common element exists or if the numbers vary greatly in magnitude), primary consideration should be given to the visual aspects of the entire table and the type of material being presented.

Rules in Tables: When typeset in AMA journals, formal tables usually have 3 horizontal rules: a "heavy" rule, such as a 3-point rule, between the table title and the column headings; a thin rule, such as a 1-point rule, between the column headings and the data field; and another 3-point rule between the field and the footnotes. For tables with cut-in headings, a 1-point rule is used above the cut-in headings. Complex tables, such as those with numerous rows and/or complex indentations, may require additional components (such as horizontal rules or shaded screens) to separate rows of data and enhance readability. Horizontal rules that appear in tables in *JAMA* are hairline rules that may be full width (ie, from one side of the table to the other) or partial width (when used to separate subentries under a stub).

Horizontal rules generally are not used in tables with only 2 columns or 2 rows because the size of the table allows the information to be visually accessible without using rules. However, when stub entries have runover lines or subentries, horizontal hairline rules may be helpful to facilitate ease of readability across columns. Vertical rules generally are not used in AMA publications.

Footnotes: Explanatory footnotes may contain information about the entire table, portions of the table (eg, a column), or a discrete table entry. The order of the footnotes is determined by the placement in the table of the item to which the footnote refers. The symbol for a footnote that applies to the entire table (eg, one that explains abbreviations used throughout the table or crediting previous publication of the table) should be placed after the table title. A footnote that applies to 1 or 2 columns or rows should be placed after the column heading(s) or stub heading(s) to which it refers. A footnote that applies to a single entry in the table or to several individual entries should be placed at the end of each entry to which it applies.

Footnotes are listed at the bottom of the table, each with a paragraph indent. Footnotes may be phrases or complete sentences and should end with a period. Any operational signs, such as <, >, or =, are abbreviations for inflected verbs and imply a verb even though the verb is not spelled out. For example, $P < .01$ is considered a complete sentence ("P is less than .01.") when used as a table footnote. Footnotes are indicated by symbols or letters, which should be set as superscripts before colons and semicolons and after commas and periods. Symbols should appear before and are set close to the footnote text.

For tables or figures with 10 or fewer explanatory footnotes, the following symbols are used in the order shown:

* (asterisk)

† (dagger)

‡ (double dagger)

§ (section mark)

‖ (parallel mark)

¶ (paragraph symbol)

\# (number sign)

** (asterisk [repeated])

†† (dagger [repeated])

‡‡ (double dagger [repeated])

For tables in which the number of footnotes exceeds 10, superscript lowercase letters should be used to denote the footnotes. Footnote symbols and footnote letters should not be used together in the same table. For tables in which superscript numbers and superscript letters are used to display data, care should be taken to ensure that superscript footnote symbols and letters are distinguished clearly from those used for data elements.

If several tables share a detailed or long footnote that explains several abbreviations or methods, this footnote may appear in the first table for which it is applicable, and a footnote in each succeeding table for which the footnote also is applicable may refer the reader to the first appearance of the detailed information:

> Abbreviations are explained in the first footnote to Table 1.

The reader also may be referred to a relevant discussion in the text by a footnote:

> See "Methods" section for a description of this procedure.

Several of the most common uses of footnotes include the following:

- To expand abbreviations:

  *OR indicates odds ratio; CI, confidence interval.

- To designate reporting of numerical values:

  *Values are expressed as mean (SD).

- To provide information on statistical analyses or experimental methods:

  *Adjusted for age, smoking status, and body mass index.

- To indicate a discrepancy in numerical data:

  *Because of rounding, percentages may not all total 100.

- To cite references for information used in the table. References are given as in the text and are designated with superscript arabic numbers:

  **International Classification of Health Problems in Primary Care.*[45]

- To acknowledge that data in the table were taken from or are based on data from another source:

  *Data from Kaufman and Bernstein.[42]

- To acknowledge credit for reproduction of a table. If the table has been reprinted with permission from another source, credit should be given in a table footnote:

  *Reprinted with permission from Montgomery and Stevens.[52]

References used in tables and figures are numbered and listed in order of their first mention. References for information in the table or figure should be considered in order as if this information were part of the text. For instance, if the source from which the material referred to in the table or figure is one of the references used in the text, and has been listed and numbered in the text before the first mention of the table or figure, that reference number should be used in the table or figure. If the source from which the material referred to in the table or figure is taken is first used for the table or figure (ie, the source is cited in the text, but after its first mention in the table or figure) or the reference pertains only to the table or figure (ie, the source is not cited elsewhere in the text), the reference should be listed and numbered according to the first mention of the table or figure in the text. That reference number also should be used for subsequent use of that citation in the text or in other tables or figures (see 2.12.6, Citation).

2.13.5 ***Units of Measure.***—AMA journals use Système International (SI) units as the primary reporting format for units of measure (see 11.12, Abbreviations, Units of Measure, and 15.1, Units of Measure, SI Units). In tables, units of measure, including the variance of the measurement if reported, should follow a comma in the table column heading or stub. The following are examples of stub entries with units of measure:

Age, mean (SD), y

Systolic blood pressure, mm Hg

Systolic blood pressure, mean (SD), mm Hg

Body mass index, mean, kg/m^2

Duration of hypertension, mean (SD) [median], y

Table 1. Lipid and Lipoprotein Analysis*

	Prerace	Postrace	Change	% Change	*P*
Cholesterol, mmol/L (mg/dL)	4.94 ± 0.88 (190.8 ± 3.8)	4.50 ± 0.79 (173.8 ± 30.6)	−0.44 ± 0.43 (−17.0 ± 16.4)	−9	<.001
Triglycerides, mmol/L (mg/dL)	1.58 ± 0.83 (139.6 ± 73.6)	0.97 ± 0.68 (85.8 ± 60.5)	−0.61 ± 0.77 (−53.8 ± 68.4)	−39	<.001
LDL-C, mmol/L (mg/dL)	2.59 ± 0.77 (100.1 ± 29.9)	2.30 ± 0.86 (88.7 ± 33.3)	−0.30 ± 0.49 (−11.4 ± 18.8)	−11	.02
HDL-C, mmol/L (mg/dL)	1.39 ± 0.29 (53.7 ± 11.1)	1.43 ± 0.33 (55.3 ± 12.8)	0.04 ± 0.16 (1.6 ± 6.3)	+3	.29
Apo A-I, g/L (mg/dL)	1.57 ± 0.23 (156.7 ± 22.9)	1.57 ± 0.31 (157.1 ± 21.2)	0.005 ± 0.11 (0.47 ± 10.9)	+0.3	.83
Apo B, g/L (mg/dL)	0.91 ± 0.20 (90.7 ± 20.0)	0.82 ± 0.18 (82.0 ± 17.9)	−0.088 ± 0.10 (−8.8 ± 9.6)	−10	<.001

*All values are expressed as mean±SE. LDL-C indicates low-density lipoprotein cholesterol; HDL-C, high-density lipoprotein cholesterol; Apo A-I, apolipoprotein A-I; and Apo B, apolipoprotein B.

Table 2. Baseline Characteristics of Survivors and Decedents, Men and Women, Aerobics Center Longitudinal Study, 1970 Through 1989*

	Men		Women	
Characteristic	Survivors (n = 24 740)	Decedents (n = 601)	Survivors (n = 6991)	Decedents (n = 89)
Age, y	42.7 (9.7)	52.1 (11.4)	42.6 (10.9)	53.3 (11.2)
Follow-up, y	8.4 (4.9)	7.1 (4.2)	7.5 (4.8)	7.6 (4.7)
Body mass index, kg/m^2	26.0 (3.6)	26.3 (3.5)	22.6 (3.9)	23.7 (4.5)
Blood pressure, mm Hg				
Systolic	121.1 (13.5)	130.4 (19.1)	112.6 (14.8)	122.6 (17.3)
Diastolic	80.7 (9.5)	84.8 (11.8)	75.4 (9.6)	79.9 (9.2)
Total cholesterol				
mmol/L	5.5 (1.1)	5.9 (1.2)	5.2 (1.0)	5.9 (1.1)
mg/dL	213.1 (40.6)	228.9 (45.4)	202.7 (40.5)	228.2 (40.8)
Fasting glucose				
mmol/L	5.6 (0.9)	6.0 (1.8)	5.2 (0.8)	5.6 (1.4)
mg/dL	100.4 (15.3)	108.1 (32.0)	94.4 (14.5)	99.9 (25.0)
Current or recent smoker, %	26.3	36.9	18.5	30.3
Family history of coronary heart disease, %	25.4	33.8	25.2	27.0
Healthy, %	77.3	48.1	83.2	66.3

*Data are given as mean (SD) except where noted. Low fitness indicates least fit 20%; moderate fitness, next 40%; high fitness, most fit 40%; family history of coronary heart disease, either parent dead of coronary heart disease; healthy, no chronic illness and no abnormal electrocardiogram. Recent smokers had quit smoking within 2 years of baseline.

EXAMPLE T12 Dual-reporting of laboratory measurements in SI units and conventional units along with variance (SD). Values are presented in SI units with values in parentheses given in conventional units (Table 1). Values for SI units and conventional units also may be presented in "stacked" arrangement beneath the analyte of interest (Table 2). Adapted from *JAMA*. 1996;276:223, and *JAMA*. 1996;276:206.

For laboratory values that are dual-reported (see 15.5.2, Units of Measure, Dual Reporting), SI units should be given first, followed by conventional units in parentheses. For measurements given with indicators of variance, dual-reported values also should include the respective variance measures (Example T12). The following are examples of stub entries for dual-reported values:

Total cholesterol, mmol/L (mg/dL)
(Value expressed with SI and conventional units)

Total cholesterol, mean (SD), mmol/L [mg/dL]
(Value expressed as mean [SD] with SI and conventional units)

Total cholesterol, mean (SD)
mmol/L
mg/dL
(Stacking of values in stub entries may be helpful for layout and space considerations.)

2.13.6 ***Capital Letters.***—For table titles and column headings, capitalization style follows that used for titles (see 2.1.6, Capitalization). For each column or row entry, the first word is capitalized. If the first word is preceded by a numeral, lowercase Greek letter, or percent sign, the first letter of the first word should be capitalized (eg, 10% Concentration, β-Blocker). However, in row entries for numerical designations in which the first word after the numeral is not a whole word but an abbreviation (eg, 36-mo), the first letter of the abbreviated word is not capitalized.

2.13.7 ***Punctuation.***—As with numbers and abbreviations, rules for punctuation may be less restrictive in tables in the interest of saving space (see 6.0, Punctuation.) For example, virgules may be used to present dates (eg, 10/18/96 for October 18, 1996) and hyphens may be used to present ranges (eg, 60-90 for 60 to 90) (see 16.0, Numbers and Percentages).

2.13.8 ***Abbreviations.***—Within the body of the table and in column headings, units of measure and numbers normally spelled out may be abbreviated for space considerations (see 15.0, Units of Measure; 16.0, Numbers and Percentages; and 11.12, Abbreviations, Units of Measure.) However, spelled-out words should not be combined with abbreviations for units of measure. For example, "First Week" or "1st wk" or "Week 1" may be used as a column heading, but not "First wk." Abbreviations or acronyms should be explained in footnotes.

2.13.9 ***Numbers.***—Additional digits (including zeros) should not be added (eg, after the decimal point) to provide all data entries with the same number of digits. Doing so may indicate more precise results than actually were calculated or measured. A percentage or decimal quotient should contain no more than the number of digits in the denominator. For example, the percentage for the proportion 9 of 28 should be reported as 32% (or decimal quotient 0.32), not 32.1% (or 0.321) (see 17.3, Statistics, Significant Digits and Rounding Numbers). Values reporting laboratory data should be provided and rounded off, if appropriate, according to the number of digits that reflects the precision of the reported results and to eliminate reporting results beyond the sensitivity of the procedure performed (see 15.4.1, Units of Measure, Expressing Quantities).

Values for reporting statistical data, such as *P* values and confidence intervals, also should be presented and rounded appropriately (see 17.3, Statistics, Significant Digits and Rounding Numbers). Although some publications[17] suggest use of specific designations for levels of significance (eg, a single asterisk in the table to denote values for entries with $P < .05$, a double asterisk for $P < .01$), exact *P* values are preferred, whether statistically significant or not. In most cases, *P* values should be expressed to 2 digits to the right of the decimal point, unless the first 2 digits are zeros (ie, *P* values less than .001 should be designated as "$P < .001$," rather than using exact values, eg, $P = .00006$), in which case 3 digits to the right of the decimal place should be provided (eg, $P = .002$). For study outcomes, statistically significant values should not be expressed as "$P < .05$" either in the table or in the table footnote, and nonsignificant *P* values should not be expressed as "NS" (not significant). For confidence intervals, the number of digits should correspond to the number of digits in the point estimate. For instance, for an odds ratio reported as 2.45, the 95% confidence interval should be reported as 1.32 to 4.78, not as 1.322 to 4.784.

2.13.10 ***Tables That Contain Supplementary Information.***—Tables that contain important supplementary information that is too extensive to be published in the journal article (usually because of length considerations) may be made available from other sources. These tables may be available in printed form (eg, from the author), in digital form (eg, online database, CD-ROM), or from the National Auxiliary Publications Service (NAPS) (see 2.10.6, National Auxiliary Publications Service [NAPS]) or Availability of Materials in Other Forms or Databases).

The American Society for Information Science provides a repository for supplemental materials, such as extensive tables, figures, bibliographies, computer printouts, or complex descriptions (such as detailed descriptions of laboratory methods or formulas) that are adjuncts to articles published in scholarly or technical journals but are too lengthy to be published in full. If an article is accepted for publication and the supplemental materials are appropriate for deposit in NAPS, the journal or other publication usually will arrange the deposit and may pay the deposit fee. Published articles for which supplementary material is deposited with NAPS contain a statement (usually in the acknowledgment section of the article) that includes the NAPS document number, the address for requesting materials, and the cost for the retrieval and receipt of a copy of the document.

2.13.11 ***Guidelines for Preparing and Submitting Tables.***—Authors submitting tables in a scientific article should consult the publication's instructions for authors for specific requirements and preferences regarding table format. Although details about preferred table presentation vary among journals, several general guidelines apply. Each table should be submitted on a separate sheet of standard paper (8.5 × 11 in [21.5 × 27.5 cm]). Each horizontal line of the table should be double-spaced. Reduced type should not be used. If a table is too large to be contained on 1 page, the table should be continued on another page with the table title and the column headings repeated; the abbreviation (*cont*) should follow the title on the subsequent page. Alternatively, if the table is large or exceedingly complex, the author should consider separating the data into 2 or more simpler tables. Tables should not be submitted on oversized paper or as photographic prints.

The availability of word processor, spreadsheet, and database programs that generate tables has simplified the creation of tables for authors and has enhanced the ability of editors and publishers to use electronic files submitted by the author for editing and incorporating tables into production software. However, because of the considerations involved in importing, converting, and incorporating author-generated tables into digital files or files with required codes suitable for electronic production programs, authors should consult the editorial office of the individual publication for information on preferred and compatible formats for submission of electronic files for tables.

2.14 ■ **FIGURES.**—The term *figure* refers to any graphical display of measured quantities by means of the combined use of points, lines, a coordinate system, numbers, symbols, words, shading, or color to create illustrative material used to present information or data.[16] Figures include a variety of displays, such as graphs, charts, maps, algorithms, line drawings, computer-generated images, and photographs. Figures may be used to clarify or explain methods, to present results or other information that supports the results, to highlight trends and comparisons among data, to provide information that aids in the understanding of complex concepts,

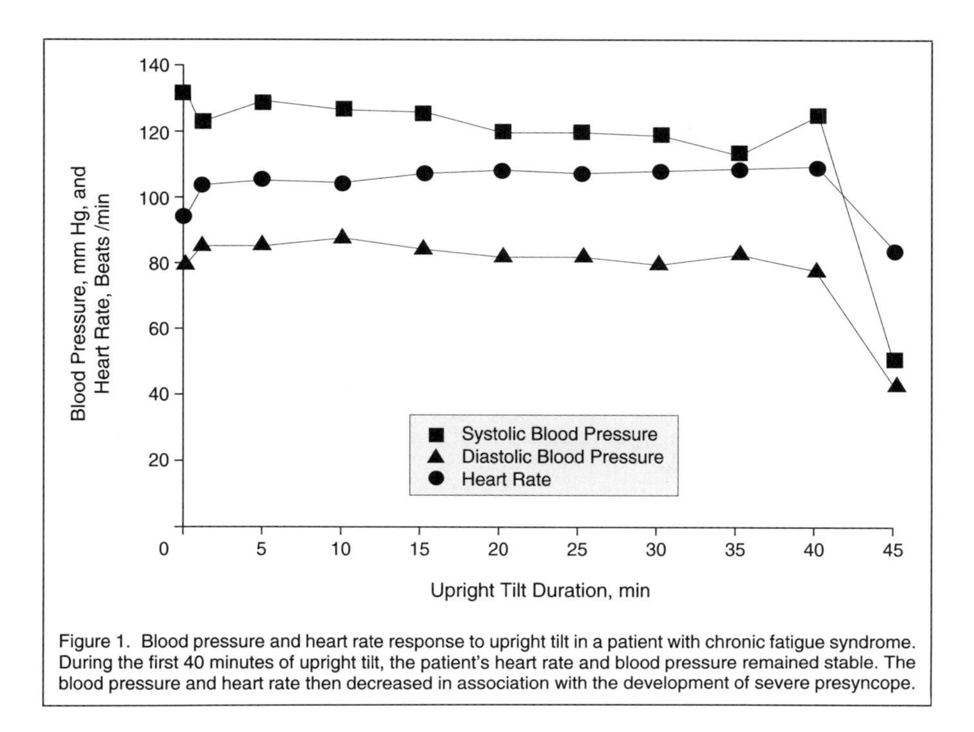

Figure 1. Blood pressure and heart rate response to upright tilt in a patient with chronic fatigue syndrome. During the first 40 minutes of upright tilt, the patient's heart rate and blood pressure remained stable. The blood pressure and heart rate then decreased in association with the development of severe presyncope.

EXAMPLE F3 Line graph. The independent variable is plotted on the horizontal axis and the dependent variable on the vertical axis. Symbols clearly distinguish the variables of interest and are explained in the figure key. Adapted from *JAMA*. 1995;274:963.

or to illustrate items or procedures under discussion. In all cases, the objective of the figure is to provide information in an accurate, clear, and concise manner.

2.14.1 ***Types of Figures.***—In scientific articles, selection of a particular type of figure depends on the intended purpose and on the type of information being displayed. Many types of figures are available to authors; some of the most commonly used figures in biomedical publications are discussed herein.

In scientific articles, figures frequently are used to illustrate the findings of a study. Graphs that contain data are the most common type of figure used for displaying quantitative information. Graphs can demonstrate values of numerical data; depict changes, trends, or patterns in data; and show relationships among variables being analyzed. The type of graph selected should be appropriate for the type of data being displayed.

Line Graph: A line graph is a 2-axis graph on which data points or curves demonstrate the relation between 2 or more quantitative variables. The line graph depicts trends, such as changes over time, rather than magnitude. Line graphs usually are designed with the dependent variable on the vertical axis (y-axis) and the independent variable on the horizontal axis (x-axis).[21] By linking at least 2 variables, the graph encourages the reader to assess the relationships visually among the plotted variables (Example F3, Example F4).

Bar Graph: A bar graph is a 1-axis graph used to compare amounts, frequencies, or magnitude for categories of discontinuous data. A bar graph may be vertical, ie, a column chart (Example F5), or horizontal, ie, horizontal bar chart (Example F6), with each category represented by a bar. Bars should have the same width and should be wider than the space between them. Bar lengths are proportional to frequency. Frequencies or relative frequencies usually are placed on the vertical

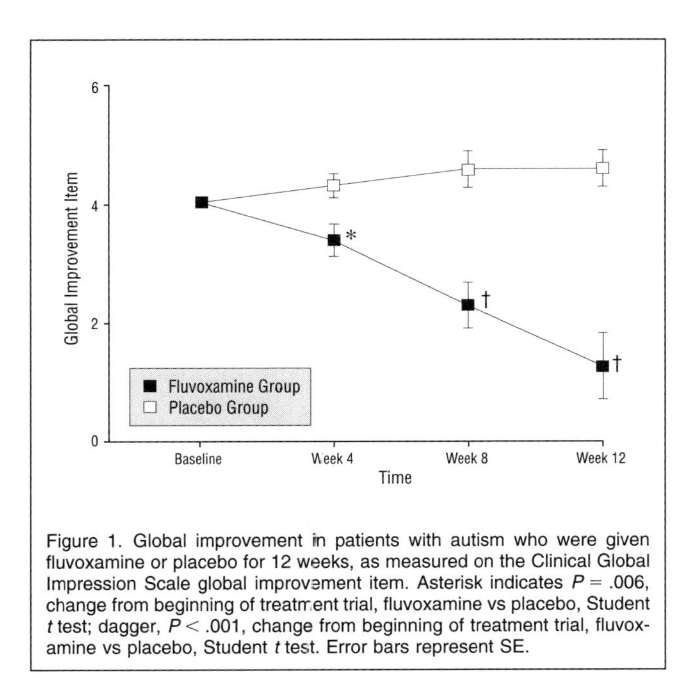

Figure 1. Global improvement in patients with autism who were given fluvoxamine or placebo for 12 weeks, as measured on the Clinical Global Impression Scale global improvement item. Asterisk indicates $P = .006$, change from beginning of treatment trial, fluvoxamine vs placebo, Student t test; dagger, $P < .001$, change from beginning of treatment trial, fluvoxamine vs placebo, Student t test. Error bars represent SE.

EXAMPLE F4 Line graph. Data for active treatment group shown as black square and placebo group shown as white square. Error bars show variance of measurement. Statistical tests and significance levels are given in the legend. Adapted from *Arch Gen Psychiatry.* 1996;53:1005.

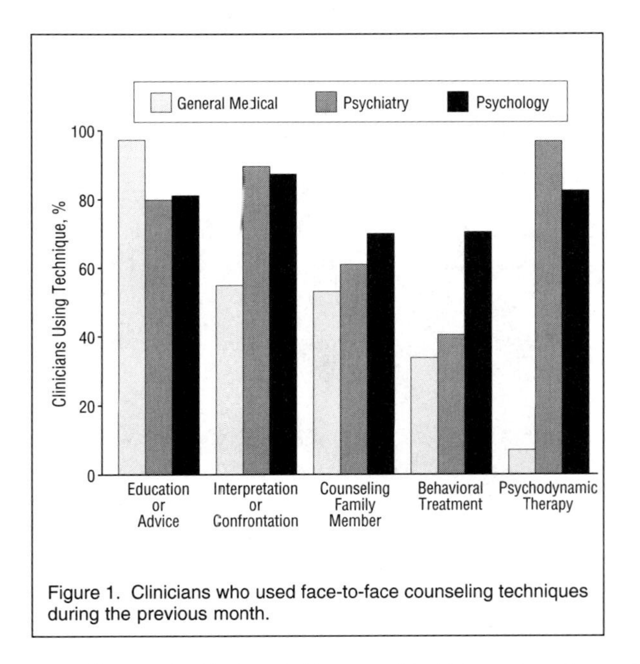

Figure 1. Clinicians who used face-to-face counseling techniques during the previous month.

EXAMPLE F5 Vertical bar graph. Shading (white, gray, black) is used to distinguish the 3 groups that are compared. Adapted from *Arch Gen Psychiatry.* 1996;53:910.

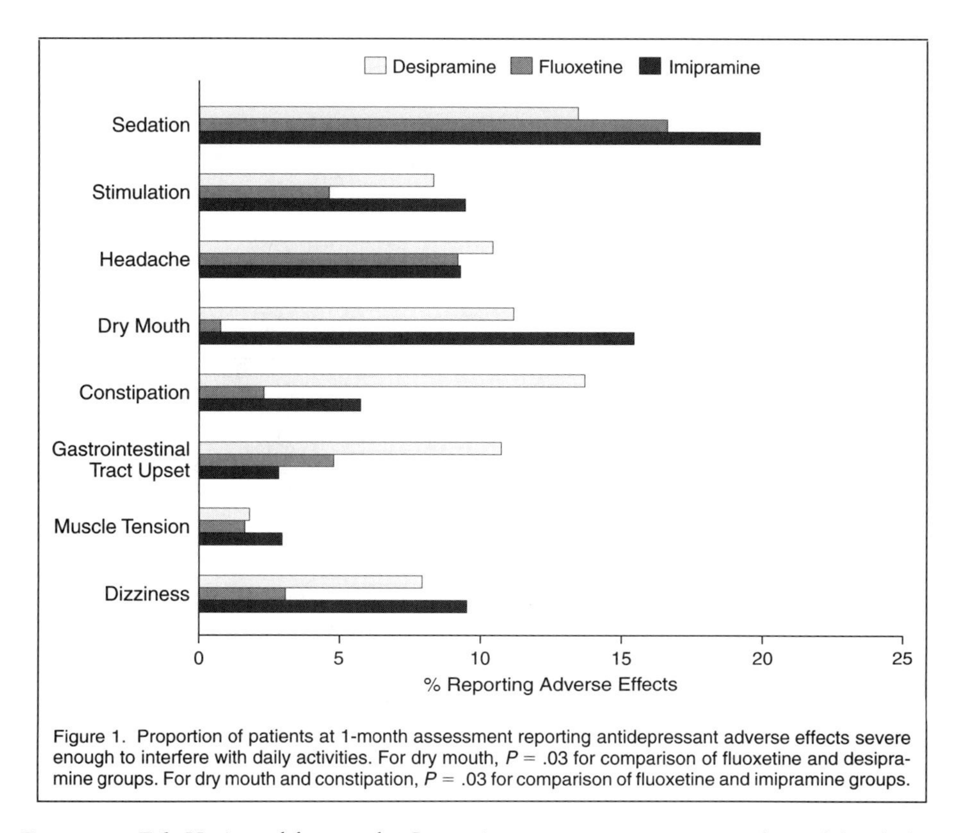

Figure 1. Proportion of patients at 1-month assessment reporting antidepressant adverse effects severe enough to interfere with daily activities. For dry mouth, $P = .03$ for comparison of fluoxetine and desipramine groups. For dry mouth and constipation, $P = .03$ for comparison of fluoxetine and imipramine groups.

EXAMPLE F6 Horizontal bar graph. Comparisons among groups are emphasized by shading characteristics. Adapted from *JAMA*. 1996;275:1899.

axis, which should generally include zero. Categories of ordinal data should be presented in logical order. The horizontal baseline of a vertical bar graph is not an axis and therefore should not contain tick marks.

GROUPED BAR GRAPH. A grouped (or paired) bar graph may display grouped or paired data, such as independent series of data over time (Example F5, Example F6). In most cases, the number of bars in a grouped bar graph generally should not exceed 3. Colors or tones used for each bar within the group should be distinct. To ensure that bars in black-and-white figures are distinguishable, a contrast in shading of at least 30% for adjacent bars is suggested. Patterns and cross-hatching (eg, diagonal lines) on bars should be replaced with color, or shades of gray or another color. Specific areas on the graph should be labeled with words rather than encoded with additional variations in shading or hatching.

DEVIATION BAR GRAPH. A deviation bar graph displays and compares positive and negative data values relative to a centrally located zero baseline (Example F7).

COMPONENT BAR GRAPH. A component bar graph (or subdivided bar graph) compares totals, proportions, or sums of proportions (Example F8). Individual components are designated by shading.

100% BAR GRAPH. A 100% bar graph compares the components of a whole, usually at a given point in time. If data for the components are shown in 100% bar graphs for 2 or more points in time, the degree of change in the components during those time periods can be observed (Example F9). The component of most interest is usually positioned nearest to the baseline. Lines connecting the similar sections of two 100% bar graphs may help to facilitate comparisons.

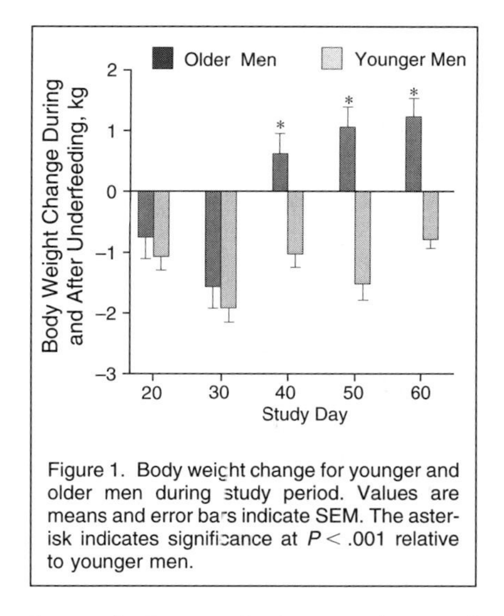

Figure 1. Body weight change for younger and older men during study period. Values are means and error bars indicate SEM. The asterisk indicates significance at $P < .001$ relative to younger men.

EXAMPLE F7 Deviation bar graph. Horizontal rule at 0, indicative of no weight change, provides baseline from which to compare weight gain or loss during the study period. Adapted from *JAMA.* 1994;272:1605.

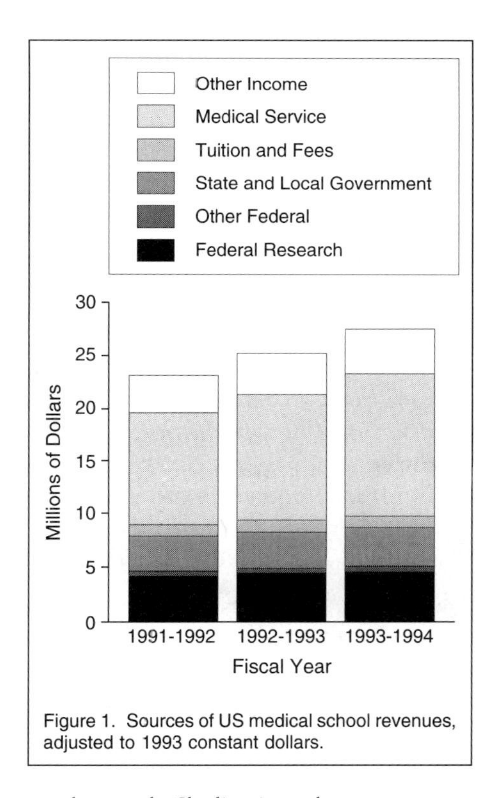

Figure 1. Sources of US medical school revenues, adjusted to 1993 constant dollars.

EXAMPLE F8 Component bar graph. Shading is used to represent components. Plots of values over time allow for comparison of trends of revenue sources. Adapted from *JAMA.* 1995;274:729.

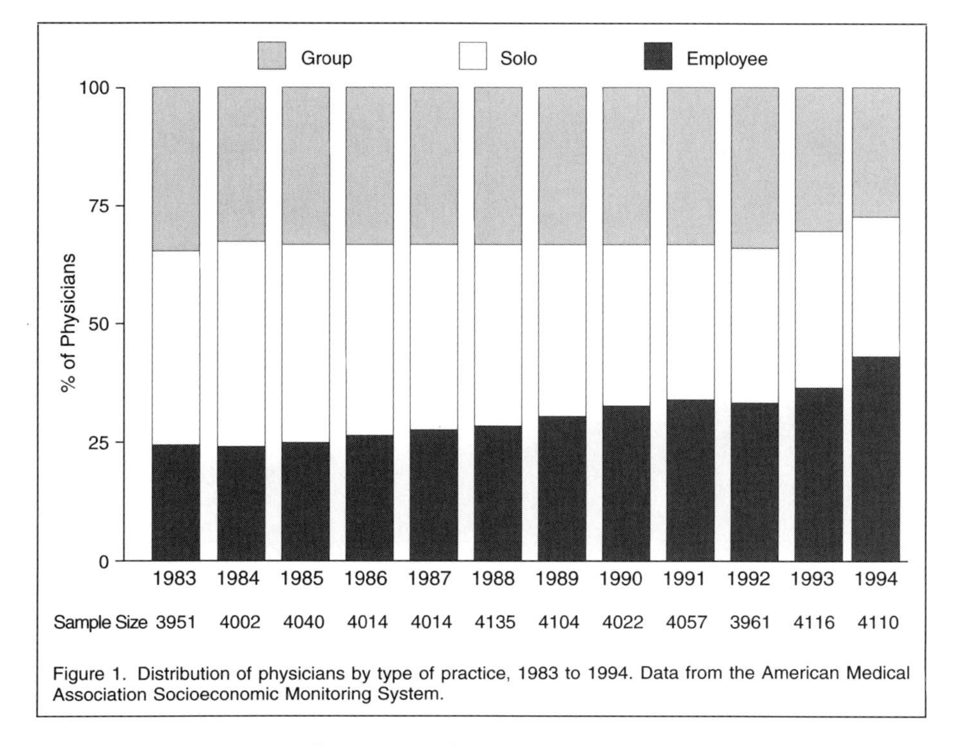

Figure 1. Distribution of physicians by type of practice, 1983 to 1994. Data from the American Medical Association Socioeconomic Monitoring System.

EXAMPLE F9 100% Bar graph. Proportional composition of variables over time is shown. Variable of most interest (changes in proportion of physicians as employees) is plotted nearest the horizontal axis. The sample size for each year also is shown. Adapted from *JAMA*. 1996;276:556.

Individual-Value Graph: An individual-value graph depicts changes in individual data points, most commonly involving paired data for a single subject. The direction of change is demonstrated by lines connecting the data points (Example F10).

Histogram: A histogram is a 2-axis graph that shows a frequency distribution by use of a series of contiguous rectangles. Histograms display grouped data when the groups are characterized by numerical values. The rectangles in a histogram should be of equal width, with the position of the rectangle along the x-axis corresponding with the location of the interval within the group.[22] The height and area of the rectangle corresponds to the frequency within the group (Example F11).

Frequency Polygon: A frequency polygon uses data points joined by lines to show 2 or more overlapping frequency distributions or a single frequency distribution.[22] Data points are plotted at the midpoint of the frequency for each data class and the midpoints are joined by lines (Example F12).

Survival Plot (Survival Curve): A survival plot presents life-table data and allows the estimation of an experience over time (eg, survival, disease-free state) of 1 or more groups of individuals with variable follow-up periods.[23] The vertical axis shows the percentage survival (usually from 0% to 100%), and the horizontal axis depicts follow-up time for each individual beginning from entry into the study. The number of individuals followed for each time interval usually is displayed, most commonly just above or just below the horizontal axis (see Figure 2 in Statistics, 17.0).

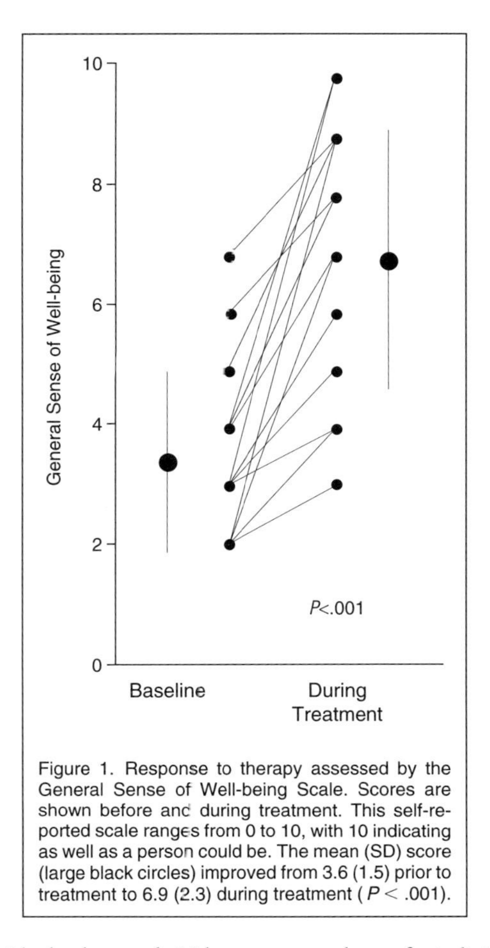

Figure 1. Response to therapy assessed by the General Sense of Well-being Scale. Scores are shown before and during treatment. This self-reported scale ranges from 0 to 10, with 10 indicating as well as a person could be. The mean (SD) score (large black circles) improved from 3.6 (1.5) prior to treatment to 6.9 (2.3) during treatment ($P < .001$).

EXAMPLE F10 Individual-value graph. Values represent change for individual subjects. Summary value (mean) along with variance (SD) illustrates overall changes for the study group. Adapted from *JAMA*. 1995;274:966.

Scatterplot and Scattergram: A scatterplot or scattergram is a 2-axis graph with plots of individual data points that determine whether the data fit a mathematical function. If a relationship exists between independent and dependent variables, the regression line through the data points illustrates how the variables are correlated. By convention, the independent variable is plotted on the x-axis and the dependent variable is plotted on the y-axis. The correlation coefficient should be provided as part of the figure or in the legend (Example F13).

Pie Chart: A pie chart compares relationships among component parts. Categories are represented by sections, with area of the section proportional to the relative frequency of each category. Pie charts are used commonly in publications intended for lay audiences, but should be avoided in scientific publications.[24] In the majority of instances, data depicted in pie charts can be summarized in the text or in a table. Moreover, for comparisons of components of 2 or more wholes contained in 2 or more pie charts, the angular areas of the individual components of pie charts may be difficult to compare. If a figure is necessary, the data typically presented in a pie chart often may be presented more effectively in another type of figure that allows easier comparisons of data, such as in component bar graphs.

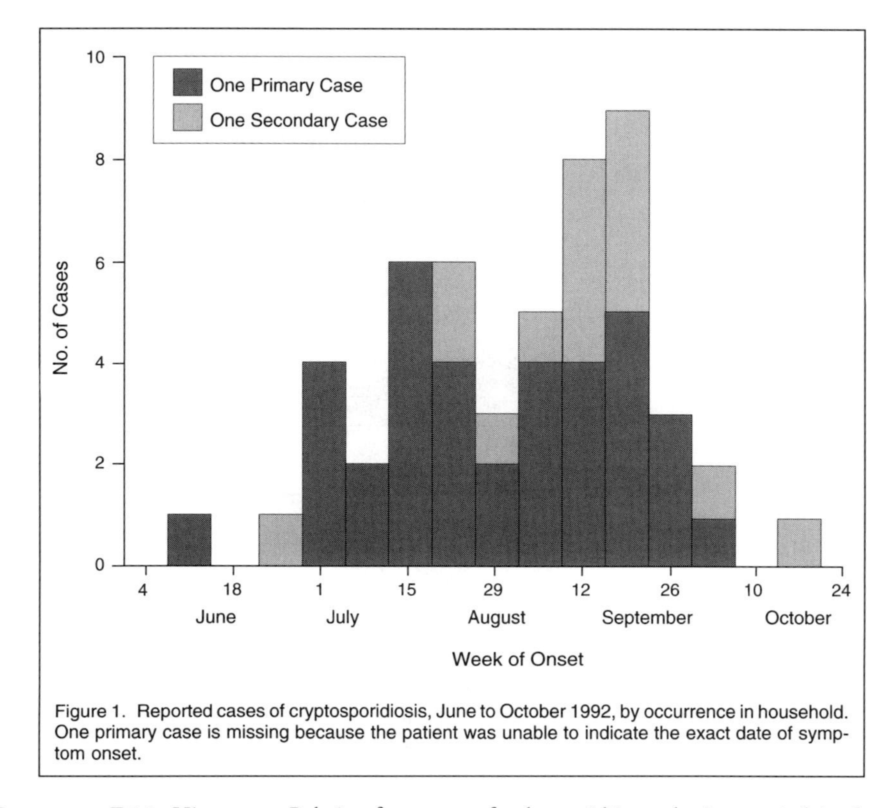

Figure 1. Reported cases of cryptosporidiosis, June to October 1992, by occurrence in household. One primary case is missing because the patient was unable to indicate the exact date of symptom onset.

EXAMPLE F11 Histogram. Relative frequency of values within each time period is shown. Column widths are the same, and the height represents the number of cases for each interval. Adapted from *JAMA*. 1994;272:1598.

Flowchart: A flowchart demonstrates the sequence of activities, processes, events, operations, or organization of a complex procedure or an interrelated system of components. Flowcharts are useful to illustrate flow patterns, to summarize complex or detailed descriptions, to depict study protocol or interventions (Example F14), or to demonstrate subject recruitment and follow-up such as in a randomized controlled trial[25] (Example F15, and Figure 1 in Statistics, 17.0).

Decision Tree: A decision tree is an analytical tool used in decision analysis.[26] The decision tree displays the logical and temporal sequence in clinical decision making

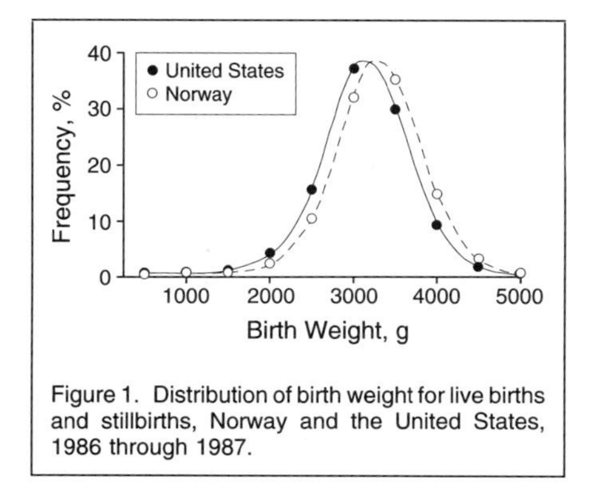

Figure 1. Distribution of birth weight for live births and stillbirths, Norway and the United States, 1986 through 1987.

EXAMPLE F12 Frequency polygon. Adapted from *JAMA*. 1995;273:710.

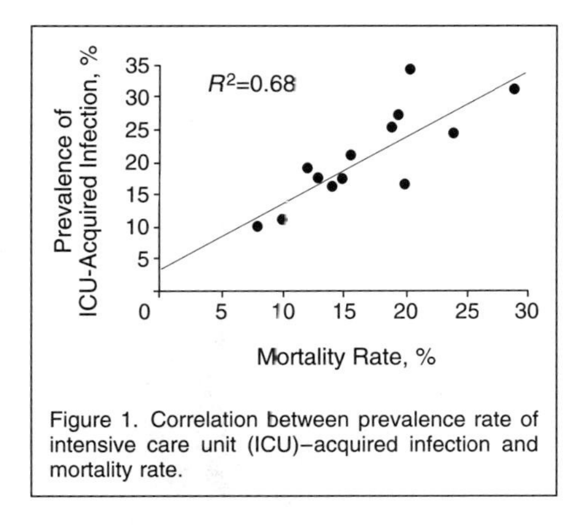

Figure 1. Correlation between prevalence rate of intensive care unit (ICU)–acquired infection and mortality rate.

EXAMPLE F13 Scatterplot (scattergram). Correlation between variables is shown and the strength of the correlation is indicated by the correlation coefficient, which may be included in the figure or in the legend. Adapted from *JAMA*. 1995;274:642.

and usually progresses from left to right. A decision node is the point in the decision tree at which several alternatives can be selected and, by convention, is designated by a square. A chance node (probability node) is a point in the decision tree at which several events, determined by chance, may occur and, by convention, is designated by a circle (see 17.0, Statistics, and Figure 2 in Statistics).

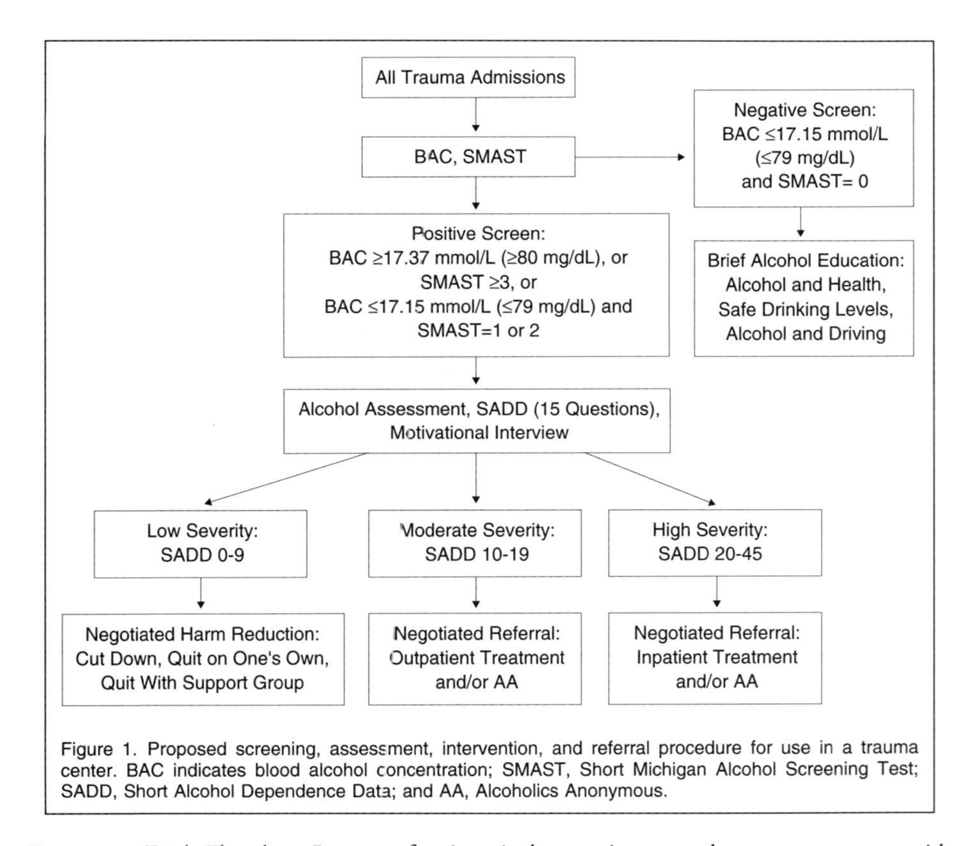

Figure 1. Proposed screening, assessment, intervention, and referral procedure for use in a trauma center. BAC indicates blood alcohol concentration; SMAST, Short Michigan Alcohol Screening Test; SADD, Short Alcohol Dependence Data; and AA, Alcoholics Anonymous.

EXAMPLE F14 Flowchart. Progress of patients is shown using top-to-bottom arrangement with arrows indicting sequence of activities. Adapted from *JAMA*. 1995;274:1046.

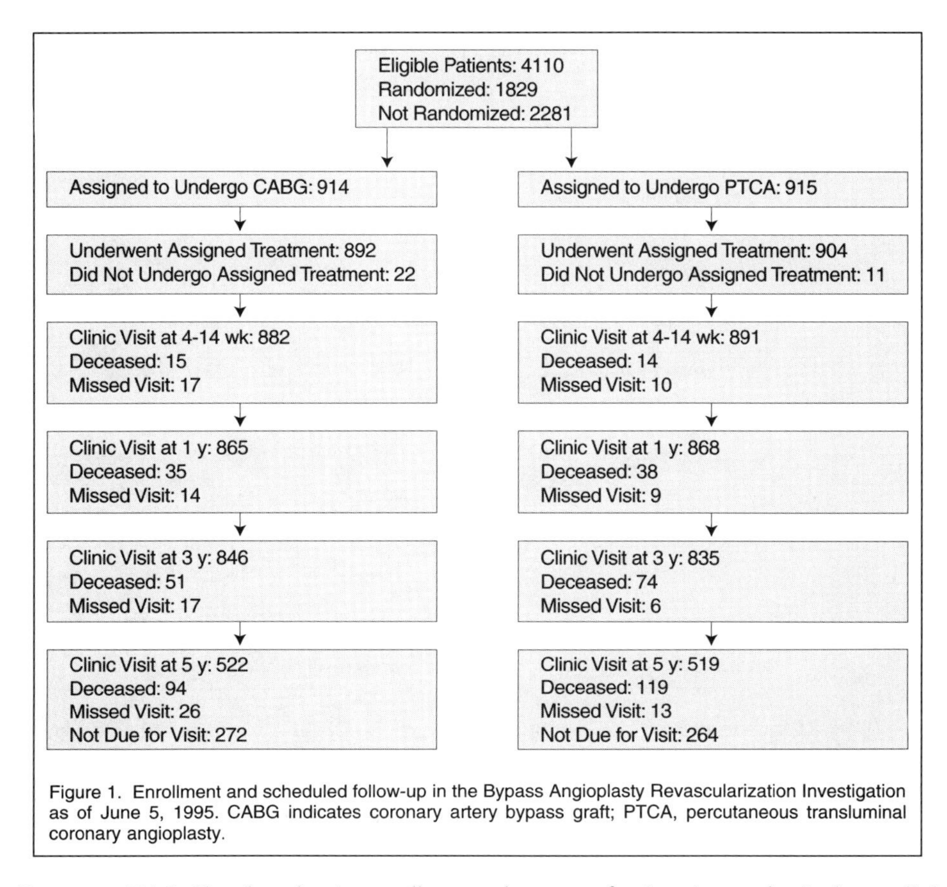

Figure 1. Enrollment and scheduled follow-up in the Bypass Angioplasty Revascularization Investigation as of June 5, 1995. CABG indicates coronary artery bypass graft; PTCA, percutaneous transluminal coronary angioplasty.

EXAMPLE F15 Flowchart showing enrollment and progress of patients in a randomized controlled trial. Reasons for dropout or lack of follow-up are shown. All patients should be accounted for at each step shown. Adapted from *JAMA*. 1997;277:717.

Figures for Pooled Data: Figures in meta-analyses and other studies that involve combining data or pooling results from individual studies are used to present data from individual studies as well as an overall pooled estimate or effect size (see 17.2.7, Statistics Meta-analysis). In these figures, the individual studies are identified and their point estimates or effect size, as well as the corresponding variance (eg, confidence interval or SD) for the outcome of interest, are shown (Example F16).

Map: A map is useful to demonstrate relationships or trends that involve location and distance. Maps may be used to demonstrate geographic relations (eg, spread of a disease). Choropleth maps depict quantitative data (eg, relative frequencies by county, state, country, province, or region), with differences in numerical data, such as rates, shown by shading or colors (Example F17).

Despite the increasing availability of graphics software, maps remain a source of potential error, which may include misspelled or incorrect names, deleted features, distorted geographic relationships, misplaced or missing cities, and misplaced boundaries. Authors should use an accurate, current atlas to verify details on computer-generated maps.

Diagram: A diagram is used to display the components of a complex system or process and to demonstrate the interrelationships of these components (Example F18).

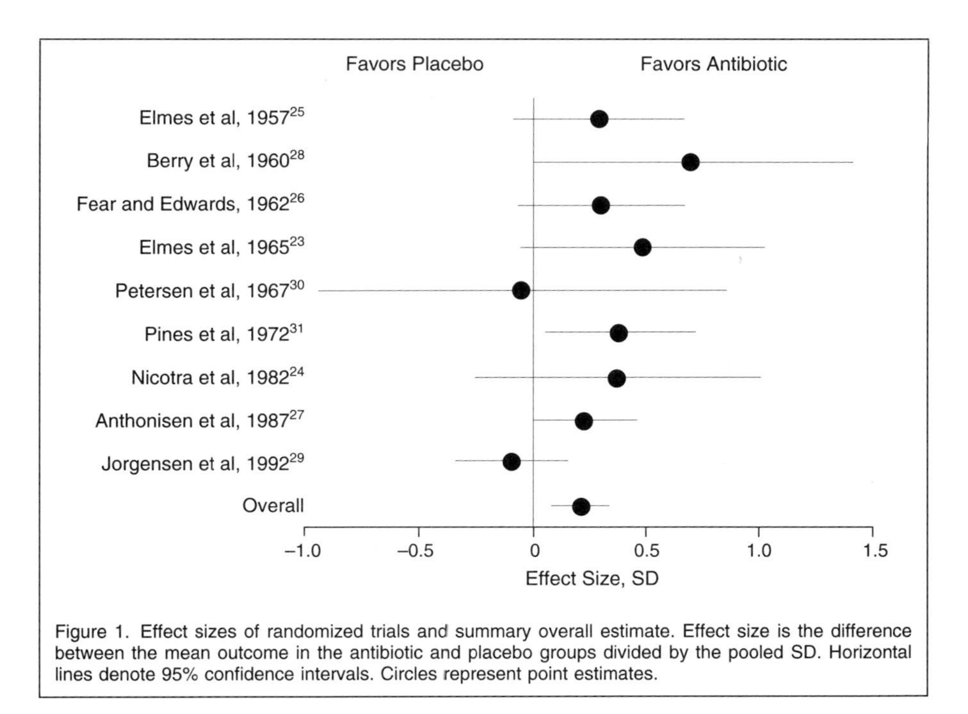

Figure 1. Effect sizes of randomized trials and summary overall estimate. Effect size is the difference between the mean outcome in the antibiotic and placebo groups divided by the pooled SD. Horizontal lines denote 95% confidence intervals. Circles represent point estimates.

EXAMPLE F16 Display of individual effect sizes and summary estimate using point estimates and 95% confidence intervals, along with study author, year of publication, and reference number. The vertical line at 0 (ie, no effect) allows for visual evaluation of direction and magnitude of effect favoring the treatment options studied. Adapted from *JAMA*. 1995;273:959.

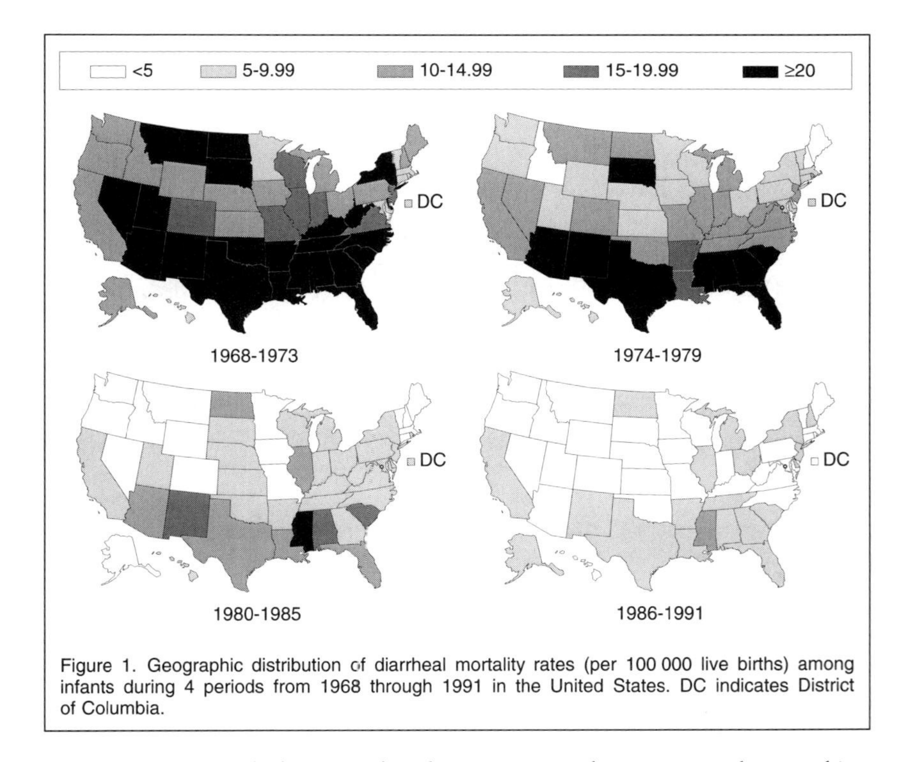

Figure 1. Geographic distribution of diarrheal mortality rates (per 100 000 live births) among infants during 4 periods from 1968 through 1991 in the United States. DC indicates District of Columbia.

EXAMPLE F17 Maps. Shading is used to depict rates according to state and geographic trends over time. Adapted from *JAMA*. 1995;274:1147.

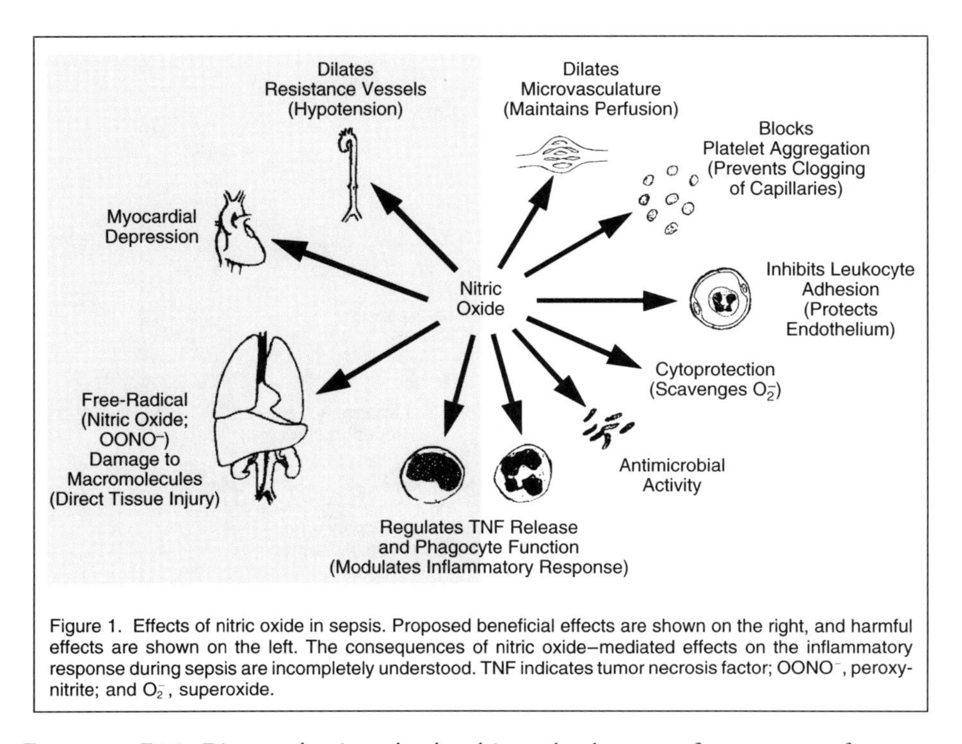

EXAMPLE F18 Diagram showing related and interrelated aspects of components of a system. Positioning and shading are used to distinguish beneficial and harmful effects. Adapted from *JAMA*. 1996;275:1193.

Photographs and Computer-Generated Images: Photographs and computer-generated images in biomedical articles are used to depict subjects, results, or procedures performed.

The availability of computer photography and digital imaging has provided the capability for enhancing images of photographic scientific data, such as clinical images or gel electrophoresis bands.[27] The result of such digital manipulation may render findings and images that never existed. Although specific guidelines have not been established, some publications require that authors who submit digital images clearly indicate the software and hardware used for producing digital photographs.[27]

2.14.2 ***Components of Figures.—****Data Display:* Clear display of data or information is the most important aspect of any figure. For figures that display quantitative information, data values may be represented by dots, lines, curves, area, length, or shading, based on the type of graph used.

Scales for Graphs: The horizontal scale (x-axis) and the vertical scale (y-axis) indicate the values of the data plotted in a graph. In most graphs, values increase from left to right (on the x-axis) and from bottom to top (on the y-axis).

RANGE OF VALUES. The range of values on the axes should be slightly greater than the range of values being plotted, so that the entire data set can appear within the graph and most of the possible range of values on the axes will be used. Ideally, the range should include 0 on both axes, if 0 is a possible value for the variable being plotted. If a large range of values is necessary but cannot be depicted with a continuous scale, discontinuity in the axis should be indicated with paired

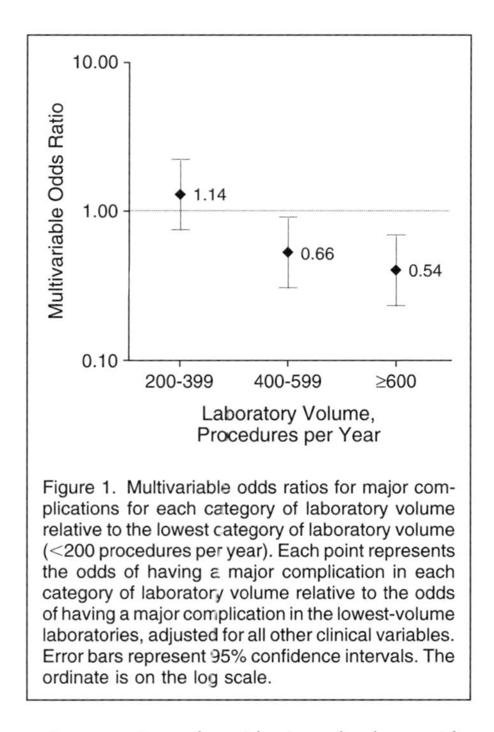

Figure 1. Multivariable odds ratios for major complications for each category of laboratory volume relative to the lowest category of laboratory volume (<200 procedures per year). Each point represents the odds of having a major complication in each category of laboratory volume relative to the odds of having a major complication in the lowest-volume laboratories, adjusted for all other clinical variables. Error bars represent 95% confidence intervals. The ordinate is on the log scale.

EXAMPLE F19 Point estimates using a logarithmic scale along with error bars indicting 95% confidence intervals. Adapted from *JAMA*. 1995;274:1141.

diagonal lines that signify a missing portion of the range (–//–).[28] Numerical data on 2 sides of a scale break should not be connected to avoid the implication that data on either side of the discontinuity are linear.

TICK MARKS. Divisions of the graph axes should be indicated by intervals chosen to be appropriate, simple multiples of the quantity plotted, such as multiples of 2, 5, or 10.[28] The intervals on the axes are indicated by interval marks (tick marks) located left of and abutting the vertical axis and below and abutting the horizontal axis. Numbers that represent the values on the axis scale are centered on their respective tick marks. Unlabeled tick marks to indicate intervals between numbered marks usually are not necessary.

SCALING FUNCTIONS. For linear scales, the axis must appear linear, with equal intervals and equal spacing between tick marks. However, logarithmic scales may be useful to show proportional rates of change (Example F19) and to emphasize the change rate rather than the absolute amount of change when absolute values or baseline values for data series vary greatly.

AXIS LABELS. Axis labels identify the variable plotted on the axis. In line graphs, each axis should be labeled with the type of data plotted and the unit of measure used. Data may represent numerical values, percentages, rates, or nominal categories. For numerical data, customary units of measure and their respective abbreviations or symbols should be used. However, if the only axis label in a figure is an abbreviation, the label should be spelled out (eg, "Seconds" or "Time, s" instead of "s"; "Dollars," or "Cost, \$" instead of "\$"; "Degrees," or "Temperature, °C" instead of "°") for ease of readability.

2.14.3 ***Legends.***—The figure legend or caption is printed below or next to the figure and contains information that identifies and describes the figure. The legend should provide sufficient detail to make the figure comprehensible without reference to the text. Although the recommended maximum length for figure legends is 40 words, longer legends may be necessary for figures that require more detailed explanations.

Figure Designations: Figure legends are set flush left and begin with the figure designation (Figure 1, Figure 2, etc) followed by a period. If the article has only 1 figure, the legend begins flush left without using the designation "Figure."

Title: The figure title follows the designation "Figure" and does not appear in the figure itself. The title is a phrase or a sentence that identifies the specific topic of the figure or describes what the data show. The title should be succinct, is capitalized in sentence style, usually should not contain abbreviations, ends with a period, and is immediately followed by the rest of the legend.

Titles of figures, including diagrams, photographs, and line drawings, generally should not begin with a phrase identifying the type of figure.

Avoid: Photograph showing prominent physical signs of familial hypercholesterolemia.

Better: Prominent physical signs of familial hypercholesterolemia.

However, a description of the type of figure may be required in certain circumstances to provide context and avoid confusion.

Figure 3. Fluorescein angiogram showing widespread retinal capillary nonperfusion and marked optic nerve head leakage.

Figure 4. Autoradiograph demonstrating loss of heterozygosity at the 3p25 locus in preneoplastic foci and corresponding invasive cancer.

Figure 7. Electron micrograph of area positive for terminal deoxynucleotidyl transferase-mediated biotinylated deoxyuridine triphosphate labeling.

Composite Figures: Composite figures consist of several parts and should have a single legend that contains necessary information about each part. If the parts share much of the same explanation, parenthetical mention of each part is appropriate.

Each component of the figure usually is described by a separate sentence beginning with the designation for the part, followed by a comma. Such information should be clearly specified by designations corresponding to the figure components. However, such designations must be consistent in all legends. For figures with 2 parts, designators such as "left, right" or "top, bottom" may be used, depending on layout. In the legend, reference to each of the figure components must be clear and should use a consistent format.

Avoid: Left, Abnormal tissue from gallbladder and liver (right).

Better: Abnormal tissue from gallbladder (left) and from liver (right).

For composite figures with more than 2 parts, reference to individual parts by their position in the figure (eg, left, middle, right; or top left, top right, bottom left, bottom right) may create confusion or become cumbersome. In these cases, capital letters (A, B, C, D, etc) should be used to label the parts of the figure. These letters should be placed in a small insert box that is positioned in the lower left corner of each figure. The figure legend should refer to each of the figure components and the letter designators in a clear and consistent format.

2.14.4 ***Abbreviations.***—Abbreviations in figures should be consistent with those used in the text. Abbreviations specific to a figure should be defined in the legend or in a key as part of the figure. Abbreviations may be expanded individually in the text of the legend or may be expanded collectively at the end of the legend.

> Figure 2. Correlations between changes in renal blood flow (RBF), mean arterial pressure (MAP), and cardiac output (CO) during dopamine infusion.

> Figure 5. Distribution of amipyrine breath test and antithrombin III values in patients with liver disease and controls. S indicates steatosis; SF, steatofibrosis; LC, liver cirrhosis; AH, acute hepatitis; and CH, chronic hepatitis.

If several illustrations share many of the same abbreviations and symbols, full explanation may be provided in the first figure legend, with reference to that legend in subsequent legends.

2.14.5 ***Symbols, Line or Bar Patterns, Shading Characteristics.***—Symbols, line or bar patterns, and shading characteristics used in the figure must be explained. If this information is brief, it may be included in the legend; alternatively, this information may be included in a key within the figure. For a series of figures within an article, the types of symbols, line or bar patterns, and shading characteristics should be used consistently. For instance, if data for the intervention group and for the control group are designated as a solid line and as a dashed line, respectively, then these same patterns should be used for similar data for these groups in subsequent similar figures.

When data points are plotted, symbols should be distinguished easily by shape and color (white or black). For example, if 2 symbols are needed, the recommended symbols are ○ and ●,[28] although △ and ▲ or □ and ■ may be used. For data displays that require 3 symbols, ○, △, and □; ●, ○, and ▲; or ●, ○, and △ may be reasonable choices. The shading or color of the symbols also can be used to designate specific types of data. For instance, ○ may be used to indicate data obtained before an intervention or the placebo group, and ● may signify data obtained after the intervention or from the treatment group.

2.14.6 ***Information About Methods and Statistical Analyses.***—Statements regarding experimental details are unnecessary for each figure if this information is provided in the "Methods" section of the article and the text that refers to the figure clearly indicates the source of the data. Reference to the "Methods" section or to other figures that contain this information may be appropriate. At times, brief inclusion of experimental details in the figure legend may be necessary for easy understanding of the figure.

For data that have been analyzed statistically, pertinent analyses and significance values may be included in the figure or its legend.[29] Values for data displayed in the figure (eg, mean or median values) should be indicated in the figure or in the legend. For plotted data, error bars (depicting SD, SEM, range, interquartile range, or confidence intervals) are a convenient way to display variability in the data.[30] The meaning of error bars should be explained clearly and specified in the legend (Example F19).

2.14.7 ***Arrows, Arrowheads, and Other Markers.***—Arrows, arrowheads, and other markers used to draw attention to specific areas in a figure should be explained in the legend (Example F20).

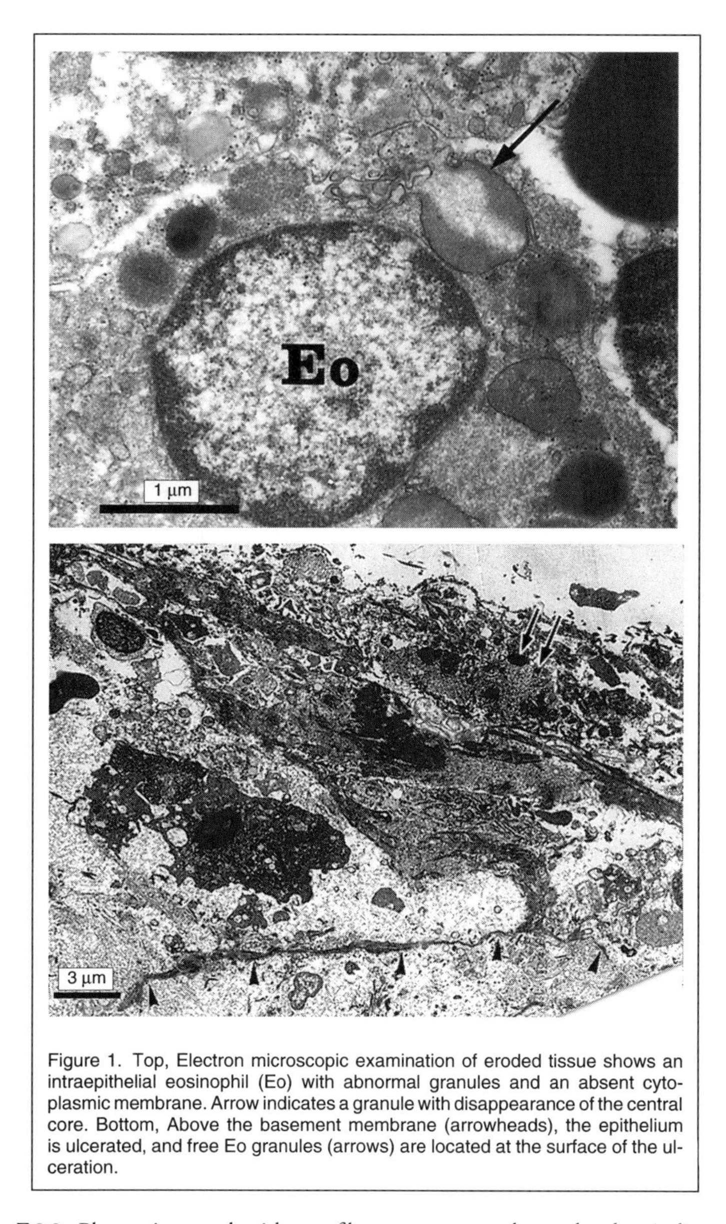

Figure 1. Top, Electron microscopic examination of eroded tissue shows an intraepithelial eosinophil (Eo) with abnormal granules and an absent cytoplasmic membrane. Arrow indicates a granule with disappearance of the central core. Bottom, Above the basement membrane (arrowheads), the epithelium is ulcerated, and free Eo granules (arrows) are located at the surface of the ulceration.

EXAMPLE F20 Photomicrograph with use of letters, arrows, and arrowheads as indicator elements. The reference bars in the lower left corners are marked clearly and provide the measure of dimension for the figures. Adapted from *Arch Dermatol.* 1996;132:537.

2.14.8 ***Photomicrographs.***—Legends for photomicrographs should include details about the type of stain used and the degree of magnification. If the original illustration has been modified (enlarged or reduced), the original magnification should be noted.

> Figure 1. Eosinophilic deposition of amyloidosis in the biopsy specimen indicated as green birefringence with polarizing light (Congo red, original magnification ×30).

Electron micrograph legends may specify magnification, without information about the stain.

Figure 1. Complete reepithelialization of the surface with normal ciliated epithelium in the stamp graft group 2 weeks after operation (top, scanning electron microscopy, original magnification ×20; bottom, corresponding photomicrograph, ×1000).

In figures with 2 or more parts, the stains or magnifications relevant to each individual part should be noted after its description.

Figure 1. Histological examination of the glans penis of patient 1. Left, Mucosal erosion covered by fibrin and neutrophils and dense inflammatory infiltrate in the lamina propria (hematoxylin-eosin, original magnification ×100). Right, Infiltrate in the laminia propria with numerous eosinophils, some of them degranulated (arrows) (May-Grunwald-Giemsa, original magnification ×250).

2.14.9 ***Visual Indicators in Illustrations or Photographs.***—Visual indicators provided in illustrations or photographs, such as a reference bar denoting a measure of dimension (eg, length) in a photomicrograph, should be clearly defined in the figure (eg, dimension and unit of measure) or described in the figure legend (Example F20).

2.14.10 ***Placement of Figures in the Text.***—In the published article, figures should be placed as close as possible to their first mention in the text. Figures should be cited in consecutive numerical order in the text, and references to figures should include their respective numbers. For example:

Patient participation and progress through the study is shown in Figure 2.

Figure 2 shows patient participation and progress through the study.

Patient participation and progress through the study were monitored by the investigators (Figure 2).

Given the potential for variability in the page layout process, the text should not refer to figures by position on the page or by other designators, such as "the figure opposite," "the figure on this page," or "the figure above."

2.14.11 ***Figures Reproduced or Adapted From Other Sources.***—For reproduction or modification of figures, illustrations, photographs, or any other graphical materials that have been published previously, written permission to reproduce them must be obtained from the copyright holder (usually the publisher). Some suggest, as a courtesy, also obtaining permission from the author. The original source should be acknowledged in the legend. If the original source in which the illustration has been published is included in the reference list, the reference may be cited in the legend, with the citation number for the reference corresponding to its first appearance in the text, tables, or figures (see 2.13.4, Table Components, Footnotes, and 2.12.6, Citations). It may be necessary to include additional information to comply with specific language required by the organization (usually a publisher) granting permission to republish the figure.

Reprinted with permission from *Nature*.[40] Copyright 1994, Macmillan Magazines Ltd.

2.14.12 ***Guidelines for Preparing and Submitting Figures and Legends.***—The preferred format for submitting figures varies among scientific journals.[31] Authors who submit figures with a scientific article should consult the instructions for authors of the publication for specific requirements. The following guidelines apply for figures submitted to AMA journals.

Graphs, line art, diagrams, charts, and other black-and-white figures should be drawn professionally and should be submitted as unmounted, glossy, sharp (in focus) photographic prints. Computer-generated graphics produced by high-quality laser printers (with at least 600 dpi) are also acceptable.

Photographs, photomicrographs, or radiographs should be submitted as high-contrast, right-reading glossy prints. Color illustrations should be submitted as 3×5-in color transparencies or 35-mm color slides along with corresponding color prints. For 35-mm transparencies, Kodachrome or similar film or a slow-speed Fujichrome, Ektachrome, or similar film should be used. Transparencies should not be submitted in glass slides, as breakage can cause severe damage. If color prints are submitted, the print should be made oversized, and the negative of the print also should be provided. Polaroid-type prints and dot-matrix prints should not be used for reproduction because the results inevitably are poor.

Crystal-clear, sharp images are essential for accurate reproduction. Dust and scratches usually can be removed, but if details are blurred in the original, details will remain blurred in reproduction. Good exposure is another important consideration in providing the best-quality prints and transparencies. If necessary, several different exposures of the same image may be submitted, and the best candidate for image reproduction will be selected.

Four sets of figures should be submitted, and all figures should be numbered according to their citation order in the text. A label with the figure number, name of the first author, short form of the manuscript title, and the proper orientation (eg, "top") should be affixed to the back of the print. Writing directly on the back of the print should be avoided as this may cause detrimental show-through in the live image area.

Proper locations for visual indicators (eg, arrows indicating the area of interest in an illustration or photograph) should be identified clearly. This can be accomplished by providing (in addition to the required clean, unmarked copies of the illustration or photograph or copies of the 35-mm slide) an extra paper copy of the illustration or photograph with locations for indicators marked directly on the paper copy.

Legends for figures should be double-spaced on a separate page and should not appear on the illustrations.

The availability of computer software for generating figures, such as statistical or graphic design programs, has simplified the creation of figures in digital format. However, the ability of publishers to use author-generated electronic files containing figures for importing, reproducing, and incorporating into production software varies considerably. Authors should consult the editorial office of the publication for information about preferred and compatible formats for submission of figures in electronic files.

2.14.13 ***Consent for Identifiable Subjects.***—For photographs in which the subject can be identified, the author should obtain and submit a signed statement of informed consent from the identifiable person that grants permission to publish the photograph. Previously used measures to conceal the identity of a patient in a photograph, such as placing black bars over the patient's eyes, are not always effective and should not be used for masking (see 3.8.2, Ethical and Legal Considerations, Rights to Privacy and Anonymity).

For figures that depict genetic information, such as pedigrees or family trees, informed consent is required from all persons who can be identified. Authors should not modify the pedigree, eg, by changing the number of persons in the generation, varying the number of offspring in families, or masking the sex of pedigree members, in an attempt to avoid potential identification (see 3.8.3, Ethical and Legal Considerations, Rights in Published Reports of Genetic Pedigree Studies).

ACKNOWLEDGMENTS

Principal authors: Cheryl Iverson, MA, for sections 2.0 through 2.12; Phil B. Fontanarosa, MD, for sections 2.13 and 2.14

The authors thank Linda Knott, director of Electronic Production for AMA Scientific Publications, and Charl Richey, manager of Color and Graphics for AMA Scientific Publications, for their assistance in obtaining and processing the figures used as examples in this chapter.

REFERENCES

1. International Committee of Medical Journal Editors. Uniform Requirements for Manuscripts Submitted to Biomedical Journals. *JAMA.* 1997;277:927-934.
2. *JAMA* Instructions for Authors. *JAMA.* 1997;278:68-76.
3. Haynes RB, Mulrow CD, Huth EJ, Altman DG, Gardner MJ. More informative abstracts revisited. *Ann Intern Med.* 1990;113:69-76.
4. Yankauer A. The accuracy of medical journal references. *CBE Views.* April 1990;13:38-42.
5. Broadus RN. An investigation of the validity of bibliographic citations. *J Am Soc Information Sci.* 1983;34:132-135.
6. Evans JT, Nadjari HI, Burchell SA. Quotational and reference accuracy in surgical journals: a continuing peer review problem. *JAMA.* 1990;263:1353-1354.
7. Shenoy BV. Peer review [letter]. *JAMA.* 1990;264:3142.
8. Schofield EK. Accuracy of references [letter]. *CBE Views.* June 1990;13:68.
9. Patrias K. *National Library of Medicine Recommended Formats for Bibliographic Citation.* Bethesda, Md: National Library of Medicine, Reference Service; 1991.
10. *List of Journals Indexed in Index Medicus: 1996.* Washington, DC: National Library of Medicine; 1996. NIH publication 96-267.
11. *Books in Print: 1995-96.* New Providence, NJ: RR Bowker; 1995;1-9.
12. Williams MA. Citing electronic information. *CBE Views.* 1995;18:60.
13. Guernsey L. Cyberspace citations: scholars debate how best to cite research conducted on the Internet. *Chron Higher Educ.* January 12, 1996:A18, 20-21.
14. Li X, Crane NB. *Electronic Styles: An Expanded Guide to Citing Electronic Information.* Medford, NJ: Information Today; 1996. Examples available at: http://www.uvm.edu/~xli/reference/estyles.html.
15. Ivey KC. Citing Internet sources. *Editorial Eye.* August 1996:10.
16. Council of Biology Editors Style Manual Committee. *Scientific Style and Format: The CBE Manual for Authors, Editors, and Publishers.* 6th ed. New York, NY: Cambridge University Press; 1994.
17. *The Chicago Manual of Style.* 14th ed. Chicago, Ill: University of Chicago Press; 1993.
18. *The Bluebook: A Uniform System of Citation.* 15th ed. Cambridge, Mass: The Harvard Law Review Association; 1991.
19. Rubens P, ed. *Science and Technical Writing: A Manual of Style.* New York, NY: Henry Holt & Co Inc; 1992.
20. Sutcliffe AJ, ed. *The New York Public Library Writer's Guide to Style and Usage.* New York, NY: HarperCollins Publishers Inc; 1994.

21. Huth EJ. *How to Write and Publish Papers in the Medical Sciences.* 2nd ed. Baltimore, Md: Williams & Wilkins; 1990.

22. Zieger M. *Essentials of Writing Biomedical Research Papers.* New York, NY: McGraw-Hill Book Co; 1991.

23. Riegelman RK, Hirsch RP. *Studying a Study and Testing a Test.* 2nd ed. Boston, Mass: Little Brown & Co; 1989.

24. Tufte ER. *The Visual Display of Quantitative Information.* Cheshire, Conn: Graphics Press; 1983.

25. Begg C, Cho M, Eastwood S, et al. Improving the quality of reporting of randomized controlled trials: the CONSORT statement. *JAMA.* 1996;276:637-639.

26. Sox HC, Blatt MA, Higgins MC, Marton KI. *Medical Decision Making.* Boston, Mass: Butterworths; 1988.

27. Anderson C. Easy to alter digital images raise fears of tampering. *Science.* 1994;263:317-318.

28. Scientific Illustration Committee of the Council of Biology Editors. *Illustrating Science: Standards for Publication.* Bethesda, Md: Council of Biology Editors; 1988.

29. Singer PA, Feinstein AR. Graphical display of categorical data. *J Clin Epidemiol.* 1993;46:231-236.

30. Cleveland WS. *The Elements of Graphing Data.* Rev ed. Summit, NJ: Hobart Press; 1994.

31. Squires BP. Illustrative material: what editors and readers can expect from authors. *Can Med Assoc J.* 1990;142:447-449.

ADDITIONAL READING AND GENERAL REFERENCE

Hall GM, ed. *How to Write a Paper.* London, England: BMJ Publishing Group; 1994.

CHAPTER 3

If we are to live with this information explosion, let us not be terrified into dropping all our standards of the natures and ethics of scholarship and science.

Derek J. de Solla Price[1]

3.0 ETHICAL AND LEGAL CONSIDERATIONS

This chapter is intended to provide guidance to authors, editors, reviewers, and publishers in the fields of biomedicine, health, and the life sciences. The discussion focuses on ethical and legal issues involved in publication.

According to Lundberg,[2] human behavior is regulated by 3 forces: morality, ethics, and law. If personal morality does not regulate acceptable and appropriate behavior, we can rely on ethics. Ethical behavior is determined by norms, principles, guidelines, and policies. This chapter cites examples of the determinants of ethical behavior as they relate to scientific publication. If ethics do not regulate behavior, we are forced to rely on public laws. Examples of cases involving scientific publication when laws have been invoked or enforced are also provided in this chapter.

Those ethical and legal considerations and dilemmas most commonly encountered in scholarly scientific publication are the focus of this chapter. References to sources for additional guidance and information not discussed in this chapter are also provided within the text and at the end of each subsection.

Acknowledgments

Principal author: Annette Flanagin, RN, MA

I wish to thank the following for reviewing and offering critical suggestions for major improvements in this section: Carol Cadmus, ELS, John H. Dirckx, MD, David Goldblatt, MD, Elizabeth Knoll, PhD, Carol Kornblith, PhD, Roy Pitkin, MD, and Drummond Rennie, MD. The following people also reviewed the manuscript and offered minor suggestions for improvement: Susan R. Benner, MLS, Marjorie A. Bowman, MD, MPA, Veda Britt, JD, Helene M. Cole, MD, Lois Ann Colianni, David S. Cooper, MD, Lois DeBakey, PhD, Faith T. Fitzgerald, MD, Phil Gunby, Wayne Hoppe, JD, Colleen M. Hubona, Leonard A. Levin, MD, PhD, Peter M. Marzuk, MD, Faith McLellan, ELS, Brian Pace, MA, Don Riesenberg, MD, Lee Ann Riesenberg, RN, MS, Povl Riis, MD, DHonC, Jennifer Sperry, MA, Joan Stephenson, PhD, and Chris Zielinski.

References

1. de Solla Price DJ. Ethics of scientific publication. *Science*. 1964;144:655-657.
2. Lundberg GD. II. Perspective from the editor of *JAMA, The Journal of the American Medical Association*. *Bull Med Libr Assoc*. 1992;80:110-114.

Some judge of authors' names, not works, and then
Nor praise nor blame the writings, but the men.

Alexander Pope[1]

3.1 ■ **AUTHORSHIP RESPONSIBILITY.**—More than 4 decades ago, Richard M. Hewitt, MD, then head of the Section of Publications at the Mayo Clinic, described the ethics of authorship in a *JAMA* article entitled "Exposition as Applied to Medicine: A Glance at the Ethics of It."[2] This may have been just a glance (3 years later he published an entire book on writing and editing), but the following excerpts from Hewitt's article demonstrate a deep appreciation of the basic ethical responsibilities of authorship and point to the basic ethical obligations of authorship:

> Authorship cannot be conferred; it may be undertaken by one who will shoulder the responsibility that goes with it.
>
> The reader of a report issued by two or more authors has a right to assume that each author has some authoritative knowledge of the subject, that each contributed to the investigation, and that each labored on the report to the extent of weighing every word and quantity in it.
>
> If we would define publication of unoriginal, repetitious medical material as a violation of medical ethics, and would officially reprove it as such, the tawdry author would be silenced and the genuine one helped.
>
> The by-line, then, is not merely a credit-line. He who took some part in the investigation, be it ever so minor, is entitled to credit for what he did. . . . Further, the generous chap who would bestow authorship on another, perhaps without even submitting the manuscript to him, may do his colleague no favor. For the investigation is one thing, the report of it another, and, sad the day that this must be admitted: The investigation may have been excellent but the report, bad.
>
> Since all of us necessarily adopt and absorb the ideas of others, we must be scrupulous in maintaining the spirit of acknowledgment to others. Fundamentally, your integrity is at stake. Unless you make specific acknowledgment, you claim the credit for yourself for anything that you write. In general, it is better to say too much about your sources than too little.
>
> The author who paraphrases or refers to an article should have read it.

3.1.1 ***Authorship: Definition and Criteria.***—Authorship offers significant professional and personal rewards, but these rewards are accompanied by substantial responsibility. During the 1980s, biomedical editors began requiring contributors to meet specific criteria for authorship. These criteria were first developed for medical journals under the initiative of Edward J. Huth, MD,[3] then editor of the *Annals of Internal Medicine,* who cited Hewitt's[2] work during discussions at the 1984 meeting of the International Committee of Medical Journal Editors (ICMJE). The ICMJE guidelines were first published in 1985[4] and are now part of the Uniform Requirements for Manuscripts Submitted to Biomedical Journals[5] (see 2.0, Manuscript Preparation). The first requirement in these guidelines states:

> Each author should have participated sufficiently in the work to take public responsibility for the content.

To take public responsibility, an author must be able to defend the content and conclusions of the article if publicly challenged. Sufficient participation means that substantial contributions have been made in *each* of the following areas[5]:

1. conception and design **or** analysis and interpretation of the data;

and

2. drafting the manuscript **or** revising it critically for important intellectual content;

and

3. approving the version of the manuscript to be published.

The first criterion, "conception and design or analysis and interpretation of the data," may be interpreted broadly. For example, an author of a nonresearch paper may not have analyzed data per se, but may have analyzed literature, events, theories, arguments, or opinions. What is important is that each of the 3 criteria is met in some manner by all authors.

The phrase "substanital contribution" has not been adequately defined (perhaps to allow for broader interpretation of the ICMJE criteria for authorship). The following might be useful for those seeking an explanation of "substantial contribution":

A substantial contribution is an important intellectual contribution, without which the work could not have been completed or the manuscript could not have been written and submitted for publication.

The ICMJE statement on authorship also considers the following contributions, which, standing alone, may not justify authorship[5]:

> Participation solely in the acquisition of funding or the collection of data does not justify authorship. General supervision of the research group is not sufficient for authorship.

(See also 3.1.2, Guest and Ghost Authors, Guest [Honorary] Authors.)

To remind authors of these responsibilities, many journals require contributors to attest in writing how they qualify for authorship. The AMA journals require authors to sign a statement of authorship responsibility based on the ICMJE guidelines. For example, all *JAMA* authors must sign the following statement of authorship criteria and responsibility:

> All persons who meet the *JAMA* criteria for authorship are listed as authors, and all authors certify that they meet the following criteria: I have participated sufficiently in the conception and design of this work or the analysis of the data (when applicable), as well as the writing of the manuscript, to take public responsibility for it. I believe the manuscript represents valid work. I have reviewed the final version of the submitted manuscript and approve it for publication. Neither this manuscript nor one with substantially similar content under my authorship has been published or is being considered for publication elsewhere, except as described in an attachment. If requested, I shall produce the data on which the manuscript is based for examination by the editors or their assignees.

According to the ICMJE, "any part of an article critical to its main conclusions must be the responsibility of one author." In addition, editors may request an explanation of the specific contributions of each author and this information may be published in the article.

Deceased or Incapacitated Authors: In the case of death or incapacitation of an author during the manuscript submission and review or publication process, a family member or an individual with power of attorney can sign the authorship form for the deceased or incapacitated author (see also 2.0, Manuscript Preparation).

Author vs Contributor: Recent proposals to replace the current system of authorship with a system of unambiguous credits for specific contributions have been given considerable attention.[6] Such a system would require each contributor to state explicitly who did what, rather than grouping all authors collectively as "authors." Whether a contributor system will replace the long-standing current system of authorship remains to be seen.

3.1.2 ***Guest and Ghost Authors.***—The ICMJE guidelines state that at least 1 author must be responsible for any part of an article critical to its main conclusions[5] and that everyone listed as an author must have made a significant contribution to that specific article. As described in section 3.1.1, many journals require authors to sign statements of authorship responsibility. The first phrase in *JAMA*'s authorship statement is intended to eliminate guest authors and "flesh out" ghost authors[7,8] (see below for the definitions of *guest authors* and *ghost authors*):

> All persons who meet the following criteria for authorship are listed as authors, and all authors certify that they meet the following criteria. . .

Guest (Honorary) Authors: Traditionally, supervisors, department chairs, and mentors have been given guest, or honorary, places in the byline even though they have not met all of the criteria for authorship. This custom is no longer acceptable because it devalues the meaning of authorship.[7,9] The ICMJE guidelines state specifically that "general supervision of the research group is not sufficient for authorship" and that "participation solely in the acquisition of funding or the collection of data does not justify authorship."[5] Such supervision and participation should be noted in an acknowledgment (see 3.2, Acknowledgments). Guest authors have also included well-known persons in a particular field accepting money or other compensation to have their names attached to a manuscript that has already been researched and prepared by or for an organization with a commercial interest in the subject of the paper.[8,10] Such practice clearly is deceitful.[7]

Ghost Authors: Ghost authors have participated sufficiently in the research or analysis and writing of a manuscript to take public responsibility for the work but are not named in the byline or listing of collaborative authors. In biomedical publication, ghost authors have included clinical research associates at pharmaceutical companies, medical writers, marketing and public relations writers, and junior staff writing for elected or appointed officials.[7] As described elsewhere, ghost writers have been hired by firms with commercial interests to write reviews of specific subjects after agreeing not to be named as authors.[7-11]

Ghost writers are not necessarily ghost authors. For example, a writer may not have participated in the research or analysis of a study but may have been given the data to write a report for publication. If participants in the project do not meet all of the criteria for authorship, but have made substantial contributions to the research, writing, or editing of the manuscript, those persons and their relevant institutional affiliation should be named, with their permission, in the acknowledgments (see 3.2, Acknowledgments). As suggested in 1994 by Morton F. Goldberg, MD[12] (then editor of the *Archives of Ophthalmology*), to give proper credit to medical writers and author's editors, journal editors should require authors to identify those persons who have participated substantially in the writing or editing of the manuscript. Substantial editing or writing assistance should be disclosed to the editor at the time of manuscript submission and mentioned in the acknowledgment. Journals that follow this policy should state it clearly in their instructions for authors. Journal editors and copy editors who substantially edit a manuscript do not have to be specifically acknowledged when their names appear in the journal's masthead.

3.1.3 ***Unsigned Editorials, Anonymous Articles, Pseudonymous Authors.***—The practice of publishing unsigned or anonymous editorials provides ''vituperative editorialists''[13] protection from the enemies they might make when taking unpopular stands in the pages of their journals. However, without named authors and affiliations, readers lack information to judge the objectivity and credibility of the articles. Although this practice is the norm for newspaper editorial pages, it has fallen out of use in most peer-reviewed journals. One rationale for anonymity has been that editorials, whether signed or not, represent the official opinion of the publication or the owner of the publication. For many years, *JAMA* published unsigned editorials, but since 1970 all *JAMA* editorials have been signed by their authors. The *BMJ* began signing its editorials in 1981.[14] As of this writing, the *Lancet* continues to publish unsigned editorials[15] (see 1.5, Types of Articles, Articles of Opinion).

Journals that publish unsigned editorials and signed scientific articles may give contradictory messages to their readers about the merits and responsibility of authorship. Authors who submit scientific papers must publicly stand by what they write, while unsigned editorialists can hide behind a journal's masthead. Unattributed editorials may also allow the publisher or owner of the journal and influential organizations to compromise the journal's editorial independence (see 3.10, Editorial Freedom and Integrity). As a result, all editorials in AMA peer-reviewed journals are signed.

Occasionally, an author requests that his or her name not be used in publication. If the reason for this request is judged to be important (such as concern for personal safety; fear of political reprisal, public humiliation, or job loss; or concern for colleagues, patients, family, or friends), then the article can be published without that author's name. The phrase ''Name withheld on request'' or the word ''Anonymous'' could be used in place of the author's name (see 2.2, Manuscript Preparation, Bylines and End-of-Text Signatures).

Pseudonyms are inappropriate in bylines of scientific reports, as they are misleading and cause problems for literature citations. For those scientific journals that also publish literary or fictional articles, a pseudonym may be acceptable but should be used rarely and with caution.

In AMA publications, if anonymity or a pseudonym is used, the author must still sign statements of authorship responsibility and copyright transfer (using his or her actual name), and those records are kept confidential as part of the manuscript file. For the extremely rare case in which withholding of an author's name is justified, the author's name should be withheld from peer reviewers as well as readers. However, both reviewers and readers should be informed that the author has requested anonymity or is using a pseudonym.

3.1.4 ***Number of Authors.***—The number of authors whose names appear in the byline of scientific papers has increased steadily during the last century.[16,17] Most of this increase occurred as a result of specialization and the need for multidisciplinary collaboration. However, authorship "inflation" has diluted the meaning of authorship responsibility. For example, which authors in a byline that contains more than 100 names can state that they actually wrote the paper or that they participated sufficiently to take public responsibility for the work? To address this problem, suggestions have been made to limit the number of authors listed in the byline, as well as reference lists and database citations.[18-20] Most of the AMA journals, following the recommendations of the US National Library of Medicine and the ICMJE,[5] limit the number of authors to appear in a reference citation to 25 (see 2.12.7, Manuscript Preparation, References, Authors, and 3.1.6, Group and Collaborative Authorship).

3.1.5 ***Order of Authorship.***—Although many journals and databases limit the number of listed authors to 3, 6, 10, or 25, the first through sixth slots in a byline can carry substantial weight. For example, AMA publications list the first 6 authors in a reference citation when the authors number 6 or less, and if there are more than 6 authors, the first 3 are listed followed by "et al" (see 2.12.7, Manuscript Preparation, References, Authors). Guides for determining order of authorship have ranged from simple alphabetical listings to mathematical formulas for assessing specific levels of individual contribution levels.[21,22] Alphabetical listings are not equitable, and even the most systematic calculations of contribution levels will require some measure of subjective judgment. The following guidelines may help determine order of authorship[23]:

1. Only those individuals who meet the criteria for authorship may be listed as authors.
2. The first author has contributed the most to the work, and the last author has contributed the least.
3. Decisions about the order of authors should be made as early as possible (eg, before the manuscript is written) and reevaluated later by consensus.
4. Disagreement about order should be resolved by the authors, not the editor.
5. Authors may provide a publishable footnote explaining the order of authorship, if there is a compelling reason.
6. Editors may request documentation of authors' specific contributions.

3.1.6 ***Group and Collaborative Authorship.***—Group or collaborative authorship usually involves multicenter study investigators, members of working groups or consensus conferences, and official or self-appointed expert boards, panels, or committees. These groups can comprise hundreds of participants, and therefore, decisions about listing group authorship pose several problems for editors and authors[24,25] (see 11.9, Abbreviations, Collaborative Groups, and 2.2.3, Manuscript Preparation, Multiple Authors, Group Authors). First, it is doubtful that all members of a very large group would be able to meet all the criteria for authorship. Frequently, a writing team is named as the author for a group, or a writing team is identified in the acknowledgment when a group name is used in the byline.

Second, without a single person named as author, no individual person can take responsibility and be held accountable for the work (ie, what Rennie et al[6] call the "guarantor"). For this reason, at least 1 individual (eg, the corresponding author or the principal investigator) should be named on the title page in the author affiliation footnote (see also 2.0, Manuscript Preparation). For papers with group authorship, the guidelines that follow may help authors and editors determine who should be listed and where they should be listed[24]; however, controversy exists regarding how strictly they should be followed.

Entire Group as Author: If authorship is attributed to a group, all members of the group must meet all criteria for authorship (as described in 2.2.3, Manuscript Preparation, Multiple Authors, Group Authors, and 3.1.2, Guest and Ghost Authors). In this case, the byline might read:

The Carotid Atherosclerosis Study Group

At the editor's discretion, the individual members of the study group may be listed separately (perhaps in a box or set off by rules) or in the acknowledgment section. However, a long list of investigators and affiliated centers could occupy several journal pages and would be of questionable value to readers.[24,25] If the group list has been published previously in an indexed and retrievable journal, the editor may choose to cite that publication in an affiliation footnote or acknowledgment rather than to republish the entire list (see 3.2, Acknowledgments).

If the group name appears in the byline, it is recommended that at least 1 person, usually the corresponding author, be named as an individual who will coordinate questions about the article. This person can be named in the byline or affiliation footnote. In this case, the byline might read:

James S. Smith, MD; and the Carotid Atherosclerosis Study Group

And the affiliation footnote might read:

A complete list of the collaborators in the Carotid Atherosclerosis Study Group appears at the end of this article.

Corresponding author: James S. Smith, MD, Department of Neurology, University of Chicago Medical School, 555 S Main St, Chicago, IL 60615.

See also 2.3.3, Manuscript Preparation, Author Affiliations, and 2.3.8, Manuscript Preparation, Reprint or Correspondence Address.

Part of the Group as Author: One or more authors may take responsibility for a group (as the author or writing team). Note that the difference here is the use of the conjunction *for* rather than *and*. Those members of the group who do not qualify for authorship would not be listed in the byline. In this case, the byline might read:

John Smith, MD; Louise Crane, PhD; for the Carotid Atherosclerosis Study Group

or

The Writing Committee for the Carotid Atherosclerosis Study Group

The group members may then be listed separately in the acknowledgment, depending on the length of the list and whether it has been published previously (see 3.2, Acknowledgments).

Study group participants should not be promised authorship status and a place in the byline merely for cooperating in a study, collecting data, attending a working conference, or lending technical assistance. Editors and authors should assess the need to publish lengthy lists of authors and participants in acknowledgments on an individual basis, and journals should publish their policies about group authorship in their instructions for authors.

REFERENCES

1. Pope A. *An Essay on Critcism*. Part Ib, line 212. 1711.
2. Hewitt RM. Exposition as applied to medicine: a glance at the ethics of it. *JAMA*. 1954;156:477-479.
3. Huth EJ. Guidelines on authorship of medical papers. *Ann Intern Med*. 1986;104: 269-274. See also Huth EJ. Guidelines on authorship. In: *How to Write and Publish Papers in the Medical Sciences*. 2nd ed. Baltimore, Md: Williams & Wilkins; 1990:229-230.
4. International Committee of Medical Journal Editors. Guidelines on authorship. *BMJ*. 1985;291:722.
5. International Committee of Medical Journal Editors. Uniform Requirements for Manuscripts Submitted to Biomedical Journals. *JAMA*. 1997;277:927-934.
6. Rennie D, Yank V, Emanuel L. When authorship fails: a proposal to make contributors accountable. *JAMA*. 1997;278:579-585.
7. Rennie D, Flanagin A. Authorship! authorship! guests, ghosts, grafters, and the two-sided coin. *JAMA*. 1994;271:469-471.
8. Flanagin A, Rennie D. Acknowledging ghosts. *JAMA*. 1995;273:73.
9. Smith J. Gift authorship: a poisoned chalice? *BMJ*. 1994;309:1456-1457.
10. Brennan TA. Buying editorials. *N Engl J Med*. 1994;331:673-675.
11. DeBakey L. Rewriting and the by-line: is the author the writer? *Surgery*. 1974;75: 38-48.
12. Instructions for authors. *Arch Ophthalmol*. 1994;112:12-15.
13. Morgan P. *An Insider's Guide for Medical Authors and Editors*. Philadelphia, Pa: ISI Press; 1986.
14. Lock S. Signed editorials. *BMJ*. 1981;283:876.
15. The Lancet. Signed—The Lancet. *Lancet*. 1993;341:24.
16. Fye WB. Medical authorship: traditions, trends, and tribulations. *Ann Intern Med*. 1990;113:317-325.
17. Stossel TP. Volume: papers and academic promotion. *Ann Intern Med*. 1987;106: 146-149.
18. Burman HD. "Hanging from the masthead": reflections on authorship. *Ann Intern Med*. 1982;97:602-605.
19. Epstein RJ. Six authors in search of a citation: villains or victims of the Vancouver convention? *BMJ*. 1993;306:765-767.
20. Shapiro DW, Wenger NS, Shapiro MF. The contributions of authors to multiauthored biomedical research papers. *JAMA*. 1994;271:438-442.
21. Schmidt RH. A worksheet for authorship of scientific articles. *Bull Ecol Soc Am*. 1987;68:8-10.
22. Davis PJ, Gregerman RI. Parse analysis: a new method for the evaluation of investigators' bibliographies. *N Engl J Med*. 1969;281:989-990.

23. Riesenberg D, Lundberg GD. The order of authorship: who's on first? *JAMA*. 1990; 264:1857.

24. Glass RM. New information for authors and readers: group authorship, acknowledgments, and rejected manuscripts [published correction appears in *JAMA*. 1993;269:48]. *JAMA*. 1992;268:99.

25. Kassirer JP, Angell M. On authorship and acknowledgments. *N Engl J Med*. 1991;325:1510-1512.

> *We recently accepted a manuscript with an acknowledgment section that listed 63 institutions and 135 physicians, the number of patients each institution had contributed (some as few as one), the 51 members of seven different committees, their institutions and their specialties, and the secretaries in the trial office. The paper was 12 pages long, the acknowledgments took up 5 pages.*
>
> Jerome P. Kassirer, MD, and Marcia Angell, MD[1]

3.2 ■ **ACKNOWLEDGMENTS.**—Acknowledgments are typically used to list grant support, donors of equipment or supplies, technical assistance, and important specific contributions from individuals who do not qualify for authorship (see 2.10, Manuscript Preparation, Acknowledgments, and 3.1.1, Authorship: Definition and Criteria). Contributions commonly recognized in an acknowledgment are shown in Table 1.

Acknowledgments should also identify medical writers and author's editors who made substantial intellectual contributions to manuscripts but do not meet the criteria for authorship (see 3.1.2, Guest and Ghost Authors). *JAMA* requires the corresponding author to identify such assistance in an acknowledgment. The acknowledgment encourages authors to give public credit to all persons who have made substantial contributions to the work and to identify all important writing or editorial assistance.[2]

> All persons who have made substantial contributions to the work reported in the manuscript (including writing and editing assistance), but are not authors, are named in the Acknowledgment and have given me their written permission to be named.
>
> If I do not include an Acknowledgment, that means I have not received substantial contributions from nonauthors.

A list of participants in a collaborative group may also be included in the acknowledgment (see 3.1.6, Group and Collaborative Authorship). However, a lengthy

TABLE 1. CONTRIBUTIONS COMMONLY RECOGNIZED IN AN ACKNOWLEDGMENT

- General advice, guidance, or supervision
- Critical review of the manuscript
- Critical review of study proposal, design, or methods
- Data collection
- Data analysis
- Participation in clinical trial
- Statistical assistance or advice
- Technical assistance or advice
- Research assistance or advice
- Writing assistance or collaboration
- Editorial assistance or collaboration
- Bibliographic assistance
- Clerical assistance
- Manuscript preparation
- Financial support
- Material support
- Grant support

acknowledgment may occupy an excessive amount of journal space. Some editors have proposed arbitrary limits on the length of an acknowledgment (eg, 1 column of a journal page or 600 words of reduced type).[1] The need to credit assistance from individuals, especially in large multicenter clinical trials, varies considerably. Thus, the editor and corresponding author should determine the length of published acknowledgments on a case-by-case basis.[3] If published previously, long lists of collaborative participants can be cited in the affiliation footnote or acknowledgment as follows:

> A list of the members of the Carotid Atherosclerosis Study Group and participating study centers was published in *JAMA* (1995;275:220-223).

Other options include publishing the list in an electronic database.

Nonspecific group acknowledgments, such as "the house staff" or "the nurses in the emergency department," would require permission from all identifiable persons in the group. Since these types of acknowledgments rarely provide useful information, it might be better to avoid them. Acknowledgment of unidentifiable groups, such as "the anonymous peer reviewers," is not problematic but is uninformative.

3.2.1 ***Permission to Name Individuals.***—Identification of individuals in an acknowledgment may imply their endorsement of the article's content. As a result, persons should not be listed in an acknowledgment without their knowledge and consent. For this reason, the International Committee of Medical Journal Editors (ICMJE) and *JAMA* require the corresponding author to obtain written permission from any individuals named in the acknowledgment and to certify in writing to the editor that such permission has been obtained.[3,4]

Personal Communication and Credit Lines: Following the rationale that including a person's name in an acknowledgment may imply endorsement of a manuscript's content, citing an individual's name in a personal communication citation may carry the same implication. The ICMJE recommends that authors who name an individual as a source for information in a personal communication, be it through conversation, a letter, e-mail, or telephone call, should obtain written permission from the named individual.[4] *JAMA* follows the ICMJE recommendation and requires authors to forward copies of all personal communication permissions to the editorial office. The same policy might apply to identifying names in credit lines in the legends of illustrations and photographs; however, obtaining such permission from the owner of the illustration or photograph usually falls under the auspices of copyright law (see 3.6.6, Copying, Reproducing, and Adapting).

REFERENCES

1. Kassirer JP, Angell M. On authorship and acknowledgments. *N Engl J Med.* 1991;325: 1510-1512.

2. Flanagin A, Rennie D. Acknowledging ghosts. *JAMA.* 1995;273:73.

3. Glass RM. New information for authors and readers: group authorship, acknowledgments, and rejected manuscripts [published correction appears in *JAMA.* 1993;269:48]. *JAMA.* 1992;268:99.

4. International Committee of Medical Journal Editors. Uniform Requirements for Manuscripts Submitted to Biomedical Journals. *JAMA.* 1997;277:927-934.

> *Wasteful publication includes dividing the results in a single study into two or more papers ("salami science"); republishing the same material in successive papers (which need not have identical format and content); and blending data from one study with additional data to extract yet another paper that could not make its way on the second set of data alone (meat extenders).*
>
> Edward J. Huth, MD[1]

3.3 ■ **DUPLICATE PUBLICATION.**—Duplicate publication is the simultaneous reporting or subsequent reporting—***unbeknownst to the editors and readers***—of essentially the same information, article, or major components of an article 2 or more times in 1 or more form of media (either print or electronic format).[2-9] Duplicate publication is also commonly known as ***redundant publication,*** which the Editorial Policy Committee of the Council of Biology Editors proposed as a more inclusive term.[6] Both terms apply to both published and unpublished works and, for example, may include 1 or more manuscripts under consideration by a journal. Other terms used to describe this practice include prior, repetitive, multiple, fragmented, fractionally divided, and topically divided publication.[3,8,9]

Duplication occurs when there is substantial overlap in 1 or more elements of an article or manuscript. For reports of research, this includes the design, materials and methods, graphic and illustrative material, discussion, or conclusions. A widely accepted quantification of the amount of overlap that is considered duplicative does not exist. This is an area in which authors and editors often disagree. Researchers in 2 studies of duplicate publication classified an article as duplicative of another if 10% or more of the content was identical or highly similar.[7,10]

Duplication also occurs in other types of articles (eg, reviews, case reports, opinion pieces, and letters to the editor). Duplicate publication or the submission of duplicate material is not necessarily unethical, but failure to disclose the existence of duplicate articles, manuscripts, or other material is unethical and may represent a violation of copyright law.[7] Reports of the same data in multiple articles waste publishing resources (ie, that of editors, reviewers, and readers as well as journal pages), pollute the literature, and cause problems for researchers and those who conduct meta-analyses.[1,7,8]

A number of bibliometric studies of duplicate publication in various fields have found that as many as 12% to 28% of published articles may be classified as duplicative of other articles.[7,8,10-12] In addition, these studies have concluded that as many as 9% to 11% of duplicative articles do not include a citation or reference to the original or primary article.[7,12]

Following the recommendations of the International Committee of Medical Journal Editors (ICMJE),[2] a policy that prohibits duplicate publications does not preclude consideration of manuscripts that have been presented orally or in abstract or poster form at a professional meeting. However, publication of complete manuscripts in proceedings of such meetings may preclude consideration for publication in a primary-source journal. Press reports that cover presentations of data at scheduled professional meetings would not necessarily violate this policy, but authors should avoid distributing copies of their complete manuscripts, tables, and illustrations during such meetings. Preliminary release of information directly to the media, usually through press conferences or news releases, may jeopardize an author's chances for publication in a primary-source journal. However, exceptions are made when a government health agency determines that there is an immediate public need for such information[8] (see 3.13.1, Release of Information to the Public). See Table 2 for examples of duplicate articles that may be acceptable and necessary.

TABLE 2. DUPLICATE ARTICLES THAT MAY BE ACCEPTABLE*

Summaries or abstracts of findings printed in conference proceedings
Editors do not discourage authors from presenting their findings at conferences or scientific meetings, but they recommend that authors refrain from distributing complete copies of their papers, which might later appear in some form of publication without their knowledge.

News media reports of author's findings
Editors do not discourage authors from reporting their findings at conferences covered by the press, but they do discourage authors from distributing their full papers, tables, or figures, which might later appear printed in a newspaper, newsletter, or the news section of a magazine. Editors do not discourage authors from participating in interviews with the press after a paper has been accepted but before it is published. Reporters should be reminded, however, that most journals prohibit media coverage of the article before it is published. A preliminary report of an author's findings disseminated widely in the news media may preclude subsequent publication of the full report in a journal.

Fragments or sequential reports of studies
Editors make decisions about these types of duplicative research articles on a case-by-case basis. For all such papers, editors ask that authors properly reference previously reported parts of a study and send copies of these papers or articles along with their submitted manuscript.

Detailed reports previously distributed to a narrow audience
The scope of this audience would determine whether editors would publish a duplicative paper. For example, a study previously reported in a hospital newsletter that was distributed to all staff nurse practitioners would have a better chance of subsequent publication in a nurse practitioner journal than would a study previously published in a newsletter that is mailed to all nurse practitioners in the country.

Reports from government documents or reports in the public domain
Large government reports that have been summarized for publication in a journal are handled on a case-by-case basis. Decisions regarding subsequent duplicate publication are based on the importance of the message, priority for the journal's readers, and availability of the information. For example, many journals publish reports from the US Centers for Disease Control and Prevention that were initially published in the *Morbidity and Mortality Weekly Report.*

Translations of reports in another language; translated articles or same-language reprints published in a journal's international edition
These are usually acceptable as long as they give proper attribution to the original publication. (see 3.3.1, Secondary Publication).

For each of these cases, a query to the editorial office is recommended, asking if any previous publication or release of information jeopardizes a chance for subsequent publication in a specific journal.

**Reprinted and adapted with permission of* IMAGE: Journal of Nursing Scholarship.[6] *Copyright 1995, Sigma Theta Tau International.*

3.3.1 ***Secondary Publication.***—Secondary publication is the subsequent republication, or simultaneous publication (sometimes called dual or parallel publication), of an article in 2 or more journals (in the same or another language) by mutual consent of both editors. Secondary publication can be beneficial. For example, the editors of an English-language journal and a non–English-language journal may agree to secondary publication in translated form for the benefit of audiences who speak different languages. The ICMJE approves secondary publication if each of the following conditions are met[32]:

1. The editors of both journals approve of the second article; the editor of the second journal must have a copy of the original article as it was published in the first journal.
2. The secondary publication appears at least 1 week after the primary publication in the first journal (except as specifically negotiated in advance by both editors).
3. The secondary publication is intended for a different audience; an abbreviated version of the first article could suffice.
4. The secondary version does not alter the data or interpretations of the primary version.
5. A footnote on the title page of the secondary publication refers to the primary publication with a complete citation.

In addition, authors should be notified of plans for secondary publication that they themselves did not initiate. *JAMA* notifies all authors of accepted manuscripts that their published article might be selected for publication in one of *JAMA*'s international editions.

3.3.2 ***Editorial Policy for Preventing and Handling Allegations of Duplicate Publication.***—Duplicate publication violates the ethics of scientific publishing and may constitute a violation of copyright law. Editors have a duty to inform prospective authors of their policies on duplicate publication, which should be published in their instructions for authors. Reviewers should notify editors of the existence of duplicate articles discovered during their review. Authors should send copies of all duplicate articles, including news media coverage, with their submitted manuscripts. Authors should also include citations to highly similar articles under their authorship in the reference list of the submitted manuscript. When in doubt about the possibility of duplication or redundancy of information in articles based on the same study or topic, authors should inform and consult the editor.

The editors of *JAMA* and the AMA *Archives* Journals have adopted the following policies to prevent the practice of duplicate publication:

> At the time a manuscript is submitted, the author must inform the editor in the event that any part of the material (1) exists elsewhere in an unpublished form; (2) is under consideration by another journal; or (3) has been or is about to be published elsewhere. In the case of a highly similar published article, the author should provide the editor with a copy of the other article, so that the editor can determine whether the contents of the manuscripts or articles are in fact duplicative.

All authors are required to sign an authorship criteria and responsibility statement, which includes the following declaration:

> Neither this manuscript nor another manuscript with substantially similar content under my (our) authorship has been published or is being considered elsewhere for publication, except as described in an attachment.

In addition, all authors are required to sign a copyright release statement, transferring ownership of the manuscript to the publisher in the event that it is published (see 3.6.4, Copyright Assignment or License). In the case of duplicate submission, copyright is held by the first journal to publish the manuscript.

Duplicate Submission: If duplicate submission of a manuscript is suspected, before publication, the editor should notify the author and ask to see a copy of the potentially duplicative material. After reviewing all material, the editor will then decide whether to continue consideration and possible publication of the submitted manuscript.

Duplicate Publication: If an editor suspects duplicate publication, the editor (possibly with the benefit of additional expert opinion) should consult the editor of the other journal in which the material appeared. If both editors agree that duplication has occurred, the editor of the second journal to publish the article should inform the author and ask for an explanation. That editor may then elect to publish a notice of duplicate publication in a subsequent issue of the journal.

The notice of duplicate publication should be published on a numbered editorial page and listed in the table of contents of the journal to ensure that the notice will be indexed appropriately in literature databases. The US National Library of Medicine recommends that such notices be published as correspondence and labeled "correction" or "erratum" (Lois Ann Colianni, written communication, July 8, 1996). It is preferable to publish an explanation from the author of the duplicate article with the notice, but this is not always possible or necessary. The words *Duplicate Publication* should be included in the title of the notice, which should include complete citations to all duplicate articles (since there may be more than 1). Figure 1 provides an example of such a notice (wording would

Correction: Notice of Duplicate Publication

The article "Prevalence of Measles in Day-Care Centers" by I. M. Shadey, MD, published in the November 4, 1994, issue of THE JOURNAL,[1] is virtually identical to an article by the same author, describing the same 3 cases in similar words, published in the *Journal of New Results*, September 1994.[2]

In June 1994, the author had sent a signed statement of authorship responsibility stating that his manuscript had not been published and was not under consideration for publication elsewhere. He also signed a document that transferred all copyright ownership to the publisher. Well before either publication, Dr Shadey received a letter of acceptance from THE JOURNAL reminding him of our policy on duplicate publication.

1. Shadey IM. Prevalence of measles in day-care centers. *JAMA*. 1994;270:2004-2008.
2. Shadey IM. Measles in children attending day care: an epidemiological assessment. *J New Results*. 1994;32:150-154.

The following response was received from Dr Shadey after he was informed that the above notice would be published.—ED.

In Reply.—I offer my sincere apologies to the readers of *JAMA*. I did not understand that my 2 manuscripts would be considered duplicative at the time I submitted them. I thought that since the 2 journals are read by different groups, some overlap in wording would be acceptable.

I. M. Shadey
State University
Chicago, Ill

FIGURE 1 Example of a notice of duplicate publication.

Correction 146
Notice of Duplicate Publication Prevalence of Measles in Day-Care Centers—I. M. Shadey

FIGURE 2 Example of a duplicate publication notice listing in the table of contents.

depend on the circumstances in each case) and Figure 2 an example of a table of contents listing.

The Editorial Policy Committee of the Council of Biology Editors recommends that all journals develop and publish a policy on duplicate publication.[5] In addition, journals should develop a process to evaluate potential violations and actions to be taken once a violation has been determined to have occurred. Some journals in a specific field (eg, anesthesiology) have decided to notify each other about cases of proved duplicate publication and ban the offending author(s) from publishing in their journals for a specified period. Other measures include legal action for copyright infringement and notification of the author's dean, director, or supervisor.

REFERENCES

1. Huth EJ. Irresponsible authorship and wasteful publication. *Ann Intern Med*. 1986;104:257-259.
2. International Committee of Medical Journal Editors. Uniform Requirements for Manuscripts Submitted to Biomedical Journals. *JAMA*. 1997;277:927-934.
3. Broad WJ. The publishing game: getting more for less. *Science*. 1981;211:1137-1139.
4. Angell M, Relman AS. Redundant publication. *N Engl J Med*. 1989;320:1212-1214.
5. Flanagin A, Glass RM, Lundberg GD. Electronic journals and duplicate publication: is a byte a word? *JAMA*. 1992;267:2374.
6. Editorial Policy Commitee, Council of Biology Editors. Redundant publication. *CBE Views*. 1996;19(4):76-77.
7. Blancett SS, Flanagin A, Young RK. Duplicate publication in the nursing literature. *IMAGE J Nurs Scholarship*. 1995;27(1):51-56.
8. Huston P, Moher D. Redundancy, disaggregation, and the integrity of medical research. *Lancet*. 1996;347:1024-1026.
9. Susser M, Yankauer A. Prior, duplicate, repetitive, fragmented, and redundant publication and editorial decisions. *Am J Public Health*. 1993;83:792-793.
10. Bailey BJ. Duplicate publication in otolaryngology-head and neck surgery. In: *Proceedings of the First International Congress of Peer Review and Biomedical Publication*. Chicago, Ill: American Medical Association; May 10-12, 1989. Abstract.
11. Waldron T. Is duplicate publishing on the increase? *BMJ*. 1992;304:1029.
12. Barnard H, Overbeke JA. Duplicate publication of original articles in and from the *Nederlands Tijdschrift voor Geneeskunde (Dutch Journal of Medicine)*. Presented at the Second International Congress on Peer Review and Biomedical Publication; September 11, 1993; Chicago, Ill.

Pressure to publish is a lame excuse for scientific fraud. No real evidence exists that it has impaired the ability of researchers to distinguish right from wrong.

Patricia K. Woolf[1]

3.4 ■ **SCIENTIFIC MISCONDUCT.**—In scientific publication, the phrase *scientific misconduct* (commonly known as fraud) has both ethical and legal connotations. Legal determinations of scientific misconduct are uncommon, yet a number of allegations that do not result in an official finding of misconduct raise important ethical concerns.

Various definitions of scientific misconduct have been suggested by US government agencies and academic institutions since highly publicized incidents of fraudulent research began to surface in the mid 1970s and early 1980s.[2-4] In 1989, the US Public Health Service released the following definition of scientific misconduct[5]:

> Fabrication, falsification, plagiarism, or other practices that seriously deviate from those that are commonly accepted within the scientific community for proposing, conducting, or reporting research.

This definition (commonly known as FFP for fabrication, falsification, and plagiarism) was considered a practical tool for recognizing and dealing with allegations of scientific misconduct during the manuscript submission, review, and publication processes.[6] However, controversy grew over various interpretations of the definition (eg, how narrow or broad should the definition be? does the definition address intent or levels of seriousness of offense? can the definition stand up in court?).

In the wake of this controversy, the US Public Health Service appointed a Commission on Research Integrity in 1993. One of the charges of the commission was to develop a better definition of scientific misconduct. In 1995, the commission released a detailed report that included a recommendation that the definition be amended to include specific offenses that constitute research misconduct: misappropriation, interference, and misrepresentation (MIM).[7] This definition replaces the word *plagiarism* with the broader term *misappropriation*; replaces the words *fabrication* and *falsification* with the term *misrepresentation*; and adds the term *interference*. The term *interference* was added to address instances "in which a person's research is seriously compromised by the intentional and unauthorized taking, sequestering, or damaging of property he or she used in the conduct of research."[7] In this context, *property* includes apparatus, reagents, biologic materials, writings, data, and software.

The 2 abbreviated definitions, FFP and MIM, are essentially the same except that MIM is broader. The commission's definition was not adopted by the US Public Health Service because the government is striving for a definition that will work for all governmental departments (eg, both the US Public Health Service and the National Science Foundation).

Note: None of the definitions of scientific misconduct include honest error or differences in interpretation. Nor do they include violations of human or animal experimentation requirements, financial mismanagement or misconduct, or other acts covered by existing laws, such as sexual harassment.[4-6]

3.4.1 ***Misrepresentation: Fabrication, Falsification, and Omission.***—Misrepresentation in biomedical publication includes fabrication, falsification, and the omission of facts as part of deliberate attempts to deceive.[6,7] Fabrication includes stating or presenting a falsehood and making up data, results, or "facts" that do not exist. Falsification is changing data, results, or facts. Omission is the act of not presenting certain information that results in a distortion of the truth. Data fabrication, falsification, and deliberate omission can occur when an investigator or author creates, alters, selects, or presents information for a desired outcome.

3.4.2 ***Misappropriation: Plagiarism and Breaches of Confidentiality.***—Misappropriation in scientific publication includes plagiarism and breaches of confidentiality during the privileged review of a manuscript.[7] In plagiarism, an author presents as his or her own ideas, language, data, graphics, or even scientific protocols created by someone else, whether published or unpublished, without giving appropriate credit.[6] Plagiarism of published work may violate copyright law (if the violation is shown to be legally actionable) as well as standards of honesty and collegial trust and may be subject to penalties imposed by a court should the holders of the copyright bring suit (see 3.6.6, Copying, Reproducing, and Adapting).

Four common kinds of plagiarism have been identified[8]:

1. Direct plagiarism: Verbatim lifting of passages without enclosing the borrowed material in quotation marks and crediting the original author.

2. Mosaic: Borrowing the ideas and opinions from an original source and a few verbatim words or phrases without crediting the original author. In this case, the plagiarist intertwines his or her own ideas and opinions with those of the original author, creating a "confused, plagiarized mass."

3. Paraphrase: Restating a phrase or passage, providing the same meaning but in a different form without attribution to the original author.

4. Insufficient acknowledgment: Noting the original source of only part of what is borrowed or failing to cite the source material in such a way that a reader will know what is original and what is borrowed.

The common characteristic of all these kinds of plagiarism is the failure to attribute words, ideas, or findings to their true authors. Such failure to acknowledge a source properly may on occasion be caused by careless note taking or ignorance of the canons of research and authorship, and coincidences of ideas certainly can occur. The best defense against charges of fraud and plagiarism is careful note taking and documentation of all data observed and sources used. Those who review manuscripts that are similar to their own unpublished work may be especially at risk for charges of plagiarism. Reviewers who foresee such a potential conflict of interest should consider returning the manuscript to the editor unreviewed. This recommendation may be stipulated in the letter that accompanies each manuscript sent for review (see 4.0, Editorial Assessment and Processing, and 3.11.6, Editorial Responsibility for Peer Review).

3.4.3 ***Editorial Policy for Detecting and Handling Allegations of Scientific Misconduct.***—Detection of scientific misconduct in publishing is often the result of the alertness of coworkers, editors, peer reviewers, other authors of the same manuscript, or readers. Table 3 lists examples of scientific misconduct in publishing.

If an allegation of scientific misconduct is made in relation to a manuscript under consideration or published, the editor has a duty to ensure that the allegation is pursued in a confidential and timely manner. According to the International Committee of Medical Journal Editors (ICMJE),[10] the editor may need to contact the person about whom the allegation is made, but the editor is not responsible for conducting an investigation. If the allegation is made about a particular manuscript or author, the responsibility to conduct an investigation lies with the author's supervisor at the institution where the work was done, with the funding agency, or with a national agency charged to investigate such allegations, such as the

TABLE 3. EXAMPLES OF SCIENTIFIC MISCONDUCT IN PUBLISHING*

By authors
- Describing data or artifacts that do not exist
- Describing documents or objects that are known to have been forged
- Misrepresenting data or deliberately distorting or suppressing evidence or data
- Presenting another's ideas or text without attribution (plagiarism), including violation of copyright
- Misrepresenting authorship by omitting an author
- Misrepresenting authorship by including a noncontributing author
- Misrepresenting publication status

By reviewers
- Misrepresenting facts or lying in a review
- Unreasonably delaying review to achieve personal gain
- Making public use of confidential information to achieve personal gain
- Stealing ideas or text from a manuscript under review

By editors, editorial advisors, or editorial staff
- Forging or fabricating a reviewer's report
- Lying to an author about the review process
- Making use of confidential information to achieve personal gain
- Stealing ideas or text from a manuscript under review

**Adapted from Lafollette.*[9]

Office of Research Integrity in the United States and the Danish Committee on Scientific Dishonesty in Denmark. The editor should take great care to maintain confidentiality during any communication about the allegation. However, the editor may need to identify the name of the person for whom the allegation is made when contacting the relevant authority to request an investigation (see 3.7.2, Confidentiality in Allegations of Scientific Misconduct). If the editor does not receive a satisfactory or timely reply (eg, within 6 months) from the investigational authority, the editor should consider contacting the authority again to request follow-up information.

Allegations Involving Manuscripts Under Editorial Consideration: In the case of a manuscript under consideration that is not yet published in which misrepresentation or plagiarism is suspected and for which some persuasive evidence exists, the editor should ask the corresponding author for a written explanation. If an explanation is not provided or is unsatisfactory, the editor may contact the author's dean, director, or other supervisor to request an investigation. If the author's explanation or a formal investigation demonstrates misconduct, the editor should promptly reject the paper. If the author's explanation or institutional investigation demonstrates that the misconduct did not occur, the editor should continue to consider the manuscript on its own merits.

Allegations Involving Published Work and Retraction: Because scientific misconduct violates the trust that must underlie all scientific communication, editors of the AMA journals will respond strongly to proved evidence of misappropriation or misrepresentation. In the case of published work, the journal should promptly publish a retraction, preferably but not necessarily signed by the offending authors. *JAMA*'s policy is to publish retractions in the correspondence column. The retraction should include a complete citation to the original article and should indicate the reason the original article is being retracted. The validity of other work published in the journal by the offending authors should also be questioned. The retraction should also be listed in the table of contents and printed on a numbered page so that it will be identified easily by indexers and included in literature databases (see 22.3, Resources, Online Resources). Figures 3 and 4 show examples of a retraction notice and listing in the table of contents, respectively.

In the first example shown in Figure 3, the authors hedged their culpability by saying "we discovered errors in the reporting of some subjects." Some authors may not want to explain the reason for the retraction in a forthright manner. Editors should work with authors of retractions to make these notices as accurate as possible, understanding that some authors may want to soften the misconduct. In such cases, publishing an author's evasive statement might be better than publishing nothing from the author, and the editor could add an explanatory note if needed.

Retraction: Falsification of Data

To the Editor.—After reanalyzing the data we reported in the article "The Effects of Low-Fat Diet on Risk for Breast Cancer,"[1] published in the January 3, 1995, issue of THE JOURNAL, we discovered errors in the reporting of some subjects. Twelve subjects in the low-fat diet group were erroneously classified as not having breast cancer. Had these subjects been correctly classified, our multivariate analysis would not have shown statistically significant results. For this reason, we believe we must retract the article. However, based on our previous publications,[2,3] which contain accurate data and valid results, we continue to believe that a low-fat diet reduces a woman's risk of breast cancer. We regret any problems our recent article may have caused.

I. M. Shadey
R. U. Certain
State University
Chicago, Ill

1. Shadey IM, Certain RU. The effects of low-fat diet on risk for breast cancer. *JAMA*. 1994; 242:135-139.
2. Shadey IM, Certain RU. Diet and breast cancer in high-risk women. *JAMA*. 1992;238:3004-3009.
3. Certain RU, Shadey IM. Risk factors for breast cancer in postmenopausal women. *JAMA*. 1989;236:250-255.

Retraction: Plagiarism

To the Editor.—We regret that the first 3 paragraphs in the "Discussion" section of our article, "The Effects of Low-Fat Diet on Risk for Breast Cancer,"[1] published in the January 3, 1995, issue of THE JOURNAL, were taken from another source without proper attribution. We should have cited the following article as the original source of the information contained in those paragraphs: Scott RB. Low-fat diets and cancer risk. *J Med Nutr Diet.* 1990;20:1450-1455.

I. M. Shadey
R. U. Certain
State University
Chicago, Ill

1. Shadey IM, Certain RU. The effects of low-fat diet on risk for breast cancer. *JAMA*. 1994; 242:135-139.

FIGURE 3 Examples of published retraction notices.

Correction 405
Retraction: Plagiarism The Effects of Low-Fat Diet on Risk for Breast Cancer—
I. M. Shadey, R. U. Certain

FIGURE 4 Listing of a retraction notice in the table of contents.

If an author of a fraudulent article, or any institutional authority, refuses to submit an explanation for publication as a retraction, the journal is obligated to publish a retraction after a formal investigation has been conducted and has determined that fraud has occurred.

Allegations Involving Unresolved Question of Scientific Misconduct: Cases may arise when an allegation requires the journal editor to have access to the data on which the manuscript or article in question was based. *JAMA*'s authorship statement includes the following language:

> If requested, I shall produce the data on which the manuscript is based for examination by the editors or their assignees.

Editors may want to add a reasonable time limit for which authors should keep their data (see 3.6.1, Ownership and Control of Data).

If an author refuses a request for access to the original data, or if the author or the author's institution refuses to comply with the journal's request for information about the allegation, the journal and its editor may be left in a precarious situation. Some editors have recommended that a statement be published indicating that the journal withdraws its aegis from an article that has such serious unresolved questions.[11,12] A withdrawal of aegis means that the journal no longer vouches for the validity of the contents of an article and that the article received an "incomplete peer review" before publication. Horton[13] has argued that withdrawal of aegis may be seen "as a belated attempt by embarrassed editors to cover up the inadequacies of the journal's peer review system." The ICMJE recommends that journals publish an expression of concern detailing the unresolved questions regarding an act of scientific misconduct in their publications rather than publish a notice of withdrawal of aegis, which implies that all other articles in the journal retain some kind of official editorial endorsement. This notice of concern should be listed in the table of contents, published in the correspondence column, and include complete citation to the article(s) in question.[10]

REFERENCES

1. Woolf PK. "Pressure to publish" is a lame excuse for scientific fraud. *Chron Higher Educ*. September 23, 1987:A52.
2. Relman AS. Lessons from the Darsee affair. *N Engl J Med*. 1983;308:1415-1417.
3. Knox R. The Harvard fraud case: where does the problem lie? *JAMA*. 1983;249: 1797-1807.
4. Rennie D, Gunsalus CK. Scientific misconduct: new definition, procedures, and office—perhaps a new leaf. *JAMA*. 1993;269:915-917.
5. Responsibilities of awardee and applicant institutions for dealing with and reporting possible misconduct in science: final rule, 54 *Federal Register* (1989).
6. National Academy of Sciences. *Responsible Science: Ensuring the Integrity of the Research Process*. Washington, DC: National Academy Press; 1992.
7. Commission on Research Integrity. *Integrity and Misconduct in Research*. Washington, DC: Office of Research Integrity; 1995.
8. *Some Notes on Plagiarism and How to Avoid It* [handout]. Evanston, Ill: Northwestern University. Based on: *Sources: Their Use and Acknowledgment*. Hanover, NH: Dartmouth College.
9. Lafollette MC. *Stealing Into Print: Fraud, Plagiarism, and Misconduct in Scientific Publishing*. Los Angeles: University of California Press; 1992.

10. International Committee of Medical Journal Editors. Uniform Requirements for Manuscripts Submitted to Biomedical Journals. *JAMA*. 1997;277:927-934.

11. Hammerschmidt DE, Gross AG. Withdrawal of aegis? so what's that? *J Lab Clin Med*. 1994;123:792-794.

12. Jackson G. The betrayers. *Br J Clin Pract*. 1995;49:115-116.

13. Horton R. Revising the research record. *Lancet*. 1995;346:1610-1611.

Of all the causes which conspire to blind
Man's erring judgment, and misguide the mind,
What the weak head with strongest bias rules,
Is pride, the never-failing vice of fools.

Alexander Pope[1]

3.5 ■ CONFLICTS OF INTEREST.

—A conflict of interest occurs when an individual's objectivity is compromised by a desire for prominence, professional advancement, or financial gain. Conflicts of interest that arise from personal relationships, academic competition, and intellectual passion are expected in science.[2] However, a number of scandals involving scientific investigators' undisclosed financial relationships to the results of their research have put journal editors, academic institutions, and funding agencies on guard.[3-5]

Recognizing that there is a difference between an actual conflict of interest and a perceived conflict,[6,7] the AMA journals require authors to submit written disclosure to the editors of all relevant, potential conflicts of interest to preserve trust in the integrity of the publication process and to allow readers to judge an author's potential for bias.[2] Financial interests include employment, consultancies, stock ownership, honoraria, expert testimony, royalties, patents, grants, and material or financial support from industry, government, or private agencies. Nonfinancial interests include personal or professional relationships, knowledge, or beliefs that might reduce one's objectivity.

Many biases are detected during the editorial assessment and peer review of a manuscript (eg, clever use of rhetoric, conclusions that go beyond a study's results) or are obvious from the author's affiliation or area of expertise, but financially motivated biases are less easily detected.[2] Therefore, many biomedical journals require authors to disclose any financial interests in the subject of their manuscript. Authors typically include information about financial support from grant and funding agencies in their submitted manuscripts, primarily because the funding agencies have required them to do so. It is not common for authors to disclose other financial interests unless such information has been requested.

The AMA journals require disclosure of financial interest from everyone involved in the publication process: authors, reviewers, editorial board members, and editors. The International Committee of Medical Journal Editors (ICMJE) supports this policy.[2] Many publishers also require employees who have access to material during the review and publication processes to comply with policies on conflicts of interest.

3.5.1 *Author's Disclosure.*

—An author's statement of financial disclosure should be held confidential during the review process. Individual financial disclosure statements should not be sent to peer reviewers.

JAMA requires all authors to sign and submit the following financial disclosure statement:

> I certify that any affiliations with or financial involvement in any organization or entity with a direct financial interest in the subject matter or materials discussed in

> the manuscript (eg, employment, consultancies, stock ownership, honoraria, expert testimony) is disclosed below. Any financial project support of this work is identified in an acknowledgment in the manuscript.

This includes financial involvement with a product or service that is in direct competition with a product or service described in the manuscript

If a manuscript is accepted for publication, the editor should decide, if necessary in consultation with the author, whether any relevant financial interests should be disclosed to the readers. Information about relevant financial interest can be published on the title page of the article near the author's affiliation or in the acknowledgment section at the end of the article (before information about grants and financial or material support). If the financial disclosure is listed in the acknowledgment, a note should be included in the title page affiliation footnote to alert readers to the existence of a financial disclosure (see Figure 5).

Placement in the author affiliation footnote

From the Department of Cardiology, Ambrose University Hospital, Boston, Mass (Dr Jones and Smith), and Wyler Laboratories, Geneva, Switzerland (Dr Jaques and Mr Dube).

Dr Jones has served as a paid consultant to Wyler Laboratories. Dr Jaques owns stock in Wyler Laboratories.

Reprints: John J. Jones, MD, Department of Cardiology, Ambrose University Hospital, 444 N State St, Boston, MA 01022.

Placement in the acknowledgment section

Dr Jones has served as a paid consultant to Wyler Laboratories. Dr Jaques owns stock in Wyler Laboratories.

This study was funded in part by Wyler Laboratories, Geneva Switzerland.

Figure 5 Examples of financial disclosure listings in published articles.

3.5.2 ***Peer Reviewer's Disclosure.***—*JAMA* reviewers are sent a letter along with each manuscript in which they are asked to return the manuscript unreviewed if they believe they have a conflict of interest that would prevent them from providing an unbiased review. If a potential conflict of interest exists (financial or otherwise), but the reviewer can provide an objective assessment, *JAMA* requests the reviewer to disclose the specific conflict. Page 1 of The Journal's confidential review form provides space for the reviewer to disclose such information. This information is not revealed to authors or other reviewers. Reviewers should never use information obtained from an unpublished manuscript to further their own interests.[2] *JAMA* includes the following instructions regarding conflicts of interest in its reviewer letter:

> We recognize that most conflicts of interest are not disqualifying, but request that you indicate any conflict in the space provided on the review form. If you perceive that you have a disqualifying conflict of interest, either financial or otherwise, please return the manuscript unreviewed. . . . This will not affect your reviewer status in any way.

See also 4.1, Editorial Assessment and Processing, Editorial Assessment, and 3.11, Editorial Responsibilities, Procedures, and Policies.

3.5.3 ***Editor's Disclosure.***—Editors have also had their objectivity biased by financial conflicts of interest (see Figure 6). For example, *JAMA* editors and editorial board

A MEDICAL EDITOR'S RESIGNATION

DR CYRUS EDSON has resigned from the editor's chair of the *Doctor of Hygiene,* of New York. At least he is reported as saying that his name will not appear again as responsible for its management. The journal was formerly known as the *Doctor,* but soon after its change of name and the entry of DR EDSON, then the Sanitary Superintendent and later a Commissioner of the Health Department, the make-up of the paper became such as to attract attention. . . . Various schemes of a sanitary nature sought the columns of that paper, with the intention apparently of taking shelter under the roof of this bright project. A water-filter company at the head of which DR EDSON'S name figured, was among these. The imputation, however, that the position of the latter as a health official was liable to misuse for private gain, led him to withdraw from the company. . .

JAMA. 1893;21:582

FIGURE 6 Report of an editor's conflict of interest.

members sign statements of financial disclosure annually. *JAMA* editors, as employees of the AMA, complete and sign a conflict of interest disclosure statement that is kept confidential in the Human Resources office. Editorial board members also complete and sign the following conflict of interest and financial disclosure statement that is kept confidential in the editorial office.

> I agree that I will promptly disclose all potentially conflicting financial and policy interests pertaining to *JAMA,* in writing, to the Editor of *JAMA* during the course of my service as a board member on the *JAMA* Editorial Board. (Attach or describe below any current potential conflicts of interest.) Financial interests can include, but are not limited to honoraria, employment, stock ownership, consultancies, expert witness activities, large gifts, or entertainment.
>
> I agree that I will not disclose or use any confidential information obtained from my activities with *JAMA* for my profit or advantage or that of anyone else, whether or not I remain a member of the *JAMA* Editorial Board.

Editors and editorial board members should refrain from making any decisions or recommendations about manuscripts in which they have a financial interest. An editor with a financial interest in a particular manuscript should assign that manuscript to another editor or a member of the editorial board in the event that the editor works alone. Editors and editorial board members should never use information obtained during the review process for personal or professional gain[2] (see 3.11, Editorial Responsibilities, Procedures, and Policies).

3.5.4 ***Editorial Policy for Failure to Disclose Financial Interest.***—Some journals may not accept articles from authors with financial interest in the subject of the manuscript.[8-10] Editors of the *New England Journal of Medicine,* for example, believe that disclosure is not enough for editorials and reviews. Unlike scientific reports, editorial and reviews are not "self-contained," contain no primary data, and offer an evaluation of a topic from a selection and interpretation of the literature. According to the *New England Journal of Medicine*'s policy, editorialists and authors of review articles, who should be experts in the subject of the editorial or review, are expected to provide an unbiased and authoritative perspective, which they may not be able to do if they have financial ties to the products or services related to their work. However, such policies may be overly restrictive and may even be viewed as scientific censorship.[11]

AMA journal policy recognizes that conflicts of interest are ubiquitous, inevitable, and in some cases necessary (for example, a critical reviewer with an opposing viewpoint). This policy prefers complete disclosure from all authors rather than selective banning of some authors. However, an author's failure to disclose a relevant financial interest could result in a published notice of conflict of interest and the failure to disclose it.

For Manuscripts Not Yet Published: In the event that an undisclosed financial interest on the part of an author is brought to the editor's attention (usually during the review process), the editor should remind the author of the journal's policy and ask the author if he or she has anything to disclose. The author's reply should not affect the editorial decision on whether to publish the manuscript.

For Published Articles: If an editor receives information (usually from a reader) alleging that an author has not disclosed a financial interest in the subject of an article that has been published, the editor should contact the author and ask for an explanation. If the author admits that he or she failed to disclose the existence of a financial interest in the subject of the article, and if that author had previously submitted a signed financial disclosure statement that indicated no personal financial interest, the editor should request a written explanation from the author and publish it as a notice of financial disclosure in the correspondence column (see Figures 7 and 8).

As with other types of allegations of wrongdoing (eg, scientific misconduct), editors are not responsible for investigating unresolved allegations of financial interest in an article or manuscript. That responsibility lies with the author's institution, the funding agency, or a national independent agency. If the editor deems the author's reply to the allegation inappropriate or incomplete, the editor may need to break confidentiality and inform the author's supervisor. Editors should refrain from discussing identifying details of the case with others (although the editor may need to seek advice from other editors, publishers, or lawyers), and the editor should not disclose the name of the informant to the author. Such disclosures may occur, if necessary, as part of due process during an official investigation.

In AMA journals, the discovery of an undisclosed financial interest on the part of peer reviewers, editors, or editorial board members is grounds for dismissal.

Notice of Financial Interest
To the Editor.—I regret that at the time I submitted my manuscript, "Effective Vaccine Strategies for Pertussis,"[1] published in the March 17, 1996, issue of THE JOURNAL, I failed to disclose that I have served as a paid expert witness in several diphtheria-pertussis-tetanus vaccine injury-related lawsuits. I had signed THE JOURNAL's financial disclosure statement, but I did not actually read it closely, and I did not know that expert testimony was considered a potential conflict of interest. I do not believe that my involvement in those legal proceedings biased me in any way, and I believe the statements made in my article are both credible and objective.

V. W. Brazen, MD
Virginia State University
Arlington

1. Brazen VW. Effective vaccine strategies for pertussis. *JAMA*. 1996;274:440-441.

FIGURE 7 Example of a notice of financial interest.

Correction 1520
Notice of Financial Interest Effective Vaccine Strategies for Pertussis—V. W. Brazen

FIGURE 8 Listing of notice of a financial interest in the table of contents.

REFERENCES

1. Pope A. *An Essay on Criticism.* Part II, lines 1-4. 1711.
2. International Committee of Medical Journal Editors. Conflicts of interest. *Ann Intern Med.* 1993;118:646-647.
3. Relman AS. Dealing with conflicts of interest. *N Engl J Med.* 1984;310:1182-1183.
4. Rennie D, Flanagin A, Glass R. Conflicts of interest in the publication of science. *JAMA.* 1991;266:266-267.
5. Koshland DE. Conflict of interest policy. *Science.* 1992;257:595.
6. Cook RR. Code of ethics for epidemiologists. *J Clin Epidemiol.* 1991;44(suppl I):135S-139S.
7. American Federation for Clinical Research Guidelines for Avoiding Conflict of Interest. *Clin Res.* 1990;38:239-240.
8. Relman AS. New "information for authors"—and readers. *N Engl J Med.* 1990;323:56.
9. Kassirer JP, Angell M. The journal's policy on cost-effective analyses. *N Engl J Med.* 1994;331:669-670.
10. Angell M, Kassirer JP. Editorials and conflicts of interest. *N Engl J Med.* 1996;335:1055-1056.
11. Rothman KJ. Conflict of interest: the new McCarthyism in science. *JAMA.* 1993;269:2782-2784.

> Will copyright survive the new technologies? *That question is about as bootless as asking whether politics will survive democracy. The real question is what steps it will take to ensure that the promised new era of information and entertainment survives copyright. History offers a clue.*
>
> Paul Goldstein[1]

3.6 ■ INTELLECTUAL PROPERTY: OWNERSHIP, RIGHTS, AND MANAGEMENT.

3.6 ■ INTELLECTUAL PROPERTY: OWNERSHIP, RIGHTS, AND MANAGEMENT.—Intellectual property is a legal term for that which results from the creative efforts of the mind (intellectual) and that which can be owned, possessed, and subject to competing claims (property).[2] Three legal doctrines govern intellectual property: copyright (the law protecting authorship and publication), patent (the law protecting invention and technology), and trademark (the law protecting words and symbols used to identify goods and services in the marketplace).[1] This section focuses primarily on intellectual property and copyright law.

3.6.1 ***Ownership and Control of Data.***—Conceptual application of the term *property* to scientific knowledge is not new, but the evolving nature of scientific research and technological advances has fueled numerous recent disputes over ownership, control, and access to original data.[1-3] With the exception of commercially owned information, scientific data are viewed as a public good, allowing others to benefit from knowledge of and access to the information without decreasing the benefit received by the individual who originally developed the data.[4] Ideally, research data would become a public good, regardless of the source of funding, after publication or public presentation.[5] However, financial and proprietary interests can often interfere with the altruistic goals of data sharing.

Ownership of Data: For purposes herein, data include but are not limited to written and digital laboratory notes, project records, experimental materials (eg, reagents, cultures), descriptions of collections of biological specimens (eg, cells, tissue, genetic material), descriptions of methods and processes, patient or subject records and measurements, illustrative material and graphics, analyses, surveys, questionnaires, responses, and databases. In scientific research, 3 primary arenas exist for ownership of data: the government, the private commercial sector, and academic or private institutions or foundations.[6] Data developed by a scientist without a relationship to the government, a commercial entity, or an academic institution are owned by that scientist.

Any information produced by an employee of the US federal government in the course of his or her employment is owned by the government. In the United States, access to some government-owned data may be obtained through the Freedom of Information Act (FOIA). The FOIA, first signed in 1966 and revised in 1974, is intended to ensure public access to government-owned information (except trade secrets, financial data, national defense information, and personnel or medical records protected under the Privacy Act).[2]

Data produced by employees in the commercial sector (eg, a pharmaceutical company, health insurance company, or for-profit hospital or managed care organization) are most often governed by the legal relationship between the employee and the commercial employer, granting all rights of data ownership and control to the employer. However, such data may be obtained by an outside party through use of the FOIA (only if the data are used to secure a government grant or contract) or by court-ordered subpoenas.[3,6]

According to guidelines established by Harvard University in 1988 and subsequently adopted by other US academic institutions, data developed by employees of academic institutions are owned by the institutions.[7] This policy allows access to data by university scientists and allows departing scientists to take copies of data with them, but the original data remain at the institution. The US National Institutes of Health (NIH) supports this policy with a set of guidelines for all research conducted at NIH. The guidelines state, "Research data and supporting materials, such as unique agents, belong to the NIH, and should be maintained in the laboratory in which they were developed. . . . Any responsible scientist seeking further information is to be shown the data promptly and completely, once the findings have been made public."[8]

Access to Data and Length of Storage: The notion that data should be shared with others for review, criticism, and replication is a fundamental tenet of the scientific enterprise. Sharing research data encourages scientific inquiry, permits reanalyses, promotes new research, and helps maintain the integrity of the scientific record.[2,4] Yet the practice of data sharing has varied, and it was not until recently that guidelines for storage and access by others were developed.

A number of scientific journals (eg, *Science, Nature*) require authors to submit certain data (eg, DNA sequences) to archival data banks as a condition of publication. Some journals require authors to have data available on request for examination by peer reviewers or by the editors (see 3.4, Scientific Misconduct). *JAMA* requires all authors to sign the following as part of their authorship responsibility statement:

> If requested, I shall produce the data on which the manuscript is based for examination by the editors or their assignees.

Most journals have not proposed terms for length of data storage, choosing instead to follow the norms set by academic and research institutions. A number of proposals prescribe the optimal length of time to keep data. The NIH requires its funded scientists to keep data for a minimum of 5 to 7 years after publication.[8]

The NIH also gives the right of data management, including the decision to publish, to the principal investigator.[8]

In 1985, the US Committee on National Statistics (part of the National Research Council)[9] released a report on data sharing that serves as a useful guide for authors and editors. Among the committee's recommendations, those listed in Table 4 have specific relevance for scientific publication.

TABLE 4. DATA SHARING AND SCIENTIFIC PUBLICATION*

- Data sharing should be a regular practice.
- Initial investigators should share their data by the time of the publication of initial major results of analyses of the data except in compelling circumstances, and they should share data relevant to public policy quickly and as widely as possible.
- Investigators should keep data available for a reasonable period after publication of results from analyses of the data.
- Subsequent analysts who request data from others should bear the associated incremental costs and they should endeavor to keep the burdens of data sharing to a minimum. They should explicitly acknowledge the contribution of the initial investigators in all subsequent publications.
- Journal editors should require authors to provide access to data during the peer review process.
- Journals should give more emphasis to reports of secondary analyses and to replications.
- Journals should require full credit and appropriate citations to original data collections in reports based on secondary analyses.
- Journals should strongly encourage authors to make detailed data accessible to other researchers (although some may view this as outside the purview of a journal's responsibilities).

**Adapted from Fienberg et al.*[9]

Although the intrinsic benefits of data sharing are essential for research, the costs of data sharing may result in restrictions on certain data imposed by the owner or initial investigator. The potential costs to the owner or initial investigator include technical and financial obstacles for storage, reproduction, and transmission; loss of financial reward or commercial profit; unwarranted or unwanted criticism; the risk of future discovery or advance by a competitor; the discovery of error or fraud; and breaches of confidentiality. The discovery of error or fraud and breaches of confidentiality have important relevance in scientific publishing. Discovery of error or fraud, if corrected or retracted in the literature, is clearly beneficial, and for research involving human subjects, epidemiologic and statistical procedures are available to maintain confidentiality for individual study participants[5,9-11] (see 3.4, Scientific Misconduct, and 3.8, Protecting Individuals' Rights in Scientific Publication).

Manuscripts Based on the Same Data: On occasion, an editor may receive 2 or more manuscripts based on the same data (with concordant or contradictory interpretations and conclusions). If the authors of these manuscripts are not collaborators and the data are publicly available, the editor should consider each manuscript on its own merit (perhaps asking reviewers to examine the manuscripts simultaneously).

Authors should attempt to resolve disputes over contradictory interpretations of the same data before submitting manuscripts to journals. When more than 1 manuscript is submitted by coworkers or former collaborators who disagree on the analysis and interpretation of the same unpublished data, the recipient editors are faced with a difficult dilemma.[12] The International Committee of Medical Journal Editors (ICMJE) has stated that since peer review will not necessarily resolve the discrepant interpretations or conclusions, editors should decline to consider competing manuscripts from coworkers until the dispute is resolved by the authors or the institution where the work was done.[12] Arguments against publishing both papers include that doing so could confuse readers and waste journal pages. However, publishing the competing manuscripts with an explanatory editorial may allow readers to see and understand both sides of the dispute. Alternatively, publishing the paper deemed of higher quality could result in biasing the literature and postponing publication of legitimate research.

3.6.2 ***Copyright: Definition, History, and Current Law.***—Copyright law provides for the protection of rights of parties involved in the creation and dissemination of intellectual property. Copyright is not merely an esoteric branch of the law that because of its complexity should be left to legal experts.[13] While a variety of people or entities derive benefits from copyright laws (authors, publishers, editors, composers, artists, and the producers of television and radio programs, films, video, computer programs, and software), few thoroughly understand the law and its basic applications. This section discusses current copyright laws and applications in scientific publishing.

Copyright Resources: Additional information about copyright law may be obtained from several sources. For a detailed legal account, consult any of the 6 volumes of *Nimmer on Copyright.*[14] Other useful texts include *The Copyright Book: A Practical Guide*,[15] *The Chicago Manual of Style* chapter "Rights and Permissions,"[16] *Kirsch's Handbook of Publishing Law*,[17] and *Copyright's Highway: The Law and Lore of Copyright From Gutenberg to the Celestial Jukebox.*[1] Specific information, guides,[18] and forms may be obtained free of charge from the US Copyright Office:

US Copyright Office
Library of Congress
Madison Building
101 Independence Ave SE
Washington, DC 20559-6000
Phone: (202)707-3000
URL: http://lcweb.loc.gov/copyright/

Additional information can also be obtained from the Association of American Publishers:

Association of American Publishers
1718 Connecticut Ave NW
Washington, DC 20009
Phone: (202)232-3335
Fax: (202)745-0694
URL: http://www.publishers.org

Information on international copyright treaties can be obtained from the World Intellectual Property Organization (WIPO) (see 3.6.11, International Copyright).

Copyright is a form of legal protection provided to the author of published and unpublished original works.[18,19(p9§102)] The author, or anyone to whom the author transfers copyright, is the owner of the work. Current law gives the owner of the work the exclusive right to

Reproduce the work in copies
Prepare derivative works based on the copyrighted work
Distribute, perform, or display the work publicly

A copyrightable work must be "fixed in a tangible form of expression" and includes the following[18,19(p9§102)]:

- Literary works (which include computer software and works produced in digital formats)
- Musical works
- Dramatic works
- Pantomimes and choreographic works
- Pictorial, graphic, and sculptural works
- Motion pictures and other audiovisual works
- Sound recordings
- Architectural works

The following are not protected by copyright, although they may be covered by patent and trademark laws[18] (see 3.6.13, Patent, and 3.6.14, Trademark):

- Works not fixed in tangible form of expression (eg, speeches or performances that have not been written or recorded)
- Titles
- Names
- Short phrases
- Slogans
- Familiar symbols or designs
- Typographic lettering or coloring
- Listings of ingredients or contents
- Ideas, procedures, methods, systems, processes, concepts, principles, discoveries, devices
- Works consisting entirely of information that is common property and containing no original authorship (eg, calendars, height and weight charts, rulers, and chemical structures)

Note: Although ideas or procedures may not be protected by copyright, the written or published expression of ideas and procedures may benefit from copyright protection.

There are a number of exceptions and provisions to current US copyright law. Some of the more common provisions and problems encountered by scientific authors, editors, and publishers are discussed in sections 3.6.3 through 3.6.10.

History of Copyright Law: Copyright law evolved after Gutenberg's movable type reduced the cost and labor required to make copies of written and printed works.[1,14] During the early 18th century, copyright became the mediator between the author or publisher and the marketplace. In 1710, England created the first copyright act for exact copies only. Article 1, section 8, of the US Constitution serves as the foundation for US copyright law. Since 1789, the US law has undergone significant revision 4 times. In 1790, the United States created the first copyright law to cover magazines and books, but again, this was only for exact copies. During the 19th century, copyright law was extended to translations and works made for hire[1,14] (following the 1834 Supreme Court ruling in *Wheaton v Peters,* in which the court decided that copyright law was not intended to "enrich authors and editors" but "to promote science and useful arts"[20]). The US Copyright Act of 1909 added formal requirements to ensure protection, such as use of copyright notice, official registration, and renewal of copyright terms.[17]

US Copyright Act of 1976: Before 1978, 2 systems of copyright coexisted in the United States. Common law copyright, regulated by individual states, protected works from creation until publication, and a separate federal law protected works from publication until 28 years thereafter (with options to renew the 28-year term).[18] The Copyright Act of 1976, which became effective January 1, 1978, contained the first major revisions of US copyright law in almost 70 years. This act, reversing many of the formalities required by the 1909 act, remains in force today. Thus, for all works created after 1978, current law automatically provides protection to the creator of the work at the time it is created, whether written, typewritten, or entered into a computer; whether or not the work is published; and whether or not the work bears a copyright notice. In addition, the 1976 act changed the terms of copyright duration, with most terms equaling the life of the author plus 50 years. However, several exceptions complicate the "life plus 50" rule (see 3.6.3, Types of Works and Copyright Duration).

Berne Convention: In 1886, the Berne Convention was created by 10 European nations to protect copyright across national boundaries. The United States did not sign on to the Berne Convention until 1989. Today, most industrial and many developing countries subscribe to the Berne Convention (for more details, see 3.6.11, International Copyright).

Copyright and New Technology: Throughout the 20th century, technologic advances have challenged copyright law: photographs, motion pictures, radio, and television, photocopying, cable television, computers, databases, new media, and the Internet.[1,14]

The most recent challenge began in the 1990s with the increase of electronic publishing and new media. Although copyright law was designed to be technology neutral, it applied only to tangible copies and to the physical distribution of these copies. Although early users of the Internet sent e-mail messages and posted information on listservs and bulletin boards without much concern for ownership and copyright of their digital communications, editors and publishers grew concerned about maintaining the integrity, quality, and ownership of their intellectual property once copies were digitized and transmitted via computer disks, CD-ROMs, and the Internet.

To address these and other concerns, the US Working Group on Intellectual Property Rights[21] issued a white paper, *Intellectual Property and the National Information Infrastructure,* in September 1995, recommending revisions in the language of the current copyright law. The proposed revisions, which caused much debate and were not adopted, included the following:

- Distribution rights to include digital transmission
- Copyright management information to govern permissions and licensing of electronic copies
- Public performance rights for sound recording as it would apply, for example, to CD-ROM and the World Wide Web
- Fair use exemptions for visually impaired persons

Since 1996, a number of proposals have been debated by the US Congress and WIPO to address the vulnerability of databases, especially electronic databases, to piracy. The concerns arose after the 1991 Supreme Court ruling in *Feist v Rural Telephone*.[20,22] In this case, a regional telephone company used a local telephone company's directory without its permission. The local company sued for copyright violation and lost the case. The court held that the "data" in the directory (collections of public telephone numbers) had no substantial originality or creativity and that comprehensive collections of data arranged in conventional formats do not merit copyright protection.[20] Thus, database compilers and owners believed they needed a law in addition to current copyright law to protect them from piracy. Although no one seems to doubt the problems facing database compilers, several important public policy concerns, not simply legal concerns, arise from this specific issue and the relevant provisions of current law and international treaties. Proposals to protect digital databases will be the subject of much future debate (see 3.6.11, International Copyright, International Treaties and Emerging Technology).

3.6.3 ***Types of Works and Copyright Duration.***—The phrase "life plus 50," meaning an author's life plus 50 years, describes the usual term of copyright duration for works created in the United States[18,19] and many other nations that adhere to the Berne Convention. However, exceptions to the "life plus 50" provision exist. The length of copyright protection depends on several factors: when the work was created (key dates are before or after January 1, 1978), the number of authors, and the type of work (eg, work made for hire or owned by the federal government).

Works by a Single Author: To be protected by copyright law, a work must be original. For works created by a single author, copyright belongs to that author from the instant of its creation and for 50 years after the author's death.[19(p87,§302)] Several different rules apply to works published before 1978. For most of these works, the copyright can be extended to 75 years.[19(p91,§304)]

Joint Works: A joint work is a work prepared by 2 or more authors with the intention that their contributions be merged into inseparable or interdependent parts of a unitary whole. This provision is particular to US law. For such works, the 50-year term begins after the death of the last surviving author.[19(p87,§302)]

Works Made for Hire: Works created by an individual who is paid specifically by another for such work are covered by a different provision of the copyright law. In these cases, the law recognizes the employer or the party contracting for the work as the owner of the copyright to the work.[22(p78,§201)] Works made for hire generally fall into 2 categories.

The first category is a work prepared by an employee within the scope of his or her employment duties, such as a journal editorial written by an editor who is employed full-time by the journal's owner.

The second category comprises certain specially ordered or commissioned works. Examples include a news story written by a freelance journalist or an index prepared by an individual under contract. In these cases, although a written copyright assignment is not necessary, the parties must sign a written agreement before the work is produced specifying that the work should be considered a work made for hire.

Copyright duration for works made for hire is 75 years from the year of first publication or 100 years from the date of the work's creation, whichever is less.[19(p87,§302)]

Works Created by Anonymous and Pseudonymous Authors: The same terms of copyright duration that apply to works made for hire apply to works published by anonymous or pseudonymous authors—75 years from the year of first publication or 100 years from the date the work was created, whichever is shorter. If 1 or more authors' names are disclosed and registered with the US Copyright Office before the 75-year or 100-year term expires, the term changes to 50 years after the last surviving author's death.[19(pp87-88,§302)]

Works in the Public Domain or Created by the US Government: After copyright expires, works enter the public domain and can be used freely by anyone. Currently, the law stipulates that works created by US federal government employees in the course of their employment are also in the public domain (see 3.6.1, Ownership and Control of Data, and 3.6.4, Copyright Assignment or License, Exception—US Government Works). However, works produced by state and local governments are not part of the US public domain and are subject to copyright protection. Works created by other national governments are subject to the copyright laws of their countries or the Berne Convention and other international treaties (see 3.6.11, International Copyright).[19(pp2-3,§101)]

Collective Works: A collective work (or series) comprises a number of independent contributions, usually from many authors, such as journals, magazines, anthologies, multiauthored books, and encyclopedias.[19(p3,§101)] Copyright of the independent contributions is separate from copyright of the work as a whole and initially belongs to the individual authors until they transfer copyright to the owner of the collective work, usually a publisher.

Except for authors of articles from the US federal government (eg, reports from the Centers for Disease Control and Prevention), all authors must transfer ownership of copyright to the AMA to publish their articles in AMA journals and Web sites. For example, both the individual articles (independent works) and the journals (collective works) published by the AMA are copyrighted by the AMA and are the property of the AMA.

Compilations: According to US copyright law, compilations are works "formed by the collection of preexisting materials or data that are selected, coordinated, and arranged in such a way that the resulting work as a whole constitutes original work of authorship."[19(p3,§101)] The term *compilation* includes collective works. Other examples of compilations include catalogs and directories.

Derivative Works: Derivative works are those based on 1 or more preexisting works, such as republication in a different format, language, or media.[19(pp4-5,§101)] Examples of derivative works include the following:

- Editorial revisions, annotations, and elaborations of previously published work (see "Revised Editions")
- Compendiums of previously published articles on a similar topic
- Abridgments or collections of abstracts of previously published articles
- Selected articles republished for a different readership (eg, an international or student edition)
- Translated articles, republished individually or collected with others in an international edition
- Author reprints
- Commercial reprints in print or digital formats
- CD-ROM articles and editions
- Online articles and editions
- Full-text articles on literature databases and available from document delivery services

- Assemblages of photocopied material for educational purposes (course packs) (see also 3.6.9, Standards for Commercial Reprints, and 3.6.10, Standards for Licensed International Editions)

Publishers who own copyright to individual articles can receive royalties from the distribution and sale of derivative works. For this reason, scientific publishers typically request that authors exclusively transfer all rights to their work. Whether authors will continue to transfer all rights to publishers without an agreement that they receive a percentage of future royalties from derivative sales is the subject of current debate (see 3.6.4, Copyright Assignment or License).

Some authors have begun to request a joint copyright agreement, in which both the publisher and the author, or the author's institution, are free to disseminate the article without permission from the other. Currently, most journals, including the AMA journals, do not accept requests for joint copyright but may grant authors permission to use their articles for noncommercial purposes (eg, education). Thus, an author who has transferred copyright to a journal publisher may not include his or her article in another publication or place the article on the Internet without the publisher's permission.

Revised Editions: A revised edition of a previously copyrighted work may be copyrighted again if there is substantial original new work in the new edition. *The Chicago Manual of Style* defines *substantial* as change that occurs in 1 or more of the essential elements of the work: text, introduction, notes, appendixes, or tables and illustrations (if they are integral to the work).[16(p10)] Thus, a new foreword or preface, the addition of a few references, or corrections to the original text do not constitute a revised edition, but they may be included in subsequent printings with an explanation on the copyright notice page. For example, this edition of the *American Medical Association Manual of Style* constitutes a major revision that requires new copyright. For revised editions, any unaltered material that is retained in a subsequent edition is not protected by the new copyright (it remains protected under the original copyright), and copyright of the new material does not extend the duration of copyright of the old material.

The Chicago Manual of Style recommends that publishers use standard language to designate specific editions: 2nd edition, 3rd edition, 4th edition, and so on.[16] If the new edition is simply printed in a different format, eg, in paperback or in a different language through a licensing agreement, the status can be designated as "Paperback edition 1995" or "Japanese-language edition, Mainichi Newspapers, 1994" (see 2.12.33, Manuscript Preparation, Edition Numbers).

Some publishers list the various dates of revisions on the copyright page as a record of publishing history. The publishing history follows the copyright notice. For example, this manual has had 8 previous editions:

> 1998, *American Medical Association Manual of Style: A Guide for Authors and Editors,* 9th ed (Iverson et al)
> 1989, *American Medical Association Manual of Style,* 8th ed (Iverson et al)
> 1981, *Manual for Authors & Editors,* 7th ed (Barclay et al)
> 1976, *Stylebook/Editorial Manual of the AMA,* 6th ed (Barclay)
> 1971, *Stylebook/Editorial Manual of the AMA,* 5th ed (Hussey)
> 1966, *Stylebook and Editorial Manual,* 4th ed (Talbott)
> 1965, *Stylebook and Editorial Manual,* 3rd ed (Talbott)
> 1963, *Stylebook and Editorial Manual,* 2nd ed (Talbott)
> 1962, *Style Book* (Talbott)

3.6.4 ***Copyright Assignment or License.***—Current law provides that copyright of a work vests initially with the author of the work. An author may transfer rights in either an exclusive assignment or a nonexclusive license.[14,16] An owner of an exclusive assignment may produce derivative works and sublicense specific rights to others (eg, the owner may grant a French publisher the rights to publish and distribute a French-language edition). An owner of a nonexclusive license may have a one-time right to reproduce a work in a specified manner (eg, permission given to photocopy articles for distribution during a presentation or class, or permission given to a pharmaceutical company to reprint and distribute a specific article) (see 3.6.6, Copying, Reproducing, and Adapting, and 3.6.9, Standards for Commercial Reprints).

Publishers who make substantial investments in their products typically request exclusive assignments from authors of written works.[14,16] However, few visual artists or professional photographers will agree to such a request and more commonly license nonexclusive rights to publishers who want to include their works. In addition, some policies encourage authors to transfer nonexclusive rights of their work to commercial publishers solely for educational and research purposes.[23] In such cases, a publisher must request permission from each author before republishing the work in any derivative format. The increased emphasis on authors' rights and incentives portends much future debate.

Common arguments for an author to transfer exclusive copyright to the publisher include the following[24]:

- The publisher must have the opportunity to publish or license the publication of the work in other forms to recoup or justify the expense of the publication and distribution of the original work.
- The publisher, with business and legal expertise and resources, has better ability to protect and distribute the work.
- The publisher is capable of taking advantage of new technologies and media.
- The publisher is better equipped to invest in the work and take the risk that the work may not be successful.
- The publisher helps serve the author's interest in self-promotion and professional advancement.

Common arguments favoring the author's retaining copyright include the following[23]:

- Authors should retain ownership of their works and distribute their works themselves or through institutional libraries (perhaps electronically via the Internet) to avoid the spiraling subscription costs of scientific journals.
- Authors' investments in their works should be financially rewarded for both the original publication and any subsequent republication or dissemination.
- New technology encourages theft of intellectual property, rendering copyright obsolete.

(See also 3.6.12, Moral Rights.)

Written Assignment of Copyright: As a condition to considering a work for publication, most publishers of scientific journals require authors to transfer copyright in the event that the work is published. Since the transfer of copyright may not actually occur until the work is published, editors may choose to consider manuscripts submitted without a statement of copyright transfer from the author and then ask for it if a revision is requested or the manuscript is to be accepted. However, to simplify the submission process, AMA journals request authors to submit a statement of copyright assignment before their work is reviewed. The author of the work must affirm that the work submitted

Manuscript Title ____

____

Copyright.—In consideration of the American Medical Association (AMA) taking further action in reviewing and editing your submission, each author must sign a copy of this form before manuscript review may proceed. Such signature shall evidence the mutual understanding between the AMA and the undersigned author(s) thereby transferring, assigning, or otherwise conveying all copyright ownership, including any and all rights incidental thereto, exclusively to the AMA.

In consideration of the action of the AMA in reviewing and editing this submission, the author(s) undersigned hereby transfer(s) or otherwise convey(s) all copyright ownership to the AMA in the event that such work is published by the AMA.

Authors(s) Signature(s)	Date Signed
______________________	______________________
______________________	______________________
______________________	______________________

US Federal Employees: I was an employee of the US federal government when this work was conducted and prepared for publication; therefore, it is not protected by the Copyright Act and there is no copyright; thus, ownership cannot be transferred.

Authors(s) Signature(s)	Date Signed
______________________	______________________
______________________	______________________
______________________	______________________

FIGURE 9 Example of copyright transfer form used by AMA journals.

has not been previously transferred or assigned to a third party and that the work has not been otherwise encumbered[21(p78,§201)] (see 3.3, Duplicate Publication). In the event that the work is published by the AMA, the author agrees to transfer copyright to the AMA. If the AMA does not publish the work, the copyright reverts to the author.

The authors of a joint work are co-owners of copyright in the work. To transfer copyright of a joint work to a US publisher, a copyright assignment must be signed by each of the authors.

A sample of copyright transfer language appears in Figure 9. Although this language is used by *JAMA* and the AMA *Archives* Journals, it may not be appropriate in all circumstances and should be modified as needed.

Exception—US Federal Government Works: Because copyright cannot be obtained in works created by the federal government, no assignment from the author is necessary.[21(p18,§105)] What constitutes a work of a government employee as part of the person's official duties is not always clear. Journals should obtain a signed statement from the author or authors representing that a work is a federal government work (Figure 9). When some authors of a joint work are employed by the federal government and other authors are not, each government-employed author must sign the government waiver and all other authors must sign the standard copyright transfer agreement.

Exception—Institutional Owners of Copyright: On occasion, a manuscript from an author or authors from a single institution may be submitted with a copyright transfer signature from the agent for the institution, rather than individual signatures from each author. In such cases, the institution has a written agreement with the authors, following the work-for-hire provision of the copyright law, that all work done while the authors are employees of the institution is owned by the institution. As a result, the agent of the institution may sign the copyright transfer form (see 3.6.3, Types of Works and Copyright Duration, Works Made for Hire).

3.6.5 ***Copyright Notice and Registration.***—Although use of a copyright notice is not required under copyright law, the US Copyright Office strongly recommends use of the copyright notice to ensure copyright preservation in a particular work.[18] A copyright notice for all visual copies of a work should contain the following 3 elements[18]:

The word "Copyright," or abbreviation "Copr," or the symbol ©
The year of first publication of the work
The name of the copyright owner

Example: Copyright 1998, American Medical Association

All copyright notices should be placed in such a "manner and location as to give reasonable notice of the claim of copyright."[18,19(p96,§401)] Such placement equally applies to print and digital works.

Registration and deposit of a work with the Copyright Office in Washington, DC, are provided for under the provisions of the 1976 act. According to the US Copyright Office, "registration is a legal formality intended to make a public record of the basic facts of a particular copyright."[18] Registration is not required for copyright protection, and failure to register a work does not affect the copyright owner's rights in that property. However, registration is a prerequisite to bringing suit for copyright infringement in US courts. The current filing fee for registration is $20. (See 3.6.2, Copyright: Definition, History, and Current Law, for information on how to contact the Copyright Office.)

3.6.6 ***Copying, Reproducing, and Adapting.***—To copy or reproduce an entire work without authorization from the copyright owner constitutes copyright infringement. However, a reasonable type and amount of copying of a copyrighted work is permitted under the "Fair Use" provisions of US copyright law.[19(p22,§107)]

Fair Use: What constitutes fair use of copyrighted material in a given case depends on the following 4 factors[19(p13,§107)]:

1. Purpose and character of the use, including whether such use is of a commercial nature or is for nonprofit educational purposes
2. Nature of the copyrighted work
3. Amount and substantiality of the portion used in relation to the copyrighted work as a whole
4. Effect of the use on the potential market for or value of the copyrighted work

Although each of these factors may provide a safe haven for use of copyrighted works without permission from the owner, the fourth factor, the market value of the original work, has been considered important by the courts in copyright infringement cases.

Fair use purposes include "criticism, comment, news reporting, teaching (including multiple copies for classroom use), scholarship, or research."[19(p21,§107)] This allows authors to quote, copy, or reproduce small amounts of text or graphic material. Authors should not quote out of context, giving a different meaning to the original text. Appropriate credit should always be given to the original source. In the case of a direct quote, quotation marks or setting off the quoted material, with an appropriate reference or footnote to the original source, will suffice (see 3.4.2, Misappropriation: Plagiarism and Breaches of Confidentiality).

- *Text.* The amount of text subject to fair use is determined by its proportion of the whole, but this proportion is not measurable by word length. Contrary to popular belief, no absolute number of words is acceptable. The so-called 300-word rule is often cited erroneously to justify quoting passages of text without permission. This erroneous rule probably originated with the custom of sending out review copies of books and allowing reviewers to quote passages of 300 words or less in a published review.[17]

  In 1985, the *Nation* magazine lost a landmark suit for copyright infringement after publishing a 300-word excerpt from then President Gerald Ford's 200 000-word unpublished memoirs, which were to be published as a book by Harper & Row (*Harper & Row Publishers, Inc v Nation Enterprises*).[25] In this case, the trial court ruled that the excerpt "was essentially the heart of the book."

  The Chicago Manual of Style recommends that a quote never extend more than a "few contiguous paragraphs" and that quotes, even if interrupted by original text, should not "overshadow the quoter's own material."[16] The length quoted should never be such that it would diminish the potential market for or value of the original work.
- *Tables and Illustrations.* Fair use of graphic or tabular material is more difficult to assess. Although 1 or 2 lines of information from a table might be used without permission, reprinting the entire table without permission could be seen as copyright infringement. The same applies to illustrations. The AMA requests all authors to obtain permission to adapt a part of or reprint an entire table or illustration that has been previously published.
- *Photographs and Works of Art.* Photographs and works of art may not be reproduced, enhanced, or altered without permission of the copyright owner, who may be the photographer or artist, a museum or gallery, an academic institution, a commercial entity, or a previous publisher. For example, the AMA obtains permission from owners of works of art, typically museums and galleries, to reproduce the art on the cover of *JAMA*. In this case, the AMA receives a nonexclusive one-time right to reproduce the art on the journal's cover (see also "Digital Images" later in this section).
- *Unpublished Works.* Authors should not rely on the fair use provision to justify quoting from unpublished manuscripts and letters.[16,17] In several recent cases, the US courts have taken a conservative view toward use of extensive quotations and paraphrasing from unpublished works without permission, making it difficult to justify such use. In *J. D. Salinger v Random House, Inc*,[26] the Second Court of Appeals ruled that inclusion of extensive quotes from Salinger's unpublished letters in Hamilton's unauthorized biography of Salinger was improper. In a subsequent case, *New Era Publications International, ApS v Henry Holt and Company, Inc*,[27] the trial court ruled that quotation from unpublished work was not fair use "even if necessary to document serious character defects of an important public figure."

- *Correspondence and Reviews Regarding Manuscripts and the Editorial Process.* All correspondence regarding a manuscript and the editorial process is considered unpublished and thus should not be used without knowledge of the owner of the correspondence. In the case of a letter, the owner is the letter writer. In the case of a manuscript review, the owner is the reviewer, unless the reviewer was contracted under a work-for-hire provision. Thus, authors and journals have no legal right to publish extensive quotes or paraphrases of reviews without the reviewer's knowledge (see 3.7.1, Confidentiality in Peer Review) or of letters, not submitted for publication, without the letter writer's permission (see "Quotes and Paraphrases From Oral and Written Communications"). In addition, to date, the courts have not allowed attempts to gain access to confidential peer review records (see, 3.7.1, Confidentiality in Peer Review).
- *Quotes and Paraphrases From Oral and Written Communications.* Many journals accept citations to oral and written communications (see 2.12.47, Manuscript Preparation, Unpublished Material). Court decisions regarding use of unpublished works[26,27] indicate that written communication, such as a letter or a memorandum (whether handwritten, typed, printed, or in digital format), if unpublished, may require permission from the letter or memo writer to be cited in a published work. Unless recorded, an oral communication, such as a personal or telephone conversation, cannot be copyrighted, and permission is not required. Although not a requirement, authors should obtain permission to use quotes from oral and written communications in their manuscripts and should inform the editor that such permission has been obtained. Following the recommendations of the ICMJE, *JAMA* requires authors to obtain written permission from any individual cited in the text as providing oral or written communication.
- *Works in the Public Domain.* Works in the public domain (which are not copyrightable) may be quoted from freely, with proper credit given to the original source. Examples of works in the public domain include those funded completely by the US government and those works for which a copyright term has expired.
- *Abstracts.* One widely debated application of fair use is the reproduction of abstracts of journal articles in other publications or databases without permission from the copyright owner (usually a publisher). In such cases, the abstracts are agreed to be a fair use portion of an entire article that is reproduced to educate readers and that does not diminish the market value of the original article. Such use might even enhance the value of the journal in which the abstract was originally published. Secondary publication and use of abstracts as derivative works on the Internet have generated even more debate about the market value of abstracts. As a result, what is accepted as fair use of abstracts may be constricted by commercial interests.[26]
- *Digital Works.* Fair use provisions apply also to reproductions of copyrighted material published in digital format. As of this writing, what is considered fair use in the print domain is fair use in the electronic world. Likewise, copyright infringement is a violation of the law—whether the pirated work is photocopied, printed, or copied electronically (see 3.6.2, Copyright: Definition, History, and Current Law).
- *Digital Images.* All digital images (eg, digitally produced or reproduced photographs, slides, radiographs, scans, and chromatographs) are protected under copyright law and require permission from the copyright owner to be reproduced in a publication. With high-performance computer technology, digital images can be manipulated to enhance communication. However, digital adjustments could also be used to bias findings or to deceive.

Journals should have guidelines for submission, enhancement, and publication of digital photographs that require authors to submit the names of the software and hardware used as well as a record of how the original image was obtained and manipulated.[28] Some journals may require the submission of the original photograph or slide along with the altered digital image for editorial and peer review. Some journals may place a symbol in the published photograph to indicate that it has been altered. In an online publication, such a symbol could link to the original unaltered image. Editors of some journals have proposed the use of standards for color, brightness, and scale. Publishers concerned about users' downloading digital images from their online publications can protect their images by encoding them.

Fair Use Exclusions: If a portion of a copyrighted work is to be used in a subsequent work and such use is not fair use, written permission must be obtained from the copyright owner (see 3.6.8, Reprint Permissions). Examples of such portions include the text and illustrations, such as charts, diagrams, or photographs. It is not permissible to use an entire article unless permission to do so is obtained in writing. In all cases, the material should carry a proper credit line and copyright notice (Figure 10). If there is doubt about the copyright status of a particular work, an inquiry should be directed to the author, publisher, or national copyright office.

Data adapted from table and used in subsequent article:

Table 1 is adapted from Garland JS, Buck RK, Allred EN, Leviton A. Hypocarbia before surfactant therapy appears to increase bronchopulmonary dysplasia risk in infants with respiratory distress syndrome. *Arch Pediatr Adolesc Med.* 1995;149:617-622. Copyright 1995, American Medical Association.

Reprinting entire article:

Reprinted with permission from *Archives of Pediatric & Adolescent Medicine* (1995;149:617-622). Copyright 1995, American Medical Association.

FIGURE 10 Examples of adaptation and reprinted with permission notices.

3.6.7 ***Publishing Discussions From Symposia and Conferences.***—When symposium papers are published, transcripts of discussion (which consist of questions posed to the presenters of papers and the presenters' responses) often accompany them and are printed at the end of the article in a separate section entitled "Discussion." The named discussants' comments and questions also require copyright transfer (see Figure 11). Publishing discussions from online bulletin boards, "chat rooms," or listservs requires permission from individual discussants and the online service provider.

3.6.8 ***Reprint Permissions.***—The copyright owner has the right to attach conditions to giving permission, such as requiring proper credit and copyright notice (Figure 10). The copyright owner may refuse permission altogether. Permission is usually granted by most publishers without charge, or with a small processing fee, to use portions (text, figures, or tables) of articles or other works, when such use will not result in commercial gain.

Manuscript title ____
____

In consideration of the American Medical Association (AMA) reviewing and editing the transcript and text of my discussion on the subject of

____

given at the

____,

and other good and valuable consideration, receipt of which is hereby acknowledged, I do hereby represent that I am the owner of the copyright of the text of my discussion and that it has not been previously published, assigned, or otherwise encumbered and I hereby transfer such copyright to the AMA and irrevocably authorize the AMA, its successors, and assignees and licensees, to edit, copyright, use, publish and sell for any lawful purpose whatsoever, the transcript and/or text of my discussion.

________________________ ________________________

Author signature Date signed

Address ____
____

City ______________________ State/province ______________
Country ____________________ ZIP/postal code ____________
Phone _____________________ E-mail ____________________

FIGURE 11 Copyright transfer form for discussant.

Publishers usually charge a significant fee or royalty for secondary use for commercial gain. Some publishers require submission of a letter of consent from the author when permission is requested to republish a part of an article or an entire article. If the publisher owns the copyright exclusively, such a letter is not required but is a reasonable courtesy to the author.

Permission to reprint an article from an AMA publication, in either a print or digital publication, must be obtained from the AMA even by the original author. Request for permission should be sent in writing with the following information included[16]:

- Title and complete citation to the original work
- Information about the secondary use or publication in which the work will appear (including commercial or noncommercial use, method of dissemination, and intended audience)
- Type and nature of the rights requested (eg, exclusive or nonexclusive right to reproduce or adapt the original)

The copyright owner will respond to the request either by returning an approved copy of the request letter or by sending a permission form. Information about fees or royalties should be included in such communications.

3.6.9 ***Standards for Commercial Reprints.***—Pharmaceutical and device companies typically purchase nonexclusive rights to reprint scientific articles, as either single articles or collections of articles, to help market their products. These industry-sponsored materials often are produced and distributed by custom publishing companies and marketing agencies. To ensure the quality of these reprints and to protect the integrity of the scientific journals that originally published the articles, the AMA has developed standards for industry-sponsored collections of republished articles and reprints, which include the following[29]:

- The publisher has absolute control over the scientific and editorial content.
- Financial sponsors may not write, edit, or otherwise attempt to direct or influence the content of a reprint or collection.
- Independent project editors with no financial ties to the sponsoring company should be appointed by the publisher.
- The project editor selects all authors and reviewers without influence from the sponsoring company.
- The project editor bases all decisions to include an article in a collection on a work's independence, objectivity, fair balance, and scientific rigor without influence from the sponsoring company.[30]
- The publisher retains all copyright; citation to the original publication must appear on each copy.
- All articles must be reprinted verbatim (incorporating any published corrections).
- New or original scientific material may not appear under the journal's name in special collections or as part of a single reprint.
- Acknowledgment of financial support or sponsorship must appear on each copy.

3.6.10 ***Standards for Licensed International Editions.***—A publisher may license others to publish international editions of its scientific journals. For example, agreements between the AMA and international licensees give these publishers the right to print and disseminate AMA-owned intellectual property (namely, scientific articles) in specific markets (countries or regions) and in specific languages (English or translations). To ensure the quality of these editions, the AMA developed editorial standards that include the following[31]:

- Each issue must contain a minimum number of pages (eg, 48 pages).
- Articles republished from *JAMA* and the *Archives* Journals must account for a minimum of 50% of each issue's total pages. The remaining 50% of total pages may include local editorial material and local commerical content (eg, advertisements).
- Commercial sponsors of advertisements, special advertising sections, and "advertorials" should be clearly identified on each page.
- The licensed publisher will appoint an editorial director to select articles from the original edition to be republished in the international edition and review the quality of translations.
- Each republished article must include a complete citation to the original article (ie, journal, year, volume number, inclusive page numbers) and complete original titles, author bylines, and author affiliations.
- International editions may include local editorial material that cannot constitute more than 50% of total pages. Local editorial includes the cover (if the original journal cover is not used), masthead, table of contents, editorial indexes, brief news reports, summaries of conferences, meeting calendars, announcements, commentaries, editorials, letters, and explanations of original articles.
- Local editorial does not include (1) any original clinical or scientific articles (ie, quantitative or qualitative research reports or analyses, case descriptions, clinical or product reviews, product or therapeutic comparisons, scientific abstracts) or (2) any articles previously published by non-AMA journals.

- All authors of all local editorial should have their complete names, appropriate medical degrees or credentials, and professional affiliations published with each article.
- Commercial content shall not be presented to appear as editorial content. Layout, artwork, and format shall be of such a nature as to avoid confusion with the editorial content of the publication.

3.6.11 ***International Copyright.***—Copyright laws do not automatically protect an author's work throughout the world.[32] Most countries offer protection to works from other nations. For a detailed discussion of the copyright laws of individual countries, consult *World Intellectual Property Organization (WIPO): General Information.*[33] The WIPO can be contacted at the following address:

World Intellectual Property Organization
34 chemin des Colombettes
PO Box 18
CH-1211 Geneva 20, Switzerland
Phone: 41-22-730-9111
Fax: 41-22-733-5428
URL: http://www.wipo.org

The Berne Convention and the Universal Copyright Convention: Two principal international copyright conventions currently protect works in many countries: the Berne Union for the Protection of Literary and Artistic Property (commonly called the Berne Convention) and the Universal Copyright Convention (UCC) (see also 3.6.2, Copyright: Definition, History, and Current Law). The Berne Convention was originally signed by 10 European countries in 1886 in Berne, Switzerland, to protect copyright across their national borders.[14] The Berne Convention is administered by WIPO (which is under the auspices of the United Nations) in Geneva, Switzerland.

For many years, the United States refused to sign the Berne Convention because of its lack of formality and minimalist approach. For example, the Berne Convention does not require the use of a copyright notice, which was in conflict with previous US copyright law. To accommodate the US need for a minimum set of standards, the UCC was created in 1952. Under the UCC, works created in the United States could have multilateral protection without forfeiting the US requirement for copyright notice.[14] The UCC is administered by the United Nations Educational, Scientific, and Cultural Organization (UNESCO).

After amending its copyright law by eliminating the requirement for copyright notice, the United States signed the Berne Convention in 1989. Most industrialized nations and many developing countries subscribe to this convention.[32,34] As of 1996, 199 nations had signed the Berne Convention.[35] The Berne Convention has no formal requirements. However, each signatory country agrees to protect the copyright of works (both published and unpublished) created in other member countries. According to the US Copyright Office, "members of the Berne Union agree to treat nationals of other member countries like their own nationals . . . therefore, US authors will often receive higher levels of protection than the guaranteed minimum."[32,36]

Under the UCC, protection in all participating nations can be obtained by publication in any one of them provided the proper copyright notice is used (the symbol ©, the year of first publication, and the name of the copyright owner) and placed in a manner and location that gives reasonable notice of the claim of copyright. Although the United States does not mandate the use of copyright notice, the US Copyright Office still encourages voluntary use (see 3.6.5, Copyright Notice and Registration).

Other International Agreements on Copyright: The General Agreement on Tariffs and Trade (GATT), signed in December 1993, after 45 years of negotiations, provides specific international protection for intellectual property under the Uruguay Rounds Agreement on Trade-Related Aspects of Intellectual Property Rights (TRIPs). This code specifies minimum standards for copyright protection, duration, enforcement measures, and dispute resolution procedures and is consistent with the Berne Convention.[13,14]

Regionally, the North American Free Trade Agreement (NAFTA), signed in 1993 by Canada, Mexico, and the United States, sets standards for copyrighted works in these 3 countries. Similar protection is offered for European members of the European Economic Union.[14]

The World Trade Organization also may help to enforce national laws and international treaties governing copyright.[1] However, piracy cannot be contained through laws and treaties alone, and, regrettably, theft of intellectual property is considerable.[13] Thus, copyright laws and conventions must be supported by member governments and judicial systems. In addition, national laws must be updated. During the last 10 years, laws in many countries have been revised.

International Treaties and Emerging Technology: In 1996, WIPO held a Diplomatic Conference on Certain Copyright and Neighboring Rights Questions. During this conference, 2 new international treaties were adopted: the WIPO Copyright Treaty and the WIPO Performances and Phonograms Treaty.[22,35] Both treaties resulted from concerns about digital technology and the Internet. Both treaties contain provisions that address technological measures of protection and the management of electronic information rights. Additional proposals are likely to be debated in the future. For more details, contact WIPO.

3.6.12 ***Moral Rights.***—Most European countries legally recognize the "moral rights" of artists and writers, a doctrine of copyright law intended to protect individual creators' investments in their work regardless of copyright ownership or transfer.[14,36,37] This doctrine is endorsed by most member countries of the Berne Convention. Under the Berne Convention, an author also has the right to object to any "mutilation or other modification" of the work that could harm the author's reputation.[36]

Although the United States is a member of the Berne Convention, US law does not provide for moral rights, except for certain visual works of art to protect them from mutilation or misattribution. A quasi-moral right is provided to US authors to discourage false attribution.[16,19] Under this provision, US editors and publishers may not give authorship credit to someone who has not written the work. Similarly, editors and publishers may not credit an author of a written work without the author's permission (see 3.1.2, Guest and Ghost Authors).

3.6.13 ***Patent.***—Patent law protects invention and technology. A patent is a grant of property right by the government to protect a newly created idea on the basis of its technical and legal merit.[38] In biomedicine, patents are commonly applied and approved for new products, such as pharmaceuticals, reagents, assays, devices, and equipment, and less commonly for procedures and methods. Patent law is intended to encourage discovery and investment into research of new technology by awarding an inventor a monopoly on the right to market the new product. This law restricts others from manufacturing, selling, or using the new product without the patent holder's permission for a period of 14 to 20 years, depending on the type and date of the patent grant.[38]

In the United States, patents are awarded by the US Patent and Trademark Office (PTO). For more details, instructions, and copies of trademark forms, contact the PTO:

Patent and Trademark Office
Department of Commerce
Washington, DC 20231
Phone: (703)308-4357 or (800)786-9199
Fax: (703)305-7786
URL: http://www.uspto.gov

For information about international treaties on patents and trademarks, contact WIPO.

Much recent controversy over claims for patents of naturally occurring substances, medical and surgical methods, and even genetically altered cells and gene fragments has appeared in the scientific literature.[39-41] Lure of financial profits and commercial success has even resulted in authorship disputes, delaying the publication of important medical information.[42] For this reason, editors should request that authors disclose ownership of patent grants and information about pending applications for patent grants in their financial disclosures to journals (see 3.5, Conflicts of Interest).

3.6.14 ***Trademark.***—Trademark and unfair competition laws are designed to prevent a competitor from selling goods or services under the auspices of another. Trademark law, not copyright law, protects trademarks, service marks, and trade names.[43,44] *Trademarks* are legally registered words, names, symbols, slogans, or any combination of these items that are used to identify and distinguish goods from those of others and to indicate the source or origin of the goods. A *service mark* is a type of trademark used to distinguish services, not goods, of a specific provider. *Trade names* are the names given by manufacturers or businesses to specific products or services (see 12.4.3, Nomenclature, Proprietary Names). Trade names are not legally protected in the same manner as are trademarks.

Trademark law provides legal protection for titles, logos, fictional characters, pseudonyms, and unique groupings of words, symbols, or graphics.[17,44] Whereas copyright law protects an authored work, trademark law protects the words and symbols used in the marketing of that work. Examples of commonly recognized trademarks include *Time* magazine, Mickey Mouse, and Coca-Cola.

Trademarks are classified into 5 categories in order of their increasing distinctiveness: generic, descriptive, suggestive, arbitrary, and fanciful.[37] Suggestive, arbitrary, and fanciful marks are more likely to receive trademark protection than are generic or descriptive marks.[37] An example of an arbitrary mark (a common word that has no specific connection to its product) is the *Nova* television series; an example of a fanciful mark (created solely for use as a trademark) is Kodak.[37] To receive trademark status, a mark must be distinctive (ie, not similar to other marks) and should not be generic or merely descriptive of a category of products. For example, trademark status was not awarded to *World Book* or the *Farmers Almanac* because both were considered "merely descriptive of the contents of each publication,"[17] and *Software News* magazine was not considered protectable because it referred to a class of products of which the magazine is a member (ie, it was generic).[37]

Titles: Book titles are rarely protected under trademark law because of judicial reluctance to protect titles that are used only once.[37] A few exceptions to this norm have occurred with book titles that have engendered common secondary meanings, ie, become widely recognized and associated with the name of the author or publisher (eg, *Gone With the Wind*).[17] The title of a series of creative works (eg, book series, journals, magazines, newspapers, television series, or software) can more easily receive trademark protection than can the title of a single creative work.[17,37]

Logos: Designs or symbols can also receive trademark protection if they distinguish particular goods or services and identify the source of those goods and services. Examples of such logos include the Bantam publishing house rooster, Apple computer's apple, the *JAMA* and *Archives* Journals logo, and the *BMJ* Publishing Group logo (Figure 12).

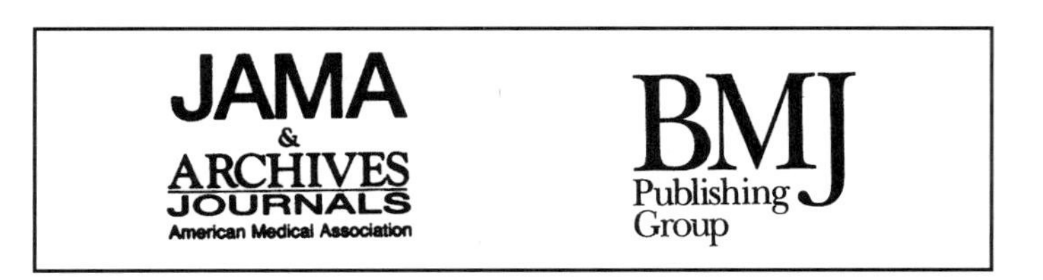

FIGURE 12 Examples of trademarked publishing logos.

Fictional Characters and Pseudonyms: Fictional characters can be protected by trademark if they achieve secondary meaning and are widely recognized (eg, Mickey Mouse). Under similar application of the law, a pseudonym, but not an author's name, can be given trademark status.

Trade Dress: Trade dress is the visual or physical appearance of a product, which, if distinct from that of other similar products, can be protected under trademark law (eg, the dust jacket of a dictionary or the cover of a medical journal).[17] Trade dress includes graphic elements and design, typography, shape, and color. For example, the designs, including the borders, of the covers of the *National Geographic* and *Time* magazine have been awarded trademark status.[17,37]

Application and Registration for Trademark Protection: In the United States, application for a trademark registration can be made under both federal and state laws. A legal expert should be consulted for information about registering trademarks in other countries. However, registering a trademark is not sufficient; actual use of the trademark in a given market ensures protection (ie, the longer the actual use of the trademark, the stronger the legal protection).[17,37,44] Typically, the rights to a trademark belong to the first user in a specific geographic market.

Trademark protection is also governed by the national laws of individual countries and international treaties, such as the Agreement of Trade-Related Aspects of Intellectual Property. In the United States, an application to register a trademark must be filed with the PTO.[44] Applying for trademark protection is more complicated than applying for copyright protection. The PTO requires a formal application to be submitted along with a drawing of the mark, samples of the mark as it has been used, and a filing fee. The PTO conducts a formal review of the application. The office may deny the request for registration if the mark is judged to be generic, merely descriptive, or similar to another registered mark (or a mark for which another application is under review). Registration may also be denied if the mark is not used or intended for use in interstate or international commerce.[17,44] If the application is approved internally by the PTO, a notice is published in the *Official Gazette* to make the application publicly known. During the 30 days following the *Official Gazette* notice, any third party can file a formal opposition to the application (only 3% of all applications are so opposed).[17]

If the application is approved, the PTO will issue a certificate of registration if the mark is in use. If the mark is not yet in use, the applicant will need to file a statement describing the mark's intended use.

Trademark Symbols: Once registered, the mark is entitled to carry the trademark symbol ®. Only those marks that are officially registered by the PTO can use the official symbol ®. Marks that are under review can use the symbol ™, but it does not have any legal significance.

Duration of Trademark Protection: After registration, a trademark remains registered for 10 years and can then be renewed every 10 years for an indefinite period—as long as the mark remains in use. Between the fifth and sixth years of the initial term, however, 2 additional forms must be filed with the PTO to ensure complete legal protection.[17,37,44]

Loss of Trademark Rights of Protection and Antidilution Law: A mark can lose its legal protection if the owner discontinues using it (this is called trademark abandonment), if the trademark is sold, if the owner does not file a statement that the trademark is still in use between the fifth and sixth years of the initial term, or if the owner does not renew the registration by the end of the 10-year registration period.[17,37,44]

Trademark protection can also be forfeited if a mark becomes too generic or loses its ability to identify its sole owner (ie, the mark becomes "diluted"). In legal terms, trademark dilution results from the use of another's mark in a manner that may cause the value of the original mark to diminish and lose its distinctive meaning.[44,45] For example, *Webster's* is no longer a registered trademark because the name lost its ability to identify a specific publisher of dictionaries, and "zipper" used to be a commercial name for "slide fastener."

For this reason, owners of trademarks will often send letters to editors and publishers objecting to misuse of their trademarks in publication. Such demands are intended to keep trademarks from being "diluted" by common use. For example, authors and editors should not use trademark names as generic verbs, nouns, or modifiers (eg, use "photocopied" rather than "xeroxed").

Use of Trademark Names in Publication: Under the recent US Federal Dilution Trademark Act,[44,45] restricted use of trademark names applies mainly to commercial use of trademarks, not to editorial use in publication. For example, a photography magazine could not use the word "Kodak®" as part of its cover design and a computer manufacturer could not place the word "Kodak®" on the front of a computer. However, an author or editor could include the word "Kodak"—without the trademark symbol—in an article about cameras and film development without risking trademark infringement.

Note: The symbol ® is not required in running text, but the initial letter of a trademarked word should be capitalized.

On occasion, the owner of a trademark name will request that their trademark name appear in all capital letters or a combination of capital and lowercase letters.

Authors and editors are not required by law to follow such requests. It is preferable to use an initial capital letter followed by all lowercase letters (eg, Xerox, Lexis, Kodak) unless the trademark name is an abbreviation (eg, IBM, *JAMA*) (see also 11.0, Abbreviations). Online databases, if trademarked, can be listed in all capital letters (eg, MEDLINE, EMBASE, CINAHL).

REFERENCES

1. Goldstein P. *Copyright's Highway: The Law and Lore of Copyright From Gutenberg to the Celestial Jukebox*. New York, NY: Hill & Wang; 1994.
2. Nelkin D. *Science as Intellectual Property: Who Controls Scientific Research?* New York, NY: Macmillan Publishing Co; 1984.
3. Mishkin B. Urgently needed: policies on access to data by erstwhile collaborators. *Science*. 1995;270:927-928.
4. Straf ML. Who owns what in research data? In: Bailar JC III, Angell M, Boots S, et al, eds. *Ethics and Policy in Scientific Publication*. Chicago, Ill: Council of Biology Editors Inc; 1990:130-137.
5. Fienberg SE. Sharing statistical data in the biomedical and health sciences: ethical, institutional, legal, and professional dimensions. *Annu Rev Public Health*. 1994;15: 1-18.
6. Riseberg RJ. Custody and responsibility for research data. In: Bailar JC III, Angell M, Boots S, et al, eds. *Ethics and Policy in Scientific Publication*. Chicago, Ill: Council of Biology Editors Inc; 1990:126-130.
7. National Academy of Sciences. *Responsible Science: Ensuring the Integrity of the Research Process.* Washington, DC: National Academy Press; 1993;2:127-128.
8. US Department of Health and Human Services, Public Health Service. *Guidelines for the Conduct of Research at the National Institutes of Health*. Rockville, Md: US Dept of Health and Human Services; March 20, 1990:1-5.
9. Fienberg SE, Martin ME, Straf ML. *Sharing Research Data*. Washington, DC: National Academy Press; 1985.
10. Duncan DT, Pearson RB. Enhancing access to microdata while protecting confidentiality: prospects for the future. *Stat Sci*. 1991;6:219-239.
11. Fienberg SE. Conflict between the needs for access to statistical information and demands for confidentiality. *J Off Stat*. 1994;10:115-132.
12. International Committee of Medical Journal Editors. Uniform Requirements for Manuscripts Submitted to Biomedical Journals. *JAMA*. 1997;277:927-934.
13. de Freitas D. *The Fight Against Piracy*. Geneva, Switzerland: International Publishers Copyright Council; 1994.
14. Nimmer MB, Nimmer D. *Nimmer on Copyright*. Vol 1-6. New York, NY: Mathew Bender & Co Inc; 1996.
15. Strong WS. *The Copyright Book: A Practical Guide*. 4th ed. Cambridge, Mass: MIT Press; 1992.
16. Rights and permissions. In: *The Chicago Manual of Style*. 14th ed. Chicago, Ill: University of Chicago Press; 1993:125-154.
17. Kirsch J. *Kirsch's Handbook of Publishing Law*. Venice, Calif: Acrobat Books; 1995.
18. US Copyright Office, Library of Congress. *Copyright Basics*. Washington, DC: US Government Printing Office; 1994.

19. US Copyright Office, Library of Congress. *Copyright Law of the United States*. Washington, DC: US Government Printing Office; September 30, 1996. Circular 92.

20. Godwin M. Copyright crisis. *Internet World*. March 1997:100-102.

21. US Information Infrastructure Task Force, Working Group on Intellectual Property Rights. *Intellectual Property and the National Information Infrastructure*. Washington, DC: Library of Congress; September 1995.

22. Platt J. Two global copyright treaties adopted by WIPO. *AAP Monthly Rep*. 1997;14:2-3.

23. The Copyright Policy Task Force of the Research Triangle Libraries Network. Model university policy regarding faculty publication in scientific and technical scholarly journals. *Scholarly Publishing Today*. 1993;2(4/5):15-16.

24. Perlmutter S. Who should own copyright? the author. *Scholarly Publishing Today*. 1993;2(4/5):5-7.

25. *Harper & Row Publishers, Inc. v Nation Enterprises,* 471 US 539 (1985).

26. *J. D. Salinger v Random House, Inc,* 811F2d 90 (2d Cir 1987).

27. *New Era Publications International, ApS v Henry Holt and Company, Inc,* 695F Supp 1493, 1524-1525 (SD NY 1988).

28. Anderson C. Easy-to-alter digital images raise fears of tampering. *Science*. 1994;263: 317-318.

29. Springer M. *American Medical Association Standards for Reprinted and Republished Articles From AMA Scientific Journals*. Chicago, Ill: American Medical Association; June 1, 1992.

30. Kessler DA. Drug promotion and scientific exchange. *N Engl J Med*. 1991;325:201-203.

31. Flanagin A. *Editorial Standards for International Editions*. Chicago, Ill: American Medical Association; February 1995.

32. US Copyright Office, Library of Congress. *International Copyright Relations of the United States*. Washington, DC: US Government Printing Office; 1994. Circular 38a.

33. General Information. World Intellectual Property Organization (WIPO) Web site. Available at: http://www.wipo.org. Accessed March 13, 1997.

34. US Copyright Office, Library of Congress. *Highlights of US Adherence to the Berne Convention*. Washington, DC: US Government Printing Office; 1989. Circular 93.

35. WIPO press release No. 106. Geneva, Switzerland: World Intellectual Property Organization; December 20, 1996. Available at: http://www.wipo.org. Accessed March 13, 1997.

36. Berne Convention for the Protection of Literary and Artistic Works. World Intellectual Property Organization (WIPO) Web site. Geneva, Switzerland; 1886. Available at: http://www.wipo.org. Accessed March 13, 1997.

37. Perle EG, Williams JT. *The Publishing Law Handbook*. 2nd ed. Englewood Cliffs, NJ: Aspen Law & Business; 1995;2(suppl).

38. US Department of Commerce, Patent and Trademark Office. *Basic Facts About Patents*. Washington, DC: US Government Printing Office; October 1995.

39. Patenting nature now. *Nature*. 1995;377:89-90.

40. Borzo G. Method patent fails. *American Medical News*. 1996;39(15):1, 90-91.

41. Patents for what genes? *Nature*. 1995;374:350.

42. Marshall E. Dispute slows paper on "remarkable" vaccine. *Science*. 1995;268:1712-1715.

43. US Department of Commerce, Patent and Trademark Office. *Basic Facts About Registering a Trademark*. Washington, DC: US Government Printing Office; October 1995.

44. Finn M. New law strengthens trademark protection. *Am Journalism Rev*. 1996;18(3):43-49. Special advertising section.

45. Pub L No. 104-98, Jan 16, 1996.

Confidentiality promises are widely recognized as an ethical obligation, regardless of the legal duty accompanying them. . . . maintenance of confidentiality promises fall within editorial descretion.

Jeffrey A. Richards[1]

3.7 ■ **CONFIDENTIALITY.**—The author-editor relationship is a privileged alliance founded on the ethical rule of confidentiality. Confidentiality occurs when a person discloses information to another with the understanding that the information will not be divulged to others without permission.[2] In the context of scientific publication, this rule provides primarily for authors' rights to have the information they submit to a journal, whether in manuscript form or in communications to the editorial office, kept confidential. The rule also provides for editors and reviewers to maintain their obligations to ensure that any information concerning a submitted manuscript be kept confidential.

3.7.1 ***Confidentiality in Peer Review.***—Strict confidentiality regarding the review and evaluation of submitted manuscripts and all relevant correspondence and other forms of communication is essential to the integrity of the editorial process (see 4.1, Editorial Assessment and Processing, Editorial Assessment). Authors must feel free to submit manuscripts that contain information that may enhance their reputations or careers or that may be proprietary in nature. Thus, editors and reviewers have an ethical duty to keep information about a manuscript confidential, and authors have a right to expect confidentiality to be maintained.[3] The very existence of a submission should not be revealed (or confirmed) to anyone other than the editorial and publishing staff and peer reviewers unless and until the manuscript is published. Even after publication, communications concerning the manuscript or the editorial process—including reviewers' comments—should not be made public without permission of the author, editor, and reviewer (see 3.6.6, Copying, Reproducing, and Adapting).

Since journals do not own unpublished works (ie, copyright is typically transferred in the event of publication), editors should not keep copies of rejected manuscripts (they should be returned to the author or destroyed). In addition, editors should refrain from discussing any aspect of the peer review process or unpublished manuscripts with anyone except the authors, reviewers, and editorial staff.

Similarly, reviewers should not keep copies of the manuscripts they are asked to assess. Reviewers should return manuscripts to the editorial office or destroy them. The practice of reviewers' using manuscripts as teaching tools or in journal club discussions is inappropriate.

Journals should publish their methods of peer review with specific reference to confidentiality in their instructions for authors, and editors should inform all reviewers of the confidential nature of peer review (see 3.11, Editorial Responsibilities, Procedures, and Policies).

Requirements During a Blinded (Masked) Peer Review Process: Journals should inform reviewers in explicit terms what they mean by "confidentiality" and "privileged information."[4] Journals should also inform reviewers and authors if the review process is single-blinded (ie, only the reviewers' identities are masked) or double-blinded (ie, both the reviewers' and the authors' identities are masked). AMA journals use a single-blind review process.

For a detailed discussion of the various mechanisms of peer review (eg, single-blinded vs double-blinded), see 4.1, Editorial Assessment and Processing, Editorial Assessment.

JAMA reviewers receive a cover letter and a statement stamped on the manuscript sent to them to remind them to maintain confidentiality (see 4.1, Editorial Assessment and Processing, Editorial Assessment). Reviewers are required to return manuscripts sent to them for review or destroy them after review, and they are instructed not to keep copies of manuscripts. Reviewers are also instructed to refrain from discussing the information in the manuscript with others. However, reviewers may enlist the aid of colleagues to assist with the review as long as confidentiality is maintained. Reviewers should inform editors if such consultation has occurred. Some journals prohibit additional consultation, and other journals require permission be sought in advance of the consultation. In any case, if a reviewer is uncertain of a journal's policy, the reviewer should contact the editorial office. Reviewers who participate in blind-review processes should never contact authors directly to discuss their review without explicit permission from the editor.

After an initial editorial decision (eg, rejection or revision) is made on a reviewed paper, *JAMA* provides copies of the unnamed reviewers' comments to the corresponding author. Comments to the editor, which include recommendations of acceptance, revision, or rejection, are not shared with the authors. However, comments directed to the editor may be summarized or excerpted and included in a letter to the author if necessary. To provide reviewers with constructive feedback, *JAMA* editors send reviewers copies of other unnamed reviewers' comments along with a copy of the editorial decision letter. Editors should inform reviewers how their reviews will be used and who will have access to the reviews and their identities (see 4.1, Editorial Assessment and Processing, Editorial Assessment).

In blinded peer review, reviewers have a right to expect that their identities will be protected. Thus, names and identifiers (eg, fax numbers and initials of names) should be removed from the pages containing reviewer comments before dissemination to the authors or other reviewers.

Occasionally an editor may choose not to send a reviewer's comments to the author if, for example, the comments are considered libelous or hypercritical. Similarly, an editor may choose to remove or mask any unhelpful or derogatory comments from an otherwise valuable review.

Signed Reviews: Occasionally, reviewers will sign their reviews, even though they know the process is blinded. Although such signature, perhaps at the bottom of a page of comments directed to the author, might imply that the reviewer has waived the right to anonymity, it does not relieve the editor or the reviewer of the duty to maintain confidentiality. The Editorial Policy Committee of the Council of Biology Editors[5] has recommended that even when journals permit identification of reviewers, any communication between authors and reviewers should occur through the editorial office and with the editor's permission.

The wider use of online and postpublication review will focus greater attention on the use of signed reviews. Editors disagree over the merits and problems associated with allowing reviewers to sign their reviews. Members of the AMA Style Manual Committee considered the following potential problems:

Reviewers who sign their reviews to disclose their identities could cause confusion. It could encourage author-reviewer communication that bypasses the editorial office. If reviewers are made known to authors, authors may dispute an editor's choice of reviewer, potentially setting the stage for an extended, acrimonious debate about perceived bias and allegations of reviewer incompetence. Reviewers may inadvertently sign reviews, not realizing that their signed comments will be sent to the authors and that their identities will be revealed.

Because of these concerns, journals that use a blind-review process should develop a policy for dealing with signed reviews. The following may be a useful guide for editors and reviewers:

If editors wish to disclose the identities of reviewers who sign their reviews, the editor should first contact the reviewer to determine that the reviewer actually intends to be revealed. The editor should remind the reviewer and the author that any communication about the manuscript should occur through the editorial office.

If editors do not want to disclose any reviewer identities, reviewers who sign their reviews should be contacted, informed that their signature will be removed from the review, and offered the opportunity either to continue reviewing for the journal anonymously or not to review for that journal.

Acknowledging and Crediting Reviewers: An author may want to credit the help of peer reviewers in an acknowledgment. According to the Editorial Policy Committee of the Council of Biology Editors,[5] public acknowledgment of reviewers is not necessary or appropriate because peer review is part of a reviewer's commitment to the scientific enterprise. However, some journals will honor authors' requests to thank anonymous reviewers.

Many journals also publish a list of people who reviewed for the journal during the previous year to thank them publicly.

Rarely, an editor may receive a request from an author to include an anonymous reviewer as an author. If the author's request appears justified (ie, the reviewer meets all the criteria for authorship as defined in 3.1.1, Authorship: Definition and Criteria), the editor should contact the reviewer to discuss the author's request and, if appropriate, the author and the reviewer should communicate directly. For such a case to occur, it must be early in the process (ie, before a major revision or complete rewrite). Such a scenario is unlikely to occur with reports of original research.

3.7.2 ***Confidentiality in Allegations of Scientific Misconduct.***—Another area in which the rules of confidentiality must be carefully considered includes allegations of fabrication, falsification, and plagiarism. In cases of alleged fraud, confidentiality may need to be breached[6] (eg, an editor may need to contact an author's institutional authority to request a formal investigation) (see 3.4, Scientific Misconduct).

3.7.3 ***Confidentiality in Selecting Editors and Editorial Board Members.***—When editors or editorial board members are interviewed and evaluated for a prospective position with a journal, all participants in the selection process should be reminded that all discussions should remain confidential. Such reminders may seem unnecessary, but without them, professional reputations and the journal's relationship with influential academic and political leaders may be jeopardized[7] (see 3.10, Editorial Freedom and Integrity).

3.7.4 ***Confidentiality in Legal Petitions and Claims for Privileged Information.***— After the 1993 US Supreme Court ruling on *Daubert v Merrell Dow Pharmaceuticals,*[8] concerns arose that attempts to breach the confidential nature of the editorial process would increase through subpoenas of journal records.[9] In 1994, a legal precedent was set regarding confidentiality and protection from attempts to invade the privileged nature of the editorial process.[10] In *Cukier v American Medical Association,* an author whose manuscript had been rejected by *JAMA* sued to compel the journal to disclose the identity of a third party responsible for providing the editors with alleged defamatory statements concerning the author's financial interest. Citing the confidential nature of the peer review process, the editors refused to disclose the source of this information. The Illinois Circuit Court of Cook County ruled that editors were not required to disclose this information based on the Illinois Reporter's Privilege Act, which states that members of the news media (in this case, journal editors) cannot be compelled to disclose sources unless the information cannot be obtained elsewhere and such disclosure is essential to the protection of the public interest. This decision was supported by the Illinois Appellate Court, and the Illinois Supreme Court declined to hear the case.

Other recent cases that have supported the confidential nature of the peer review process include *Henke v US Department of Commerce and the National Science Foundation*[11] (decided in May 1996) and *Cistrom Biotechnology Inc v Immunex Corp*[12] (settled out of court in October 1996).

References

1. Richards JA. Note: confidentially speaking: protecting the press from liability for broken confidential promises. *67 Wash L Rev 501* (1992).
2. Beauchamp TL, Childress JF. *Principles of Biomedical Ethics*. 3rd ed. New York, NY: Oxford University Press; 1989.
3. Glass RM, Flanagin A. Communication, biomedical II, scientific publication. In: Reich WT, ed. *Encyclopedia of Bioethics.* 2nd ed. New York, NY: Macmillan Publishing Co; 1995:428-435.
4. Marshall E. Suit alleges misuse of peer review. *Science*. 1995;270:1912-1914.
5. Editorial Policy Committee, Council of Biology Editors. *Ethics and Policy in Scientific Publication*. Chicago, Ill: Council of Biology Editors Inc; 1990.
6. International Committee of Medical Journal Editors. Uniform Requirements for Manuscripts Submitted to Biomedical Journals. *JAMA*. 1997;277:927-934.
7. Bishop CT. *How to Edit a Scientific Journal*. Philadelphia, Pa: ISI Press; 1984.
8. *Daubert v Merrell Dow Pharmaceuticals, Inc*, 113 S Ct 27866 (1993).
9. Gold JA, Zaremski MJ, Lev ER, Shefrin DH. *Daubert v Merrell Dow:* the Supreme Court tackles scientific evidence in the courtroom. *JAMA*. 1993;270:2964-2967.
10. *Cukier v American Medical Association,* 630 NE 2d 1198 (Ill App 1 Dist 1994).
11. *Henke v US Department of Commerce and the National Science Foundation,* 83 F 3d 1445 (US App 1996).
12. Peer review in the courts. *Nature*. 1996;384:1.

> *The right of the research subject to safeguard his or her integrity must always be respected. Every precaution should be taken to respect the privacy of the subject and to minimize the impact of the study on the subject's physical and mental integrity and on the personality of the subject.*
>
> World Medical Association[1]

3.8 ■ **PROTECTING INDIVIDUALS' RIGHTS IN SCIENTIFIC PUBLICATION.**—Contemporary rules for protecting the rights of individuals, namely, patients and research subjects, in scientific publication have their foundations in doctrines developed during the mid-20th century: the Nuremberg Code,[2] the World Medical Association's Declaration of Geneva,[3] and the World Medical Association's Declaration of Helsinki.[1]

Editors and authors have a specific ethical duty to follow the principles outlined in these doctrines (namely, respect for persons or autonomy, beneficence, and justice) when making decisions about publishing studies that involve human experimentation.[1,4] Numerous historical examples exist of medical journals that have published the results of unethical studies. In a 1966 pioneering article on ethics and clinical research,[5] Henry Beecher, MD, identified 50 unethical studies involving human subjects that were published in medical journals. Beecher concluded that "an experiment should be ethical at its inception and is not made ethical by publication" and that "failure to obtain publication would discourage unethical experimentation."[5]

In addition, the US Privacy Act and legal privacy doctrines in other countries protect an individual's right to privacy. A legal claim for invasion of privacy (eg, publishing details from which a private individual can be identified without his or her permission) could penalize a journal for publishing otherwise truthful statements about an individual.[6] Privacy law differs from defamation law in that truth may not be used as a defense for invasion of privacy (see 3.9, Defamation, Libel).

3.8.1 ***Informed Consent and Ethics Review Committees.***—To protect the safety and dignity of human subjects in experimental investigations, academic institutions and grant agencies require that the nature and purpose of all procedures, and their attendant possible risks, be fully explained to potential subjects in advance and that subjects fully comprehend the nature of the participation and voluntarily agree to such participation. In addition, the study protocol must be reviewed by a formal ethics board or committee.

Journal Policies and Procedures: In accordance with these requirements, journals should request authors of manuscripts that describe experimental investigation of human subjects to state explicitly in the methods section of the manuscript that informed consent was obtained from all participating adult subjects and from parents or legal guardians for minors or incapacitated adults and that an appropriate ethics committee or institutional review board approved the project. Approval for research involving animal subjects should also be adequately described. If the approval process raises concerns among the researchers or the reviewing board/commitee members, the author may want to explain the resolution of those issues for the readers.

As recommended by the International Committee of Medical Journal Editors,[7] specific guidelines regarding documentation of informed consent and formal ethical review should be included in a journal's instructions for authors.

Additional Regulations and Principles: For US investigators who do not have access to formal ethics review committees, the principles described in the Belmont Report[8] or the Department of Health and Human Services (DHHS) Regulations for the Protection of Human Subjects[9] may be followed. Many non-US institutions and investigators cite the Declaration of Helsinki in addition to their national regulations as an ethical standard.[1] In addition to requiring researchers to obtain study subjects' "freely given informed consent, preferably in writing," and to have the protocol describing the study reviewed by a "specially appointed committee independent of the investigator and sponsor," the Declaration of Helsinki specifies that reports of experimentation not in accordance with the basic principles described in the Declaration "should not be published."[3]

Reports of Unethical Studies: If the author of a report of an experimental investigation that involves human or animal subjects did not obtain formal ethical review and informed consent from human subjects, the editor should reject the manuscript and inform the author of the reason for the rejection. Publication of an investigation that raises ethical dilemmas may be warranted if such publication would encourage professional and public debate and reform. Such publication should be accompanied by an editor's note or editorial describing the ethical issues and concerns. Research that violates established ethical principles should not be published.

Even when complete approval from an ethics committee or review board has been obtained, the ethics of the reported research may be questioned by reviewers and editors. In such cases, editors are obliged to question the situation and unless the author can provide satisfactory reassurance, editors may choose to reject the manuscript in question.

3.8.2 ***Patients' Rights to Privacy and Anonymity.***—Historically, medical journals have taken steps to protect patients' rights to privacy and anonymity, including the deletion of patients' names, initials, and assigned numbers from case reports; removal of identifying information from x-ray films, digital images, and laboratory slides; and deletion of identifying details from descriptions of patients or subjects in published articles.

Until the late 1980s, placing black bars over the eyes of patients in photographs was accepted as a way to mask the identities of patients when consent to publish their photographs was not or could not be obtained. However, bars across eyes do not always mask identities and should not be used.[10]

Patients also have recognized themselves in medical articles that describe them in the text without accompanying photographs and even after "superfluous social details" have been removed.[11] To protect an individual's right to anonymity, identifying data (eg, sex, age, occupation) may be removed from a manuscript. However, omitting certain details may be problematic.[12,13] For example, omitting a patient's occupation from a case report might seem reasonable at first, but this information may be needed later during an occupational exposure assessment or during an epidemiologic investigation.

Authors and editors should not alter details in case descriptions to secure anonymity because doing so allows falsified data to enter the medical literature.[7,13] For example, changing the city in which the patient lived may seem innocuous, until another investigator subsequently cites the case report and the erroneous city in an epidemiologic analysis of locations of disease outbreaks.

Therefore, when photographs of faces or identifiable body parts or detailed case descriptions are included in a manuscript, authors should obtain written permission from the identifiable subject (or a legally authorized representative) to publish the photograph or case description, and send a copy of the permission to the journal.[7]

3.8.3 ***Rights in Published Reports of Genetic Pedigree Studies.***—The rules for obtaining informed consent apply to studies of genetic pedigrees. However, obtaining written informed consent from all members of a large pedigree (many of whom may be deceased or unaware of the collection of family data) may be difficult or impossible.[14] Proposals for obtaining some form of group consent and for avoiding the publication of information about identifiable family members who will not give their permission have been debated, but these issues remain unresolved.[14]

Following the ethical rule that patients have a right to privacy and anonymity in scientific publication, unnecessary identifying information should be removed from pedigree reports if possible.[14,15] However, pedigree data should not be altered. In pedigree charts, triangles can be used instead of squares and circles if the sex of family members is not essential to the report (eg, if the disease is known not to be sex linked).

REFERENCES

1. World Medical Association Declaration of Helsinki. Recommendations guiding medical doctors in biomedical research involving human subjects. *JAMA*. 1997;277: 925-926.
2. The Nuremberg Code. *JAMA*. 1996;276:1691.
3. World Medical Association Declaration of Geneva, 1948. In: Reich WT, ed. *Encyclopedia of Bioethics*. 2nd ed. New York, NY: Macmillan Publishing Co; 1995:2646-2647.
4. Rennie D. The ethics of medical publication. *Med J Aust*. 1979;2:409-412.
5. Beecher HK. Ethics and clinical research. *N Engl J Med*. 1966;274:1354-1360.
6. Kirsch J. *Kirsch's Handbook of Publishing Law*. Los Angeles, Calif: Acrobat Books; 1995.
7. International Committee of Medical Journal Editors. Uniform Requirements for Manuscripts Submitted to Biomedical Journals. *JAMA*. 1997;277:927-934.
8. National Commission for the Protection of Human Subjects of Biomedical and Behavioral Research. The Belmont Report: ethical principles and guidelines for the protection of human subjects of research, 1979. In: Reich WT, ed. *Encyclopedia of Bioethics*. 2nd ed. New York, NY: Macmillan Publishing Co; 1995:2767-2773.
9. DHHS Regulations for the Protection of Human Subjects (45 CFR 46) June 18, 1991. In: Reich WT, ed. *Encyclopedia of Bioethics*. 2nd ed. New York, NY: Macmillan Publishing Co; 1995:2773-2794.
10. Slue WJ. Unmasking the Lone Ranger. *N Engl J Med*. 1989;321:550-551.
11. Riis P, Nylenna M. Patients have a right to privacy and anonymity in medical publication. *JAMA*. 1991;265:2720.
12. Riis P, Nylenna M. Identification of patients in medical publications: need for informed consent. *BMJ*. 1991;302:1182.
13. Smith J. Keeping confidence in published papers: do more to protect patient's rights to anonymity. *BMJ*. 1991;302:1168.

14. Glass RM, Flanagin A. Communication, biomedical II. scientific publication. In: Reich WT, ed. *Encyclopedia of Bioethics.* 2nd ed. New York, NY: Macmillan Publishing Co; 1995:428-435.

15. Knoppers BM, Chadwick R. The Human Genome Project: under an international ethical microscope. *Science.* 1994;265:2035-2036.

Truth is generally the best vindication against slander.
Abraham Lincoln[1]

3.9 ■ **DEFAMATION, LIBEL.**—Defamation is the act of harming another's reputation by libel or slander and thereby exposing that person to public hatred, contempt, ridicule, or financial loss.[2-5] Libel is "a method of defamation expressed by print, writing, pictures, or signs."[2] Technically, libel differs from slander in that slander is defamation by oral expressions or gestures. With the advent of digital publications and the mix of print, audio, and video images, the distinction between these terms has become blurred.[3]

Defamatory statements about groups of individuals are usually not legally actionable suits if the group is so large that no individual can be identified. Convention holds that those cases in which defamation has been proved typically involve groups comprising 25 or fewer individuals.[3]

In US courts, truth is considered an absolute defense against libel in most cases (see 3.9.7, Defense Against Libel). However, libel law is complex, and it is difficult for an author or an editor to know with certainty if the text of a specific manuscript could be defended successfully in a libel suit.[6] Libel law requires courts to balance 2 competing values: freedom of expression vs protection of personal reputation.[7]

Freedom of expression has its foundation in the First Amendment of the US Constitution, and this freedom has been nearly guaranteed to authors, journalists, and editors since a landmark Supreme Court decision in 1964 (*New York Times Co v Sullivan*).[8] Yet recently, libel suits have been used to silence those with opposing viewpoints and censor the free flow of information.[7] For example, some commercial entities have filed a new form of suit, Strategic Lawsuit Against Public Participation (SLAPP), in an attempt to intimidate their opponents from publishing information that could expose wrongdoing on the part of a particular industry or corporation. Even if the suit is groundless, a protracted and expensive legal battle may ensue.

The final judgment in a 1989 case, *Moldea v New York Times Co,*[9] upheld the balance between the right to freedom of expression and the right to protect personal reputation (see 3.9.4, Editorials, Letters, and Reviews, for more details about this case).

Publication is an essential element for a legal action of libel. For example, in the 1993 suits *Paine v Time, Inc* and *Paine v The Washington Times,* a claim of defamation could not be made of a manuscript written and mailed by authors to various newspapers throughout the United States until the article was actually printed, or "published."[3] Libel may be actionable at the point of printing whether or not the publication has been distributed to readers.

A publication is considered defamatory when it includes each of the following[5,6]:

- A false statement concerning another
- An unprivileged (ie, not confidential) publication to a third party

- Fault amounting at least to "negligence" (ie, failing to meet the minimum standards that a reasonable person would have been expected to meet in researching, fact checking, writing, reviewing, and publishing the statement) or "actual malice" (ie, publishing with knowledge that the statement was false or with reckless disregard for the truth of the statement)
- Actionability of the statement (ie, that which is subject to a lawsuit)

A statement is actionable in the following ways[3]:

- *actionable per se:* the words are damaging in and of themselves
- *actionable per quod:* the words are innocent but are made damaging in a specific context

3.9.1 ***Living Persons and Existing Entities.***—A statement may not be libelous unless it is "of and concerning" a living person or existing entity (eg, corporation, institution, or organization).[3] According to a 1992 case, *Gugliuzza v KCMC, Inc,* "once a person is dead, there is not extant reputation to injure or for the law to protect."[10] Even when the living person or entity is not named in the statement, if the person or corporation's identity can be determined from other published facts, a case for libel can be made. In 1992, a court declined to dismiss the Church of Scientology's complaint against Time-Warner, because of the publication of allegedly defamatory statements concerning a "Los Angeles-based church."[3,11]

3.9.2 ***Public and Private Figures.***—A public figure is a person who assumes a role of prominence in society, such as an elected official, a celebrity, or an infamous criminal. In cases of alleged libel, public figures are afforded less legal protection than private individuals. In a 1964 case, *New York Times Co v Sullivan,*[8] the US Supreme Court determined that for a public official to prove defamation, the official must demonstrate that the alleged defamatory statement was made with "actual malice" (ie, with knowledge that the statement was false or with disregard for the truth of the statement). A private individual needs only to establish negligence. Answers to the following questions may aid in determining public or private status of an individual and vulnerability to a claim of defamation when a personal statement about an individual is published[3,6]:

- Is the person described a public or a private figure?
- Does the subject of the statement pertain to a matter of public controversy or public concern?
- If the statement refers to a public figure, does it contain references to the individual's job performance or public behavior?
- If the statement refers to a public figure, will the connection between such references and the individual's public status be evident to a reasonable reader?
- If the reference is completely peripheral, does it involve nonrelevant, highly intimate, or embarrassing facts?

3.9.3 ***Statements of Opinion.***—Statements that contain opinion (ie, subjective judgment) are not actionable because an idea cannot be considered false.[3,5] However, an opinion that includes, asserts, or implies facts that are false and defamatory could result in legal action. Similarly, publication of an expression of opinion made about a public figure is protected under the "fair comment" doctrine. This doctrine also protects publications that contain fair and accurate reports of defamatory statements based on official action or public proceedings.[6]

Opinion vs Fact: The Publishing Law Handbook[3] offers the following questions for distinguishing statements of fact from statements of opinion:

- Can the statement be proved true or false?
- Are the facts on which the opinion is based fully disclosed to the reader?
- If not, are the facts on which the opinion is based obvious to a reasonable reader or readily available to the reader from other sources?
- Are both the disclosed and undisclosed facts on which the opinion is based substantially true?
- Does the context of the opinion suggest to a reasonable reader that it represents opinion and not fact?
- Have the statements that contain opinions been clearly demarcated to inform the readers that they deal with opinion, commentary, or criticism (eg, a clearly identified editorial or opinion page)?

3.9.4 ***Editorials, Letters, and Reviews.***—In some publications, such as newspapers and popular magazines, editorials, correspondence, and critical reviews tend to alert the reader that the content is opinion. However, this is not always the case for scientific journals. In any case, editors and publishers should be cautious about statements made in editorials, letters, and reviews. Use of such phrases as "in my opinion" will not indemnify against an action of libel. Editors and publishers should consider obtaining legal review of all material being considered for publication that contains potentially libelous statements (see also 3.9.7, Defense Against Libel).

Book Reviews: For book reviews, conventional wisdom holds that critical comments about a specific book are acceptable, but critical comments about an author (ie, a private figure) should be avoided. In *Moldea v New York Times Co,*[9] Dan Moldea, the author of a book that received an unfavorable review in the *New York Times,* sued the paper for libel. The book review included the statement that Moldea's book contained "too much sloppy journalism to trust the bulk of this book's 512 pages."[9] This comment was supported with specific examples of misspellings and mischaracterization of events.[7] After an initial decision in favor of the *New York Times,* an appeal that favored Moldea's claim, and an unusual reversal by the appeals court, Moldea's libel suit was dismissed. The final decision in this case reaffirmed impunity from libel suits for opinion pieces and provided a "workable test for analyzing allegedly defamatory statements of opinion."[7]

3.9.5 ***Works of Fiction.***—Fictional accounts are not actionable for defamation unless a reasonable reader believes that the story is depicting factual events and can identify the person bringing suit in the story.[3-6] Humor, satire, and parody may be exempt from defamation suits as long as they are clearly works of fiction.[6]

3.9.6 ***Republication and News Reporting.***—A publisher can be held liable for republishing a defamatory statement. For example, if a publisher reprinted a defamatory statement about a public figure knowing that the statement was false, the publisher may be held liable. Similarly, if the republished statement was about a private figure, the publisher may be held liable for negligence.

Under the privilege of "fair reporting," an author can repeat a previously published defamatory statement if it was part of official proceedings (eg, a congressional debate or press conference) as long as the account is fair and accurate.[6] Under the privilege of "neutral reporting," an author may repeat a previously published defamatory statement as long as the second account is a neutral or balanced report of a public controversy or matter of legitimate public concern (see also 3.9.3, Statements of Opinion).

Quotations: Since the decision in *New York Times Co v Sullivan,* journalists have been protected from libel suits for inadvertent or negligent quotations by the requirement that the plaintiff demonstrate deliberate reckless conduct on the part of the defendant. In *Masson v New Yorker Magazine, Inc,*[12] the Ninth Circuit Court of Appeals determined that a journalist may even alter quotations provided that the quotations are reasonable interpretations of the statements made by the person quoted. In this case, Janet Malcolm altered quotations of what she believed to be ambiguous remarks made by Jeffrey Masson during a series of interviews that Malcolm tape-recorded and of which she took notes. The altered quotations were published in an article in the *New Yorker,* and subsequently, Masson filed a libel suit against Malcolm, the *New Yorker,* and the publisher. The court determined that there was no evidence of actual malice in Malcolm's actions and that the altered quotations were not libelous.

3.9.7 ***Defense Against Libel.***—In the United States, truth is a defense against claims of libel in most cases. In addition to proof of falsity, some states also require evidence of a motive to harm another's reputation.[3,6] Editors should query authors about any statements that criticize or imply criticism of individuals or corporate entities. If an editor cannot determine the veracity of a statement, obtaining a legal review (vetting) as part of the process of peer review is recommended. The legal review should be performed by an attorney with knowledge of the field under consideration. Even though legal review may result in delay and several requests for revision, it may protect a publisher from a libel action.

According to some pundits, fear of libel suits has kept some editors from meeting their ethical duties to their readers. For example, during the 1980s a number of medical journals declined to reprint retractions of articles by 2 separate researchers, Robert Slutsky and Stephen Breuning (even though the articles had been proven to be fraudulent and even after Breuning's federal indictment), because of fear that they would be liable for publishing statements impugning Slutsky's and Breuning's work.[13]

Such "defensive" editorial practices should be undertaken with caution as they may impair the integrity of the journal. For example, allowing Slutsky's and Breuning's fraudulent articles to stand unretracted was an injustice to the readers of those articles.[14] Biomedical editors and publishers can rely on the statement on retractions from the International Committee of Medical Journal Editors for protection against claims of defamation after publishing a retraction of an article proved to be fraudulent[15] (see 3.4.3, Editorial Policy for Detecting and Handling Allegations of Scientific Misconduct).

A claim involving the *Journal of Alcohol Studies* demonstrates the need for an editor's awareness of the risks of libel and the need for legal review of potentially defamatory material before acceptance for publication.[16] In this case, an author sued the *Journal of Alcohol Studies* for breach of contract after the journal did not publish an "accepted" paper. The editor had determined the paper to be libelous after accepting it but before publication. The journal agreed to publish the paper in an agreement with the plaintiff author that he would drop his lawsuit. The editor said he had no choice in light of the mounting legal fees. Ironically a libel suit was never filed after publication of the article because the person about whom the potentially libelous statements were made believed that readers could determine that the statements made about him were not truthful.[16]

3.9.8 ***Other Liability Concerns.***—There are numerous sources of legal problems for publishers and editors that are beyond the scope of this manual. *The Publishing Law Handbook*[3] and *Kirsch's Handbook of Publishing Law*[6] are good resources for information on preventing and resolving many of these problems, including issues related to the following: copyright, patent, and trademark (see 3.6, Intellectual Property: Ownership, Rights, and Management), privacy (see 3.8, Protecting Individual's Rights in Scientific Publication), advertising and liability (see 3.12, Advertisements, Advertorials, and Sponsored Supplements), circulation audits, subscription list fraud, taxation and accounting issues, employment issues, and postal rates and regulations.

REFERENCES

1. Lincoln A. Letter to Secretary Stanton, refusing to dismiss Postmaster General Montgomery Blair, July 18, 1864. In: Bartlett J. *Familiar Quotations.* 15th ed. Boston, Mass: Little Brown & Co Inc; 1980:523.
2. *Black's Law Dictionary*. St Paul, Minn: West Publishing Co; 1990.
3. Perle EG, Williams JT. *The Publishing Law Handbook*. Englewood Cliffs, NJ: Prentice Hall Law & Business; 1994.
4. Libel and slander. In: *American Jurisprudence*. Vol 50. 2nd ed. Rochester, NY: Lawyers Cooperative Publishing; 1994:205-206.
5. Stubbs SE, Boyce WJ. The risks of libel in medical publishing. *Ann Allergy*. 1994;72:101-103.
6. Kirsch J. *Kirsch's Handbook of Publishing Law*. Los Angeles, Calif: Acrobat Books; 1995.
7. Hershey J. Casenote: if you can't say something nice, can you say anything at all? *Moldea v New York Times Co* and the importance of context in First Amendment law. *67 U Colo L Rev 705* (Summer 1996).
8. *New York Times Co v Sullivan,* 376 US 254, 280 (1964).
9. *Moldea v New York Times Co,* 793 F Supp 335, 337 (DDC 1992); *Moldea I, supra* note 12; *Moldea II, supra* note 12.
10. *Gugliuzza v KCMC, Inc,* 606 So2d 790, 20 Media La Rptr 1866 (La 1992).
11. *Church of Scientology Int'l v Time Warner, Inc,* 806 F Supp 1157, 20 Media La Rptr 2047 (SD NY 1992).
12. *Masson v New Yorker Magazine, Inc,* 686 F Supp 1396, 1398 (ND Cal 1987); *Mason,* 895 F 2d 1535 (9th Cir 1989).
13. LaFollette MC. *Stealing Into Print: Fraud, Plagiarism, and Misconduct in Scientific Publishing*. Los Angeles: University of California Press; 1992.
14. Whitely WP, Rennie D, Hafner AW. The scientific community's response to evidence of fraudulent publication. *JAMA*. 1994;272:170-173.
15. International Committee of Medical Journal Editors. Uniform Requirements for Manuscripts Submitted to Biomedical Journals. *JAMA*. 1997;277:927-934.
16. MacDonald KA. Rutgers journal forced to publish paper despite threats of libel suit. *Chronicle Higher Educ*. September 13, 1989:A5.

The freedom of the press is one of the greatest bulwarks of liberty.
George Mason[1]

3.10 ■ **EDITORIAL FREEDOM AND INTEGRITY.**—Editorial freedom implies a range of independence, from complete absence of external restraint and coercion to the mere avoidance of unnecessary interference or hindrance.[2] The First Amendment of the US Constitution affirms several freedoms, including the freedom of the press. Thus, communicating through the US press or other media is a constitutionally guaranteed right that should not be interfered with by the government, other institutions, or individual persons.[3] Yet history is full of examples of journalists and editors battling incursions from many human, social, and economic forces. Editors have been dismissed from their posts and journals have ceased publication after a mere "stroke of the editorial pen."[4]

One example of a medical editor credited for his struggles to maintain editorial freedom is Hugh Clegg, editor of the *BMJ* from 1944 to 1965. In 1956, Clegg wrote an unsigned editorial entitled "The Gold-headed Cane," in which he attacked the president of the Royal College of Physicians for taking office for the seventh successive year. He also admonished the college for its failure to recognize the modern welfare state and its lack of attention to postgraduate medical education.[4] With much difficulty, Clegg kept his editorial position and freedom and published a reply from the president that rebutted all of Clegg's criticisms. Clegg believed that medical editors are the protectors of the conscience of the profession, and he is well known for his assertion that editors who maintain this ideal will often find themselves in trouble. This trouble may come in the form of incursions into editorial freedom, which editors must be able to defend.

In scientific publishing, editors must have complete authority for determining the editorial content of their publications.[5-8] Editors must be free from restraint or interference from the publication's owner, publisher, advertisers, sponsors, subscribers, authors, editorial board or publication committee members, reviewers, and readers. Owners, publishers, boards, and publication committees may have the right to select and dismiss the editor, but they should not interfere with editorial decisions and policies.

Without a clear delineation of editorial freedom and the authority to maintain this freedom, an editor cannot ensure the integrity of the publication. Thus, owners, publishers, advertisers, authors, and reviewers must recognize and accept the editor's authority,[5] and editors should not comply with any external pressure that may compromise their autonomy or their journal's integrity. Examples of such pressures include an advertiser's request to insert an advertisement next to an article about its product, an owner or politically powerful individual's pressure to avoid publishing certain types of articles, or a request from a group of authors to bypass peer review and fast-track the publication of their manuscript. Editors may need to educate and remind the publication's various constituents of the fundamentals of editorial freedom and its direct relation to the publication's integrity.

3.10.1 ***Policy on Editorial Freedom.***—Since 1983, *JAMA* has operated under a set of goals and objectives developed by editor George D. Lundberg, MD, and the journal's editorial staff and approved by the editorial board (see Table 5). These goals and objectives have protected the editor on several occasions from external pressures to restrict the journal's editorial freedom, and in 1993 the AMA House of Delegates passed a resolution reaffirming editorial independence for all of its scientific journals.[9]

TABLE 5. *JAMA's* EDITORIAL MISSION: KEY AND CRITICAL OBJECTIVES

Key objective

To promote the science and art of medicine and the betterment of the public health.

Critical objectives

1. To publish original, important, well-documented, peer-reviewed clinical and laboratory articles on a diverse range of medical topics.
2. To provide physicians with continuing education in basic and clinical science to support informed clinical decisions.
3. To enable physicians to remain informed in multiple areas of medicine, including developments in fields other than their own.
4. To improve public health internationally by elevating the quality of medical care, disease prevention, and research provided by an informed readership.
5. To foster responsible and balanced debate on controversial issues that affect medicine and health care.
6. To forecast important issues and trends in medicine and health care.
7. To inform readers about nonclinical aspects of medicine and public health, including the political, philosophic, ethical, legal, environmental, economic, historical, and cultural.
8. To recognize that, in addition to these specific objectives, THE JOURNAL has a social responsibility to promote the integrity of science.
9. To report American Medical Association policy, as appropriate, while maintaining editorial independence, objectivity, and responsibility.
10. To achieve the highest level of ethical medical journalism and to produce a publication that is timely, credible, and enjoyable to read.

The following may help editors develop a policy on editorial freedom for their publications:

- The editor should have a written contract or job description that clearly defines the editor's duties, rights, term of appointment, relation to the publication's owner, and mechanism for conflict resolution.[6]
- The editor should have direct access to the highest level of management in the organization or company that owns the publication.[6]
- All publications should have a mission statement that includes reference to editorial freedom.
- An independent editorial advisory board may help the editor establish and maintain policy on editorial freedom.[6]
- The journal should publish a prominently placed disclaimer that identifies and separates a publication's owner and sponsor from the editorial staff and content. *JAMA* regularly publishes 2 such disclaimers, separating it from its owner, the American Medical Association. The following appears on the masthead of each issue:

> All articles published, including editorials, letters, and book reviews, represent the opinions of the authors and do not reflect the official policy of the American Medical Association or the institutions with which the author is affiliated, unless this is clearly specified.

In addition, the following notice appears at the top of the editorial opinion page:

> Editorials represent the opinions of the authors and THE JOURNAL and not those of the American Medical Association.

- Editors should publish articles on editorial freedom when appropriate.
- Editors should inform board members, committee members, publishers, and new staff of the journal's policies on editorial freedom.

- Editors should alert the international medical community to major transgressions against editorial freedom.[6]

REFERENCES

1. Mason G. *Virginia Bill of Rights*. Article 12. June 12, 1776.
2. *Merriam-Webster's Collegiate Dictionary*. 10th ed. Springfield, Mass: Merriam-Webster Inc; 1993.
3. Edwards RB, Erde EL. Freedom and coercion. In: Reich TW, ed. *Encyclopedia of Bioethics*. Vol 2. New York, NY: Macmillan Publishing Co; 1995:883.
4. Death of a journal. *Lancet*. 1987;2:1442.
5. Booth CC. The *British Medical Journal* and the twentieth-century consultant. In: Bynum WF, Lock S, Porter R, eds. *Medical Journals and Medical Knowledge*. New York, NY: Routledge Chapman Hall Inc; 1992:259-260.
6. International Committee of Medical Journal Editors. Uniform Requirements for Manuscripts Submitted to Biomedical Journals. *JAMA*. 1997;277:927-934.
7. Editorial Policy Committee, Council of Biology Editors. Cross cutting issues. In: *Ethics and Policy in Scientific Publication*. Chicago, Ill: Council of Biology Editors Inc; 1990:102-105.
8. Lock S. Editorial freedom: a modest proposal to Dublin. *BMJ*. 1988;296:733-734.
9. Lundberg GD. House of Delegates reaffirms editorial independence for AMA's scientific journals. *JAMA*. 1993;270:1248-1249.

I believe the editor is the primary source for ethical responsibility among professional publications.

George D. Lundberg, MD[1]

3.11 ■ EDITORIAL RESPONSIBILITIES, PROCEDURES, AND POLICIES.—Coupled with the autonomy that comes with editorial freedom is responsibility. Editors are responsible for maintaining procedures and creating and enforcing editorial policies that allow the publication to meet its mission and goals effectively, efficiently, and ethically[2,3] and in a fiscally responsible manner.

3.11.1 *The Editor's Responsibilities.*—An editor's primary responsibility is to inform and educate readers. Thus, editors are obliged to make rational, clear, and consistent editorial decisions and select papers for publication that are appropriate for their readers.[4-6] The editor's duty to the readers often outweighs obligations to others with vested interest in the publication and may require actions that may not appear fair or suitable to authors, reviewers, owners, or advertisers.

Some editors envision a broad, ethically based, social responsibility for themselves (eg, editors-in-chief of major medical or scientific journals),[2,3] whereas other editors' responsibilities are more focused and technical (eg, copy editors, managing editors). These responsibilities, regardless of their scope, should be clearly delineated in the editor's job description and supported by the publication's editorial mission statement (see 3.10, Editorial Freedom and Integrity).

Bishop,[6] Morgan,[7] and Riis[8] have identified 5 additional requisites of an editor: competence, fairness, confidentiality, expeditiousness, and courtesy (described in greater detail below).

Competence: Competence requires editors to possess a general scientific knowledge of the fields covered in their publications and to be skilled in the arts of editing, negotiation, and diplomacy. In addition, editors should consider joining professional societies in their respective scientific fields as well as professional organizations for editors (eg, Council of Biology Editors, European Association of Science Editors, American Medical Writers Association [see 22.2, Resources, Professional Writing, Editing, and Communications Organizations and Groups]). Editors who publish original research, or summaries or interpretations of research, should be familiar with the scientific methods used, including the general principles of statistics.[8] Editors should also rely on the expertise of others (eg, editorial board members, peer reviewers, statistical consultants) for advice and guidance, with the recognition that the editor has the ultimate authority for all editorial decisions. A competent editor will make rational editorial decisions, within a reasonable period, and communicate these decisions to authors in a clear and consistent manner.[4,6-8] A competent editor (whether editor-in-chief or copy editor) will also be skilled in the art of rhetoric[9] to recognize the tools of linguistic persuasion and identify and remove hyperbole, inconsistent arguments, and unsupported assertions and conclusions from otherwise promising manuscripts. Finally, as Bishop[6] suggests, a sense of humor should not be regarded as a trivial characteristic for an editor, as a bit of humor can often avoid, or at least soften, potential conflicts between authors, reviewers, and editors.

Fairness: Fairness requires editors to act impartially and honestly.[5,8] Because editors are human, they cannot avoid the influence of all biases. Using peer review and consulting other editors during the editorial process may help control some personal biases.[4] Editors of peer-reviewed journals are responsible for maintaining the integrity of the peer review process, for developing policies regarding the peer review process, and for seeing that staff are properly trained in the procedures involved. Editors should document factors relevant to editorial decisions and keep copies of reviewers' comments so they will be prepared to deal with appeals or complaints. However, editors should not keep copies of rejected manuscripts. In resolving disputes, editors should consider all sides of an issue and should avoid favoritism toward friends and colleagues. To avoid external pressure, editors should not have financial interests in any entity that might influence editorial evaluations and decisions[4] (see 3.5, Conflicts of Interest).

Confidentiality: Confidentiality requires editors to ensure that information about a submitted manuscript is not disclosed to anyone outside the editorial office, other than the peer reviewers (see 3.7, Confidentiality). This requires editors to create and maintain policies about confidentiality. Editors must also ensure that all current and new staff (editorial and production), reviewers, and editorial board members are sufficiently educated about the principles of confidentiality. The following statement may be useful when handling inquiries about manuscripts under consideration or previously rejected:

"We can neither confirm nor deny the existence of any manuscript unless and until such manuscript is published."

Expeditiousness: Although the length of time it takes to evaluate a manuscript depends on many factors (eg, number of submitted manuscripts, resources of the editorial office, time allocated for peer review, frequency of the journal's publication, and pages allotted for editorial material), an author has a right to expect to receive a decision within a reasonable period of time.[7,8] Ideally, the initial editorial evaluation of a manuscript should not exceed 6 to 8 weeks, including 3 to 4 weeks for peer review.[5,8] If the review and evaluation are delayed beyond 8 weeks, notifying the author of the reason for the delay is appropriate. Authors have a right to contact the editorial office to inquire about the status of their manuscripts.

Editors should plan to accept papers with knowledge of the number of accepted manuscripts in abeyance awaiting publication and the approximate number of pages and articles that can be published during a year. Morgan[7] argues that a journal that accepts more papers than it can publish within the time span observed by other journals in the same field is suppressing, not disseminating, information.

On occasion, an editor will receive a request from an author or a suggestion from a reviewer to fast-track publication of a specific manuscript. The quickened pace of scientific discovery and heightened competition among scientists and journals have fostered an increase in requests for rapid publication, and technologic advances have changed the facility to do so.[10] Yet editors should approach such requests with caution. A policy should be developed to allow for rapid publication of appropriate manuscripts (eg, those with important and urgent implications for public health) that does not compromise the peer review process and that does not result in the premature publication of an incomplete or inaccurate article (see 3.13, Relations With the News Media).

Courtesy: More than a mere extension of etiquette and convention, editorial politeness requires editors and all editorial staff to deal with authors and reviewers in a respectful, fair, and courteous manner.[6-9] Diplomacy, tact, empathy, and negotiation skills will help editors maintain positive relationships with authors, even those whose work the editor rejects.

3.11.2 ***Editorial Responsibility for Rejection.***—Rejecting manuscripts may be the most important responsibility of an editor. By rejecting papers appropriately, an editor sets standards and defines the editorial content for the journal.[7] A rejection letter must be carefully worded to avoid offending the author and should express regret for the outcome, but it also must not raise false hopes about the merits of an unsuitable paper. Many editors avoid use of the word *rejection* in any letters, opting instead for phrases such as "we are unable to accept," or "your paper is not acceptable for publication." However, editors should be certain that the intent of a letter of rejection is clear. If the letter sounds too much like a request for revision, the author may subsequently resubmit an irrevocably flawed manuscript; or worse, the author may resubmit a rejected manuscript, essentially unchanged, with the hope that the editor will not notice.[7]

An editor should determine whether a standard rejection letter (form letter) or a personal letter explaining the specific deficiencies of the manuscript should be sent to the author on a case-by-case basis. Some editors argue that for a paper rejected for "reasons of editorial choice (usually without outside editorial peer review), the editor has no obligation to give the author any explanation beyond the statement that the manuscript was not considered appropriate."[4] Other editors suggest that every author should be provided a specific reason for rejection of their manuscript. Clearly, a form letter that turns down a good manuscript without any sort of explanation is inappropriate. Conversely, a form letter accompanied by copies of detailed reviewer comments is sufficient for many papers that are rejected.

Editors should develop specific policies for the rejection process, including how to handle previously rejected manuscripts resubmitted with an appeal for reconsideration. If the author's appeal provides reasonable justifications, the editor should carefully consider the appeal (see 4.1.7, Editorial Assessment and Processing, Appealing a Rejection).

Returning Rejected Manuscripts: Once a common act of courtesy, the practice of returning all copies of rejected manuscripts has become obsolete.[11] While the replacement of the typewriter and carbon copies by the personal computer and disk copies have made generating new copies much easier, increased postal rates rendered this practice costly and unnecessary for many publications. Journals that do not return manuscripts should make this clear to all authors. However, original illustrations, photographs, slides, and other artwork should be returned, as should any manuscripts an author specifically requests be returned. Disk copies of manuscripts should be treated like print copies and need not be returned unless specifically requested. This policy is listed in *JAMA*'s instructions for authors and included in its rejection letters. Because journals do not own unpublished works (ie, copyright is typically transferred in the event of publication), journal offices should not keep copies of rejected manuscripts; they should be destroyed or recycled (see also 3.6.4, Copyright Assignment or License, Written Assignment of Copyright).[11]

3.11.3 ***Acknowledging Manuscript Receipt.***—Many journals send a notice to authors to acknowledge receipt of their manuscripts and provide names and telephone numbers of relevant editorial staff. Major journals that receive thousands of contributions are unable to acknowledge receipt of all submissions (eg, letters to the editor). This policy should be disclosed to prospective contributors in the publication's guide for authors. For example, *JAMA* does not send an acknowledgment for receipt of letters sent by mail or fax because of the high volume of letters submitted. (Authors of letters sent by e-mail receive an automatic computer-generated acknowledgment.) Authors of all letters receive a final disposition letter after a decision regarding publication has been made.

3.11.4 ***Editorial Responsibility for Revision.***—Courtesy assumes a major role in an editor's request for revision. According to Morgan,[7] "in letters requesting revision the editor should use an impersonal tone in criticizing." All such correspondence is best if the tone is neutral and objective. Editors must be skilled in arbitrating reviewer disagreements and contradictory recommendations, which may result from reviewers having diverse backgrounds, different expectations of the journal, and variable levels of competence, diligence, or interest in the subject of the manuscript.[7] Authors object to receiving inconsistent or contradictory comments from reviewers and editors as well as new and different criticisms of the revised manuscript submitted in response to the initial review. Although editors can never be certain that new issues will not surface at the time of resubmission, they are obliged to evaluate all reviewer comments, address any inconsistencies or unreasonable criticisms, censor any inappropriate criticisms, and guide authors in preparing their revisions.[4] Editors who make decisons about publication should never relegate themselves to the role of manuscript traffic controllers; they are obligated to use sound editorial judgment in requesting a revision.

Some editors feel uncomfortable asking an author to revise a manuscript if there is a possibility the revision will not be published. Here, an editor's responsibility to readers may outweigh the desire to publish the author's revised manuscript. Editors should develop specific policies regarding requests for revisions, and every revision letter should state explicitly whether the author can expect publication of the revised manuscript. For example, *JAMA* editors include language similar to the following in their revision letters:

> If you decide to revise your paper along these lines, there is *no guarantee* that it will be accepted for publication. That decision will be based on our priorities at the time and on the quality of your revision.

The rejection of a revised manuscript is probably best handled with a personal letter tactfully describing why the revision did not develop into an acceptable paper. Editors should avoid requests for multiple revisions of a paper without explicit justification.

3.11.5 ***Editorial Responsibility for Manuscript Assessment.***—Depending on the nature of a journal's editorial resources and the number of manuscripts received annually, the editor may rely on a triage system to evaluate all manuscripts before peer review. Not all manuscripts will be appropriate for the journal, and after an initial assessment the editor may decide to reject some papers without sending them for external peer review. For example, *JAMA* editors reject about 50% of the approximately 4000 manuscripts received annually without seeking peer review. In such cases, the editor's duty to the author is outweighed by duties to reviewers (by not wasting their time on a manuscript that has no chance of publication), to owners (by not wasting resources), and to other authors who have submitted papers to the journal (by maintaining efficient processes) (see 4.0, Editorial Assessment and Processing).

Occasionally, an editor will need to make a decision on 2 or more manuscripts covering the same topic that are submitted simultaneously by different authors. Editors may then send more than one manuscript on the same topic to the same reviewers and ask them to indicate whether one manuscript is better than the other. Another common dilemma for editors occurs when a new manuscript is received after a different manuscript on the same topic was just rejected. Here again, the editor may rely on the peer reviewers of the previously submitted manuscript to evaluate the current submission.

3.11.6 ***Editorial Responsibility for Peer Review.***—Editors are obliged to be courteous to peer reviewers. Many journals publish lists of reviewers' names to praise and thank them publicly for their work. Editors and reviewers should have a mutual understanding about the number of manuscripts they may be expected to review during a year. Editors should remember not to share a specific review with anyone outside the editorial office, other than the authors and the other reviewers (see 3.6.6, Copying, Reproducing, and Adapting). Editors should provide feedback to reviewers. Such feedback can include notifying reviewers of the manuscript's final disposition, sharing copies of other reviewer comments of the same manuscript, and providing regular assessments of the quality of the reviewers' work. Editors should develop a specific policy regarding who has access to copies of a review, and this policy should be clearly communicated to all persons involved in the review process (see 4.0, Editorial Assessment and Processing, and 3.7.1, Confidentiality in Peer Review).

Many journals develop databases of reviewers, including their addresses and affiliations, areas of expertise, turnaround times, and quality ratings for each manuscript review. Editors and publishers are obliged not to exploit the information in the database for their personal use or profit without the prior consent of the reviewers (eg, selling a mailing list).

3.11.7 ***Editorial Responsibility for Acceptance.***—Editors should inform authors of acceptance of their manuscripts in a letter that describes the subsequent process of publication, including substantive editing, copyediting, and what material the author will be expected to review and approve. Editors may also provide an approximate timetable for the publication process. If authors are given an expected date of publication, they should be informed of the likelihood of the date changing.

Authors should avoid making substantial editorial changes after acceptance of a manuscript, unless correcting an error, answering an editor, responding to a copy editor's or a proofreader's query, or providing an essential update. Likewise, editors should review manuscripts before acceptance and ask authors for substantial changes during the revision process.

If circumstances (eg, an unanticipated decrease in the number of pages allotted for publication or clustering of certain papers for a special issue) cause a delay beyond the average time between acceptance and publication, editors should inform the corresponding author of the reason for the delay. The acceptance letter should also remind authors of any policies regarding duplicate submissions or the prepublication release of information to the public or the media (see 3.3, Duplicate Publication, and 3.13, Relations With the News Media).

An example of editorial discourtesy in handling accepted manuscripts occurred when an editor "unaccepted" a paper that his journal had accepted unconditionally 20 months earlier. The reason provided to the authors for this editorial change of heart was that the journal's inventory of accepted papers had grown too large.[12] If a new editor inherits from a previous editor a large inventory of accepted manuscripts deemed outdated or inappropriate, the editor's responsibility to the readers may outweigh the responsibility to publish those manuscripts. However, any decisions not to publish previously accepted papers should be made carefully and should not be made without consulting the publisher, the journal's legal adviser, and the editorial board or publications committee.

Provisional Acceptance: Some editors will grant authors a "provisional acceptance," offering to publish their papers if certain conditions or minor requirements are met. Some journals use provisional or conditional acceptances for revision requests when they are fairly certain that the revision will be accepted for publication. However, use of a provisional acceptance as a request for revision can cause problems if the revised manuscript is not suitable for publication. By policy, *JAMA* editors use provisional acceptances with caution, offering them, for example, to authors of manuscripts that may be missing 1 of several coauthors' signatures on a copyright transfer form or that may require minor content editing—and only if a manuscript is otherwise ready for complete acceptance. Likewise, if a new editorial policy requires a new condition for publication to be met by authors who submitted papers before the policy took effect, a provisional acceptance can be used to permit these papers to move forward without unnecessary delay.

3.11.8 ***The Role of the Correspondence Column and Corrections.***—A biomedical journal should provide a forum for readers and authors to exchange important information, especially with regard to articles published in the journal.[13] A common place for such exchange is the correspondence, or letters to the editor, column. Here, journal readers have the opportunity to offer relevant comments, query authors, and criticize published articles. Authors of articles being criticized should always be given the opportunity to respond. The critical comments and the author's reply should be published in the same issue to enable readers to evaluate the arguments presented. If an author chooses not to submit a reply for publication, the journal may publish a statement similar to the following after the critical letter:

> Dr Smith was shown this letter and declined to comment.

Editors should establish policies and procedures for handling letters just as they have done for handling manuscripts, and these should be published in the journal's instructions for authors or as part of the regular correspondence column. Many journals have strict limits on the number of words and references allowed in letters submitted for publication (eg, 500 words or less and no more than 5 references). Some journals will publish small tables or figures in letters, space permitting.

Many journals also set a limit on the amount of time in which a letter sent in response to a published article must be received. For example, *JAMA* editors allow readers 4 weeks to submit a letter in response to a published article. With fax machines and e-mail, this amount of time is sufficient for readers throughout the world to submit timely letters.

Some journals treat letters as minimanuscripts. A submitted letter undergoes an initial assessment, at which point it may be rejected, sent for peer review, or accepted without external peer review. Letters on the same topic or in response to the same article that are accepted for publication are then grouped, sent to the author of the original article for reply (if necessary), and published in the same issue under one general title. Like authors of manuscripts, authors of letters accepted for publication should sign statements of authorship responsibility, financial disclosure, and copyright transfer.

Some journals also publish short reports (eg, <500 words) of original research or novel case reports in the correspondence column. These reports should be handled as regular manuscripts, with peer review and revision, if necessary. They may benefit from a letter in reply (eg, a letter from a pharmaceutical company in reply to a letter reporting an adverse drug reaction not previously reported).

Corrections: All journals need to publish corrections following errors made by authors or introduced by editors, copy editors, production staff, or printers. According to the International Committee of Medical Journal Editors, journal editors have a duty to publish corrections in a timely manner.[13] In addition, corrections should be published on a numbered editorial page and listed in the journal's table of contents. It is preferable to publish corrections in a consistent place in the journal, such as at the end of the correspondence column.

If easily identified, corrections will then be included in literature databases, such as MEDLINE, and appended to digital citations to the original article that contains the error. Corrections should also be appended to all derivative publications (eg, reprints, collections of articles, international editions, online editions, CD-ROMs). If major errors are actually corrected in derivative publications, an indication should be made at the point of correction, explaining what has taken place or linking to an official correction.

3.11.9 ***Disclosure of Editorial Practices, Procedures, and Policies.***—Underlying the ethics of editorial responsibility is the need for disclosure of editorial procedures and policies to authors, reviewers, and readers. Typically, these are listed, and explained if necessary, in the publication's guide for authors, which should be published and available on request. Table 6 lists items that should be considered for inclusion in a biomedical journal's guide for authors.

When an important editorial policy is first created or undergoes a major revision, it should be announced to all prospective authors, reviewers, and readers. The simplest way to accomplish this is to publish an editorial note or

TABLE 6. ITEMS THAT SHOULD BE CONSIDERED FOR INCLUSION IN A BIOMEDICAL JOURNAL'S GUIDE FOR AUTHORS

Information about the journal
- Name, address, telephone and fax numbers, and e-mail address or uniform resource locator (URL), if available for online submission, of editor and editorial office
- Policies on editorial assessment, review, and processing (eg, single-blind, double-blind, or open peer review process; acknowledging receipt of submissions; returning rejected manuscripts; editing and copyediting of accepted manuscripts; ordering reprints)
- Types of manuscripts suitable for submission

Requirements for manuscript submission
- Name, address, telephone and fax numbers, and e-mail address, if available, of corresponding author; list of all coauthors with their relevant academic degrees and institutional affiliations
- Number of copies of manuscripts, tables, and artwork required
- Style and format of manuscript text, tables, artwork, references, and abstracts
- Manuscript submission checklist
- Methods and requirements for submitting manuscripts electronically

Requirements for manuscript consideration
- Policy on submission of duplicate or redundant papers
- Policies on authorship, acknowledging assistance, financial disclosure, and copyright transfer
- Specific requirements for categories of manuscripts (eg, reports of original research, structured reviews, consensus statements)
- For experimental investigations involving human or animal subjects, policy on informed consent and approval by ethics committee
- Policy on including identifiable descriptions or photographs of persons
- Policies on obtaining permission for reprinting or adapting previously published material
- Payment responsibility for publication of color reproduction (if applicable)

an editorial. Editors should also draw attention to major changes in policy and procedures in the journal's instructions for authors and correspondence with authors.

Editors should also ensure that all individuals responsible for contributing to the publication are properly identified, typically in the masthead (eg, editorial and publishing staff, editorial board members, and advisers). Other items that should be disclosed include the name(s) of the owner(s) of the publication and sources of financial support.

3.11.10 ***Editorial Audits and Research.***—Many journals conduct internal assessments, audits, and research into various aspects of the editorial process. For example, a journal may produce monthly or annual reports from the database to track work flow and efficiency. (These reports typically contain average time intervals, reflecting trends rather than absolute numbers.) Trends from these reports can help editors determine the number and types of papers to accept for publication, assess staffing needs, track reviewer performance, and determine when to institute corrective action. For example, *JAMA,* the *BMJ,* and the *Lancet* publish annual editorial audits that include the number of manuscripts received the previous year, acceptance rates, and the average time it takes for a manuscript to be reviewed, accepted or rejected, and published. The AMA *Archives* Journals publish dates of acceptance with each article.

In addition, some journals systematically analyze information from submitted manuscripts as part of research to improve the quality of the editorial or peer review processes. All identifying information should remain confidential during such assessments, and any research conducted should not interfere with the review process or the ultimate editorial decision. For example, in its instructions for authors, *JAMA* notifies prospective authors that information related to their submissions may be subject to such analysis and that confidentiality will be maintained. If a research project involves change in the journal's usual review process (eg, random assignment to a different review procedure), authors should be informed and given the opportunity to choose whether they want their manuscripts to be included in the study.

3.11.11 ***Editorial Quality Review.***—A final editorial procedure that should be a part of every publication's operation is quality review. After publication, editorial and production staff and advisers should review each issue for content errors (which, if detected, should be considered for publication as corrections), problems in presentation and format, and general appearance. All editorial and publishing staff should have the opportunity to participate in the quality review process, and all errors, problems, and suggestions for improvement should be communicated to management as well as those directly involved in editing and producing the publication.

REFERENCES

1. Lundberg GD. II. Perspective from the editor of *JAMA, The Journal of the American Medical Association. Bull Med Libr Assoc.* 1992;80:110-114.
2. Behlmer GK. Ernest Hart and the social thrust of Victorian medicine. *BMJ.* 1990;301:711-713.
3. Lundberg GD. The social responsibility of medical journal editing. *J Gen Intern Med.* 1987;2:415-419.
4. Relman AS. Publishing biomedical research: role and responsibilities. *Hastings Cent Rep.* May/June 1990:23-27.
5. Schiedermayer DL, Siegler M. Believing what you read: responsibilities of medical authors and editors. *Arch Intern Med.* 1986;146:2043-2044.
6. Bishop CT. *How to Edit a Scientific Journal.* Philadelphia, Pa: ISI Press; 1984.
7. Morgan P. *An Insider's Guide for Medical Authors and Editors.* Philadelphia, Pa: ISI Press; 1986.
8. Riis P. The ethics of scientific publication. *Science Editors' Handbook.* January 1994;B3:1-4.
9. Horton R. The rhetoric of research. *CBE Views.* 1995;18(1):3.
10. Roberts L. The rush to publish. *Science.* 1991;251:250-263.
11. Glass RM. New information for authors and readers: group authorship, acknowledgments, and rejected manuscripts [published correction appears in *JAMA.* 1993;269:48]. *JAMA.* 1992;268:99.
12. Chusid MJ, Casper JT, Camitta BM. Editors have ethical responsibilities, too. *N Engl J Med.* 1984;312:658-659.
13. International Committee of Medical Journal Editors. The role of the correspondence column. In: Uniform Requirements for Manuscripts Submitted to Biomedical Journals. *JAMA.* 1997;277:927-934.

The uncertain romance between scholarly journals and the drug industry has long been like a marriage of convenience between partners who became friends ultimately, not because they were very fond of each other originally, but because they needed each other.

Robert H. Moser, MD[1]

3.12 ■ **ADVERTISEMENTS, ADVERTORIALS, AND SPONSORED SUPPLEMENTS.**—Advertising provides a major source of revenue for many scientific publications and allows publishers to set lower subscription rates than would otherwise be possible. Thus, editors and readers often treat advertising as a necessary evil. A cynic might say that generating revenue is the ultimate goal of both advertisers and editors—advertisers want to sell more products, and editors want to maintain the economic viability of their journals as well as their esteemed positions. But editors have a larger ethical responsibility to their readers. Readers must be able to rely on the editor to ensure that the journal's integrity remains intact and that the information contained in the publication is valid and objective. Although editorial responsibility typically does not include review and approval of advertisements, editors should help develop and evaluate advertising policy for their journals.

3.12.1 ***Advertisements.***—For biomedical publications, advertisements typically include the following:

- Advertisements that promote professional or trade-related products (primarily pharmaceuticals and medical equipment in biomedical publications), services, educational opportunities or products, or announcements; these are typically called display advertisements
- Display advertisements that promote products and services not specifically related to a profession or trade (such as an ad for an automobile or an airline in a medical journal)
- Classified or recruitment advertisements (listings of employment opportunities, educational courses, workshops, announcements, or other services)

In most cases, advertisers pay to place advertisements for their products and services in publications. Those advertisements for which a publisher does not charge a fee include public service announcements and "house ads," which promote a product or service provided by the owner of the publication.

Do paid advertisements and other forms of sponsorship invite infringements on editorial independence, or do they represent opportunities for journals in increasingly competitive markets? The answer lies somewhere in between these 2 questions. The key to maintaining editorial integrity is to achieve a balance between these seemingly opposing forces and to maintain a recognizable separation between the functions and decisions of editorial and advertising departments. For example, advertising sales staff for *JAMA* and the AMA *Archives* Journals do not know the editorial content of these journals until after they are published.

Although the primary function of most journals is to provide education and information in a neutral manner and that of advertisements is to educate and inform in a promotional manner, advertisers and editors share a common goal—to influence the behavior of readers.[2]

Obvious differences between editorial text and ad copy exist. Editorial material typically comprises text and black-and-white tables, charts, and graphs, whereas advertisements contain bold, colorful statements and eye-catching graphics. Editorial material, with the aid of a good editor, is intended to be objective, whereas advertisements are intended to be biased and persuasive. Problems arise when the means to achieve the common goal—of influencing behavior—fall outside expected norms or violate specific regulations and standards.

In many countries, advertisers must meet specific criteria established by the regulatory agencies of their countries. For example, drug ads must follow regulations produced by the Food and Drug Administration in the United States, the Association of the British Pharmaceutical Industry in the United Kingdom, or the Pharmaceutical Advertisement Advisory Board in Canada. The Pharmaceutical Advertisement Advisory Board must preview drug advertisements before they can be published, and many of these organizations are also assessing advertorials and supplements.[3] The World Health Organization and the International Federation of Pharmaceutical Manufacturers Associations, both based in Geneva, Switzerland, have guides for pharmaceutical marketing practices that may be helpful for anyone living in a country without well-defined regulations.[4,5] However, each of these regulatory agencies is commonly criticized for lacking the ability to enforce its regulations.[1,6,7]

3.12.2 ***Criteria for Advertisements Directed to Physicians and Other Health Care Professionals.***—Typical complaints about the content of advertisements include concerns that they are misleading, inappropriate, stereotypical, racist, or sexist. The AMA has developed a list of general eligibility requirements and guidelines for advertising copy to ensure that advertisements published in AMA-owned journals are appropriate (see Tables 7 and 8).[8] The American Society of Magazine Editors also has developed a useful guide (Table 9).[9]

The following criteria for pharmaceutical ads are adapted from the guidelines prepared by the World Health Organization and the International Federation of Pharmaceutical Manufacturers Associations[4,5]:

1. Advertising text should be presented legibly.
2. Pharmaceutical ads must include
   a. the name of the product, typically the trade (brand) name.
   b. the active ingredients, using either the international nonproprietary names or the approved generic name of the drug.
   c. the name and address of the manufacturer or distributor.
3. Full advertisements, those that include promotional claims for the use of a product, must also include prescribing information in the form of an approved indication or indications for use with the dosage and method of use and a succinct statement of the contraindications, precautions, side effects, major interactions, and major adverse drug reactions.
4. Reminder advertisements, those that contain no more than a simple statement of indications to designate the therapeutic category of the product, do not have to include prescribing information provided that they include a statement that further information is available on request.
5. When published studies are cited in promotional material, standard references with complete bibliographic information to these should be included (see also 2.12, Manuscript Preparation, References). Quotations from medical literature or from personal communications must not change or distort the intended meaning of the author or the clinical investigator or the significance of the relevant work or study.

TABLE 7. ELIGIBILITY REQUIREMENTS TO ADVERTISE IN AMA PUBLICATIONS

1. Products or services eligible for advertising in the Scientific Publications shall be germane to, and useful in (*a*) the practice of medicine, (*b*) medical education, or (*c*) health care delivery, and should be commercially available.
2. In addition to the above, products and services that are offered by responsible advertisers and that are of interest to physicians as a business, physicians, other health professionals, and consumers are also eligible for advertising.
3. Pharmaceutical products for which approval of a New Drug Application by the Food and Drug Administration is a perquisite for marketing will not be eligible for advertising until such approval has been granted.
4. Institutional advertising germane to the practice of medicine and public service messages of interest to physicians may be considered for inclusion in all AMA publications.
5. Alcoholic beverages and tobacco products may not be advertised.
6. Apparatus, instruments, and devices: the Publishing Group determines the eligibility of advertising for products intended for preventive, diagnostic, or therapeutic purposes.
7. Complete scientific and technical data concerning the product's safety, operation, and usefulness may be required. These data may be either published or unpublished. Samples of apparatus, device, equipment, or instruments should not be submitted. The AMA reserves the right to decline advertising for any product that is involved in litigation with a governmental agency with respect to claims made in the marketing of the product.
8. Food products:
   A. General purpose foods, such as bread, meats, fruits, and vegetables are eligible.
   B. Special purpose foods (eg, foods for carbohydrate-restricted diets and other therapeutic diets) are eligible when their uses are supported by acceptable data.
   C. Dietary programs: only those diet programs prescribed and controlled by physicians may be advertised.
9. Vitamin preparations: Advertisements for nutritional supplements and vitamin preparations are not eligible unless the product is approved for marketing by the Food and Drug Administration for its efficacy and safety and substantiated by clinical studies acceptable to the AMA.
10. Books: A book may be requested for review so that its eligibility may be determined.
11. Miscellaneous products and services: Products or services not in the above classifications may be eligible for advertising if they satisfy the general principles governing eligibility for advertising in AMA publications.

Peer review and editorial evaluation usually eliminate problems associated with misleading or inappropriate information from published articles, but editors usually do not review ads before they are published. Some editors do have formal review processes to assess the validity of claims made in ads.[10,11] Although other journals, including AMA publications, prefer to keep editorial and advertisement review separate,[12] the line between editorial and advertising responsibilities is not always well defined. Many opportunities exist for both collusion and reasonable collaboration between editors and advertisers.

The International Committee of Medical Journal Editors (ICMJE) released a general statement on advertising that may help guide editors and publishers through the gray areas.[13] Specifically, advertising (ie, advertising representatives and promotional material) must not be allowed to influence editorial decisions. Editors should also consider publishing letters that criticize advertising content, in the same way that they publish critical letters about articles, and should ask for a reply from the advertiser. The ICMJE also recommends that editors have full responsibility for advertising policy. This does not mean that editors have to review

TABLE 8. GUIDELINES FOR ADVERTISING COPY IN AMA PUBLICATIONS

1. The advertisement should clearly identify the advertiser of the product or services offered. In the case of drug advertisements, the full generic name of each active ingredient shall appear.
2. Layout, artwork, and format shall be such as to avoid confusion with the editorial content of the publication. The word *advertisement* may be required.
3. Unfair comparisons or unwarranted disparagements of a competitor's products or services will not be allowed.
4. Advertisements will not be acceptable if they conflict with the *Principles of Medical Ethics of the American Medical Association* or the advertising guidelines in *Current Opinions of the Council on Ethical and Judicial Affairs of the American Medical Association.*
5. It is the responsibility of the manufacturer to comply with the laws and regulations applicable to marketing and sale of its products. Acceptance of advertising in AMA publications should not be construed as a guarantee that the manufacturer complies with such laws and regulations.
6. Advertisements may not be deceptive or misleading.
7. Advertisements will not be accepted if they are offensive in either text or artwork, or contain attacks of a personal, racial, sexual, or religious nature, or are demeaning or discriminating toward an individual or group.

TABLE 9. AMERICAN SOCIETY OF MAGAZINE EDITORS' GUIDELINES FOR AD PAGES*

1. Any page of advertising that contains text or design elements that have an editorial appearance must be clearly and conspicuously identified with the words *advertising* or *advertisement* horizontally at or near the top of the page in type at least equal in size and weight to the publication's normal editorial body typeface. The word *advertorial* should not be used.
2. The layout, design, and typeface of advertising pages should be distinctly different from the publication's normal layout, design, and typefaces.
3. No advertisement or advertising section may be promoted on the front cover of the magazine or included in the editorial table of contents. The publication's name or logo should not appear on any advertising pages except that normal running feet may be used at the bottom of each page in the magazine's usual style.
4. Advertising pages should not be placed adjacent to editorial material in a manner that implies editorial endorsement of the advertised products or services. Similarly, an advertiser's name or logo may not be used on any editorial pages to suggest advertising sponsorship of those pages, nor should any editorial page be labeled as "sponsored" or "brought to you" by an advertiser.
5. For the publication's chief editor to have the opportunity to monitor compliance with the guidelines, advertising pages should be made available to the editor in ample time for review and to recommend any necessary changes.

**Adapted and reprinted with permission from the American Society of Magazine Editors.[9] Copyright 1996, American Society of Magazine Editors.*

or approve ads, but rather that editors should be involved in developing advertising policy as it relates to editorial material.

Five issues should be addressed in any policy on advertising:

1. Advertising-to-editorial page ratio
2. Advertising interspersion
3. Ad juxtaposition (adjacency)
4. Editorial calendars
5. Appropriate advertising content

Advertising-to-Editorial Page Ratio: For those publications that have an abundance of advertising, setting an ad page ratio (ie, limiting the advertising content to no more than a certain percentage of total annual pages) may help protect the perceived integrity of the publication.[14] Relevant postal regulations may also need to be examined if the number of ad pages exceeds the number of editorial pages.

Advertising Interspersion: Placing ads between or in the middle of articles may help attract advertisers, but this too may affect the perceived credibility of the publication—especially if the ads make it difficult to read or find editorial content.[3,14] Many publications group, or stack, their ads in the front and back of their journals, leaving an editorial "well" in the middle of the publication for major articles that are not interspersed with ads. Stacking can cause some advertisers to go elsewhere because they want their ads to be placed next to editorial material. For that reason, some journals place popular editorial features (including news articles and correspondence) in the front and back of the journal to allow for ad interspersion and maintain an ad-free editorial well for the original research and other major articles. Ads should not appear on the journal's front cover or in the table of contents.

Ad Juxtaposition (Adjacency): Advertisers may request placement of their ads next to related editorial pages to help promote their products. Although commonly seen in consumer publishing, this practice is increasingly discouraged in scientific publishing.[3] Allowing ad juxtaposition may be an impediment to readers and it may diminish the perceived integrity of a scholarly publication.[2,9] To avoid the occurrence of ad juxtaposition, even by chance, the editors of *JAMA* review the entire makeup (imposition) of the journal after the ad deadlines have closed and before the journal is printed. If an ad is scheduled to appear next to an article on the same topic, the editors ask the production staff to move the ad or the article.

Editorial Calendars: Providing advertising sales representatives with editorial calendars of upcoming issues invites pressure for ad juxtaposition and even attempts from industry to interfere with editorial decisions. The ICMJE states that advertising should not be sold on the condition that it will appear in the same issue as a particular article.[13] Journal editors can respond to industry pressure by reminding advertisers of the importance of the journal's integrity.[3] Advertisers understand this issue, because without integrity, a publication will have few readers, and without readers, the advertiser cannot sell products. For this reason, advertising sales staff for *JAMA* do not see the journal's contents until after publication.

Appropriate Advertising Content: Appropriate ads must meet the following requirements[3,4,7,15]:

- No false claims
- No implied false claims
- No omissions of important facts
- Ability to substantiate claims
- Good taste (although this is not objectively defined)
- Clear identification of the advertiser of the product or services being offered
- Layout, artwork, and format that differ from those of the editorial content so that readers can clearly distinguish the advertising and editorial content

Biomedical journals typically publish disclaimers in an attempt to separate the claims made by advertisers from the views of the journals' owners. For example, AMA journals include the following in their mastheads:

> ADVERTISING PRINCIPLES—Advertisements in this issue have been reviewed to comply with the principles governing advertising in AMA publications. A copy of these principles is available on request. The appearance of advertising in AMA publications is

not an AMA guarantee or endorsement of the product or the claims made for the product by the manufacturer.

3.12.3 ***Advertorials.***—An advertorial is an ad that imitates editorial format. During the early 1990s, with the decline in the biomedical advertising market, advertorials became more common. The American Society of Magazine Editors developed guidelines for special advertising sections,[9] which may help a publication maintain its integrity if it publishes advertorials (see Table 10).

TABLE 10. GUIDELINES FOR SPECIAL ADVERTISING SECTIONS*

1. Each page of special advertising must be clearly and conspicuously identified as a message paid for by advertisers.
2. To identify special advertising sections clearly and conspicuously:
   A. The words *advertising, advertisement,* or *special advertising section* should appear prominently at or near the top of every page of such sections containing text, in type at least equal in size and weight to the publication's normal editorial body typeface. (The word *advertorial* should not be used.)
   B. The layout, design, and type of such sections should be distinctly different from the publication's normal layout, design, and typefaces.
   C. Special advertising sections should not be slugged on the publication's cover or included in the editorial table of contents.
   D. If the sponsor or organizer of the section is not the publisher, the sponsor should be clearly identified.
3. The editors' names and titles should not appear on, or be associated with, special advertising sections, nor should the names and titles of any other staff members of or regular contributors to the publication appear or be associated with special advertising sections. The publication's name or logo should not appear as any part of the headlines or text of such sections.
4. Editors and other editorial staff members should not prepare advertising sections for their own publication, for other publications in their field, or for advertisers in the fields they cover.
5. For the publication's chief editor to have the opportunity to monitor compliance with these guidelines, material for special advertising sections should be made available to the publication's editor in ample time to review and recommend necessary changes. Monitoring would include reading the text of special advertising sections *before* publication for problems of fact, interpretation, and taste and for compliance with any relevant laws.
6. To avoid potential conflicts or overlaps with editorial content, publishers should notify editors well in advance of their plans to run special advertising sections.
7. The size and number of special advertising sections within a single issue should not be out of balance with the size and nature of the magazine.

**Adapted and reprinted with permission from the American Society of Magazine Editors.[9] Copyright 1996, American Society of Magazine Editors.*

3.12.4 ***Sponsored Supplements.***—Sponsored supplements are collections of articles, usually on a single topic, published as an extra edition or a separate section of a journal, often after a meeting or symposium. Between 1960 and 1992, the number of supplements published by medical journals increased 4-fold.[16] Sponsored supplements tend to look like a regular issue of a journal, but many undergo a less rigorous form of peer review, if any at all, than the articles published in regular issues. Supplements are frequently sponsored by pharmaceutical companies, and they may have promotional attributes, such as misleading titles, focus on a single-drug topic, and use of brand names only.[16]

Supplements can, however, serve useful educational purposes, provided that the content is objective, balanced, independent, and scientifically rigorous.[17] Sponsored supplements also may provide additional revenue to publishers. Recognizing this, the ICMJE developed a set of principles to guide editors when considering the publication of sponsored supplements.[13] These principles should help avoid potential bias in the selection of content for inclusion in industry-sponsored publications:

- The journal editor must take full responsibility for policies, practices, and content of supplements. The journal editor must approve the appointment of any supplement editors and retain the authority to reject papers.
- The sources of funding for the research, meeting, and publication should be clearly stated and prominently displayed in the supplement, preferably on each page. Whenever possible, funding should come from more than 1 sponsor.
- Advertising in supplements should follow the same policies as in the rest of the journal.
- Editors should enable readers to distinguish readily between ordinary editorial pages and supplement pages.
- Editing by the funding organization or sponsor should not be permitted.
- Journal editors and supplement editors should not accept personal favors or excessive compensation from sponsors of supplements.

3.12.5 ***Advertising and Sponsorship in Digital Publications.***—The current standards for protecting editorial integrity of print publications apply to advertising in electronic publications and digital spinoff products, such as CD-ROM, Web sites, and online databases, especially for publications in clinical and health-related fields. For example, just as a print ad should not be placed next to a relevant editorial page, a digital ad should not be linked to editorial content that appears on a computer screen; and just as a print reader can choose to read an ad or skip over it, a computer user should have the same choice.

Digital ads are not restricted by the limits of a printed page. For example, a user can increase the type size of the prescribing information that appears in minitype in print pharmaceutical ads. Or an ad for a particular drug can have links to a professional version of the package insert and a version of the same information written for consumers. As the technology advances, digital advertising will provide additional opportunities and ethical dilemmas for publishers and editors.

The following rules were developed for use in AMA digital publications:

1. Digital advertisements must be readily distinguishable from editorial content.

2. Digital advertisements must be clearly labeled as such, perhaps with a prominent menu bar indicator or other consistent and readily recognizable on-screen message that identifies the content as advertising information.

3. Digital advertisements should not be juxtaposed with, appear inline or on screen with, frame, or be linked in any way with any related editorial content.

4. Digital advertisements should not appear on screen with or within the abstracts or text of major peer-reviewed scientific or clinical articles.

5. Digital advertisements, in the form of banner ads, can appear on screen with abstracts, news articles, and other editorial departments. These banner ads can be placed before or after individual abstracts; these ads can be placed before, after, and within news articles and other editorial departments. All such ads will be limited to 1 per screen.

6. Advertisements and promotional icons should not appear on the home screen (the initial screen or summary screen for a specific digital publication, which may be considered equivalent to the front cover of a print publication).

7. Advertisement banners and promotional icons may appear on the screen that contains the digital table of contents. Such ads should be limited to 1 per screen.

8. An advertising index with links to specific ads should be included as an entry in the digital table of contents menu.

9. Advertisements may not be linked to any non-AMA or commercial sites or material.

10. Digital advertisements should identify the nation or market for which the product or service advertised has been approved for marketing.

REFERENCES

1. Moser RH. Advertisements and our journal. *Ann Intern Med*. 1977;87:114-115.
2. Dixon T. Pharmaceutical advertising: information or influence? *Can Fam Phys*. 1993;39:1298-1300.
3. Chappell M. Editors and advertisers. *CBE Views*. 1994;17(5):79-80.
4. World Health Organization. *Ethical Criteria for Medicinal Drug Promotion*. Geneva, Switzerland: World Health Organization; 1988.
5. International Federation of Pharmaceutical Manufacturers Associations. *IFPMA Code of Pharmaceutical Marketing Practices*. Geneva, Switzerland: International Federation of Pharmaceutical Manufacturers Associations; 1994.
6. Kessler DA. Addressing the problem of misleading advertising. *Ann Intern Med*. 1992; 116:950-951.
7. Lexchin J, Holbrook A. Methodologic quality and relevance of references in pharmaceutical advertisements in a Canadian medical journal. *Can Med Assoc J*. 1994;151:47-54.
8. American Medical Association. *Principles Governing Advertising in Publications of the American Medical Association*. Chicago, Ill: American Medical Association; 1997.
9. American Society of Magazine Editors. *Guidelines for Special Advertising Sections*. 8th ed. New York, NY: American Society of Magazine Editors; July 1996.
10. Pitkin RM. Advertising in medical journals. *Obstet Gynecol*. 1989;74:667-679.
11. ASHP policy on the acceptance of advertising. *Am J Hosp Pharm*. 1992;49:160-161.
12. Rennie D. Editors and advertisements: what responsibility do editors have for the advertisements in their journals? *JAMA*. 1991;265:2394-2396.
13. International Committee of Medical Journal Editors. Advertising in medical journals and the use of supplements. *BMJ*. 1994;308:1692.
14. Rennie D, Bero LA. Throw it away, Sam: the controlled circulation journals. *CBE Views*. 1990;13(13):31-35.
15. Parmley WW. Has Madison Avenue become Medicine Avenue? *J Am Coll Cardiol*. 1994;23:1726-1727.
16. Bero LA, Galbraith A, Rennie D. The publication of sponsored symposiums in medical journals. *N Engl J Med*. 1992;327:1135-1140.
17. Kessler DA. Drug promotion and scientific exchange: the role of the clinical investigator. *N Engl J Med*. 1991;325:201-203.

Most people understand science and technology less through direct experience than through the filter of journalism. . . . Journalists are, in effect, brokers, framing social reality and shaping the public consciousness about science.

Dorothy Nelkin[1]

3.13 ■ RELATIONS WITH THE NEWS MEDIA.

■ RELATIONS WITH THE NEWS MEDIA.—The public is increasingly interested in matters of health, and its appetite for news about medicine and health seems insatiable. A 1993 telephone survey of 1250 US adults concluded that the majority of citizens consider news coverage of science to be as important as coverage of crime, the economy, politics, sports, and entertainment.[2] Numerous factors have changed science news journalism, including the increase in print publication and distribution costs; a concomitant decline in newspaper circulation and the disappearance of newspaper health and science sections; a dearth of investigative journalists trained as scientists and more coverage of science news by reporters who do not understand science; tabloid journalism; infotainment and infomercials; online news systems; new technology enabling the delivery of on-demand news to niche markets; and the increasingly competitive nature of the news business.[3-5]

Although many of these factors provide important opportunities, each threatens the ability of the news media to provide consistently accurate and reliable coverage of science news to the public. To gain a competitive edge in the information chain, news organizations are exchanging complexity, analysis, background, and a sense of perspective for a sense of immediacy and alarm.[6] Thus, the need for journal editors to develop and maintain viable relationships with news journalists—for all types of media—has become even more important. Journal editors have several responsibilities regarding the news media:

- Publish appropriate, accurate, reliable, timely, and accountable scientific information.
- Ensure that all journalists have equal access to the information published in the journal and the sources of that information (see 3.13.1, Release of Information to the Public).
- Inform authors of accepted manuscripts about journal policies regarding news coverage of their articles and embargoes (see 3.13.1, Release of Information to the Public).
- Evaluate the quality of news coverage of information published in the journal. For example, if a news organization has published an inaccurate report of a particular journal article, the journal editor should consider notifying the news editor of the errors in the report.

Journal editors and news journalists share a common obligation—to ensure that the public receives accurate information and is not misled.[6,7] This obligation becomes particularly important when information about risk is communicated to the public, because failure to describe health risks accurately and in proper perspective can cause undue anxiety and a loss of public trust in reporters, editors, and scientists. Tensions between journalists, editors, and scientists—often driven by self-interests—can do much to confuse the public. These tensions should be recognized and mitigated.[8] Rubin and Rogers'[7] study of the relationship between the news media and the medical community is worth reviewing. They surveyed a random sample of 4 populations: US physicians, the AMA House of Delegates, Associated Press managing editors, and the National Association of

Science Writers. From their survey findings, Rubin and Rogers determined the following:

- Physicians believe that reporters tend to sensationalize news about medicine and health care.
- Unlike reporters who cover politics or the government, reporters who cover health and medicine depend too much on press releases, do not conduct enough background research or interviewing, and often report technical details inaccurately.
- Television avoids covering complex medical topics.
- Journalists and physicians share responsibility for providing accurate information and not misleading the public.
- Editors of the leading medical journals are influential in determining which research is covered by the news media.

3.13.1 ***Release of Information to the Public.***—In many ways, biomedical journals and their editors act as gatekeepers for the release of scientific information to the public and to health professionals. However, conflicts often arise between editors (who have an ethical duty to ensure that the information they publish has been appropriately peer reviewed and assessed for quality) and authors (who want to disseminate their findings as widely and quickly as possible) and between editors and news reporters (who need to deliver information about new scientific developments to their readers as quickly as possible).[8] The announcement of "scientific breakthroughs" at press conferences or through press releases before the data that support the supposed advance have been evaluated and published in a peer-reviewed journal may cause problems for the media (who may give undue attention to an inaccurate or incomplete claim), for journal editors (who may have a policy that discourages publication of data that have already been reported in the press), and for investigators (who may forfeit their chance for publication in a reputable peer-reviewed journal by choosing to publish by press conference or through press releases).[9]

Journal editors have developed 2 policies to discourage premature release of information to the public. The first policy, based on the "Ingelfinger rule" (developed in 1969 by Franz Ingelfinger, MD, then editor of the *New England Journal of Medicine*), is an agreement extracted from authors by editors to avoid submission of a manuscript that has been submitted or reported elsewhere[10] (see 3.3, Duplicate Publication). The second policy is a news embargo (restricting news coverage of a journal article until it is published). Although some investigators and journalists disagree with the intent of both the Ingelfinger rule and the news embargo,[11,12] many journals have found that both, if applied consistently and fairly (with exceptions made in cases of public health urgency), serve well all communities interested in disseminating quality scientific information to the public.

3.13.2 ***Embargo.***—A news embargo is an agreement between editors and news reporters not to release information contained in a manuscript that has been accepted, but not yet published, until a specified date and time. For *JAMA,* this date and time is 3 PM Central time on the day before the journal's cover date. *JAMA* is printed and mailed 10 days before the cover date. During this time, the embargo is intended to provide competitive news reporters with an equal amount of time to research and prepare their news stories, and physicians can read pertinent journal articles before they are reported in the news media and before patients begin calling with questions after reading or viewing the news coverage. The AMA's monthly *Archives*

Journals share a common embargo date, usually the second or third Tuesday of each month, 3 PM Central time.

Embargo Waivers: Contrary to what many authors and news reporters believe, few findings from medical research have such significant and urgently important clinical implications for public health that the information should be released to the public before it has been reviewed and published in a journal. Calling such circumstances "exceptional," the International Committee of Medical Journal Editors (ICMJE) recommends that public health authorities should make such decisions and should be responsible for disseminating such information to health professionals and the media.[13] However, an editor may recognize the public health urgency of releasing information contained in a manuscript under consideration without prompting from the authors or relevant public health authorities. In such a case, the editor should ask the author to notify the appropriate authority to consider advance dissemination of the information. For example, recognizing that these policies and procedures may need to be waived in exceptional circumstances, the following policy was developed for AMA journals:

> In situations in which there is an immediate public health need for the information, there should be no delay in its release even if this release antedates AMA journal publication. It is the editor's responsibility to speed the peer review process and the publisher's responsibility to speed the production process for articles that have an immediate impact on patient care or disease prevention decisions.[14]

3.13.3 ***Instructions for Authors When Dealing With the News Media.***—The following guides for authors are adapted from recommendations made by the ICMJE[13] and Rubin and Rogers[7]:

- Authors should abide by agreements made with a journal not to publicize their work while their manuscript describing their work is under consideration or awaiting publication by a journal.[13]
- Authors presenting research at clinical and scientific meetings may discuss their presentations with reporters but should refrain from distributing copies of their presentations or data sheets (see 3.3, Duplicate Publication).
- Authors should inform editors of previous news coverage of their work at the time of manuscript submission[13] (see 3.3, Duplicate Publication).
- Authors should be as accessible to the media as their schedules permit, keeping reporters' deadlines in mind.[7]
- Authors who expect to be interviewed frequently by the media should have training in providing informative and accurate interviews.[7]
- Authors should establish an understanding with a reporter before the interview regarding comments on and off the record and the opportunity to review direct quotations.[7]
- Authors should inform reporters and news organizations of errors in news stories and request published corrections if necessary.[7]

In addition, journal editors should inform authors of accepted manuscripts of the journal's policies regarding relations with the news media. For example, *JAMA* reminds authors of its policies on duplicate publication and news embargoes in acceptance letters, noting that the news media should not release any information about the author's article until the specified embargo date and time. This embargo does not preclude authors from giving interviews to reporters who are preparing stories; it is meant to remind authors that any news stories resulting from such interviews should not precede publication of the authors' articles in the journal.

Some journals notify authors of projected publication dates in their acceptance letters, and some journals include a notice of the publication date on the typescript or page proof sent to authors for approval before publication. Editorial and publishing staff may also receive calls from authors requesting information about expected dates of publication. Staff and authors should not assume that such dates or their corresponding embargo dates are definite or final. Editors often rearrange the editorial content schedules of specific issues and thus, publication dates may change. When informing authors of the expected dates of publication for their accepted articles, editors should remind authors that these dates may change. Journals should include the phrase "tentative date" in all correspondence and on all typescripts and proofs seen by authors to avoid any confusion.

If authors want to coordinate media coverage of their published articles through a press conference or press release, they should first contact the journal editor to ascertain the exact date of publication. The ICMJE states that editors and publishers may want to help authors and representatives from their organizations coordinate press conferences and releases with the simultaneous publication of their articles.[13] Editors and publishers can also "help the media prepare accurate reports by providing news releases, answering questions, supplying advance copies of the journal, or referring reporters to the appropriate experts. This assistance should be contingent on the cooperation of the media in timing their release of stories to coincide with the publication of the article."[13] Advance copies of journals should be marked "Advance Copy," and such copies sent to members of the media should be marked or stamped with information about the date and time of embargo.

3.13.4 ***News Releases.***—The AMA issues press releases on selected important articles of interest to the public published in *JAMA* and the *Archives* Journals. Experienced science writers prepare the press releases after researching the articles and interviewing the authors and editor, if necessary. These releases are carefully written and reviewed, so that they may be used as a source for a news story; the AMA news releases contain key information on which to base an accurate report of a complicated or controversial medical study or opinion.

News editors, writers, and producers receive hundreds of press releases a week. Thus, a release must attract attention, but it also must conform to a familiar format and style. Table 11 contains a guide for press release format, some of which can serve for releases distributed via the Internet if the word *screen* is substituted for *page*.

News writers are taught to present facts accurately, but they may not know how to interpret biomedical statistics. Too often, statistics are cited carelessly and out of context to support an exaggerated medical claim.[15,16] To help prevent this, news writers must be provided with accurate and clearly stated statistics (see 17.1, Statistics, The Manuscript: Presenting Study Design, Rationale, and Statistical Analysis). Examples of common problems to avoid in news releases are listed below:

- Unfamiliar mathematical and statistical terms and incomprehensible numbers should be avoided.
- If the results of a survey are reported, the response rate should be provided along with a caveat that the results may not be generalizable if the response rate is low.
- Statements about statistical significance should not be quoted from an article out of context or without an explanation. Reporters and readers do not necessarily know the difference between statistical significance and clinical significance.

For example, quoting a statement that there was a trend toward a statistically significant association between treatment X and outcome Y may give undue importance to a treatment that has no real clinical value.

- If a press release mentions a specific sample that was studied or a specific number of cases, whether the number is large or small, information about the size of the total population from which the sample or cases were drawn should be included. For example, a press release about people who live near nuclear facilities in 107 counties stated that 900 000 cancer deaths were found. Unfortunately, the press release did not mention that the total combined population of these 107 counties was 19 million. Given the apparently large number of cancers reported, information about the size of the total population in which the cancers occurred helps put the findings in proper context.
- Care should be taken to avoid confusing absolute and relative risks. For example, a decrease from 2.5% to 2.0% should not be reported as a 20% reduction in risk.

Before press releases are distributed they should be proofread, and the content should be reviewed by a professional familiar with the article or report covered in the release, or by the editor.

TABLE 11. GUIDE FOR PRESS RELEASE FORMAT*

- Printed releases should be double-spaced and printed legibly on plain white paper with an identifying logo or letterhead.
- The name, address, telephone and fax numbers, and e-mail address and uniform resource locator (if available) of the releasing organization should be listed under the title "News Release" at the top of the page.
- The name, address, telephone and fax numbers, and e-mail address (if available) of the release contact person should be clearly identifiable.
- The release should be no longer than 1 to 2 pages (approximately 200-600 words). For releases that exceed 1 page, the word "—more—" should appear at the bottom of the first page.
- The time and date of the release and the embargo should appear prominently at the top of the first page.
- An easily identifiable headline (eg, boldface or underlined) that provides the essence of the release should also appear at the top of the first page.
- Before the lead sentence, the location of the release should appear in capital letters.
- The lead sentence should contain the most important information. Details should be given in later paragraphs. The name of the journal in which the article appeared should be included in the lead sentence to help facilitate mention of the journal in the story as a source of the information.
- Authors of the article should be clearly identified with complete names, academic degrees, and institutional affiliations.
- Releases should contain simple, declarative sentences and should avoid jargon and undefined abbreviations. All medical terms should be explained.
- All statistics and numbers should be properly explained and put in the proper context.

**Adapted from a handout developed by Bruce B. Dan, MD, 1989.*

REFERENCES

1. Nelkin D. Journalism and science: the creative tension. In: *Health Risks and the Press*. Washington, DC: Media Institute; 1989.

2. Science news: what does the public want: a survey by Lou Harris commissioned by SIPI. *SIPIscope*. 1993;20(2):1-10.

3. Hume E. *Tabloids, Talk Radio, and the Future of News: Technology's Impact on Journalism*. Washington, DC: Annenberg Washington Program; 1995.

4. Hard times hit science sections. *SIPIscope*. 1992;20(1):1-4.

5. Ethiel N, ed. *Medicine and the Media: A Changing Relationship*. Chicago, Ill: Robert R McCormick Tribune Foundation; 1995.

6. Garrett L. Reporting epidemics: real and unreal. Presented at the Institute of Medicine Annual Meeting: Emerging and Reemerging Infections; October 16, 1995; Washington, DC.

7. Rubin R, Rogers HL Jr. *Under the Microscope: The Relationship Between Physicians and the News Media*. Nashville, Tenn: Freedom Forum; 1993.

8. Glass RM, Flanagin A. Communication, biomedical II. scientific publication. In: Reich WT, ed. *Encyclopedia of Bioethics*. 2nd ed. New York, NY: Macmillan Publishing Co; 1995.

9. Butler D. "Publication by press conference" under fire. *Nature*. 1993;366:6.

10. Kassirer JP, Angell M. The Ingelfinger rule revisited. *N Engl J Med*. 1991;325:1371-1373.

11. Altman L. The Ingelfinger rule, embargoes, and journal peer review, part 1. *Lancet*. 1996;347:1382-1386.

12. Rosenberg S. Who's responsible to whom—and for what. In: Ethiel N, ed. *Medicine and the Media: A Changing Relationship*. Chicago, Ill: Robert R McCormick Tribune Foundation; 1994.

13. International Committee of Medical Journal Editors. Medical journals and the popular media. *N Engl J Med*. 1993;328:1283.

14. Lundberg GD, Glass RM, Joyce LE. Policy of AMA journals regarding release of information to the public. *JAMA*. 1991;265:400.

15. Hough GA. *News Writing*. 3rd ed. Boston, Mass: Houghton Mifflin Co; 1984.

16. Cohn V. *News and Numbers: A Guide to Reporting Statistical Claims and Controversies in Health and Related Fields*. Ames: Iowa State University Press; 1989.

CHAPTER 4

4.0 EDITORIAL ASSESSMENT AND PROCESSING

The principal goals of editing biomedical publications are to select, improve, and disseminate information that will advance the art and science of medicine to the eventual benefit of patients and the public health. Medical publications are a major source of information for the improvement of medical care. In addition to initial transmission to professionals at the time of publication, information from journal articles is often carried by the public media and can also be subsequently accessed by clinicians and researchers seeking information about particular topics. Published articles also influence educators and opinion leaders who transmit the information to many persons who do not read the original publications. These myriad uses of biomedical literature indicate the importance of the quality-improvement procedures involved in editorial assessment and processing.

4.1 ■ **EDITORIAL ASSESSMENT.**—The assessment process (Figure 1) consists of 2 phases: editorial review and peer review. In editorial review, editors first assess submissions for their overall quality and appropriateness for the publication's readership. Some manuscripts are rejected on the basis of this editorial "triage." Manuscripts that pass this initial step go on to the second phase. Peer review (see 4.1.3, Peer Review) involves evaluation by experts who are "peers" of the authors with regard to knowledge about the topic of the submission and may require evaluation by expert statistical reviewers (see 4.1.5, Statistical Review). The integrity of the editorial assessment process requires strict confidentiality (see 3.7.1, Ethical and Legal Considerations, Confidentiality in Peer Review).

4.1.1 ***Editorial Decisions.***—On the basis of evaluations by the editors and peer reviewers, manuscripts are either rejected or returned to authors with suggestions for improvement through revision. Authors should realize that a request for revision does not guarantee acceptance, because revised manuscripts are subject to editorial review and may also have additional peer review. Several rounds of review and revision may occur before a final decision is reached. Acceptance of articles of opinion may be based solely on editorial review, but reports of original data and other major articles almost always undergo peer review, statistical review, and revision before acceptance for publication (see 1.0, Types of Articles). Journals with more than 1 editor may hold meetings during which submissions and their

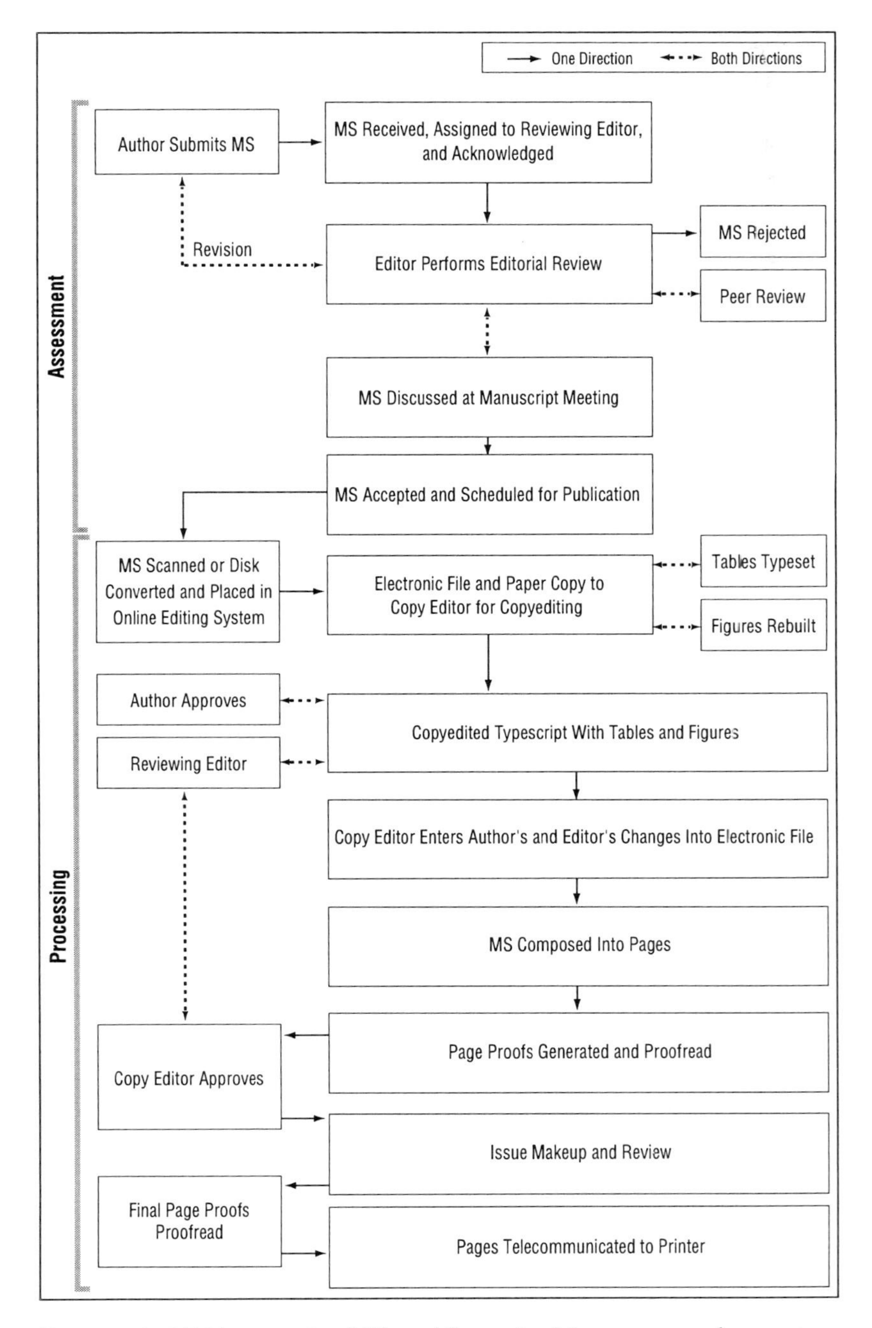

FIGURE 1 *JAMA* manuscript (MS) workflow: editorial assessment and processing.

reviews are discussed before decisions are reached regarding acceptance for publication.

The decisions for rejection, revision, and acceptance all belong to the editor, not the peer reviewers. The term *referee,* meaning a person to whom a paper is referred for review, is sometimes used synonymously with *peer reviewer*. However, in the United States *referee* can be misleading because that term often implies one who has authority for decisions. In medical publishing, editors have that responsibility, not peer reviewers, who have an important and helpful, but advisory, role.

4.1.2 ***Assessment Criteria.***—Two major criteria are central to the evaluation of manuscripts submitted for publication: importance and quality.

Importance involves an assessment of whether the work

- Represents a scientific advance (recognizing that individual articles usually convey only small advances)
- Has clinical relevance (if the journal is to be read and the information used by practicing clinicians)
- Presents new information
- Will be of interest to readers

An additional component of importance is *editorial priority,* a composite judgment made by the editor regarding the value of a particular submission relative to other submissions under evaluation at the same time, weighed in the context of the articles that journal has recently published and has scheduled for publication. The reality of limited page space is also a consideration, so short, concise papers may be given higher priority than long ones.

Evaluation of *quality* involves an assessment of how well a paper treats its topic, including how well the topic and the methods used to deal with that topic are described (see 17.1, Statistics, The Manuscript). For original research reports, assessment of quality involves consideration of whether

- The design and methods are appropriate to answer the stated research question
- The research question and the methods used to answer it are well described
- The data analysis is appropriate
- The conclusions are supported by the results
- Ethical problems exist in the ways patients or research subjects were dealt with (see 3.8, Ethical and Legal Considerations, Protecting Individuals' Rights in Scientific Publication)

The specific nature or direction of results should not be an issue in quality assessment. If a paper addresses an important question and uses high-quality methods to answer it, the results are worth publishing no matter what they are. Publication bias that results from a tendency for investigators not to submit, or editors not to accept, papers that do not report statistically significant "positive" results should be eliminated.[1] A well-done study that shows that a particular intervention is ineffective may be just as important as a study that reports a "positive" result.

4.1.3 ***Peer Review.***—Peer review was first used for biomedical publications by the Royal Societies of London and Edinburgh in the 18th century, but it evolved haphazardly and was not used consistently until after World War II.[2,3] The essence of peer review consists of asking experts: "How important and how good is this paper, and how can it be improved?" (see 4.1.2, Assessment Criteria). This use of expert consultants to advise editors about the selection and improvement of papers has become a standard quality-assessment measure in biomedical publication. Yet, the process and effectiveness of peer review have only recently come under scientific scrutiny.[4-6]

Experts in the topic of a paper are needed to assess importance and quality. However, peer review has been criticized for its reliance on human judgments that are subject to biases and conflicts of interest, and there have been few empirical documentations of the efficacy of the peer review process.[7-9] Empirical research on editorial peer review has just begun to address some of the deficiencies in knowledge about it. (See the March 9, 1990, and July 13, 1994, issues of *JAMA* for articles from the first 2 International Congresses on Peer Review in Biomedical Publication.)

Peer reviewers are usually asked to provide comments for the authors regarding the strengths and weaknesses of a paper, including suggestions for improvement. Reviewers also make recommendations to the editor, usually on a form provided by the journal (Figure 2), but specific criticisms and suggestions are more valuable than summary judgments.[7,10] It is remarkable that the peer review process depends largely on the efforts of peer reviewers who donate their time—sometimes large amounts of it.[11]

4.1.4 ***Selection of Reviewers.***—The selection of peer reviewers and the number of reviewers for a particular submission are matters of editorial judgment. Peer reviewers are selected by editors. The reviewers may be members of the editorial board, editorial staff, or a peer review panel, or they may have no other association with the journal. The editor's knowledge of experts in a particular field often determines reviewer selection. Many journals maintain a database of reviewers indexed by area of expertise and including information on review quality and turnaround time. A paper's reference list can be useful in indicating contributors to the literature on the same topic. A literature search by the editor can also be helpful in identifying potential reviewers.

Authors sometimes suggest names of possible reviewers and also may indicate persons they believe should not review their paper, usually because of perceived bias. Editors should consider such information, but the selection of reviewers belongs to the editor, who must use judgment in distinguishing valid praise or criticism from unwarranted bias for or against a particular submission. Reviewers should disclose to the editor any conflicts of interest they may have regarding a topic or an author (see 3.5.2, Ethical and Legal Considerations, Peer Reviewer's Disclosure).

4.1.5 ***Statistical Review.***—Reviewers with expertise in statistics (including the assessment of study design and research methods) are essential to evaluate the quality of original research reports. Such reviewers may serve as paid consultants to a journal. Empirical studies have shown that statistical review can be very helpful in selecting and improving scientific reports for publication.[12] Unfortunately, many published medical research articles are flawed by weaknesses in study design and methods that should have been detected by review or, far better, corrected by appropriate statistical consultation in planning the research before the manuscript was written.[13]

4.1.6 ***Concealing of Author and Reviewer Identities.***—Among the unsettled issues in peer review are efforts to conceal the identities of authors (and their affiliations) from reviewers, and the question of whether the identities of reviewers should be revealed to authors. Biomedical journals commonly use a "single-blind" review process in which authors' identities are revealed to reviewers, but the names of reviewers are not revealed to authors (see 3.7.1, Ethical and Legal Considerations, Confidentiality in Peer Review). This process recognizes the difficulty of concealing author identity, makes it easier for reviewers to detect attempts at duplicate publication by the same authors, and may encourage more candid reviews because

The Journal of the American Medical Association

Please make one copy for your files and return the original forms to the editorial office with the manuscript and original artwork. Page 1 will not be sent to authors, but it may be summarized or excerpted for them. If your comments are prepared on a word processor, you may print pages 2 and 3 on your own paper. Please provide 4 copies, if possible.

COMMENTS FOR EDITORIAL OFFICE

Manuscript Number ____________ Manuscript Classification ____________

Manuscript Title ____________

Author(s) ____________

Editor ____________

Date Sent to Reviewer ____________ **PLEASE RETURN BY** ____________

RECOMMENDATION

- ☐ Accept as is
- ☐ Accept if suitably revised
- ☐ Revise and reconsider
- ☐ Reject

QUALITY

- ☐ Superior
- ☐ Good
- ☐ Fair
- ☐ Poor

PUBLICATION TIMING

- ☐ Routine
- ☐ ASAP
- ☐ Fast track

PRIORITY

(Low) 1 2 3 4 5 (High)

CONSORTIUM MANUSCRIPT?

- ☐ *Arch Dermatol*
- ☐ *Arch Fam Med*
- ☐ *Arch Gen Psychiatry*
- ☐ *Arch Intern Med*
- ☐ *Arch Neurol*
- ☐ *Arch Ophthalmol*
- ☐ *Arch Otolaryngol Head Neck Surg*
- ☐ *Arch Pediatr Adolesc Med*
- ☐ *Arch Pathol Lab Med*
- ☐ *Arch Surg*

VALUE	YES	NO	UNCERTAIN	N/A
Material original?	☐	☐	☐	☐
Data valid?	☐	☐	☐	☐
Conclusions reasonable?	☐	☐	☐	☐
Information important?	☐	☐	☐	☐
Writing clear?	☐	☐	☐	☐
General medical interest?	☐	☐	☐	☐
Tables/figures appropriate? If not, explain.	☐	☐	☐	☐
Editorial needed?	☐	☐	☐	☐
If yes, I volunteer to write such, or I suggest ____________	☐	☐		

GENERAL COMMENTS FOR EDITOR

☐ **I disclose below my conflict(s) of interest in reviewing this manuscript.**

____

____

Reviewer Name ____________ *Reviewer Signature* ____________ *Date* ____________

PLEASE BEGIN YOUR GENERAL AND SPECIFIC COMMENTS TO AUTHOR ON PAGES 2 AND 3

FIGURE 2 *JAMA* peer reviewer comments form. N/A indicates not applicable.

the reviewers know they are anonymous to the authors, who may be their professional colleagues.

However, this single-blind tradition is controversial. Reviewers might be influenced by the identities and reputations of authors or their affiliations and thus not judge a manuscript solely on quality and importance. Furthermore, some critics believe that authors ought to know who is evaluating their work and that reviewers should stand by their critiques by signing them.[14,15]

Journal policies vary regarding concealing or revealing author and reviewer identities, but these practices should be indicated in the instructions for authors (see 3.11.6, Ethical and Legal Considerations, Editorial Responsibility for Peer Review). Authors who submit a paper to a journal that conceals author identities should remove identifying information from all parts of the manuscript. Author names, affiliations, and acknowledgments (including funding sources) should be submitted on a separate sheet of paper.

Few empirical studies of these issues have been published. One relevant finding is that attempts to conceal author identities are often not successful. Studies of medical journal peer review have found that reviewers accurately identified the authors in 27% to 46% of the masked submissions,[16-18] usually from self-references in the paper or knowledge of the authors' work. The latter is not surprising because the reviewers are experts in the authors' fields. Thus, "blind" review may not be so blind.

In a randomized trial of masking author identities, McNutt et al[16] reported that ratings of the quality of reviews tended to be higher for masked than unmasked reviews of the same 127 papers submitted to the *Journal of General Internal Medicine.* However, 27% of the reviewers of papers in which author identities were masked correctly identified authors, and the absolute differences in quality ratings were modest. In a large-scale "field trial," *The Canadian Medical Association Journal* in 1984 switched to concealing author identities but reversed this practice in 1990 after concluding that the time-consuming efforts to conceal author identities were often unsuccessful and did not improve the review process.[19]

Assessing the current status of peer review, Kassirer and Campion[10] concluded that "this fallible, poorly understood process has been indispensable for the progress of biomedical science." Further research on peer review is needed to increase our understanding and to evaluate and increase the quality of this improvement process.

4.1.7 ***Appealing a Rejection.***—If a paper is rejected, authors occasionally ask for reconsideration, usually because they believe the reviewers or the editor have misjudged the importance and quality of the submission. This situation can be viewed in 2 different ways. On the one hand, peer review and editorial decisions are based on fallible human judgments. Mistakes can be made, so perhaps the rejected manuscript merits reconsideration. On the other hand, heeding appeals for reconsideration may fulfill the adage "The squeaky wheel gets the grease." Reconsideration of papers on the basis of author complaints could be unfair to authors who have equally legitimate grounds for reconsideration but who do not appeal. Thus, some journals take the position that rejections are final. Other journals reconsider rejected submissions at the discretion of the editor who made the initial decision (see 3.11.2, Ethical and Legal Considerations, Editorial Responsibility for Rejection).

4.1.8 ***Postpublication Review.***—Evaluation does not end with publication. Postpublication review includes (1) letters to the editor that identify flaws or additional implications, (2) efforts to replicate the work, and (3) the experience of clinicians in applying the information in daily practice. Such evaluations are at least as important as prepublication review. Editors should also perform a quality review of each published issue of their journal, looking for problems in content and format that can be corrected or improved in subsequent issues (see 3.11.11, Ethical and Legal Considerations, Editorial Quality Review).

4.2 ■ **EDITORIAL PROCESSING.**—At the AMA, manuscript tracking and processing are performed electronically. Accepted manuscripts generally are received on disk and are entered into an online editing system by disk conversion, scanning of the typescript (see 2.0, Manuscript Preparation, Table 2, for specific guidelines), or keyboarding. After manuscripts have been edited and made into pages, they are transmitted electronically to the printer. Editorial and production staff track a manuscript's progress through the stages in the publishing process (Figure 1) by means of an online database.

4.2.1 ***Copyediting.***—After acceptance for publication, a manuscript is copyedited. The copy editor coordinates communication between the editor, author, and production staff. At the AMA, copy editors incorporate suggestions of the reviewing editor; correct grammar, spelling, and usage; query ambiguities and inconsistencies; verify mathematical calculations; and edit to AMA style. Tables and line art are also copyedited for style (see 2.13 and 2.14, Manuscript Preparation, Tables and Figures), accuracy, and consistency with the text and are then sent on to composition. Halftones and color figures are sized for position on the page by a production specialist. Technical deficiencies not resolved before acceptance (for instance, artwork that cannot be reproduced, values not converted to SI units, or lack of permission for material reprinted from another source) are also followed up and resolved by the copy editor. The copy editor sends the edited manuscript, with proposed additions and deletions clearly indicated (see 20.0, Copyediting and Proofreading Marks), as well as queries, along with a cover letter and the typeset art and tables, to the author for approval. After the author responds, the copy editor incorporates the author's changes. Any substantive changes requested by the author (eg, inclusion of additional case reports, requests for addition of figures or tables) are discussed with the reviewing editor, who then approves the copyedited typescript.

4.2.2 ***Composition and Page Makeup.***—Once the author's and reviewing editor's changes have been made, the manuscript is ready to be composed, or made into pages. Before the widespread use of electronic page makeup systems, galley proofs of typeset text in long columns were produced. A layout served as the model for the page, showing breaks (if any) in the title, type sizes and spacing in the text, and placement of tables, figures, and headings. The galley proofs were then cut and pasted along with the tables and art to make page proofs.

In an electronic composition system, codes must be inserted for each element (eg, title, byline) of an article according to journal style. At the AMA, the copy editor adds these codes to the electronic file. An electronic composition operator then pulls the text, tables, and art together in the electronic composition system and arranges these elements according to design and typographic specifications.

4.2.3 ***Proofreading.***—The page proofs are checked by a proofreader and by the copy editor. In a traditional publishing process, the proofreader checks the manuscript copy word for word against the typeset copy, alerting the copy editor to any discrepancies (see 20.0, Copyediting and Proofreading Marks). In electronic publishing, the role of the proofreader has changed and—in some cases—almost vanished; the proofreader may look only for line breaks and problems that arose through improper coding (eg, space problems or incorrect font) or page makeup (eg, misplaced blocks of type or improper line justification). In these cases, the copy editor, reviewing editor, and/or the author may perform the word-for-word reading once done by the proofreader. If the author has requested to see page proofs, the copy editor will send the author the proofread version. Revised page proofs are generated and checked by a proofreader.

4.2.4 ***Advertising.***—At the same time as the copyediting and composition of articles for an issue are proceeding, advertisements are scheduled for specific issues, and possibly for specific positions in an issue (eg, back cover or facing the table of contents). At the AMA, advertising is administratively separate from all editorial functions, an important separation in ensuring that there is no influence by an advertiser on an editorial decision. Staff members of the AMA responsible for issue makeup ensure that there is no inadvertent link between advertisements and articles—for instance, that no advertisement for an antihypertension medication appears next to a research report on hypertension. The AMA journals do not endorse commercial products and scrupulously avoid any editorial content or structure that could imply such an endorsement (see 3.12, Ethical and Legal Considerations, Advertisements, Advertorials, and Sponsored Supplements).

4.2.5 ***Issue Makeup and Review.***—For each journal issue, the production staff merges the editorial and the advertising material, numbers the pages, prepares the table of contents, and produces an imposition (a list that shows the sequential order of pages with placement of editorial and advertising content). For the AMA journals, the editorial content of each issue is determined by the journal editor, who considers the balance in types of articles and thematic consistency (eg, there might be several articles on related topics). The made-up issue is reviewed by editorial and production staff, and final editorial changes are incorporated. When final pages have been created, the electronic files are telecommunicated to the printer. The printer prepares photographic negatives for each page and returns final page proofs to the AMA. The production department reviews these final proofs to ensure that instructions have been followed. When all pages have been approved, the issue is printed, bound, and mailed.

4.2.6 ***Reprints.***—Authors have the option to purchase reprints of their articles. Reprints of AMA journal articles are mailed to the author approximately 6 weeks after the article appears in print. Reprints may also be sold to individuals, organizations, or companies interested in disseminating the article (see 3.6.9, Ethical and Legal Considerations, Standards for Commercial Reprints).

4.2.7 ***Corrections.***—Mistakes sometimes appear in print. Fortunately, authors or readers usually call them to the journal's attention, or they are found during the internal quality-review process, and corrections can be published. In *JAMA,* corrections are printed at the end of the Letters to the Editor section. Corrections should be indexed, with a cross-reference to the original article. This will enable online database services (such as MEDLINE) to link indexed articles with published corrections (see 3.11.8, Ethical and Legal Considerations, The Role of the Correspondence Column and Corrections).

4.2.8 ***Index.***—Indexes organized by subject and author's surname are published regularly in most medical journals. At *JAMA,* indexes created by indexing software that searches articles for key words appear at the end of each volume, in the last issues of June and December.

ACKNOWLEDGMENT

Principal author: Richard M. Glass, MD

REFERENCES

1. Chalmers TC, Frank CS, Reitman D. Minimizing the three stages of publication bias. *JAMA.* 1990;263:1392-1395.
2. Kronick DA. Peer review in 18th-century scientific journalism. *JAMA.* 1990;263:1321-1322.
3. Burnham JC. The evolution of editorial peer review. *JAMA.* 1990;263:1323-1329.
4. Rennie D. Guarding the guardians: a conference on editorial peer review. *JAMA.* 1986;256:2391-2392.
5. Lock S. *A Difficult Balance: Editorial Peer Review in Medicine.* Philadelphia, Pa: ISI Press; 1988.
6. Rennie D. Editorial peer review in biomedical publication: The First International Congress. *JAMA.* 1990;263:1317.
7. Goodman SN, Berlin J, Fletcher SW, Fletcher RH. Manuscript quality before and after peer review and editing at *Annals of Internal Medicine. Ann Intern Med.* 1994;121:11-21.
8. Lock S. Does editorial peer review work? *Ann Intern Med.* 1994;121:60-61.
9. Pierie J-PEN, Walvoort HC, Overbeke AJPM. Readers' evaluation of effect of peer review and editing on quality of articles in the *Nederlands Tijdschrift voor Geneeskunde. Lancet.* 1996;348:1480-1483.
10. Kassirer JP, Campion EW. Peer review: crude and understudied, but indispensable. *JAMA.* 1994;272:96-97.
11. Yankauer A. Who are the peer reviewers and how much do they review? *JAMA.* 1990;263:1338-1340.
12. Gardner MJ, Bond J. An exploratory study of statistical assessment of papers published in the *British Medical Journal. JAMA.* 1990;263:1355-1357.
13. Altman DG. The scandal of poor medical research. *BMJ.* 1994;308:283-284.
14. Fabiato A. Anonymity of reviewers. *Cardiovasc Res.* 1994;28:1134-1139.
15. DeBakey L. Journal peer reviewing: anonymity or disclosure? *Arch Ophthalmol.* 1990;108:345-349.
16. McNutt RA, Evans AT, Fletcher RH, Fletcher SW. The effects of blinding on the quality of peer review: a randomized trial. *JAMA.* 1990;263:1371-1376.
17. Yankauer A. How blind is blind review? *Am J Public Health.* 1991;81:843-845.
18. Fisher M, Friedman SB, Strauss B. The effects of blinding on acceptance of research papers by peer review. *JAMA.* 1994;274:143-146.
19. Squires B. Editor's page: blinding the reviewers. *Can Med Assoc J.* 1990;142:279.

STYLE

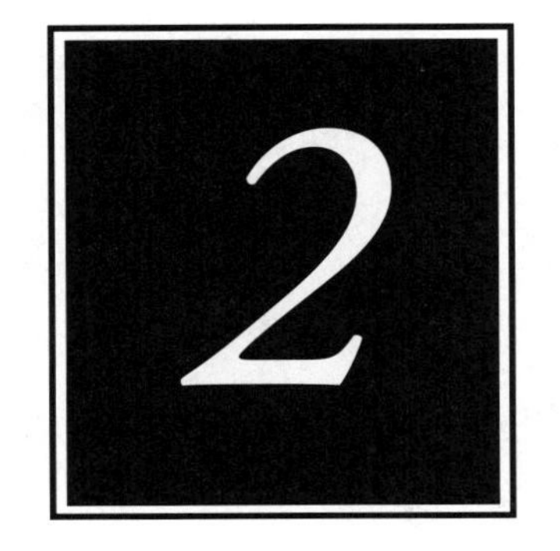

CHAPTER 5

5.0 GRAMMAR

A clear understanding of grammar is basic to good writing. Many excellent grammar books provide a detailed discussion of specific principles (see 22.1, Resources, Readings). In this section, the focus is on how to avoid common grammatical errors.

5.1 ■ **THE SENTENCE.**—A sentence must have at minimum a subject and a verb; it usually contains modifiers as well. Sentence fragments, which omit a subject or a verb, should not be used in scientific or technical writing (except for within the structured abstract; see 2.5, Manuscript Preparation, Abstract). Occasionally, writers of prose and poetry use sentence fragments intentionally, for effect:

> Dogs, undistinguishable in mire. Horses, scarcely better; splashed to their very blinkers. (Dickens, *Bleak House*)

> Her affect signaled depression. Utter depression.

In scientific writing, these fragments are likely to be unintentional and are definitely inappropriate:

> The clinical spectrum of disease varying according to the population and age group under study.

5.2 ■ **THE PARAGRAPH.**—A paragraph is a cohesive group of sentences (or, occasionally, a single sentence), one that presents a thought or several related thoughts. Each paragraph should be long enough to stand alone but short enough to hold the reader's attention and then direct that attention to the next thought.

5.3 ■ **PUNCTUATION.**—Punctuation is an important element of sentence composition and helps convey meaning by indicating groupings, divisions, pauses, and tone (see 6.0, Punctuation, for specific punctuation marks). When punctuation is incorrectly placed or omitted, the reader is given unclear signals or no signals at all.

5.4 ■ **MODIFIERS.**—Words, phrases, and clauses may all be modifiers. An adjective modifies a noun or a pronoun. An adverb modifies a verb, an adjective, another adverb, or a clause. A phrase is a group of words without a subject or predicate, usually introduced by a preposition or conjunction. A clause is a group of words with a subject and predicate within a compound or complex sentence. Clauses or phrases may serve as adjectives or adverbs.

5.4.1 ***Misplaced Modifiers.***—Misplaced modifiers result from failure to make clear what is being modified. Illogical or ambiguous placement of a word or phrase can usually be avoided by placing the modifying word or phrase appropriately close to the word it modifies.

Unclear: Dr Young treated the patients **using antidepressants.** [Who used the antidepressants? Ambiguity makes 2 meanings possible.]
Better: Dr Young treated the patients with antidepressants. *Or* [alternative meaning]: Dr Young treated the patients who were using antidepressants.

Unclear: The patient was referred to a specialist **with a severe bipolar disorder.** [Who had the bipolar disorder?]
Better: The patient with a severe bipolar disorder was referred to a specialist.

Use of the word *only* as a modifier poses particular problems. It must be placed immediately before the word or phrase it modifies for the meaning to be clear. Note the different meanings achieved depending on placement in the examples below:

Only medication can ease the pain.

Medication can **only** ease the pain.

Medication can ease **only** the pain.

5.4.2 ***Verbal Phrase Danglers.***—A participle is a verb form used as an adjective. A dangling participle implies an actor but does not specify who or what that actor is. The following examples of dangling participles illustrate the problem:

Avoid: **Organized into 13 chapters,** the reader of this book will benefit from an extensive appendix. [The participle appears to refer to "the reader"; however, it is the *book* that is organized into 13 chapters.]
Better: The reader of this 13-chapter book will benefit from its extensive appendix.
Or: Because this book is organized into 13 chapters, the reader will benefit from its extensive appendix.

Avoid: **Based on my experience,** English majors make excellent copy editors. [Are the English majors "based on my experience"? Of course not. It is the statement *about* the English majors that is based on the writer's experience.]
Better: I have found that English majors make excellent copy editors.
Or: Experience has shown that English majors make excellent copy editors.

A gerund is a verb form used as a noun. Like the dangling participle, the dangling gerund implies an actor but does not specify who or what that actor is.

Avoid: Dietary therapy slows the return of hypertension **after stopping long-term medical therapy.** [This states that dietary therapy not only slows the return of hypertension but also stops prolonged medical therapy.]

Better: Dietary therapy slows the return of hypertension after cessation of long-term medical therapy.

Or: After cessation of long-term medical therapy, dietary therapy slows the return of hypertension.

Avoid: **Before initiating an exercise program or engaging in heavy physical labor after a myocardial infarction,** a physician should review the exercise program carefully. [''A physician'' is erroneously implied to be the actor, the one initiating an exercise program or engaging in heavy physical labor.]

Better: Anyone about to initiate an exercise program or engage in heavy physical labor after a myocardial infarction should first consult a physician.

5.5 ■ PARALLEL CONSTRUCTION.

5.5 ■ PARALLEL CONSTRUCTION.—One device used to build a sentence or emphasize a point is parallel construction.

5.5.1 ***Correlative Conjunctions.***—This device may rely on accepted cues (either/or, neither/nor, not only/but also, both/and). In this usage, the correlative conjunctions are often misplaced. All elements of the parallelism that appear on one side of the coordinating conjunction should match corresponding elements on the other side.

Avoid: The compleat physician has **not only** mastered the science of medicine **but also** its art.

Correct: The compleat physician has mastered **not only** the science of medicine **but also** its art.

Avoid: Poor drug efficacy may be caused by **either** lack of absorption **or** by increased clearance.

Correct: Poor drug efficacy may be caused **either** by lack of absorption **or** by increased clearance.

Also correct: Poor drug efficacy may be caused by **either** lack of absorption **or** increased clearance.

Avoid: Three patients **either** took their medication incorrectly **or** not at all.

Correct: Three patients took their medication **either** incorrectly **or** not at all.

5.5.2 ***In Series or Comparisons.***—Parallel construction may also present a series or make comparisons. In these usages, the elements of the series or of the comparison should be parallel structures, ie, nouns with nouns, prepositional phrases with prepositional phrases.

Avoid: The text was written for residents, interns, and to help them teach their students.

Correct: The text was written to educate residents and interns and to help them teach their students.

Avoid: When an operation is designed to improve function rather than extirpation of an organ, surgical technique becomes paramount.

Correct: When an operation is designed to improve the function of an organ rather than to extirpate the organ, surgical technique becomes paramount.

Avoid: There was a long delay between the purchase of a magnetic resonance imager and when it started to be widely used.

Correct: There was a long delay between the purchase of a magnetic resonance imager and its widespread use.

Note: Using *either* or *neither* with more than 2 items is incorrect.

Incorrect: This medication can be used under either makeup, sunscreens, or moisturizers.

Correct: This medication can be used under makeup, sunscreens, or moisturizers.

Also: Avoid the use of *nor* when the first negative is expressed by *not* or *no*.

Fetuses with congenital diaphragmatic hernia who were stillborn would not have been included in this study or [not *nor*] in many previously published studies.

However, in a sentence that contains 2 independent clauses in which the negation implied by *not* is also carried over into the second element, note the inversion of the subject and the verb in the second independent clause, introduced by *nor*.

Fetuses with congenital diaphragmatic hernia who were stillborn would not have been included in this study, nor would they have been included in many previously published studies.

5.5.3 ***Lists.***—Parallel construction is also important in constructing lists, whether run in or set off by bullets or some other device (see 6.2.2, Semicolon, Enumerations, and 16.5, Numbers and Percentages, Enumerations).

5.6 ■ NOUNS.—Nouns may serve as subjects or objects.

5.6.1 ***As Modifiers (Noun Strings).***—Although in English, nouns are used as modifiers, overuse can lead to a lack of clarity. Purists may demand stricter rules on usage, but, as with the use of nouns as verbs (see 9.3, Correct and Preferred Usage, Back-formations), the process of linguistic change is inevitable, and grammatical rigor must be tempered by judgment and common sense.

Avoid	*Preferred*
diabetes patient	patient with diabetes, diabetic patient
depression episode	depressive episode, episode of depression
elderly over-the-counter drug users	elderly users of over-the-counter drugs

Bernstein,[1] in *The Careful Writer,* advises the use of no more than 2 polysyllabic modifiers per noun for the sake of clarity; however, long noun strings are sometimes difficult to avoid, and if several of the attributive nouns are read as a unit, the use of more than 2 may not compromise clarity, especially in scientific or technical communications. Thus, noun strings may be more acceptable, for the sake of brevity, if the terms have been previously defined without noun strings in the text. Some acceptable examples appear below:

community hospital program

physician provider organization

risk factor surveillance system

baseline CD4 cell counts

sudden infant death syndrome

nicotine replacement program

placebo pain medication

proficiency testing program

very low birth weight

randomized clinical trial

right ventricular ejection fraction

If there is a possibility of ambiguity, hyphens may be added for clarity (see 6.3.1, Punctuation, Hyphen, Temporary Compounds).

5.6.2 ***Modifying Gerunds.***—When a noun or pronoun precedes a gerund (a verb form ending in *-ing* that is used as a noun), the noun or pronoun takes the possessive (see also 6.7, Punctuation, Apostrophe).

> The toxicity of the drug was not a factor in the patient's dying so suddenly.

Present participles (used adjectivally) should not be confused with gerunds. In the sentence below, the objective case (*them*) is correct.

> I watched them gathering in the auditorium.

If the possessive *their* were used instead of the objective *them,* the action (gathering in the auditorium) would be emphasized, rather than the word that precedes the *-ing* word.

5.6.3 ***Referring to Time or Money.***—Nouns that refer to time or money, when used as adjectives, also take the possessive (see also 6.7.6, Punctuation, Units of Time and Money as Possessive Adjectives).

> After 2 months' therapy, the child's condition improved. [*But,* equally acceptable: After 2 months of therapy, the child's condition improved.]

> This equipment represents many thousands of dollars' worth of our annual budget.

This does not apply when the word modified is not a noun but an adjective. For example, no apostrophe should appear in "6 months pregnant" or "2 hours late."

5.7 ■ **PRONOUNS.**—Pronouns replace nouns. In this replacement, the antecedent must be clear and the pronoun must agree with the antecedent in both number and gender.

Avoid: The authors unravel the process of gathering information about diethylstilbestrol and disseminating **it.** [Antecedent unclear; does *it* refer to information or to diethylstilbestrol?]
Correct: The authors unravel the process of gathering and disseminating information about diethylstilbestrol.

Avoid: A survey was given to each medical student and **their** spouses. [Disagreement of pronoun with referent in number. The referent is *each medical student* (singular), but the pronoun used is plural (*their spouses*).]
Better: A survey was given to the medical students and their spouses.

Also, animate pronouns should not be mixed with inanimate nouns:

Avoid: The American Medical Association is having **their** annual meeting in June in Chicago, Ill.
Better: The American Medical Association is having **its** annual meeting in June in Chicago, Ill.

5.7.1 ***Personal Pronouns.***—Care must be taken with personal pronouns to use the correct case, subjective (the pronoun is the subject of the sentence) or objective (the pronoun is the object of the sentence). Difficulty often arises when pronouns are used after prepositions or after forms of the verb *to be*. Below are several examples of correct usage:

> Give the award to **whomever** you prefer. [Objective case: *whomever* is the object of the verb *prefer*.]
> Give the award to **whoever** will benefit most. [Subjective case: *whoever* is the subject of *will benefit*.]
>
> **Whom** did you consult? [Objective case: *whom* is the object of *consult*.]
> **Who** was the consultant on this case? [Subjective case: *who* is the subject of the sentence.]
>
> He is one of the patients **whom** Dr Rundle is treating. [Objective case: *whom* is the object of *is treating*.]
> He is one of the patients **who** are receiving the placebo. [Subjective case: *who* is the subject of *are receiving*.]

Do not use reflexive pronouns, those ending in *-self* or *-selves,* as subjects.

> *Wrong:* George, Patricia, and **myself** attended the lecture.
> *Correct:* George, Patricia, and **I** attended the lecture.

Note: It's and *its* are frequently erroneously interchanged. *It's* is the contraction of *it is,* and *its* is the possessive form of the pronoun *it* (see also 6.7, Punctuation, Apostrophe, and 5.8.6, Contractions).

5.7.2 ***Relative Pronouns.***—Relative pronouns may be used in subordinate clauses to refer to previous nouns. The word *that* introduces a *restrictive* clause, one that is essential to the meaning of the sentence. The word *which* introduces a *nonrestrictive* clause, one that adds more information but is not essential to the meaning. Clauses that begin with *which* are preceded by commas. Two examples of correct usage follow:

> Jimmy Carter is profiled in the 1993 Hiroshima issue of *JAMA,* **which** focuses on humanitarian aid during war and disaster. [**Nonrestrictive;** there was only one 1993 Hiroshima issue of *JAMA,* not one containing the profile of Jimmy Carter and one or more without this profile.]
>
> The issue of *JAMA* **that** contained the profile of Jimmy Carter was the 1993 Hiroshima issue. [**Restrictive;** there are thousands of issues of *JAMA*.]

A few examples of ambiguous or incorrect usage are shown below to highlight this grammatical problem:

> *Incorrect:* The high prevalence of antibodies to the 3 *Bartonella* species, **which** were examined in the present study, indicates that health care workers should be alert to possible infection with any of these organisms when treating intravenous drug users. [There are more than 3 species of *Bartonella*. Hence, the correct form here would be "the 3 *Bartonella* species **that** were examined."]
>
> *Ambiguous:* Many reports have been based on series of patients from urology practices **that** may not fully reflect the entire spectrum of illness. [Is it that urology practices *in general* may not reflect the entire spectrum of illness? If so, the correct expression is "urology practices, **which.**" If only *some* urology practices do not reflect the entire spectrum of illness, it is correct as it stands.]

Note: The omission of *that* to introduce a clause may cause difficulty in comprehension.

Avoid: This morning he revealed evidence that calls the breast cancer study's integrity into question has been verified.

Better: This morning he revealed **that** evidence has been verified that calls the breast cancer study's integrity into question.

The addition of *that* after *revealed* frees the reader from backtracking to uncover the meaning of the sentence. The use of *that* to introduce a clause is particularly helpful when the second verb appears long after the first has been introduced (above, the interval between *revealed* and *has been verified*).

Note: Although it is important to maintain these distinctions, the use of *which* in place of *that* is sometimes desirable to prevent a "that that" construction.

We often have time to do only that **which** [not *that*] is essential.

5.8 ■ **VERBS.**—Verbs express an action, an occurrence, or a mode of being. They have voice, mood, and tense.

5.8.1 ***Voice.***—In the active voice, the subject does the acting; in the passive voice, the subject is acted on. In general, the active voice is preferred, except in instances in which the actor is unknown or the interest concerns what is acted on (as in the following example of passive voice).

The 45-year-old man had been shot in the abdomen and within 10 minutes was brought to the emergency department.

If the actor is mentioned in the sentence, the use of the active is preferred over the passive.

Avoid: Data were collected from 5000 patients by physicians.

Better: Physicians collected data from 5000 patients.

5.8.2 ***Mood.***—Verbs may have 1 of 3 moods: the indicative (the most common; used for ordinary objective statements), the imperative (used for requesting or commanding), and the subjunctive. Subjunctive verbs cause the most difficulty. The subjunctive is now used primarily for expressing a wish (I wish it were *possible*), a supposition (If I *were* to accept the position, . . .), or a condition contrary to fact (If I *were* younger, . . .). The subjunctive occurs in fairly formal situations and usually involves past (*were*) or present (*be*) forms.

Past form: If we **were** to begin treatment immediately, the patient's prognosis would be excellent.

Present form: The patient insisted that she *be* treated immediately so that her prognosis would be excellent.

The subjunctive is sometimes used incorrectly, eg, where matters of fact—not supposition—are discussed. In the following examples, the indicative, not the subjunctive, is correct.

Therefore, we determined whether there **had been** [not the subjunctive, *were*] a tendency to deviate from the prescribed regimen.

We investigated whether his fractured leg **had been** [not the subjunctive, *were*] set incorrectly.

5.8.3 ***Tense.***—Tense indicates the time relation of a verb: present (*I am*), past (*I was*), future (*I will be*), present perfect (*I have been*), past perfect (*I had been*), and future perfect (*I will have been*). Choose the verb that expresses the time that is intended. It is equally important to maintain uniformity of tense. In scholarly writing, the choice of tense for referral to published papers is sometimes difficult.

The present tense is used to express a general truth, a statement of fact, something continuingly true.

> I didn't know that Pb **stands** [not *stood*] for lead.

For this reason, the present tense is often used to refer to recently published work, indicating that it is still valid.

> Kilgallen's assay results **demonstrate** the highest recorded sensitivity and specificity to date.

The present perfect may be used to refer to a report published in the recent past that continues to have intellectual importance.[2]

> Kaplan and Rose **have described** this phenomenon.

In a biomedical article, the past tense is often used to refer to the results of the study being described:

> Group 1 **had** a seropositivity rate of 50%.

> We examined him after he **was** bitten by a rat.

The past tense is also used to refer to a paper published months or years ago that is now primarily of historical value. Frequently, a date will be used in such a reference.[2]

> In their 1985 article, Northrup and Miller **reported** a high rate of mortality among children younger than 5 years.

In general, tense must be used consistently:

> *Incorrect:* There **were** no false negatives in group 1, but there **are** 3 in group 2.

However, tense may vary in a single article, as dictated by context and judgment.

> We **examined** the type of news more viewers **are** likely to watch and consider credible.

Alternatively, the past tense and the present tense may be used in the same sentence to place 2 things in temporal context:

> Although the previous report **demonstrated** a significant response, the follow-up study **does** not.

Even when tenses are mixed, however, consistency is still the rule:

> *Incorrect:* I found it difficult to accept Dr Smith's contention in chapter 3 that the new agonist **has** superior pharmacokinetics and **was** therefore more widely used.
>
> *Correct:* I found it difficult to accept Dr Smith's contention in chapter 3 that the new agonist **has** superior pharmacokinetics and **is** therefore more widely used.

5.8.4 ***Double Negatives.***—Two negatives used together constitute a double negative. The use of a double negative to express a positive is acceptable, although it yields a weaker affirmative than the simpler positive.

> Our results are **not inconsistent** with the null hypothesis.

> More direct incentives have produced substantial changes in behavior in the past, although **not without** adverse consequences.

> Rheumatologic complaints were **not uncommon** in both groups.

When the double negative is used to reinforce the negative, however, it is not grammatically acceptable, and, as in the example below, the double negative conveys the opposite of what is intended.

Incorrect: I **can't hardly** keep penicillin in stock.

Because a double negative often causes the reader to go back and reread the sentence to make sure of the meaning, it is best used with care or avoided.

5.8.5 ***Split Infinitives.***—Although some authorities may still advise the avoidance of split infinitives, this proscription—a holdover from Latin grammar, wherein the infinitive is a single word and cannot be split—has been relaxed. In some cases, moreover, clarity is better served by the split infinitive.

Ambiguous: Don vowed **to promote** exercising vigorously. [Is it the exercising or the promotion of exercising that is vigorous?]
Clearer: Don vowed **to** vigorously **promote** exercising.
Or: Don vowed **to promote** vigorous exercise.

5.8.6 ***Contractions.***—A contraction consists of 2 words combined into 1 by omitting 1 or more letters (eg, *can't, aren't*). An apostrophe shows where the omission has occurred. Contractions are usually avoided in formal writing (see also 5.7.1, Personal Pronouns).

5.9 ■ **SUBJECT-VERB AGREEMENT.**—The subject and verb must agree; use a singular subject with a singular verb and a plural subject with a plural verb. Unfortunately, this simple rule is often violated. The guidelines outlined below will help ensure proper usage.

5.9.1 ***Intervening Phrase.***—Plural nouns take plural verbs and singular nouns take singular verbs, even if a plural phrase follows the subject.

A **review** of all patients with grade 3 tumors **was** undertaken in the university hospital. [Remember, the subject in this sentence is *review.* Ignore all modifying prepositional phrases that follow a noun when determining verb agreement.]

If the intervening phrase is introduced by *together with, as well as, along with, in addition to,* or similar phrases, the singular verb is preferred if the subject is singular, as the intervening phrase does not affect the singularity of the subject.

The **editor,** as well as the reviewers, **believes** that this article is ready for acceptance.

The **patient,** together with her physician and her family, **makes** this decision.

Liver **failure,** in addition to massive hepatic enlargement and severe macrovesicular steatosis, **was** not described in HIV-positive patients before the cases reported in September 1990.

5.9.2 ***False Singulars.***—A few nouns are used so often in the plural that many have come to use the plural with a singular noun. Frequently treated erroneously in this way are the plurals *criteria, phenomena,* and *memoranda*. The distinction between singular and plural, however, should be retained; when the singular is intended, use *criterion, phenomenon,* and *memorandum*.

The treatment of the word *agenda* as a singular, however, has become acceptable.[3]

The **agenda has** been set for our next meeting.

Also, many now consider acceptable the use of *data* as a singular.[3] In this usage, *data* is thought of as a collective noun and, when considered as a unit rather than as the individual items of data that compose it, it takes the singular verb. AMA's preference, however, is to retain the use of the plural verb with *data* in all situations.

Very few **data were** [not *very little data was*] available to support our hypothesis.

The word *media* in the sense of communications media is becoming acceptable in this collective usage, although its use in this sense has not yet reached the acceptability that *agenda* has gained and *data* is close to gaining.[3] In the sense of laboratory culture media, *medium* should be used for the singular and *media* for the plural. In the sense of communications media, AMA prefers to retain the distinction between singular and plural.

Singular: Each news **medium shapes** journalism to its own constraints.
Plural: The **media give** great attention to the managed care debate. [Here *media* refers to television and newspaper coverage.]

5.9.3 ***False Plurals.***—Some nouns, by virtue of ending in a "plural" *-s* form, are mistakenly taken to be plurals even though they should be treated as singular and take a singular verb (eg, *measles, mumps, mathematics, genetics*).

5.9.4 ***Parenthetical Plurals.***—When *-s* or *-es* is added parenthetically to a word to express the possibility of a plural, the verb should be singular. However, in most instances it is preferable to avoid this construction and change to the plural noun.

The **name(s)** of the editor(s) of the book in reference 2 **is** unknown.

5.9.5 ***Collective Nouns.***—A collective noun is one that names more than 1 person, place, or thing (see also 5.9.11, Number). When the group is regarded as a unit, the singular verb is the appropriate choice:

The **couple has** a practice in rural Montana. [*Couple* is considered a unit here and so takes the singular verb.]

Twenty percent of her time **is** spent on administration. [*Twenty percent* is thought of as a unit, not as 20 individual units, and so takes the singular verb.]

The paramedic **crew responds** to these emergency calls. [*Crew* is thought of as a unit here and so takes the singular verb.]

When the individual members of the pair or group are emphasized, rather than the group as a whole, the plural verb is correct:

The **couple are** both family physicians. [*Couple* is thought of as the 2 individuals who constitute the couple, not as a unit, and so takes the plural verb.]

Ten percent of the staff **work** flexible hours. [*Ten percent* is thought of as being composed of each individual staff member, not as a unit, and so takes the plural verb.]

The surgical **faculty were** from all over the country. [*Faculty* here refers to the individual members of the faculty, rather than to the faculty as a group, and so takes the plural verb.]

The use of a phrase such as "the members of" may make this last example less jarring.

The **members** of the surgical faculty **were** from all over the country.

5.9.6 ***Compound Subject.***—When 2 words or 2 groups of words, usually joined by *and* or *or,* are the subject of the sentence, the singular or plural verb form may be appropriate, depending on whether the words joined are singular or plural and on the connectors used.

Compound subject joined by and: With *and,* a plural verb is usually preferable. A singular verb should be used if the 2 elements are thought of as a unit (bread and butter, dilation and curettage) or refer to the same person (our friend and host) or thing (vocation and avocation).

Compound subject joined by or *or* nor: With a compound subject joined by *or* or *nor,* the plural verb is correct if both elements are plural; if both elements are singular, the singular verb is correct. When one is singular and one is plural, the verb form that agrees with the closer noun is the better choice.

Both plural:	Neither staphylococci nor streptococci **were** responsible for the infection.
Both singular:	Neither a false-positive test nor a false-negative test **is** a definitive result.
Mixed:	Neither the hospital nor the physicians **were** responsible for the loss.

5.9.7 ***Shift in Number of Subject and Resultant Subject-Verb Disagreement.***—In elliptical constructions involving the verb, ie, when a verb is omitted as understood, if the number of the subject changes, the construction may be incorrect.

Incorrect:	Her tests **were** run and her chart updated.
Correct:	Her tests **were** run and her chart **was** updated.

Incorrect:	The diagnosis **was** made and physical therapy sessions begun.
Correct:	The diagnosis **was** made and physical therapy sessions **were** begun.
Or:	The diagnosis **was** made and physical therapy begun.

5.9.8 ***Subject and Predicate Nominative Differ in Number.***—When the subject and the predicate nominative differ in number, follow the number of the *subject* in selecting the singular or plural verb form.

Incorrect:	The most significant **factor** that affected the study results **were** interhospital variations in severity of illness.
Correct:	The most significant **factor** that affected the study results **was** interhospital variations in severity of illness.

Avoid this by rephrasing:

Study **results were** most affected by interhospital variations in severity of illness.

5.9.9 ***Every/Many a.***—When *every* or *many a* is used before a word or series of words, use the singular verb form.

Many a clinician **does** not understand statistics.

Every resident **has** such encounters with patients.

Better yet: Many clinicians do not understand statistics.

5.9.10 ***One of Those.***—In clauses that follow *one of those,* the plural verb form is always correct.

Dr Cotter is **one of those** researchers who **prefer** the library to the laboratory.

5.9.11 ***Number.***—*The number* is singular and *a number of* is plural (see also 5.9.5, Collective Nouns).

The number that responded **was** surprising.

A number of respondents **were** verbose in their answers.

The same is true of *the total* and *a total of.*

5.9.12 ***Indefinite Pronouns.***—Most indefinite pronouns express the idea of quantity and share properties of collective nouns (see 5.9.5, Collective Nouns). Some indefinite pronouns (eg, *each, either, neither, one, no one, everyone, someone, anybody, nobody, somebody*) always take the singular; some (eg, *several, few, both, many*) always take the plural. And some (eg, *some, any, none, all,* and *most*) may take either the singular or the plural, depending on the referents; in this case, usually the best choice is to use the singular verb when the pronoun refers to a singular word and the plural verb when the pronoun refers to a plural word, even when the noun is omitted.

Singular referent:	**Some** of my time **is** spent wisely.
Plural referent:	**Some** of his calculations **are** difficult to follow.
Singular referent:	**Most** of the manuscript **was** typed with a justified right-hand margin.
Plural referent:	**Most** of the manuscripts **are** edited electronically.
Singular referent:	Some of the manuscripts had merit, but **none was** of the caliber of last year's award winner.
Plural referent:	**None** of the demographic variables that were examined **were** found to be significant risk factors.

ACKNOWLEDGMENT

Principal author: Cheryl Iverson, MA

REFERENCES

1. Bernstein TM. *The Careful Writer: A Modern Guide to English Usage.* New York, NY: Atheneum; 1984.

2. Huth EJ. *How to Write and Publish Papers in the Medical Sciences.* 2nd ed. Baltimore, Md: Williams & Wilkins; 1990.

3. *The American Heritage Dictionary of the English Language.* 3rd ed. Boston, Mass: Houghton Mifflin Co; 1992.

ADDITIONAL READINGS AND GENERAL REFERENCES

The Chicago Manual of Style 14th ed. Chicago, Ill: University of Chicago Press; 1993.

Copy Editor: The National Newsletter for Professional Copy Editors. New York, NY: Copy Editor.

DeBakey L, DeBakey S. Syntactic orphans and adoptees: unattached participles, I: mischievous intruders. *Int J Cardiol.* 1983;3:67-70.

DeBakey L, DeBakey S. Syntactic orphans and adoptees: unattached participles, II: medical miscontructions. *Int J Cardiol.* 1983;3:231-236.

Editorial Eye. Alexandria, Va: Editorial Experts Inc.

Fowler HW. *The New Fowler's Modern English Usage.* 3rd ed. New York, NY: Oxford University Press; 1997.

Huth EJ. *Medical Style & Format: An International Manual for Authors, Editors, and Publishers.* Baltimore, Md: Williams & Wilkins; 1989.

Kilpatrick JJ. *The Writer's Art.* Kansas City, Kan: Andrews McMeel & Parker Inc; 1985.

Strunk W Jr, White EB. *Elements of Style.* 3rd ed. New York, NY: Macmillan Publishing Co Inc; 1994.

Warriner JE. *English Grammar and Composition: Complete Course.* Franklin ed. New York, NY: Harcourt Brace Jovanovich; 1982.

Webster's Dictionary of English Usage. Springfield, Mass: Merriam-Webster Inc Publishers; 1989.

CHAPTER 6

6.0 PUNCTUATION

6.1 ■ **PERIOD, QUESTION MARK, EXCLAMATION POINT.**—Periods, question marks, and exclamation points are the 3 end-of-sentence punctuation marks.

6.1.1 ***Period.***—Periods are the most common end-of-sentence punctuation marks. Use a period at the end of a declarative or imperative sentence and at the end of each footnote and each legend. Also use a period after an indirect question not requiring an answer.

> Advances in medical technology have saved many lives.
>
> Where, indeed, is the Osler of today.
>
> They asked if we found it odd that the occasion for this public outburst was the publication of a dictionary.
>
> Always listen carefully.

Placement: The period precedes ending quotation marks and reference citations.

> The child is rated in 7 areas, such as "accepts responsibility" and "interacts appropriately with peers."
>
> We followed the methods of Wilkes et al.[5]

Enumerations: Use a period after the arabic numeral when enumerating paragraphed items (see 16.5, Numbers and Percentages, Enumerations).

Decimals: Use the period as a decimal indicator (see 16.7.1, Numbers and Percentages, Decimals).

> $r = 0.75$ 0.1% .32-caliber

Multiplication: The period in raised position indicates multiplication (see 15.2.2, Units of Measure, Products and Quotients of SI Unit Symbols, and 18.6, Mathematical Composition, Expressing Multiplication and Division).

When Not to Use a Period: AMA style tends not to use periods when other style sources might. Omit the period from honorifics, scientific terms, and abbreviations (see 2.1, Manuscript Preparation, Titles and Subtitles, 2.2, Manuscript Preparation, Bylines and End-of-Text Signatures, and 11.0, Abbreviations).

> Dr Hussey George Hussey, MD *E coli* AMA

6.1.2 ***Question Mark.***—The primary use of the question mark is to end interrogative sentences.

> How long has he been practicing medicine?
>
> If this symphony were a work of the 1930s, not the 1990s, would we hear it differently today? And should we?

In Dates: Use the question mark to show doubt about specific data.

> Catiline (108?-62 BCE) lived during the time of Cato the Younger.

Placement: Place the question mark inside the end quotation mark (see 6.6.5, Quotation Marks, Placement), the closing parenthesis, or the end bracket when the question mark is part of the quoted or parenthetical material.

> The patient asked her physician of 25 years, "Why are you retiring, Doctor?"
>
> The chapter on interpretation asks the question, "Can I be wrong?"
>
> The mandate for health reform (can we agree on this?) will change practice as we know it.

In declarative sentences that contain a question, place the question mark at the end of the interrogative statement.

> Why did I bother to attend this meeting? she wondered.
>
> The first section of the book, "What Medical Advances Made Open Heart Surgery Possible?" is certain to interest medical historians.
>
> The investigators asked the question, "Have you ever injected drugs?" of every study subject.

Note: The question mark, like the exclamation point (see 6.1.3, Exclamation Point, Placement), is never combined with another question mark, exclamation point, period, semicolon, or comma; thus, the need for a comma is obviated in the last 3 examples above.

6.1.3 ***Exclamation Point.***—Exclamation points indicate emotion, an outcry, or a forceful comment. Try to avoid their use except in direct quotations and in rare and special circumstances. They are more common in less formal articles, such as book reviews or editorials, where added emphasis may be appropriate.

> Beware!
>
> If you cannot accept the "gold standard" (within reason, that is, nothing is perfect!), then you should question whether the diagnostic data are worth capturing [Sackett DL, Haynes BR, Tugwell P. *Clinical Epidemiology.* Boston, Mass: Little Brown & Co; 1985:49].
>
> I think of the noon whistle as a wake-up call: You, weeding your tomato patch, wake up!

Placement: When it completes the emphasized material, the exclamation point goes inside the end quotation mark, parenthesis, or bracket. (The exclamation point, like the question mark [see 6.1.2, Question Mark, Placement], is never combined with another exclamation point, question mark, period, semicolon, or comma; thus, there is no comma in the first example below.)

> "Let the buyer beware!" his listeners shouted back as one.
>
> The frightened child cried, "Don't leave me here all alone!"

Factorial: In mathematical expressions, the exclamation point is used to indicate a factorial (see 18.6, Mathematical Composition, Expressing Multiplication and Division).

$$5! = 5 \times 4 \times 3 \times 2 \times 1$$

6.2 **■ COMMA, SEMICOLON, COLON.**—Commas, semicolons, or colons can be used to indicate a break or pause in thought, to set off material, or to introduce a new but connected thought. Each has specific uses, and the strength of the break in thought determines which mark is appropriate.

6.2.1 ***Comma.***—Commas are the least forceful of the 3 marks. There are definite rules for using commas; however, usage is often subjective. Some writers and editors use the comma frequently to indicate what they see as a natural pause in the flow of words, but commas can be overused. The trend is to use them sparingly. A safe rule of thumb is to follow the accepted rules and use commas only when breaks are needed for sense or readability and to avoid confusion or misinterpretation.

Separating Groups of Words: The comma is used to separate phrases, clauses, and groups of words and to clarify the grammatical structure and the intended meaning.

Use a comma after opening dependent clauses (whether restrictive or not) or long opening adverbial phrases (however, a comma is not essential if the introductory phrase is short).

> If the infection recurs within 2 weeks, an additional course of antibiotics should be given.

Use commas to set off nonrestrictive subordinate clauses (see 5.7.2, Grammar, Relative Pronouns) or nonrestrictive participial phrases.

> Dr Frederick, who had been waiting on hold for more than an hour, abandoned all hope of having her questions answered.
>
> The delegates, attaining consensus, passed the resolution.
>
> The numbness, which had been apparent for 3 days, disappeared after drug therapy.

Use a comma to avoid an ambiguous or awkward juxtaposition of words.

> Outside, the ambulance siren shrieked.
>
> Peace is a daily, a weekly, a monthly process, gradually changing opinions, slowly eroding old barriers, quietly building new structures. [John F. Kennedy]

Use commas to set off appositives. (*Note:* Commas precede and follow the apposition.)

> Two colleagues, John Smith and Perry White, worked with me on this study.
>
> The battered-child syndrome, a clinical condition in young children who have suffered serious physical abuse, is a frequent cause of permanent injury or even death.

Series: In a simple coordinate series of 3 or more terms, separate the elements by commas (see 5.6.1, Grammar, Nouns, As Modifiers [Noun Strings]).

> Each patient was asked to complete a 21-item, 7-point, self-administered questionnaire.

Use a comma before the conjunction that precedes the last term in a series.

> Outcomes result from a complex interaction of medical care and genetic, environmental, and behavioral factors.
>
> The physician, the nurse, and the family could not convince the patient to take his medication daily.
>
> While in the hospital, these patients required neuroleptics, maximal observation, and seclusion.

In some instances, a series of 3 or more modifiers should not be separated by commas as the modifiers are seen as one term or entity:

> The patient has chronic progressive multiple sclerosis.
>
> Inner-city geriatric hemodialysis patients were studied.

This rule, however, will not always apply. Judgment and common sense are required in the interpretation of this rule. The clue here is, if the order of the adjectives can be rearranged, use the comma; if the adjectives modify the noun at the end of this adjectival unit, do not use commas:

> We designed a randomized, double-blind, placebo-controlled trial.
>
> The MR image showed an undescended, high, "functioning" testis.
>
> Recent large, multicenter clinical trials were analyzed.

Note: When fewer than 3 modifiers are used, avoid adding a comma if the modifiers and the noun are read as one entity:

> We used a randomized placebo-controlled trial.
>
> Multicenter clinical trials were performed.

Names of Organizations: When an enumeration occurs in the name of a company or organization, the comma is usually omitted before the ampersand. However, follow the punctuation used by the individual firm, except in references (see 2.12.35, References, Publishers).

> Farrar, Straus & Giroux Inc
>
> SmithKline Beecham Pharmaceuticals
>
> Little, Brown & Co
>
> Houghton Mifflin Co

Setting Off ie, eg, viz: Use commas to set off *ie, eg, viz,* and the expanded equivalents, *that is, for example,* and *namely*.

> The use of standardized scores, eg, *z* scores, has no effect on statistical comparisons.
>
> The most important tests, ie, the white blood cell and platelet counts, were unduly delayed.

Note: If an independent clause follows these terms or their equivalents, precede the clause with a semicolon.

> Our double-blind study compared continuous with cyclic estrogen treatment; ie, estrogens for 4 weeks were compared with estrogens for 3 weeks followed by placebo for 1 week.

Separating Clauses Joined by Conjunctions: Use commas to separate main clauses joined by coordinating conjunctions (*and, but, or, nor, for, so, yet*). But be careful not to confuse a coordinating conjunction used to link a compound predicate with the coordinating conjunction used between independent clauses.

> Plasma lipid and lipoprotein concentrations were unchanged after low-intensity training, but high-intensity training resulted in a reduction in triglyceride levels.
>
> No subgroup of responders could be identified, and differences between centers were so great that no real comparison was possible.
>
> These facilities are beginning to resemble "minihospitals" and are losing their identity as freestanding ambulatory surgery centers.

Clauses introduced by *yet* and *so* and subordinating conjunctions (eg, *while, where, since, after, whereas*) are preceded by a comma (see 9.1, Correct and Preferred Usage, Commonly Misused Words and Phrases).

> He did writing, performed careful research, and wrote thoughtful articles, yet he was denied tenure.
>
> The samples were stored at −70°C, after the proteins had denatured.
>
> I consulted the cardiology fellow, since the attending physician was not available.

If both clauses are short, punctuation can be omitted.

> The test may be useful or it may be harmful.
>
> I have Bright's disease and he has mine. [S. J. Perelman]

Setting Off Parenthetical Expressions: Use commas to set off parenthetical words, phrases, questions, and other expressions that interrupt the continuity of a sentence, eg, *therefore, moreover, on the other hand, of course, nevertheless, after all, consequently, however* (see 6.8.1, Ellipses, Omission Within a Sentence).

> The real issue, after all, was how to fund the next study.
>
> We should take care not to make the intellect our god; it has, of course, powerful muscles, but no personality. [Albert Einstein]
>
> However, much as I try, I cannot understand Bayes theorem.
> (*But:* However much I try, I cannot understand Bayes theorem.)
>
> Therefore, the authors drew the correct conclusion.
> (*But:* The authors therefore drew the correct conclusion.)

Setting Off Degrees and Titles: Academic degrees, titles, and *Jr* and *Sr* are set off by commas when they follow the name of a person.

Berton Smith, Jr, MD, and Priscilla Armstrong, MD, PhD, interpreted the radiographic findings in this study. (*But:* Marshall Field IV; Pope John Paul II [see 16.7.4, Numbers and Percentages, Roman Numerals].)

Joyce Fredrickson-Smith, MD, PhD, vice-chancellor, attended the conference on health system reform.

Addresses: Use commas to separate the elements in an address, in running text, and in affiliation footnotes. Use commas after the city and before and after the state or country name. (*Note:* In US addresses, commas are not used before the ZIP code.)

This year, the editorial board meeting will be held in the Board Room, American Medical Association, 1101 Vermont Ave NW, Washington, DC 20420.

The study was conducted at The Wilmer Institute, Baltimore, Md, in 1989.

Dates: In dates and similar expressions of time, use commas according to the following examples. Commas are not used when the month and year are given without the day.

The first issue of *JAMA* was published on Saturday, July 14, 1883.

The patient's rhinoplasty was scheduled for August 19, 1995, with postoperative evaluation on August 30.

The events of December 1941 have received intense historical scrutiny.

They were married on New Year's Day, 1967.

Numbers: In accordance with SI convention, separate digits with a space, not a comma, to indicate place values beyond thousands (see 15.4.3, Units of Measure, Number Spacing).

5034 12 345 615 478 9 473 209

Occasionally, a comma may be used to separate adjacent unrelated numerals if neither can be expressed easily in words. Usually, it is preferable to reword the sentence or spell out one of the numbers.

By December 1993, 93 282 cases of AIDS had been reported in the United States. (*Better:* By December 1993, a total of 93 282 cases of AIDS had been reported in the United States.)

NASA reported that in the year 2000, 3000 active satellites would orbit the earth. (*Better:* NASA reported that 3000 active satellites would orbit the earth in the year 2000.)

Units of Measure: Do not use a comma between 2 units of the same dimension.

3 years 4 months old 3 lb 4 oz

Placement: The comma is placed inside quotation marks (see 6.6.5, Quotation Marks, Placement) and before superscript citation of references and footnote symbols.

As a result of the "back-to-sleep campaigns," a call has been issued for a "back-to-the-bench" one.

These missed opportunities have been shown to occur during office visits,[6-9] health department appointments,[10-13] and hospitalizations.[16]

To Indicate Omission: The comma is used to indicate omission or to avoid repeating a word when the sense is clear (see 5.9.7, Grammar, Shift in Number of Subject and Resultant Subject-Verb Disagreement).

Three patients could not be studied: in 1, duration of treatment was too short; in 2, too long.

A plus indicates present; and a minus, absent.

Dialogue: Commas are used before direct dialogue or conversation is introduced.

In the middle of the laboratory examination, a student asked, "Would it be okay to take a break?"

6.2.2 ***Semicolon.***—Semicolons represent a more definite break in thought than commas. Generally, semicolons are used to separate 2 independent clauses. Often a comma will suffice if sentences are short; but when the main clauses are long and joined by coordinating conjunctions or conjunctive adverbs, especially if 1 of the clauses has internal punctuation, a semicolon is the mark to use.

Separating Independent Clauses: Use a semicolon to separate independent clauses in a compound sentence when no connective word is used. In most instances it is equally correct to use a period and create 2 sentences.

The conditions of 52% of the patients improved greatly; 4% of the patients withdrew from the study.

However, if clauses are short and similar in form, use a comma.

Seventy grafts were patent, 5 were occluded.

Use a semicolon between main clauses joined by a conjunctive adverb (eg, *also, besides, furthermore, then, however, thus, hence, indeed, yet*) or a coordinating conjunction (*and, but, or, nor, for, so, yet*) if 1 of the clauses has internal punctuation or is considerably long.

The word *normal* is often used loosely; indeed, it is not easily defined.

This consideration is important in any research; yet it is often overlooked, if not denied.

The patient's fever had subsided; however, his condition was still critical.

Enumerations: For clarity, use semicolons between items in a complex or lengthy enumeration within a sentence or in an enumeration that contains serial commas in at least 1 of the items listed. (In a simple series with little or no internal punctuation, use commas.) In less formal writing and where the last element of a series is also a series, commas are acceptable provided the clarity is retained.

A number of questions remain unresolved: (1) whether beverages that contain caffeine are an important factor in arrhythmogenesis; (2) whether such beverages can trigger arrhythmias de novo; and (3) whether their arrhythmogenic tendency is enhanced by the presence and extent of myocardial impairment.

There was, to be sure, a decent assortment of male champions: for example, Byeong-Keun Ahn, of Korea, in lightweight judo; Juha Tiainen, of Finland, in the hammer throw; and Mauro Numa, of Italy, in the men's individual foils.

We lunched on Caesar salad, French onion soup, and bacon, lettuce, and tomato sandwiches.

The photomicrographic illustrations of the gross and microscopic features of normal skin, Spitz congenital and dysplastic nevi, lentigines, and malignant melanoma demonstrated the complexity of pigmented lesions.

6.2.3 ***Colon.***—The colon is the strongest of the 3 marks used to indicate a decided pause or break in thought. It separates 2 main clauses in which the second clause amplifies or explains the first.

> We begin with a single tenet: all men are created equal.

When Not to Use a Colon: Do not use a colon if the sentence is continuous without it.

> You will need enthusiasm, organization, and a commitment to your beliefs.

Do not use a colon to separate a preposition from its object or a verb (including *to be* in all of its manifestations) from its object or predicate nominative.

> *Avoid:* The point is: do not insert the catheter at this time.

In general, try to avoid use of a colon after *because* or forms of the verb *include*.

Introducing Quotations or Enumerations: Use a colon to introduce a formal or extended quotation. (If the sentence to follow is in quotation marks, the first word is capitalized.)

> Harold Johnson, MD, chair of the committee, summarized: "The problems we face in developing a new vaccine are numerous, but foremost is isolating the antigen."

Use a colon to introduce an enumeration, especially after anticipatory phrasing such as *thus, as follows, the following.*

> The solution included the following: phosphate buffer, double-distilled water, and a chelating agent.

> Laboratory studies yielded the following values: hemoglobin, 119 g/L; erythrocyte sedimentation, 104 mm/h; calcium, 4.22 mmol/L (16.9 mg/dL); phosphorus, 1.81 mmol/L (5.6 mg/dL); and creatinine, 270 μmol/L (3 mg/dL).

If 2 or more grammatically independent statements follow the colon, they may be treated as complete sentences separated by periods, and the initial words may or may not be capitalized.

> The following rules apply to manuscript preparation: (1) Submit an original typescript and 2 high-quality copies. (2) Type all copy double-spaced on heavy-duty white bond paper. (3) Provide ample margins. (4) Do not justify the right-hand margin. (5) Do not use a dot matrix printer.

Numbers: Use a colon to separate chapter and verse numbers in biblical references, hours and minutes in expressions of time, and parts of numerical ratios.

> The reading for today is Genesis 3:28.

> Medication was given twice a day at 8:30 AM and at 8:30 PM.

> The chemicals were mixed in a 2:1.5 ratio.

> The controls and study subjects were randomized in a 2:1 ratio.

References: In references, use a colon (1) between title and subtitle; and (2) for periodicals, between volume and page numbers (see 2.12, Manuscript Preparation, References).

6.3 ■ HYPHENS AND DASHES.

6.3 ■ HYPHENS AND DASHES.—Hyphens and dashes are internal punctuation marks used for linkage and clarity of expression.

6.3.1 ***Hyphen.***—Hyphens are connectors. The hyphen connects words, prefixes, and suffixes permanently or temporarily. Certain compound words always contain hyphens. Such hyphens are called *orthographic.* Examples are seen in the compound words *merry-go-round, free-for-all,* and *mother-in-law.* For temporary connections, hyphens help prevent ambiguity, clarify meaning, and indicate word breaks at the end of a line.

When not otherwise specified, hyphens should be used only as an aid to the reader's understanding, primarily to avoid ambiguity. For capitalization of hyphenated compounds in titles, subtitles, subheads, and table heads, see 8.4.2, Capitalization, Hyphenated Compounds.

Temporary Compounds: Hyphenate temporary compounds according to current dictionary usage and the following rules:

Hyphenate a compound that contains a noun or an adverb and a participle that together serve as an adjective if they precede the noun but not if they follow the noun.

decision-making methods
(*But:* methods of decision making)

least-read work in the collection
(*But:* The work was the least read in the collection.)

Hyphenate a compound adjectival phrase when it precedes the noun it modifies but not when it follows the noun.

end-to-end anastomosis
(*But:* The anastomosis was end to end.)

Hyphenate an adjective-noun compound when it precedes and modifies another noun but not when it follows the noun.

upper-class values
(*But:* Values were upper class.)

low-quality suture material
(*But:* The suture material was low quality.)

low-density resolution
(*But:* The resolution was low density.)

Note: In most instances *middle-, high,-* and *low-* adjectival compounds are hyphenated.

For compound adjectival phrases, adverb-participle compounds, and adjective-noun compounds that have become commonplace and familiar in everyday usage, hyphenate whether these phrases or compounds precede or follow the noun they are modifying. (Follow *The Chicago Manual of Style,* 14th edition, to verify.)

long-term therapy

the commitment was long-term

up-to-date schedule

the schedule was up-to-date

Hyphenate a combination of 2 nouns used coordinately as a unit modifier when preceding the noun but not when following.

albumin-globulin ratio
(*But:* ratio of albumin to globulin)

the Binet-Simon Test
(*But:* the test of Binet and Simon)

Hyphenate a combination of 2 nouns of equal participation used as a single noun (see 6.4.1 Virgule [Solidus], Used to Express Equivalence or Duality).

player-manager   author-critic

soldier-statesman   physician-poet

actor-director   obstetrician-gynecologist

Hyphenate most compound nouns that contain a preposition. Follow the latest edition of *Merriam-Webster's Collegiate Dictionary.*

tie-in   tie-up   go-between

hand-me-down   looker-on

(*But:* onlooker, passerby, handout, workup, makeup)

Hyphenate a compound in which a number is the first element and the compound precedes the noun it modifies.

18-factor blood chemistry analysis

2-way street

ninth-grade reading level

1-cm increments

Hyphenate 2 or more adjectives used coordinately or as conflicting terms whether they precede the noun or follow as a predicate adjective.

The false-positive test results were noted.

The test results were false-positive.

We performed a double-blind study.

The test we used was double-blind.

Hyphenate color terms in which the 2 elements are of equal weight.

blue-gray eyes   blue-black lesions (lesions were blue-black)
(*But:* bluish gray lesions)

Hyphenate compounds formed with the prefixes *all-*, *self-*, and *ex-* whether they precede or follow the noun.

self-assured salesperson   all-powerful ruler

He needs self-respect.   My ex-husband called.

Note: With the prefix *vice,* follow the latest edition of *Merriam-Webster's Collegiate Dictionary,* eg, vice-chancellor, vice-consul, *but* vice president, vice admiral.

Hyphenate compounds made up of the suffixes *-type, -elect,* and *-designate.*

Hodgkin-type lymphoma

Valsalva-type maneuver

chair-elect

secretary-designate

Hyphenate most contemporary adjectival *cross-* compounds (consult the latest edition of *Merriam-Webster's Collegiate Dictionary* for absolute accuracy; there are exceptions, eg, crossbred, crosshatched, crossmatched, cross section).

cross-country race

cross-city competition

cross-eyed cat

Hyphenate *adjectival* compounds with *quasi.*

quasi-legislative group quasi-diplomatic efforts

Note: Noun compounds formed with *quasi* are not hyphenated.

quasi diplomat

Hyphenate some compounds in which the first element is a possessive. Consult the latest edition of *Merriam-Webster's Collegiate Dictionary.*

bird's-eye view crow's-feet bull's-eye

Hyphenate all prefixes that precede a proper noun, a capitalized word, a number, or an abbreviation.

anti-American demonstration pro-Israeli forces

pre-AIDS era pseudo-Christian

post-1945 clothing

Note: There is growing recognition and acceptance of the use of a stand-alone prefix with a hyphen when a contrasting unhyphenated prefix follows.

We found a need for pre- and postoperative examination.

AMA chooses *not* to follow this trend and instead would use

We found a need for preoperative and postoperative examination.

Hyphenate compound numbers from 21 to 99 and compound cardinal and ordinal numbers when written out, as at the beginning of a sentence (see 16.1, Numbers and Percentages, Use of Numerals).

Thirty-six patients were examined.

Twenty-fifth through 75th percentile rankings were shown.

One hundred thirty-two people were killed in the plane crash.

Hyphenate fractions used as adjectives.

A two-thirds majority was needed.

The flask was three-fourths full.

One-and-a-half-page essays were required of all entrants into the competition.

But: Do not hyphenate spelled-out common fractions used as nouns.

Three fourths of the questionnaires were returned.

When 2 or more hyphenated compounds have a common base, omit the base in all but the last. In unhyphenated compounds written as 1 word, repeat the base.

first-, second-, and third-grade students

10- and 15-year-old boys

Videocassettes and videodiscs were used in the presentation.

Clarity: Use hyphens to avoid ambiguity. If a term could be misleading without a hyphen, hyphenate it.

a small-bowel constriction (constriction of the small bowel)
a small bowel constriction (a small constriction of the bowel)

an old-car salesperson (a salesperson of old cars)
an old car salesperson (a car salesperson who is old)

man-eating plants (a plant that eats humans)
man eating plants (a person eating plants)

Use a hyphen after a prefix when the unhyphenated word would have a different meaning.

re-treat re-creation re-formation

Note: Do not hyphenate other forms of these words for which no ambiguity exists: retreatment.

Occasionally, a hyphen is used after a prefix or before a suffix to avoid an awkward combination of letters, such as 2 of the same vowel or 3 of the same consonant (with exceptions noted below, When Not to Use Hyphens). Follow the latest edition of *Merriam-Webster's Collegiate Dictionary.*

semi-independent	hull-less	ultra-atomic
de-emphasize	intra-abdominal	bell-like

(Some exceptions to this rule include microorganism, cooperation, reenter [see below, When Not to Use Hyphens].)

In complex modifying phrases that include suffixes or prefixes, hyphens and en dashes are sometimes used to avoid ambiguity (see 6.3.2, Dashes, En Dash).

non–self-governing	non–group-specific blood
non–brain-injured subjects	manic-depressive–like symptoms
non–English-language journals	

Expressing Ranges and Dimensions: When expressing dimensions, use hyphens and spacing in accordance with the following examples in the left-hand column when the dimension being expressed is being used as a modifier before a noun. The alternatives in the right-hand column give the expression of dimensions when they are not being used as a modifier preceding a noun.

As Modifier	*Alternative*
in a 10- to 14-day period	10 to 14 days' duration
a 3 × 4-cm strip	a strip measuring 3 × 4 cm
a 5- to 10-mg dose	a dose of 5 to 10 mg
in a 5-, 10-, or 15-mg dose	a dose of 5, 10, or 15 mg
a 3-cm-diameter tube	a tube 3 cm in diameter

In the text, do not use hyphens to express ranges, eg, in 5% to 10% of the group.

The exceptions to this rule about ranges are for (1) ranges expressing fiscal years, academic years, life spans, or a study span and (2) ranges given in parentheses.

We present results from the 1992-1997 Renal Study Group.

The patients' median age was 56 years (range, 31-92 years).

Word Division: Use hyphens to indicate division of a word at the end of a line (follow the latest edition of *Merriam-Webster's Collegiate Dictionary* or of *Stedman's* or *Dorland's* medical dictionary).

When Not to Use Hyphens: Rules also exist for when *not* to use hyphens.

The following common prefixes are not joined by hyphens except when they precede a proper noun, a capitalized word, or an abbreviation: *ante-, anti-, bi-, co-, contra-, counter-, de-, extra-, infra-, inter-, intra-, micro-, mid-, neo-, non-, over-, pre-, post-, pro-, pseudo-, re-, semi-, sub-, super-, supra-, trans-, tri-, ultra-, un-, under-.*

antimicrobial	midaxillary	posttraumatic
repossess	nonresident	coauthor
overproduction	coidentity	coexistence
coworker	postoperative	ultramicrotome
transsacral	nonnegotiable	underrepresented

Retain the hyphen if needed to avoid ambiguity or awkward spelling that could interfere with readability: co-opt, co-payment, co-twin, intra-aortic.

Retain the hyphen when the term after the prefixes *anti-, neo-, pre-, post-,* and *mid-* is a proper noun or a number (see above, Temporary Compounds).

Note: As an adjective, *mid* is a separate word meaning "in the middle [of]." In such usage, it may appear without a hyphen: the mid finger, the mid Atlantic.

The following suffixes are joined without a hyphen, with exceptions if the clarity would be obscured (see above, Temporary Compounds): *-hood, -less, -like, -wise.*

womanhood	manhood	catatoniclike
shoeless	barklike	clockwise

Some combinations of words are commonly read as a unit. As such combinations come into common usage, the hyphen tends to be omitted without a sacrifice of clarity.

birth control methods	bone marrow biopsy
public health officials	urinary tract infection
medical school students	amino acid levels
social service agency	deep vein thrombosis
primary care physician	tertiary care center
lower extremity amputation	inner ear disorder
health care system	low back pain
foreign body infiltrate	soft tissue mass
open heart surgery	

Do not hyphenate names of disease entities used as modifiers.

grand mal seizures   hyaline membrane disease

basal cell carcinoma   sickle cell trait

Do not use a hyphen after an adverb that ends in *-ly* even when used in a compound modifier preceding the word modified, because the adverb is modifying the adjective and not the noun that follows.

the clearly stated purpose   a highly developed species

Do not hyphenate names of chemical compounds used as adjectives.

sodium chloride solution   tannic acid test

Most combinations of proper adjectives derived from geographic entities are not hyphenated when used as noun or adjective formations.

Central Americans   Southeast Asia

African American   Mexican American

Pacific Rim countries   Central American customs

Far Eastern customs   Latin Americans

(*But:* Scotch-Irish ancestry. Here the hyphen is used to indicate 2 countries of origin.)

Do not hyphenate Latin expressions or non–English-language phrases used in an adjectival sense. Most of these are treated as separate words; a few are joined without a hyphen. Follow the latest edition of *Merriam-Webster's Collegiate Dictionary.*

an a priori argument   per diem employees

prima facie evidence   postmortem examination

an ex officio member   antebellum South

in vivo specimens   carcinoma in situ

café au lait spots

Do not hyphenate modifiers in which a letter or number is the second element.

grade A eggs   study 1 protocol   type 1 diabetes

Compound Official Titles: Hyphenate combination positions of office but not compound designations as follows:

secretary-treasurer   acting secretary

honorary chair

(*But:* past vice president, executive vice president, past president)

Special Combinations: Special combinations may not necessitate the use of hyphens. If clarity of concept or readability are compromised, it is preferable to add a hyphen to avoid any misinterpretation or awkwardness. Consult the latest edition of *Stedman's* or *Dorland's* medical dictionary or *Merriam-Webster's Collegiate Dictionary* (see 12.0, Nomenclature, and 14.0, Greek Letters).

T wave	T-shirt	γ-globulin	I beam (I-shaped beam)
T square	*t* test	Mann-Whitney *U* test	foreign body infiltrate
T tube	B cell	B-cell helper	soft tissue mass
T-cell marker			

6.3.2 *Dashes.*—Dashes as another form of internal punctuation convey a particular meaning or emphasize and clarify a certain section of material within a sentence. Compared with parentheses, dashes convey a less formal "aside."

There are 4 types of dashes that differ in length: the *em* dash, the most common; the *en* dash; the *2-em* dash; and the *3-em* dash. When typing a manuscript, if a dash is not available, use 2 hyphens to indicate an em dash (--) and 1 for an en dash (-), which the copy editor will mark for the typesetter.

Em Dash: Em dashes are used to indicate a sudden interruption or break in thought in a sentence. It is best to use this mode sparingly; do not use an em dash when another punctuation mark will suffice, for instance, the comma or the colon, or to imply *namely, that is,* or *in other words,* when an explanation follows.

> All of these factors—age, severity of symptoms, psychic preparation, and choice of anesthetic agent—determine the patient's reaction.

An em dash may be used to separate a referent from a pronoun that is the subject of an ending clause.

> Osler, Billings, and Apgar—these were the physicians she tried to emulate.

En Dash: The en dash is longer than a hyphen but half the length of the em dash.

The en dash shows relational distinction in a hyphenated or compound modifier, 1 element of which consists of 2 words or a hyphenated word, or when the word being modified is a compound.

> Winston-Salem–oriented group
>
> physician-lawyer–directed section
>
> anti–basement membrane glomerulonephritis
>
> phosphotungstic acid–hematoxylin stain
>
> post–World War I
>
> multiple sclerosis–like symptoms

2-Em Dash: The 2-em dash is used to indicate missing letters in a word.

> Our study began in N——, noted for its casual lifestyle.

3-Em Dash: The 3-em dash is used to show missing words.

> Each subject was asked to fill in the blank in the following statement: "I usually sleep ——— hours per day."
>
> I admire Dr ——— too much to expose him in this anecdote.

6.4 ■ VIRGULE (SOLIDUS).—The virgule is a diagonal line used to represent *per, and,* or *or* and to divide material (eg, numerator and denominator in fractions; month, day, and year in dates [only in tables and figures]; lines of poetry).

6.4.1 *Used to Express Equivalence or Duality.*—When 2 terms are of equal weight in an expression and *and* is meant between them to express this, the virgule can be retained to show this.

One needs a hot/cold environment in which to carry out the experiment.

The diagnosis and initial treatment/diagnostic planning were recorded.

When the question of duality arises, in the area of the he/she construction, change the virgule construction when the gender is to be specified; substitute the word *or* for the virgule or, preferably, rephrase to be gender neutral.

Tom and Kate said they were coming. Now I need to know whether he or she [not he/she] will be bringing the extra chairs.

Better: Now I need to know which of them will be bringing the extra chairs.

If the sex is unspecified and does not matter, retain the virgule construction.

This aspiration technique is one that any physician can master whether or not he/she has surgical expertise.

Note: The trend today is toward rephrasing such sentences and using the plural to avoid sexist language; eg, "This aspiration technique can be mastered by physicians whether or not they have surgical expertise" (see 9.10, Correct and Preferred Usage, Inclusive Language).

Although the virgule can be used to indicate alternative or combined states in the same person, such as Jekyll/Hyde personality, no ambiguity should be introduced. If there is any likelihood of ambiguity, the sentence should be reworded.

However, when 2 separate individuals are implied in a relationship, change the virgule to another punctuation mark or word.

One often reads about the physician-patient relationship in medical literature. [Here it is the relationship between the physician and the patient. The use of the virgule (physician/patient) would refer to the physician *as* patient.]

They decided to sign up for the mother-and-daughter workday.

6.4.2 ***Used to Mean* Per.**—In the "per" construction, use a virgule only when (1) the construction involves units of measure (including time) *and* (2) at least 1 element includes a specific numerical quantity *and* (3) the element immediately adjacent on each side is either a specific numerical quantity or a unit of measure. In such cases, the units of measure should be abbreviated in accordance with 11.12, Abbreviations, Units of Measure (see 16.7.3, Numbers and Percentages, Proportions and Rates).

The hemoglobin level was 140 g/L.

The $CD4^+$ cell count was 0.20×10^9/L (200/μL).

Blood volume was 80 mL/kg of body weight.

Respirations were 60/min; pulse rate was 98/min.

Do *not* use the virgule in a "per" construction (1) when a prepositional phrase intervenes between the 2 elements, (2) when neither element contains a specific numerical quantity, or (3) in nontechnical expressions.

4.5 mmol of potassium per liter
(*Avoid:* 4.5 mmol/L of potassium; instead reword: a potassium concentration of 4.5 mmol/L)

expressed in milliliters per minute

2 days per year

6.4.3 ***In Dates.***—Use the virgule in dates only in tables and figures to save space (month/day/year) (see 2.13.7, Tables, Punctuation).

6.4.4 ***In Equations.***—In equations that are set on line and run into the text rather than centered and set off (see 18.3, Mathematical Composition, Stacked vs Unstacked), use the virgule to separate numerator and denominator.

The "stacked" fraction $y = \frac{r_1 + r_2}{p_1 - p_2}$ is written as $y = (r_1 + r_2)/(p_1 - p_2)$.

When the virgule is used for this purpose, parentheses and brackets must often be added to avoid ambiguity.

6.4.5 ***In Ratios With Abbreviations.***—The virgule is used instead of a colon or a hyphen or an en dash when the ratio is between items that are abbreviations.

the SUN/Cr ratio was greater than 10:1
(*But:* the serum urea nitrogen–creatinine ratio was greater than 10:1)

6.4.6 ***Phonetics, Poetry.***—The virgule is also used to set off phonemes and phonetic transcription and to divide run-in lines of poetry.

/d/ as in *dog*

. . . cold-breathed earth/earth of the slumbering and liquid trees/earth of the mountains misty-topped.

6.5 ■ **PARENTHESES AND BRACKETS.**—Parentheses and brackets are internal punctuation marks used to set off material that is nonrestrictive or, as in the case of mathematical and chemical expressions, to alert the reader to the special functions occurring within.

6.5.1 ***Parentheses.***—*Supplementary Expressions:* Use parentheses to indicate supplementary explanations, identification, direction to the reader, or translation (see 6.3.2, Dashes, and 6.5.2, Brackets).

A known volume of fluid (100 mL) was injected.

The differences were not significant ($P > .05$).

One of us (B.O.G.) saw the patient in 1994.

Asymmetry of the upper part of the rib cage (patient 5) and pseudoarthrosis of the first and second ribs (patient 8) were incidental anomalies (Table 3).

Of the 761 hospitalized patients, 171 (22.5%) were infants (younger than 1 year).

In this issue of THE JOURNAL (p 1037), a successful transplant is reported.

The 3 cusps of the aortic valve (the "Mercedes-Benz" sign) were clearly shown on the echocardiogram.

If there is a close relationship between the parenthetical material and the rest of the sentence, commas are preferred to parentheses.

The hemoglobin level, although in the normal range, was lower than expected.

If the relationship in thought after the expressions *namely* (*viz*), *that is* (*ie*), and *for example* (*eg*) is incidental, use parentheses instead of commas.

He weighed the advice of several committee members (namely, Jones, Burke, and Easton) before making his proposal.

Punctuation Marks With Parentheses: Use no punctuation before the opening parenthesis except in enumerations (see Enumerations below).

Any punctuation mark can follow a closing parenthesis, but only the 3 end marks (the period, the question mark, and the exclamation point) may precede it when the parenthetical material interrupts the sentence. If a complete sentence is contained within parentheses, it is not necessary to have punctuation within the parentheses if it would noticeably interrupt the flow of the sentence.

> The discussion on informed consent lasted 2 hours. (A final draft has yet to be written.) The discussion failed to resolve the question.

> The discussion on informed consent lasted 2 hours (a final draft has yet to be written) and did not resolve the question.

> After what seemed an eternity (It took 2 hours!), the discussion on informed consent ended.

When the parenthetical material includes special punctuation, such as an exclamation point or a question mark, or several statements, terminal punctuation is placed inside the closing parenthesis.

> Oscar Wilde once said (When? Where? Who knows? But I read it in a book once upon a time, hence it must be true.) that "anyone who has never written a book is very learned." [Ball P. *The Unauthorized Biography of a Local Doctor: Or From Infancy Through Puberty and On to Senility, by Phil Ball.*]

Identifying Numbers or Letters: When an item identified by letter or number is referred to later by that letter or number only, enclose the letter or number in parentheses.

> You then follow (3), (5), and (6) to solve the puzzle.

If the category name is used instead, parentheses may be dropped.

> Steps 1, 2, and 3 must be done slowly.

Enumerations: For division of a short enumeration that is run in and indicated by numerals or lowercase italic letters, enclose the numerals or letters in parentheses (see 16.5, Numbers and Percentages, Enumerations).

> The patient is to bring (1) all pill bottles, (2) past medical records, and (3) our questionnaire to the first office visit.

References in Text: Use parentheses to enclose all or part of a reference given in the text (see 2.12.3, References, References Given in Text).

> The case was originally reported in the *Archives of Surgery* (1975;148:343-346).

> The legality of this practice was questioned more than 3 decades ago (*BMJ.* 1963;2:394-396).

In Legends: In legends, use parentheses to identify a case or patient and parts of a composite figure when appropriate.

> **Figure 6.** *Facial paralysis on the right side (patient 3).*

> **Figure 2.** *Fracture of the left femur (patient 7).*

The date, if given, is similarly enclosed.

> **Figure 2.** *Fracture of the left femur (patient 7, October 23, 1995).*

For photomicrographs, give the magnification and the stain, if relevant, in parentheses (see also 2.14.8, Manuscript Preparation, Photomicrographs).

> **Figure 3.** *Marrow aspiration 14 weeks after transplantation (Wright stain, original magnification ×600).*

Trade Names: If the author provides a trade name for a drug or for equipment, enclose the trade name in parentheses immediately after the first use of the nonproprietary name in the text and in the abstract (see 12.4.3, Nomenclature, Proprietary Names, and 12.5, Nomenclature, Equipment, Devices, and Reagents).

> Treatment included oral administration of indomethacin (Indocin), 25 mg 3 times a day.

Abbreviations: If used 5 or more times in the text, specialized abbreviations (as specified in 11.11, Abbreviations, Clinical and Technical Terms) are enclosed in parentheses immediately after first mention of the term, which is spelled out in full.

Explanatory Footnotes: Explanatory footnotes may be incorporated into the text within parentheses. In such instances, terminal punctuation is used before the closing parenthesis, the sentence(s) within the parentheses being a complete thought but only parenthetical to the text.

Parenthetical expressions within a parenthetical expression are enclosed in brackets.

> (Antirejection therapy included parenteral antithymocyte globulin [ATGAM], at a dosage of 15 mg/kg per day.)

But: In mathematical expressions, parentheses are placed *inside* brackets. See 6.5.2, Brackets, Within Parentheses.

Parenthetical Plurals: Parentheses are sometimes used around the letters *s* or *es* to express the possibility of a plural when singular or plural could be meant (see 5.9.4, Grammar, Parenthetical Plurals).

> The name(s) of the editor(s) of the book in reference 2 is unknown.

Note: If this construction is used, the verb should be singular because the *s* is parenthetical. Try to avoid this construction and use the plural noun instead.

6.5.2 ***Brackets.—Insertions in Quotations:*** Brackets are used to indicate editorial interpolation within a quotation and to enclose corrections, explanations, or comments in material that is quoted (see 6.6.1, Quotations, 6.8.7, Change in Capitalization, and 6.8.8, Omission of Ellipses).

> "Enough questions had arisen [these are not described] to warrant medical consultation."

> Thompson stated, "Because of the patient's preferences, surgery was *absolutely* contraindicated [italics added]."

> "The following year [1947] was a turning point."

Use *sic* (Latin for "thus" or "so") in brackets to indicate an error or peculiarity in the spelling or grammar of the preceding word in the original source of the quotation. As with apologetic quotation marks (see 6.6.8, Apologetic Quotation Marks), use *sic* with discretion.

> "The plural [*sic*] cavity was filled with fluid."

> "Breathing of the gas is often followed by extraordinary fits of extacy [*sic*]."

Within Parentheses: Use brackets to indicate parenthetical expressions within parenthetical expressions.

> A nitrogen mustard (mechlorethamine [Mustargen] hydrochloride) was one of the drugs used.

In scientific text, one often encounters complex parenthetical constructions such as consecutive parentheses and brackets within parentheses.

> Her platelet count was 100×10^9/L (100 000/mm^3) (reference range, 150 to 450×10^9/L [150 000 to 450 000/mm^3]).

In Formulas: In mathematical formulas, parentheses are generally used for the innermost units, with parentheses changed to brackets when the formula is parenthetical (see 18.3, Mathematical Composition, Stacked vs Unstacked).

> $t = d(r_1 - r_2)$
>
> The equation suggested by this phenomenon ($t = d[r_1 - r_2]$) can be applied in a variety of circumstances.

In chemical formulas, the current trend is to use only parentheses and brackets, making sure that every parenthetical or bracketed expression has an opening and closing parenthesis or bracket symbol. Consult the most recent edition of *USP Dictionary of USAN and International Drug Names* for drug formularies and *The Merck Index* for chemical compounds to verify the correct use of parentheses and brackets. If the older style of parentheses, braces, and brackets has been used by the author, retain it. The notation will be readily understood by the author's intended audience.

> An experimental drug (9-[(2-hydroxy-1-(hydroxymethyl)ethoxymethyl)]guanine) was used to treat the cytomegalovirus retinopathy in patients with AIDS (*Arch Ophthalmol.* 1986;104:1794-1800).

When a parenthetical or bracketed insertion in the text contains a mathematical formula in which parentheses or brackets appear, the characters within the formula should be left as given unless that would place 2 identical punctuation symbols (eg, 2 open parentheses) immediately adjacent to each other. To avoid adjacent identical characters, change parentheses to brackets or brackets to parentheses in the formula as needed, working from inside out, starting with parentheses, to brackets, to braces.

> $CV_t^2 = [CV_b^2 + (CV_a^2/NR)]/NS$

6.6 ■ QUOTATION MARKS.

—Quotation marks are used to indicate that material is taken directly from another source, ie, quoted material.

6.6.1 *Quotations.*

—Use quotation marks to enclose a direct quotation of no more than 4 typewritten lines from textual material or speeches (for longer material, see 6.6.14, Block Quotations). When the quotation marks enclose conversational dialogue, there is no limit to the length that may be set in run-on format.

In all quoted material, follow the wording, spelling, and punctuation of the original exactly. The only time this rule does not apply is when the quoted material, although a complete sentence or part of a complete sentence in its original source, is now used as part of another complete sentence. In this case, the capital letter in the quoted sentence would be replaced by a lowercase letter in brackets.

Similarly, in legal material any change in initial capital letters from quoted material should be indicated by placing the change in brackets (see 6.8.7, Ellipses, Change in Capitalization).

To indicate an omission in quoted material, use ellipses (see 6.8, Ellipses).

To indicate editorial interpolation in quoted material, use brackets (see 6.5.2, Brackets, Insertions in Quotations). Use [*sic*] after a misspelled word or an incorrect or apparently absurd statement in quoted material to indicate that this is an accurate rendition of the original source. However, when quoting material from another era that uses now obsolete spellings, use *sic* sparingly. Do not use *sic* with an exclamation point. (*Note:* The use of *sic* is not limited to quoted material; in other instances, it means that any unusual or bizarre appearance in the preceding word is intentional, not accidental).

The author should always verify the quotation from the original source.

6.6.2 ***Dialogue.***—With conversational dialogue, enclose the opening word and the final word in quotation marks.

> "Please don't close the door just yet."
>
> "Okay, if you insist, I won't."

6.6.3 ***Titles.***—Within titles (including titles of articles, references, and tables), centered heads, and run-in sideheads, use double quotation marks.

> The "Sense" of Humor

6.6.4 ***Single Quotation Marks.***—Use single quotation marks for quotations within quotations.

> He looked at us and said, "As my patients always told me, 'Be a good listener.' "

6.6.5 ***Placement.***—Place closing quotation marks outside commas and periods, inside colons and semicolons. Place question marks, dashes, and exclamation points inside quotation marks only when they are part of the quoted material. If they apply to the whole statement, place them outside the quotation marks.

> Why bother to perform autopsies at all if the main finding is invariably "edema and congestion of the viscera"?
>
> The clinician continues to ask, "Why did he die?"
>
> "I'll lend you my stethoscope for clinic"—then she remembered the last time she had lent it and said, "On second thought, I'll be needing it myself."

Note: Commas are not always needed with quoted material. For instance, in the following example commas are not necessary after "said" or to set off the quoted material.

> He said he had had his "fill of it all" and was "content" to leave the meeting.

6.6.6 ***Omission of Opening or Closing Quotation Marks.***—The opening quotation mark should be omitted when an article beginning with a stand-up or drop 2-line initial capital letter also begins with a quotation. It is best, however, to avoid this construction.

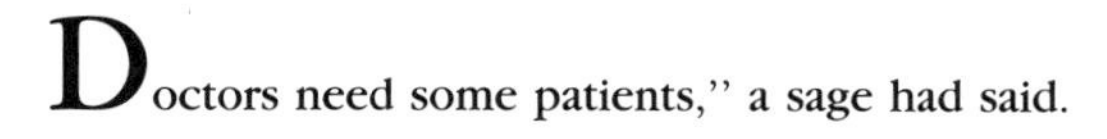
Doctors need some patients," a sage had said.

When excerpting long passages that consist of several paragraphs, use opening double quotation marks before each paragraph and closing quotation marks only at the end of the final paragraph (see 6.8, Ellipses, and 6.6.14, Block Quotations).

6.6.7 ***Coined Words, Slang.***—Coined words, slang, nicknames, and words or phrases used ironically or facetiously may be enclosed in quotation marks at first mention. Thereafter, omit quotation marks (see 19.5.2, Typography, Italics).

> We further hope that, above all, those who have been fed only "docufiction" on this matter, as if it were truth, will cease to be misled.

> *Nelson Essentials of Pediatrics* is not a . . . synopsis of or a companion to the *Nelson Textbook of Pediatrics,* although initially our associates dubbed it "Baby Nelson," "Half Nelson," and "Junior Nelson." [Behrman R, Kliegman R. *Nelson's Essentials of Pediatrics.* Philadelphia, Pa: WB Saunders; 1990.]

> It has been said that shoes and latrines are the best "medicine" for ancylostomiasis (hookworm disease).

Do not use quotation marks when emphasizing a word, when using a non-English word, when mentioning a term as a term, or when defining a term. In these instances, italics are preferred (see 19.5.2, Typography, Italics).

> The page number is called the *folio.*

> The eye associated with the greater reduction in hitting ability when dimmed by a filter was termed the *dominant eye* for motion stereopsis.

> *Pulsus paradoxus* is defined as an exaggeration of the physiologic inspiratory drop in systolic blood pressure.

6.6.8 ***Apologetic Quotation Marks.***—Quotation marks used around words to give special effect or to indicate irony are usually unnecessary.

When irony or special effect is intended, skillful preparation can take the place of using these quotes. Resort to apologetic quotation marks or quotation marks used to express irony only after such attempts have failed, keeping in mind that the best writing does not rely on apologetic quotation marks.

> Using their own finances and being informed about the economics of the approach, some may opt for the "boutique class" of health care.

6.6.9 ***So-called.***—A word or phrase following *so-called* should not be enclosed in quotation marks.

6.6.10 ***Common Words Used in a Technical Sense.***—Enclose in quotation marks a common word used in a special technical sense when the context does not make the meaning clear (see 6.6.11, Definition or Translation of Non-English Words).

> In many publications, "running feet" on left-hand pages face the "gutter" at the bottom of the page.

> "Coma vigil" (akinetic mutism) may be confused with conscious states.

6.6.11 ***Definition or Translation of Non-English Words.***—The literal translation of a non-English word or phrase is usually enclosed in quotation marks if it follows the word or phrase, whereas the simple definition of the word or phrase is not (see also 10.0, Non-English Words and Phrases; Accent Marks [Diacritics]).

> Hysterical patients may exhibit an attitude termed *la belle indifférence* ("beautiful indifference" or total unconcern) toward their condition.

6.6.12 ***Titles.***—In the text, use quotation marks to enclose titles of short poems, essays, lectures, radio and television programs, songs, the name of an electronic file, parts of published works (chapters, articles in a periodical), papers read at meetings, dissertations, theses, and parts of the same article (eg, the "Results" section) (see 8.5, Capitalization, Types and Sections of Articles, and 19.5.2, Typography, Italics).

6.6.13 ***Indirect Discourse, Discussions.***—After indirect discourse, do not use quotation marks.

> He said he would go home earlier.

Do not use quotation marks with yes or no.

> His answer to the question was no.

In interview or discussion formats when the speaker's name is set off, do not use quotation marks.

> Dr Black: Now let us review the slides of the bone marrow biopsy.
>
> Dr Smith: The first slide reveals complete absence of granulocytic precursors.

6.6.14 ***Block Quotations.***—If material quoted from texts or speeches is longer than 4 typewritten lines, the material should be set off in a block, ie, in reduced type and without the quotation marks. Paragraph indents are generally not used unless the quoted material is known to begin a paragraph. Space is often added both above and below these longer quotations.

If the block quotation appears in a section to be set in reduced type, do not reduce the type size of the quoted material further.

If another quotation appears within a block quote, use double quotation marks around the contained quotation, rather than setting off in blocks, regardless of the length.

6.7 ■ APOSTROPHE.

6.7.1 ***To Show Possession.***—Use the apostrophe to show the possessive case of nouns and indefinite pronouns in accordance with the following examples (see 13.2, Eponyms, Possessive Form):

Jones' bones (1 person named Jones)	the Joneses' bones (2 or more people named Jones)

If a singular or plural word does not end in *s*, add *'s* to form the possessive.

> a child's wants   everyone's answer
>
> men's concerns

If a proper noun or name ends in a silent *s*, *z*, or *x*, form the possessive by adding *'s*.

> Marx's theories   Jacqueline du Pres's work

6.7.2 ***Possessive Pronouns.***—Do not use -*'s* with possessive pronouns: his, hers, ours, its, yours, theirs, whose.

> The car is hers.
>
> Give the book its due.

Note: Do not confuse the contraction of *it is* [*it's*] with the possessive *its*, eg, "It's a beautiful day. The sun is at its peak."

6.7.3 ***Possessive of Compound Terms.***—Use *-'s* after only the last word of a compound term.

father-in-law's tie physician-in-chief's decision

mothers-in-law's letters secretary of health's ruling

someone else's book

6.7.4 ***Joint Possession.***—When joint possession is being shown with nouns, or with an organization's or business firm's name, use the possessive form only in the last word of the noun or name.

Food and Drug Administration's policy

Farrar, Straus & Giroux's books

Merck Sharp & Dohme's drug inserts

Centers for Disease Control and Prevention's Task Force

Hammond and Horn's study

When possession is individual, each noun takes the possessive form.

We matched the infant's and mother's records.

Note: When one of the nouns takes a possessive pronoun, the other nouns take the possessive as well.

I presented the intern's and my workup.

6.7.5 ***Using Apostrophes to Form Plurals.***—Do not use an apostrophe to indicate the plural of a name. Do not use an apostrophe in the name of an organization in which the qualifying term is used as an adjective or an attributive rather than a possessive. Of course, always follow the official name.

The Chicago Cubs

Veterans Affairs

Rainbow Babies Hospital

state parks rangers

musicians union

Use *-'s* to indicate the plural of letters, signs, or symbols spoken as such, or words referred to as words when *-s* alone would be confusing. Note the italics with inflectional ending in roman type for words, letters, and numbers but not for symbols and signs.

He uses too many *and*'s.

Mind your *p*'s and *q*'s.

There are 9 +'s on the page.

His *l*'s looked like *7*'s.

Do not use an apostrophe to form the plural of an all-capital abbreviation or of numerals (including years).

ECGs EEGs IQs WBCs RBCs

a woman in her 40s

during the late 1980s

6.7.6 ***Units of Time and Money as Possessive Adjectives.***—With units of time (minute, hour, day, month, year, etc) used as possessive adjectives, an *-'s* is added. The same holds true for monetary terms (see 5.6.3, Grammar, Nouns, Referring to Time or Money):

a day's wait

an hour's delay

5 days' hard work

a few hours' time

6 months' gestation

2 cents' worth of advice

6.7.7 ***Prime.***—Do not use an apostrophe where a prime sign is intended. Do not use a prime sign as a symbol of measurement (see 12.4.4, Nomenclature, Chemical Names, and 12.6, Nomenclature, Genetics).

The methyl group was in the 5′ position.

6.8 ■ **ELLIPSES.**—Ellipses are 3 spaced dots (. . .) generally used to indicate omission of 1 or more words, lines, paragraphs, or data from quoted material (this omission being the *ellipsis*). Excerpts from the following paragraph will be used to demonstrate the use of ellipses.

> In *Fruit Displayed on a Stand* (cover), exhibited in 1882, Caillebotte depicts a traditional subject in a manner far removed from the traditional cornucopian flow of fruit. Instead, he shows a stark, rectangular grid lit by centers of rounded forms, brilliantly colored. Vivid oranges, reds, and purples, light greens, creamy violets, and color-flecked gold are cupped within areas of crinkly blue-white paper, the cooler shades in the center separating the hotter tones, preventing them from spilling into each other. [*JAMA.* 1985;254;1000.]

6.8.1 ***Omission Within a Sentence.***—If the ellipsis occurs within a sentence, ellipses represent the omission. A space precedes and follows the ellipses.

Instead, he shows a . . . grid lit by centers of rounded forms, brilliantly colored.

In some such instances, additional punctuation may be used on either side of the ellipses if it helps the sense of the sentence or better shows the omission.

Instead, he shows a stark, rectangular grid . . . , brilliantly colored.

6.8.2 ***Omission at the End of a Sentence.***—If the ellipsis occurs at the end of a complete sentence, but before a new sentence begins, ellipses follow the final punctuation mark, the final punctuation mark being set close to the word preceding it, although this word is not the final word in that sentence in the original.

In *Fruit Displayed on a Stand* (cover), exhibited in 1882, Caillebotte depicts a traditional subject in a manner far removed from the traditional. . . . Instead, he shows a stark, rectangular grid lit by centers of rounded forms, brilliantly colored.

6.8.3 ***Omission Between Sentences.***—If the ellipsis occurs between 2 complete sentences, ellipses follow the final punctuation mark of the first sentence, the final punctuation mark being set close to the preceding word.

> In *Fruit Displayed on a Stand* (cover), exhibited in 1882, Caillebotte depicts a traditional subject in a manner far removed from the traditional cornucopian flow of fruit. . . . Vivid oranges, reds, and purples, light greens, creamy violets, and color-flecked gold are cupped within areas of crinkly blue-white paper, the cooler shades in the center separating the hotter tones, preventing them from spilling into each other.

If a sentence is omitted after a sentence that already ends in an ellipsis, no additional dots are needed; ie, the 3 spaced dots following the preceding incomplete sentence are sufficient.

> In *Fruit Displayed on a Stand* (cover), exhibited in 1882, Caillebotte depicts a traditional subject. . . . Vivid oranges, reds, and purples, light greens, creamy violets, and color-flecked gold are cupped within areas of crinkly blue-white paper, the cooler shades in the center separating the hotter tones, preventing them from spilling into each other.

6.8.4 ***Grammatically Incomplete Expressions.***—The sentence preceding as well as that following the ellipses should be a grammatically complete expression. However, 3 dots and *no* period may be used at the end of a sentence fragment to indicate that it is purposely grammatically incomplete.

> Complete the sentence, "When I retire, I plan to . . ." in 20 words or less.

6.8.5 ***Omissions in Verse.***—Use 1 line of em-spaced dots to indicate omission of a full line or several consecutive lines of verse.

> Sometimes you say it's smaller. Today
> . . . .
> you said it was a touch larger, and would change.
> [Marc Straus, MD, "Autumn"]

6.8.6 ***Omissions Between or at the Start of Paragraphs.***—With material in which several paragraphs are being quoted and omissions of full paragraphs occur, a period and 3 dots at the end of the paragraph preceding the omitted material is sufficient to indicate this omission.

> Indeed, it is no more than the just desert of Dr Theodore Schott and his late brother to attribute to them the credit of having introduced and elaborated a method capable of restoring most cases of heart disease to a state of complete compensation, after the failure of other means, such as digitalis. . . .

If the initial word(s) or the first sentence of the paragraph being quoted is omitted, begin that paragraph with a paragraph identation and 3 ellipsis dots to indicate that this is not the beginning of that paragraph.

> . . . it is no more than the just desert of Dr Theodore Schott and his late brother to attribute to them the credit of having introduced and elaborated a method capable of restoring most cases of heart disease to a state of complete compensation, after the failure of other means, such as digitalis. . . .

6.8.7 ***Change in Capitalization.***—The first word after the end punctuation mark and the ellipses should use the original capitalization, particularly in legal and scholarly documents. This facilitates finding the material in the original source and avoids any change of meaning. If a change in the original capitalization is made, brackets should be used around the letter in question (see 6.5.2, Brackets, Insertions in Quotations, and 6.6.1, Quotations).

. . . . [H]e shows a stark, rectangular grid lit by centers of rounded forms, brilliantly colored.

In the cover story, the artist is described as using "[v]ivid oranges, reds, and purples, light greens, creamy violets, and color-flecked gold" to depict "a traditional subject."

6.8.8 ***Omission of Ellipses.***—Ellipses are not necessary at the beginning and end of a quotation if the quoted material is a complete sentence from the original.

In a 1985 *JAMA* cover story, Martha Bier wrote, "Instead, he shows a stark, rectangular grid lit by centers of rounded forms, brilliantly colored."

Omit ellipses within a quotation when the omitted words occur at the same place as a bracketed editorial insertion (see 6.5.2, Brackets, Insertions in Quotations).

"[Caillebotte] shows a stark, rectangular grid lit by centers of rounded forms, brilliantly colored."

When a quoted phrase is an incomplete sentence, readers understand that something precedes and follows; therefore, ellipses are not used.

In *Place de L'Europe on a Rainy Day,* Caillebotte does not use "centers of rounded forms, brilliantly colored" but instead uses muted grays and purples to give the feel of the rain.

Ellipses are generally not needed when the first part of the introductory sentence is deleted.

Here Caillebotte "depicts a traditional subject in a manner far removed from the traditional. . . ."

6.8.9 ***Ellipses in Tables.***—In tables, ellipses may be used to indicate that no data were available, or that a specific category of data is not applicable (see 2.13.4, Tables, Table Components). An explanatory footnote should also be included if it is not clear from the context what the ellipses represent.

*Ellipses indicate no test performed.

ACKNOWLEDGMENT

Principal author: Paula Glitman

ADDITIONAL READINGS AND GENERAL REFERENCES

The Chicago Manual of Style. 14th ed. Chicago, Ill: The University of Chicago Press; 1993.

Warriner JE. *English Grammar and Composition: Complete Course.* Franklin ed. New York, NY: Harcourt Brace Jovanovich Publishers; 1982.

CHAPTER 7

7.0 PLURALS

7.1 ■ **ABBREVIATIONS.**—With units of measure, use the same abbreviation for singular and plural forms (see 11.2, Abbreviations, Units of Measure). For most all-capital abbreviations, the plural is formed by adding *s*. Do not add an apostrophe before the *s*.

RBCs   WBCs   HMOs   PSROs   EEGs   IQs   ECGs

7.2 ■ **COLLECTIVE NOUNS.**—Collective nouns may take verbs that are singular or plural, depending on the intended meaning (see 5.9.5, Grammar, Collective Nouns).

A number of subjects were unavailable for follow-up.

The number of controls was small.

The majority rules.

The majority were cured.

Note: With units of measure, always use a singular verb: Five milliliters was injected.

7.3 ■ **COMPOUND NOUNS.**—For compound nouns written as one word, add *s* to form the plural.

teaspoonful   teaspoonfuls

For compound nouns formed by a noun and a modifier, form the plural by making the noun plural. Follow the latest edition of *Merriam-Webster's Collegiate Dictionary* when in doubt.

mother-in-law	mothers-in-law
surgeon general	surgeons general
coup d'état	coups d'état
man-of-war	men-of-war

Other compound nouns form the plural by adding an *s* at the end of the compound noun.

tie-up	tie-ups
2-month-old	2-month-olds
obstetrician-gynecologist	obstetrician-gynecologists

7.4 ■ **LATIN AND GREEK VS ENGLISH.**—Follow the latest edition of *Merriam-Webster's Collegiate Dictionary* or of *Stedman's* or *Dorland's* medical dictionary. Where the dictionaries show both forms as equally acceptable, use the English form rather than the Latin or Greek, unless common usage dictates otherwise, as with *phenomenon, phenomena, phenomenons* (see 5.9.2, Grammar, False Singulars).

The following are commonly seen Latin and Greek terms and their preferred plurals:

Singular	*Preferred Plural*	*Also Acceptable Plural*
alga	algae	. . .
appendix	appendices	appendixes
cannula	cannulas	cannulae
corpus delicti	corpora delicti	. . .
cranium	crania	craniums
criterion	criteria	criterions
fistula	fistulae	fistulas
formula	formulas	formulae
genus	genera	. . .
humerus	humeri	. . .
maxilla	maxillae	maxillas
sequela	sequelae	. . .
vertebra	vertebrae	vertebras

Be aware, however, that, although rare, there may be a difference in meaning with the variant forms:

The book had both subject and author indexes.

The book was rated on numerous indices.

In mathematics, *indices* is always the preferred spelling.

7.5 ■ **MICROORGANISMS.**—Use the lowercase plural form for organisms that have a common designation. Consult the latest edition of *Stedman's* or *Dorland's* medical dictionary (see 12.12, Nomenclature, Organisms).

Bacillus	bacilli
Staphylococcus	staphylococci
Streptococcus	streptococci

For some organisms that do not have a common plural designation, add the word *organisms* or *species* to indicate a plural use (see 12.12, Nomenclature, Organisms).

7.6 ■ **OTHER PLURALS.**—For the plurals of numbers, letters, signs, and symbols, see 6.7.5, Punctuation, Using Apostrophes to Form Plurals.

Acknowledgment

Principal author: Paula Glitman

Additional Readings and General References

Dorland's Illustrated Medical Dictionary. 28th ed. Philadelphia, Pa: WB Saunders Co; 1994.

Merriam-Webster's Collegiate Dictionary. 10th ed. Springfield, Mass: Merriam-Webster Inc; 1993.

Stedman's Medical Dictionary. 26th ed. Baltimore, Md: Williams & Wilkins; 1995.

CHAPTER 8

8.0 CAPITALIZATION

Words are capitalized sparingly but conventionally in the scientific publications of the AMA.

8.1 ■ **PROPER NOUNS.**—Capitalize proper nouns; follow the most recent editions of *Merriam-Webster's Collegiate Dictionary* and *Webster's New International Dictionary.*

8.1.1 ***Geographic Names.***—Capitalize geographic names for cities, townships, counties, states, countries, continents, islands, peninsulas, straits, bodies of water, mountain chains, streets, parks, forests, canyons, dams, specific locations, accepted designations for regions, and political divisions.

the Antarctic
the Badlands
the Bay Area
the Black Forest
the British Isles
Central America
the China Sea
Cook County
Fifth Precinct
Fisherman's Wharf
the 43rd Ward office
the Great Lakes
Green Mountains
Gulf of Mexico
the High Plains
Hoover Dam
Hudson Bay
the Iron Curtain
Isle of Wight
Kettle Moraine
Kuril Islands
Lake Erie
the Loop [Chicago]
Mexico City
(*But:* Quebec city)
Mississippi River
New Trier Township
New York City
New York State
(*But:* the state of New York)
North Pole
Pacific Ocean
Province of Nova Scotia
Rocky Mountain National Park
Straits of Gibraltar
Third World
Tiananmen Square
the 23rd Congressional District
United Kingdom
Upstate New York
the West Coast

When a common noun is capitalized in the singular as part of a proper name or in a title, it is generally not capitalized in the plural.

Mississippi and Missouri rivers   Atlantic and Pacific oceans

Expanded compass directions are not capitalized when they indicate general directions or locations, although they are capitalized when used as accepted designations for regions and when part of geographic designations.

She practices medicine in the Far East, in central China. Her home is east of Chongqing (Chungking) but not as far east as Wuhan.

He is a westerner. He lives in the West, 15 miles west of Salt Lake City, Utah.

Go due north, then northwest. (*But:* ENE, SSW)

North Carolina   Eastern influence   North Korea
(*But:* southern France, northern Illinois, south Florida, northern California)

Nouns and adjectives derived from compass directions should not be capitalized.

midwesterner   southern-style cooking

8.1.2 ***Sociocultural Designations.***—Capitalize proper names of languages, peoples, races, political parties, religions, and religious denominations and sects. Do not capitalize the common nouns that follow these designations. Do not capitalize political doctrines. Do not capitalize *white* or *black* as a designation of race.

As society becomes more aware of the issue of cultural diversity, it is extremely important to be sensitive to the changing preferences of various cultural groups as to the terminology used when referring to these groups. For example, over the years, Black, Afro-American, and African American have entered the literature only to change in favor as times and attitudes changed (see 9.10, Correct and Preferred Usage, Inclusive Language).

the English language	Sanskrit	African American
Southeast Asian community	Europeans	French people
of Spanish ancestry	the Jewish people	Chiricahua Apache
Hispanic population	a Baptist church (*But:* First Baptist Church)	Protestant
Native American		

Although she has been a member of the Republican party for years, at one time she was a Democrat. She nonetheless has always endorsed the principles of democracy in our republican form of government. She is democratic in her attitudes toward social equality.

8.1.3 ***Events, Awards, Legislation.***—Capitalize the names of historical events and periods, special events, awards, treaties, and official names and specific parts of adopted laws and bills. Do not capitalize common nouns and adjectives in proposed laws, bills, or amendments that have not been passed.

Americans With Disabilities Act	Congressional Medal of Honor
Battle of Gettysburg	Declaration of Helsinki
Bill of Rights	Family and Medical Leave Act of 1993
Civil Rights Law	Geneva Convention

1949 Geneva Conventions, article 3	Physician's Recognition Award
Kentucky Derby	Public Law 89-74
Louisiana Purchase	Purple Heart
Medicaid	Russian Revolution
Medicare	Sixteenth Amendment
Medicare Act	Social Security Act
New York Marathon	Special Olympics
Nobel Prize	Title XVIII
Persian Gulf War	Vietnam War
Pfizer Biomedical Research Award	

(*But:* King-Anderson bill; Medicare law; premarital laws; the act)

8.1.4 ***Words Derived From Proper Nouns.***—Most words derived from proper nouns are not capitalized. Follow the first boldface entries in the most recent edition of *Merriam-Webster's Collegiate Dictionary* for nonmedical terms; follow the current edition of *Stedman's* or *Dorland's* medical dictionary for terms used in a medical context (see 12.12, Nomenclature, Organisms, and 12.5, Nomenclature, Equipment, Devices, and Reagents).

Addison	addisonian
Candida	candidiasis
Mendel	mendelian
Parkinson	parkinsonian
Schistosoma	schistosomiasis
plaster of paris	
india ink	
brussels sprouts	

Note: Although *Merriam-Webster's Collegiate Dictionary* is a useful standard, there are instances in which words derived from proper nouns have become part of common usage and, in contradistinction to *Merriam-Webster's Collegiate Dictionary,* are not capitalized, eg, arabic numerals, roman numerals, turkish coffee, roman candles.

8.1.5 ***Eponyms.***—When an eponym is included in the name of a disease, syndrome, sign, position, or similar designation, capitalize the eponym but not the common noun. Consult the current editions of *Stedman's* or *Dorland's* medical dictionary (see 13.0, Eponyms).

Raynaud disease	Babinski sign	Marfan syndrome
Gram stain (*But:* gram-negative specimen)	Trendelenburg position	

8.1.6 ***Proprietary Names.***—Capitalize trademarks and proprietary names of drugs and brand names of manufactured products and equipment. Do not capitalize generic names or descriptive terms. The common noun after a brand name is not capitalized (see 12.4, Nomenclature, Drugs, and 12.5, Nomenclature, Equipment, Devices, and Reagents).

Smith-Corona typewriter	Peter Pan peanut butter
Xerox copier	Macintosh computer
Dacron implant	Teflon-coated electromagnetic needle
Silastic catheter	Kleenex tissues

8.1.7 ***Organisms.***—Capitalize the formal name of a genus when used in the singular, with or without a species name. Do capitalize formal genus names but not traditional plural generic designations (eg, streptococci) or derived adjectives (streptococcal). Do not capitalize the name of a species, variety, or subspecies. Do capitalize phylum, class, order, family, and tribe (see 12.12, Nomenclature, Organisms). For capitalization of virus names, see 12.12.2, Nomenclature, Viruses.

8.1.8 ***Seasons, Deities, Holidays.***—Do not capitalize the names of the seasons. Do capitalize the designations of specific deities and personifications.

the Almighty	Nature	God	Allah
the Holy Spirit	summer	Maheo	Corn Mother

Capitalize recognized holiday and calendar events.

Easter	Passover	Fourth of July	St Patrick's Day
Rosh Hashanah	Kwanza	Yom Kippur	Hanukkah
Holy Week	Thanksgiving Day	New Year's Eve	Ramadan
Cinco de Mayo	May Day	Christmas	

8.1.9 ***Tests.***—The exact and complete titles of tests are capitalized. When the word *test* appears with the name of a test that is in a written form and that is used as a survey or tool, the word *test* is capitalized. For tests that involve a process, as is the case with most statistical tests, the word *test* is not capitalized (see 17.4, Statistics, Glossary of Statistical Terms). The word *scale* or *test* is not capitalized when used to refer to a subscale of a test. In addition, in text, figure legends, and table footnotes, any words that precede the word *subscale* or that refer to a subscale of a scale or test would also not be capitalized, eg, anhedonia subscale of the Scale for the Assessment of Negative Symptoms.

Note: There is one exception to this rule: in table stub entries where the first word of the entry takes an initial capital letter, the first word of the subscale would be capitalized.

Bayley Scales of Infant Development
(*But:* Bayley Scales consist of 3 tools: Mental scale, Motor scale, and Infant Behavior record. Only the Mental and Motor scales were used.)

Goodenough-Harris Drawing Test
(*But:* The Goodenough-Harris test was used.)

Hamilton Depression Rating Scale
(*But:* Hamilton scale)

Minnesota Multiphasic Personality Inventory
(*But:* Minnesota Multiphasic Personality Inventory Depression scale [this is a subscale of the MMPI])

Below is a list of tests or scales, statistical and nonstatistical, and the style AMA follows for capitalization:

Advanced Vocabulary Test

Beck Depression Inventory

Benton Revised Retention Test

Binet-Simon Scale (or Test)

Brief Psychiatric Rating Scale

Center for Epidemiological Studies Depression Scale

Clinical Dementia Rating Scale

Conners' Parent Rating Scale

Conners' Teacher Rating Scale

Diagnostic Interview Schedule

Draw-a-Man Test

Eysenck Personality Inventory

Farnsworth D-15 panel test

Farnsworth-Munsell 100-hue test

the Fisher exact test

General Health Questionnaire

Glasgow Coma Scale

goodness-of-fit test

Hamilton Anxiety Rating Scale

Hamilton score

Hardy-Rand-Ritler plates (or American Optical–Hardy-Rand-Ritler color plates)

Hopkins Symptom Checklist–90

Injury Severity Score

Ishihara color plates

Jaeger 5 (or J5)

Kuder-Richardson reliability (or coefficient)

Kurtzke Expanded Disability Status Scale

Kurtzke Expanded Severity Score

Likert scale

Maddox rod test

Mann-Whitney *U* test

Mental Status Examination

Michigan Alcoholism Screening Test

Mini-Mental State Examination

Minnesota Multiphasic Personality Inventory

Minnesota Multiphasic Personality Inventory–Revised

Newman-Keuls test

Object Sorting Test

Peabody Picture Vocabulary Test

Profile of Mood States depression scale

Research Diagnostic Criteria

Rorschach Test

Scale for the Assessment of Negative Symptoms

Scale for the Assessment of Positive Symptoms

Schedule for Affective Disorders and Schizophrenia

Schedule for Affective Disorders and Schizophrenia-Lifetime version

Schedule for Schizotypal Personality

Schirmer test

Southern blot

Spearman rank correlation test

Stanford-Binet Scale

Stanford Diagnostic Reading Test

Stroop color test

the Student *t* test

Structured Clinical Interview for *Diagnostic and Statistical Manual of Mental Disorders, Fourth Edition*

Symptom Checklist-90

Trail-Making Test

Yale-Brown Obsessive Compulsive Scale

Visual Retention Test

vocabulary test

Wechsler Adult Intelligence Scale

Wechsler Adult Intelligence Scale-Revised

Wechsler Intelligence Scale for Children

Westergren method

Western blot

Wide Range Achievement Test

Wilcoxon rank sum test

Wilcoxon signed rank test

Wisconsin Card Sorting Test

Worth 4-dot test

the Yates Correction for Continuity
(*But:* the Yates correction)

8.2 ■ **TITLES AND DEGREES OF PERSONS.**—Capitalize the title of a person when it precedes the person's name but not when it follows the name.

Chair John W. Smith

John W. Smith was named chair.

Prime Minister Major addressed the US Congress. Later in the week the prime minister will meet with the president.

However, institutions and organizations, when referring to themselves and their officers in abbreviated form, often use capitals (see 8.3, Official Names).

Capitalize academic degrees when abbreviated but not when written out (see 11.1, Abbreviations, Academic Degrees and Honors, and 11.6, Abbreviations, Names and Titles of Persons).

8.3 ■ **OFFICIAL NAMES.**—Capitalize the official titles of conferences, congresses, postgraduate courses, organizations, institutions, business firms, and governmental agencies, and their departments and other divisions. Do not capitalize a conjunction, article, or preposition of 3 letters or less, except when it is the first or last word in a title or subtitle. In institution names, do not capitalize *the* unless it is part of the official title.

Note: If retaining the capital *t* in *The* causes inelegance in the prose or how the sentence looks aesthetically, use a lowercase *t*, eg, "He cited the Johns Hopkins University model of medical education as exemplary."

the Ad Hoc Committee on Evaluation of Experimental Trials

Cambridge University

Chicago Board of Education

Chicago Lying-In Hospital

Congress

Congressional Budget Office

Department of Labor

Family Service Association of America

the Federal Bureau of Investigation

the Federation of State Medical Boards in the United States

the Forty-seventh World Health Assembly

the Girl Scouts of America

House of Representatives

the Illinois State Senate

the Insect Allergy Committee of the American Academy of Allergy

the International Committee of the Red Cross

the International Subcommittee on Viral Nomenclature

Interstate Commerce Commission

The Johns Hopkins Hospital

New York Academy of Sciences

Pharmaceutical Products Division, Baxter Laboratories, Inc

Quaker Oats Corporation

The Robert Wood Johnson Foundation

The Salvation Army

the Second International Congress on Peer Review in Biomedical Publication

Supreme Court (*Note:* capitalize Court when referring to the Supreme Court)

the 10th Annual Surgical Symposium of the Association of Veterans Affairs Hospitals

the Third International Congress on Poliomyelitis

Trans World Airlines

Tufts University School of Medicine

the US Army

But:

an ad hoc committee	the congresswoman
the armed forces	the department
the army	federal courts
the association	the federal government
the board of health	naval service
the board of trustees	the navy
the committee	state senators
the company	the university
congressional reports	

Often when referring to themselves and their officers in abbreviated form, institutions and organizations use capitals for the generic terms being used as abbreviations. We prefer lowercasing such generic terms. For example, at the AMA:

the American Medical Association	the association
the Board of Trustees	the board or the trustees
the Committee on Allied Health Education and Accreditation	the committee
the Council on Scientific Affairs	the council
the House of Delegates	the house or the delegates
the Department of Continuing Medical Education	the department
the president of the AMA	the president

A singular noun that is capitalized as part of the official name is usually not capitalized in the plural.

Department of Pediatrics *but* departments of pediatrics and neurology
(*Exception:* From the Departments of Medicine and Pediatrics, University of Tennessee College of Medicine, Memphis.)

However, when the plural of a common noun is part of the title of an organization or institution, it should be capitalized.

National Institutes of Health   Centers for Disease Control and Prevention

Vanderbilt University Affiliated Hospitals
(*But:* Michael Reese and Northwestern Memorial hospitals have programs on prenatal care.)

8.4 ■ **TITLES AND HEADINGS.**—Capitalize major words in titles, subtitles, and headings of publications, parts of publications, musical compositions, plays (stage and screen), radio and television programs, movies, paintings, works of art, software programs, electronic systems, and names of ships, airplanes, awards, and monuments (see 10.1.2, Non-English Words and Phrases, Accent Marks [Diacritics], Translation). Do not capitalize a conjunction, article, or preposition of 3 letters or less, except when it is the first or last word in a title or subtitle.

Note: The may be dropped from such titles if the syntax of the sentence improves without it.

> As part of the experiment, subjects stayed in a single room and were entertained by being shown the movie *The Right Stuff.*
>
> The university's theater workshop staged a production of Molière's *Le Médecin Malgré Lui,* to everyone's delight.

But

> That exhilarating *Right Stuff* liftoff scene from Cape Canaveral brought the moviegoer into the excitement of the first space shuttle launches.
>
> The current production of the witty and often ribald *Médecin Malgré Lui* by Molière is as funny and relevant today as when first performed.

the *Merrimac*
the yacht *America*[3]
Golden Globe Award
Oscar
Busse Highway
The Lasker Award
the *Journal of the American Medical Association*
the *New England Journal of Medicine*
Seurat's *Sunday Afternoon on the Grande Jatte*
Calder's *Baseball Bat*
Samuel Barber's *Adagio for Strings,* op 11
General Hospital
WordPerfect
the Tomb of the Unknown Soldier
the "EEF's Guide to the Internet" file
Truman Memorial Library
Tartuffe
the *Kitty Hawk*
Casablanca
World Wide Web
Internet
Vivaldi's *The Four Seasons*
Friends
Windows
Navy Pier

But: In a television series with separately titled episodes, use quotation marks around the episode name:

> the *Dream On* episode "Stone Cold"

In titles and headings, capitalize 2-letter verbs, for example, *go, do, am, is, be. Note:* In infinitives, the "to" is not capitalized.

> What Is Sarcoma?
>
> We Do Need to Treat Mild Hypertension
>
> Where the World Will Be in the Year 2010

With dual verbs, such as *follow up,* capitalize both parts in a title.

Following Up the Diabetic Patient

8.4.1 ***In References.***—In listed references, follow 2.12.9, Manuscript Preparation, References, Titles, 2.12.10, References, Non-English-Language Titles, and 2.12.11, References, Subtitles, for capitalization of titles and subtitles of articles, parts of books, bulletins, and pamphlets, in English or in a non-English language.

8.4.2 ***Hyphenated Compounds.***—In titles, subtitles, table heads, centerheads, sideheads, and line art, do not capitalize the second part of a hyphenated compound in the following instances:

- If either part is a hyphenated prefix or suffix (see 6.3.1, Punctuation, Hyphens, Temporary Compounds).

Re-treat	Self-preservation
Anti-infective Drugs	Intra-abdominal Surgery
Intra-arterial Embolism	Vaso-occlusive Disease

- If both parts together constitute a single word (if in doubt about hyphenation of such terms, consult the current edition of *Merriam-Webster's Collegiate Dictionary,* or of *Stedman's* or *Dorland's* medical dictionary; if necessary, extrapolate from similar words, eg, adult-onset diabetes and late-onset diabetes; corticospinal and corticosubcortical).

Long-term	Follow-up Studies
X-ray Films	Part-time Help
End-expiratory Pressure	Signet-ring Carcinoma In Situ

(*But:* Auditory Brain-Stem Response; Low-Level Radioactive Waste; Drug-Resistant Diseases; T-Cell Receptors; B-Cell Lymphoma)

Note: Capitalize the first letter of the word that follows a lowercase but not a capital Greek letter (see 14.2, Greek Letters, Capitalization After a Greek Letter), a numeral (except when an abbreviated unit of measure that never is capitalized follows), a symbol, italicized organic chemistry prefixes *trans-* and *cis-,* or a small capital letter in titles, subtitles, table heads, centerheads, sideheads, and line art.

β-Blockers	1,25-Dihydroxycholecalciferol
10% Strength	*trans*-Fatty Acid Content of Common Foods

8.5 ■ **TYPES AND SECTIONS OF ARTICLES.**—When speaking in broad terms about a type of article or a section within an article, lowercase the first letter of the category or section name.

The methods sections of articles are often inadequate.

However, when referring to a specific type of article such as "original contribution," or a section of an article within the article itself, capitalize the first letter in the words of the category or section name.

In our "Methods" section, we give a full description of each of the groups in the study.

8.6 ■ **FIRST WORD OF STATEMENT, QUOTATION, OR SUBTITLE.**—Capitalize the first word (1) of a formal statement that follows a colon (see 6.2.3, Punctuation, Colon, Introducing Quotations or Enumerations); (2) after the word *resolved* in a resolution; (3) of a direct quotation (but see 6.6.1, Punctuation, Quotations); and (4) of a question or a statement inserted in a sentence but not in quotation marks (see 6.2.1, Punctuation, Comma). (Concerning legal quotations, see 6.6.1, Punctuation, Quotations.)

In the case of a question, capitalization of the first word can be left to the author's personal style. Generally, with a more formal question, the first word will take a capital letter.

After a colon, capitalize the first word (1) in book titles (see 2.12.9, Manuscript Preparation, References, Titles; however, the first word in subtitles of journal articles is *not* capitalized) and, often, (2) in the text when the enumeration or explanation that follows contains 2 or more independent clauses (see 6.2.3, Punctuation, Colon, Introducing Quotations or Enumerations).

For capitalization in quoted material, follow the quotation exactly. Usually the first word of a direct quotation should be capitalized, especially if it is formally presented as a quotation.

> The report noted: "A candidate may be admitted after completing 2 years of medical school."

If the quotation is run into the sentence, however, a lowercase letter on the first word might be preferable (see 6.6.1, Punctuation, Quotations).

> The report noted that "a candidate may be admitted after completing 2 years of medical school."

If a sentence fragment is being quoted, do not capitalize the first word.

> The committee agrees with the report that candidate admission requires "completing 2 years of medical school."

8.7 ■ **ACRONYMS AND INITIALISMS.**—Do not capitalize the words from which an acronym or an initialism is derived (see 11.0, Abbreviations).

> prostate-specific antigen (PSA)
>
> enzyme-linked immunosorbent assay (ELISA)

Exception: When the words that form the acronym or initialism are proper names, use capitals as described in 8.3, Official Names.

> National Broadcasting Company (NBC)

8.8 ■ **DESIGNATORS.**—When used as specific designations, with or without numerals, capitalize *Table, Tables, Figure,* and *Figures.*

> as shown in the Table
>
> as seen in compact bundles (Figure)
>
> summarized in Table 2
>
> as illustrated in Figure 2 through Figure 7
>
> cultures yielded *Candida* (Figure 3)

Note: When a table or figure is cited in a paragraph with its number designation and is then referred to again in that paragraph, the capital letter as well as the numeral designation can be deleted provided no other tables or figures are cited in the intervening material.

In Table 5 one can see the distribution of the patient population. This table also shows the prevalence of disease in each group.

Do not capitalize the following words, even when used as specific designations, unless they are part of a title:

case	fraction	notes	series
chapter	grade	page	stage
chromosome	grant	paragraph	stub
column	group	part	type
control	lead	patient	volume
experiment	level	phase	wave
factor	method	section	

(*But:* Step I diet and Axis I of the *Diagnostic and Statistical Manual of Mental Disorders, Fourth Edition*)

ACKNOWLEDGMENT

Principal author: Paula Glitman

ADDITIONAL READINGS AND GENERAL REFERENCES

Anastasi A. *Psychological Testing.* 5th ed. New York, NY: Macmillan Publishing Co Inc; 1982.

The Chicago Manual of Style. 14th ed. Chicago, Ill: The University of Chicago Press; 1993.

Dorland's Illustrated Medical Dictionary. 28th ed. Philadelphia, Pa: WB Saunders Co; 1994.

Stedman's Medical Dictionary. 26th ed. Baltimore, Md: Williams & Wilkins; 1995.

CHAPTER 9

That an occasional physician should write obscurely is only to be expected.

Lester S. King, MD[1]

9.0 CORRECT AND PREFERRED USAGE

This section on correct and preferred usage is intended to help authors and editors avoid common errors and to encourage sensitivity in the use of proper language. This section is also intended to describe distinctions between and clarify the meanings of frequently misused words. Beyond that, authors should avoid words and phrases that are unnecessarily elaborate, trendy, tautologic, or euphemistic.

9.1 ■ COMMONLY MISUSED WORDS AND PHRASES.

abnormal, normal; negative, positive—Examinations and laboratory tests and studies are not in themselves abnormal, normal, negative, or positive. These adjectives apply to observations, results, or findings (see also 17.0, Statistics).

Results of cultures and tests for microorganisms and specific reactions to tests may be negative or positive. Other tests focus on a pattern of activity rather than a single feature, and in these a range of normal and abnormal results is possible. These tests include electroencephalograms and electrocardiograms and modes of imaging such as isotope scans, radiographic studies, and computed tomographic scans.

Incorrect: The physical examination was normal.
Correct: The findings from the physical examination were normal.

Incorrect: The throat culture was negative.
Correct: The throat culture was negative for β-hemolytic streptococci.

Incorrect: The electroencephalogram was positive.
Correct: The electroencephalogram showed abnormalities in the temporal regions.

Exceptions: HIV-positive patients
seronegative mothers
negative node

Note: Patients or subjects should not be classified as "normal" (or "abnormal") when one is referring to their health status.

Incorrect: All normal subjects were excluded from the analysis.

Possible: All healthy subjects were excluded from the analysis.

Or: All subjects without asthma were excluded from the analysis.

abort, terminate—*Abort* means to stop a process in the early stages. In pregnancy, *abortion* means the premature expulsion—spontaneous or induced—from the uterus of the products of conception. A pregnancy, not a fetus or a woman, may be aborted. The synonym *terminate*—to bring to an end or a halt—may also be used.

accident, injury—According to the National Center for Injury Prevention and Control of the US Centers for Disease Control and Prevention (G. Ingraham, written communication, March 14, 1995), *accident* should not be used to refer to injuries from any cause. Although *accident* implies a random act that is unpredictable and unavoidable, epidemiologic studies and injury control programs indicate that injuries may be predictable and therefore preventable. The preferred terms refer either to the external cause (injury from falls, injury from motor vehicle crashes, gunshot injury) or to the intentionality ("unintentional injury" for injuries resulting from acts that were not intended to cause harm and "violence" for any act in which harm was intended).

Accident is considered by the public health community to be imprecise and should therefore be avoided. The injury-causing event can be described as noted above or with other terms, such as *crash, shooting, immersion, collision,* or *poisoning.*

Note: Do not change *accident* if it is integral to the terminology being used, for example, in an established injury classification system (eg, Fatal Accident Reporting System, *International Classification of Diseases*). Do not change *accident* in terms that describe specific medical conditions, such as *cerebrovascular accident.*

acute, chronic—These terms are most often preferred for descriptions of symptoms, conditions, or diseases; they refer to duration, not severity. Avoid the use of *acute* and *chronic* to describe patients, parts of the body, treatment, or medication.

Avoid:
chronic dialysis
chronic heroin users
acute administration of epinephrine
chronic diagnosis

Preferred:
long-term dialysis (also: maintenance dialysis [query author])
long-term heroin users
immediate administration of penicillin
long-standing diagnosis of a chronic disease
acute cystitis
chronic obstructive pulmonary disease
acute renal failure

Exception: Acute abdomen is a specific medical condition.

A note on short- and long-term patient care: According to Kane and Kane,[2] "*acute care hospital* is preferred to *short-term care hospital. Long-term care* has come to include both an acute component (sometimes called *subacute care* or *postacute care*), which effectively provides the care formerly offered in hospitals, and the more traditional chronic component, which includes both medical and social services. As the name implies, subacute care has a shorter time frame and serves patients who are expected to recuperate or die, while the more chronic form provides more sustained supportive services."

adapt, adopt—To *adapt* means to modify to fit a particular circumstance or requirement. To *adopt* means to take and use as one's own.

> Methods for measuring health status were adapted from the Medical Outcomes Study functioning and well-being scales.

> *JAMA* and the AMA *Archives* Journals adopted Système International (SI) units as standards of measurement.

adverse effect, adverse event, adverse reaction, side effect—*Side effect* is the secondary consequence for which an agent (usually a drug) is implemented. The term is often used incorrectly when *adverse effect, adverse event,* or *adverse reaction* is intended. Since a side effect may be either beneficial or harmful, specific terminology should be used.

> Constipation, headache, nausea, and syncope were the most commonly reported adverse effects among patients in the drug treatment group.

affect, effect—*Affect,* as a verb, means to have an influence on. *Effect,* as a verb, means to bring about or to cause. The 2 words cannot be used interchangeably.

> Ingesting massive doses of ascorbic acid may affect his recovery [influence the recovery in some way].

> Ingesting massive doses of ascorbic acid may effect his recovery [produce the recovery].

Affect, as a noun, refers to immediate expressions of emotion (in contrast to *mood,* which refers to sustained emotional states). *Affect* is often used as part of psychiatric diagnostic terminology. *Effect,* as a noun, means result.

> Mr Jones' general lack of affect was considered to be an effect of the recent trauma.

age, aged, school-age, school-aged, teenage, teenaged—The adjectival form *aged,* not the noun *age,* should be used to designate a person's age. Similarly, *school-aged* and *teenaged* are preferred to *school-age* and *teenage*. However, a precise age should be given whenever possible. See also 9.5, Age and Sex Referents.

> The patient, aged 70 years, had symptoms of dementia.

> *Alternate form:* The 70-year-old patient had symptoms of dementia.

> The health program was designed for children aged 5 through 8 years.

> The teenaged patients with tinnitus had spent an average of 4½ hours a day listening to music on their stereo headphones.

> *Better:* The patients with tinnitus, aged 14, 16, and 17 years, had spent an average of 4½ hours a day listening to music on their stereo headphones.

Note: In some expressions regarding age, it is redundant to add *of age* after the number of years, since it is implied in the adjectives *younger* and *older*.

> The patient group comprised women younger than 25 years.

See also 9.2.1, Redundant Words.

aggravate, irritate—When an existing condition is made worse, more serious, or more severe, it is *aggravated* (also, *exacerbated*). When tissue is caused to be inflamed, it is *irritated*. An irritation may be aggravated, but an aggravation cannot be irritated.

although, though—Although *although* and *though* may be considered interchangeable, *although* is preferable as a complete conjunction, because *though* in this construction is an "abbreviation" and thus may be less appropriate for formal prose. *Though* is correct in the adverbial construction, though.

> Although the analysis was done correctly, the fundamental terms of the investigation were too narrow to be interesting.

Clue to usage: Although is usually placed at the beginning of a sentence, and *though* is placed elsewhere when used to link words or phrases.

among, between—*Among* usually pertains to general collective relations and always in a group of more than 2. *Between* pertains to the relation between 1 thing and 1 or more other things. For instance, a treaty may be made *between* 4 powers, since each is defining a relationship with each of the others, but peace may exist *among* them.

> The patients shared the library books equally among themselves.
>
> Between you and me [not *I*], we are certain to find the common factor among those we have examined.

apt, liable, likely—*Apt* connotes a volition or habitual tendency and should not be used in regard to an inanimate object. *Liable* connotes the possibility of risk or disadvantage to the subject. *Likely* merely implies probability and thus is more inclusive than *apt*.

> A child is apt to cry when frustrated.
>
> Patients receiving immunosuppressant drugs are liable to acquire fungal infections.
>
> The computer system is likely to crash if it is overloaded.

Note: To write "The system is apt to crash . . ." implies that the computer is capable of habitual tendencies or volitions—an implication the careful writer may wish to avoid given the present limitations of artificial intelligence.

article, manuscript, paper, typescript—An unpublished study, report, or essay—that is, the document itself—may be referred to as a *manuscript, paper,* or *typescript*. When published, it is an *article*.

> The authors thank Carolyn King for comments on earlier drafts of the manuscript.
>
> This article is one of an ongoing series sponsored by the American Heart Association.

as, because, since—Why explain the distinction? Because!

Because, since, and *as* can all be used when "for the reason that" is meant. However, in this construction, *as* should be avoided when it could be construed to mean *while*.

> *Ambiguous:* She could not answer her page as she was examining a critically ill patient.
>
> *Better:* She could not answer her page, as she was examining a critically ill patient [use comma].
>
> *Preferred:* She could not answer her page because she was examining a critically ill patient.

Similarly, *since* should be avoided when it could be construed to mean "from the time of" or "from the time that."

Ambiguous: She had not been able to answer her page since she was in the clinic.

Preferred: She had not been able to answer her page because she was in the clinic.

assure, ensure, insure—These verbs are used synonymously in many contexts, but there are distinctions. *Assure* means to provide positive information to a person or persons and implies the removal of doubt and suspense (*assure* the subjects that their results will be held in complete confidence). *Ensure* means to make sure or certain (*ensure* the statistical power of the study). *Insure* means taking precautions beforehand (*insure* his life).

because of, caused by, due to, owing to—These phrases are not synonymous, but the differences are subtle. *Due to* and *caused by* are adjectival phrases, *owing to* and *because of* adverbial phrases. The use of *due to* in both situations can sometimes alter a sentence's meaning.

Survivors of child abuse tend to enter abusive relationships due to intrapsychic conflicts.

Meaning: Survivors of child abuse tend to enter abusive relationships that are caused by intrapsychic conflicts.

Because *due to* is adjectival, "intrapsychic conflicts" describes the relationships. *Caused by* could be substituted, and the meaning would be retained. *That are* could be inserted before *due to* without changing the sentence's meaning.

Survivors of child abuse tend to enter abusive relationships owing to intrapsychic conflicts.

Meaning: Because of intrapsychic conflicts, survivors of child abuse tend to enter abusive relationships.

Because *owing to* is used adverbially, "intrapsychic conflicts" characterizes the entrance into abusive relationships. *Because of* could be substituted and the meaning would be retained. However, if *that are* is inserted before *owing to,* the sentence's meaning changes.

Clue to usage: The phrase "coughs due to colds" is a good paradigm for the use of *due to*. If "because of" sounds right, use it or "owing to"; if "caused by" is intended, use it or "due to" (or even "attributable to").

between: see **among, between**

biopsy—*Biopsy* refers to the removal and examination (usually microscopically) of tissue, cells, or fluids from the living body. The word should not be used as a verb. Observations are made on the biopsy specimen, not on the biopsy itself.

Incorrect: The mass was biopsied.
Correct: A biopsy of the mass was performed.
The surgeon performed a biopsy on the lung mass.

Incorrect: Biopsy was negative.
Correct: The results of the biopsy were negative.

breast-feed, nurse—When referring to human lactation, *breast-feeding* is preferred. This term is more specific than *nursing* and prevents any confusion with the profession of nursing.

calorie, energy—With the adoption of the Système International as the standard for reporting units of measurement, the term *calorie* has become less commonly used in scientific writing (see 15.8, Units of Measure, SI Units and Energy). Food does not contain calories but yields energy when nutrients are metabolized. *Energy* has been largely accepted as a substitute for *calorie* in referring to this metabolic concept. Following are suggested replacements:

Avoid	*Preferred*
calorie intake; caloric intake	energy intake
calorie expenditure; caloric expenditure	energy expenditure
calorie requirement	energy requirement
calorie value	energy value; specific energy
calorie balance	energy balance
isocaloric	of equal energy value; isoenergetic
low-calorie diet	controlled-energy diet
percentage of calories from fat	energy fraction from fat
protein-calorie malnutrition	protein-energy malnutrition

If an author requests the use of *calorie* or *kilocalorie* in the text because he or she considers this form of expression more familiar to readers, the values expressed in calories or kilocalories may be dual-reported after the values are first expressed in joules or kilojoules; thereafter, phrases containing *calories* and *caloric* may be retained in the text (with values still dual-reported). For example:

> To maintain his body weight, a healthy, relatively sedentary 70-kg man needs a daily energy (caloric) intake of about 7500 kJ (1800 kcal).

See also 15.5, Units of Measure, SI Units and Conventional Units.

case, client, consumer, patient, subject—In biological research, a *case* is a particular instance of a disease. A *patient* is a particular person under medical care. A *research subject* is a person with a particular characteristic or behavior, or a person who undergoes an intervention, examined in a scientific investigation. A *control subject* is a person who does not share the characteristic under study, or receive the intervention, in an investigation and provides a basis of comparison with the case patient (see 17.0, Statistics). In case-control studies, it is appropriate to refer to *cases, patients in the case group,* or *case patients;* and *controls, subjects in the control group,* or *control subjects.*

Always avoid the dehumanizing use of *case* when referring to a specific person, for example, "A 43-year-old case of diabetes. . . ."

Note: Make the distinction between *person* and *patient:*

> Many persons in the United States have diabetes [persons with diabetes regardless of care].

> Many patients in the United States have diabetes [only persons under medical care].

A *case* is evaluated, documented, and reported. A *patient* is examined, undergoes testing, and is treated. A *research subject* is recruited, selected, sometimes subjected to experimental conditions, and observed. (See **diagnose, evaluate, examine, identify;** and **follow, follow-up, observe**.)

Note: In general, patients should not be referred to as *clients* or *consumers.* However, persons enrolled in drug abuse treatment programs, for example, or persons undergoing treatment at a dialysis center are sometimes referred to as *clients*. *Client* may also be used by social workers and in some research settings where *patient* or *subject* is inappropriate. *Consumer*—one who consumes goods or services—has worked its way into the medical lexicon. Some feel the term interjects the language of business into what was once a unique relationship: that between patient and physician. Yet *consumer* may be appropriate in certain discussions. For instance, in the following example, *patient* would not fit the context:

> Unlike purchasers of VCRs, consumers of health care may have little idea what they are buying when they require care.

case-fatality rate, fatality; morbidity, morbidity rate; mortality, mortality rate—See 17.4, Statistics, Glossary of Statistical Terms.

catatonic, manic, schizophrenic—These adjectives refer to severe psychiatric disorders. It is inappropriate to trivialize the disorders by using these terms to describe normal variations of individual or group behavior, since suitable descriptors are available. For example, *contradictory* can usually be substituted for *schizophrenic, overactive* for *manic,* and *motionless* for *catatonic.*

Note: It is dehumanizing to refer to a patient as "a schizophrenic." Use "the patient with schizophrenia" or "the schizophrenic patient." See also 9.10.4, Disabilities.

cesarean delivery, cesarean section—According to the American College of Obstetricians and Gynecologists (R. D. Rinehart, written communication, November 20, 1995), the preferred terms are *cesarean delivery* (or *cesarean birth*) or *abdominal delivery* (vs *vaginal delivery*).

chronic: see **acute, chronic**

classic, classical—In most scientific writing, the adjective *classic* generally means authentic, authoritative, or typical (the *classic* symptoms of myocardial infarction include chest pain, shortness of breath, nausea, and diaphoresis). In contrast, *classical* refers to the humanities or the fine arts (a *classical* column, unlike a medieval column or pier, is strictly defined and self-sufficient).

However, some disciplines (eg, genetics, immunology) use *classical* for specific terms:

> In previous studies, the authors included patients with classical lissencephaly as well as some lissencephaly variants associated with areas of polymicrogyria or scattered calcifications; in this article, they focus on patients with the classical form.
>
> The classical and alternative pathways of complement components are described in 12.8.1, Nomenclature, Complement.
>
> Classical (frequentist) analysis is the most prevalent statistical method used, leading to the ubiquitous *P* values and confidence intervals.

Classic is also used as a noun. See also **-ic, -ical**.

clinician, practitioner—Depending on context, these terms may be used to describe health professionals in the clinical practice of such fields as medicine, nursing, psychology, dentistry, optometry, and podiatry, as distinguished from those specializing in laboratory science, research, policy, or theory. When referring to a particular type of clinician or practitioner, it is preferable to use the more descriptive term (eg, physician, nurse, dentist). See also **provider**.

compare to, compare with—One thing or person is usually compared *with* another when the aim is to examine similarities or differences in detail. An entity is compared *to* another when a single striking similarity (or dissimilarity) is observed, or when a thing of one class is likened to one of another class, without analysis.

> Rates of improvement among patients treated with the new therapy were compared with rates among those treated with conventional therapy.
>
> "Shall I compare thee to a summer's day?" [William Shakespeare]

compose, comprise—Although these 2 verbs are often used interchangeably, *compose* is not synonymous with *comprise. Comprise* means to be composed of or to include; it takes the active voice, whereas *compose* takes the passive voice. The whole is composed of its parts and comprises its parts.

> The medication is composed of several highly toxic ingredients.
>
> The medication comprises several highly toxic ingredients.

Clue to usage: Never use *of* with *comprise.*

continual, continuous—*Continual* means to recur at regular and frequent intervals. *Continuous* means to go on without pause or interruption.

> The patient with emphysema coughed continually.
>
> His labored breathing was eased by a continuous flow of oxygen through a nasal cannula.

delivery—A neonate (or newborn infant) is delivered, but a woman is delivered *of* an infant.

describe, report—Patients or cases are *described*; only cases are *reported*. (See **case, client, consumer, patient, subject; management, treatment; diagnose, evaluate, examine, identify**.)

diabetes mellitus—The types of diabetes mellitus currently recognized are as follows (note arabic numerals)[3]:

Older Terms	*Preferred Terms*
juvenile diabetes, or juvenile-onset diabetes, or insulin-dependent diabetes mellitus	type 1 diabetes mellitus
maturity-onset diabetes, or adult-onset diabetes, or non-insulin-dependent diabetes mellitus	type 2 diabetes mellitus
chemical diabetes, or borderline diabetes, or latent diabetes	impaired glucose tolerance (nondiagnostic fasting blood glucose level, glucose tolerance between normal and diabetic)
. . .	gestational diabetes mellitus

For other specific types, consult Table 1 in *Diabetes Care.*[3]

diagnose, evaluate, examine, identify—*Diagnose, evaluate,* and *identify* apply to conditions, syndromes, and diseases. Patients themselves are not diagnosed but their condition may be diagnosed. Patients are also *examined.* Patients may be *evaluated* for the possibility of a condition (eg, The patient was evaluated for possible cardiac disease). (See **case, client, consumer, patient, subject; and management, treatment**.)

dilate, dilation, dilatation—According to the American College of Obstetricians and Gynecologists,[4] *dilate* is a verb meaning to expand or open. *Dilation* means the act of dilating. *Dilatation* means the condition of being stretched or expanded.

> The patient's cervix dilated over a period of 12 hours.
>
> The patient was treated by dilation and curettage.
>
> After 4 hours of labor, the dilatation of the cervix was 3 cm.

disc, disk—For ophthalmologic terms, use *disc* (eg, optic disc); for other anatomical terms, use *disk* (eg, lumbar disk).

In discussions related to computers, use *disk* (eg, floppy disk, hard disk, disk drive, diskette) (exceptions: *compact disc, videodisc*) (see also 21.0, Glossary of Publishing Terms).

disinterested, uninterested—Although these 2 words are increasingly treated as synonyms in written and spoken language, their differences in meaning are sufficiently useful to be worth preserving. To be *disinterested* is to be free of bias or impartial; to be *uninterested* is to be unconcerned, indifferent, or inattentive: A disinterested judge is admirable; an uninterested judge is not.

doctor, physician—*Doctor* is a more general term than *physician,* since it includes persons who hold such degrees as DDS, EdD, DVM, and PharmD. Thus, the term *physician* should be used when referring specifically to a doctor of medicine, ie, a person with an MD or a DO degree (see also **clinician, practitioner; provider,** and 9.4, Jargon).

dosage, dose—A *dose* is the quantity to be administered at one time, or the total quantity administered during a specified period. *Dosage* implies a regimen; it is the regulated administration of individual doses and is usually expressed as a quantity per unit of time.

> The patient received an initial dose of 50 mg. Thereafter, his dosage was 25 mg 3 times a day for 6 days. He received a total dose of 500 mg during the course of treatment.

effect: see **affect, effect**

effective, effectiveness; efficacious, efficacy—Although all refer to effectiveness of some kind, these 4 terms have different nuances of meaning. *Efficacy* and *efficacious,* used especially in pharmacology and decision analysis, have to do with the ability of a medication or intervention to produce the desired or intended effect under ideal conditions of use. *Effective* and *effectiveness,* however, describe the ability of an intervention to produce the effect in average conditions of use.

See also 17.4, Statistics, Glossary of Statistical Terms.

eg, ie—Use *eg* (from the Latin *exempli gratia:* "for example") and *ie* (*id est:* "that is") with care.

> Persons in risk groups for endemic disease (eg, tuberculosis in immigrants or homeless persons, histoplasmosis in residents of the Mississippi and Ohio River valleys) warrant special consideration.
>
> Geographic and temporal characteristics (ie, month and time of day) were assessed to determine areas and times of greatest frequency of gang-related homicides.

Clue to usage: Do not add *etc* when using *eg,* since "for example" already indicates that the list is not inclusive. The use of *ie* implies that the items that follow are specific and inclusive. See **etc**.

endemic, epidemic, hyperendemic, pandemic—The distinction among these similar terms is important in epidemiology as well as lexicography. *Endemic* conditions or diseases are prevalent in a particular place or among a particular group of people. *Epidemic* conditions occur abruptly in a defined area and are (usually) temporary. A *hyperendemic* condition is one that has a high prevalence. A *pandemic* condition is one that is epidemic over a wide geographic area.

> Lyme disease is endemic in many regions worldwide, including the southeast coast of Sweden, southwestern Finland, and the northeastern United States.
>
> The study reported an epidemic of legionnaires disease among the participants of 8 conferences in a large midwestern city.
>
> Parasitism is hyperendemic in underdeveloped countries.
>
> The depredations of the HIV pandemic have been a humbling experience for the scientific community.

energy: see **calorie, energy**

ensure: see **assure, ensure, insure**

etc—Use *etc* (or *and so on* or *and the like*) with discretion. Such terms are often superfluous and are used simply to extend a list of examples. When, in other instances, omission would be detrimental, substitute more specific phrasing such as *and other methods* or *and other factors. Etc* may be used in a noninclusive listing when a complete list would be unwieldy *and* its content is obvious to the reader.

> *Incorrect:* A first-aid kit should include aspirin, emetics, self-adhesive bandages, etc.
> *Correct:* Cough resulting from irritation of pharyngeal mucosa can be managed with demulcents and sialagogues (hard candy, cough drops, etc).

Do not use *etc* when the listing is preceded by *eg* or *for example* (see also **eg, ie**).

Use a comma before *etc* when it is preceded by more than 1 term but not when preceded by 1 term only.

evaluate: see **diagnose, evaluate, examine, identify**

fever, temperature—*Fever* is a condition in which body temperature rises above normal. It is incorrect to say a person has a temperature if "fever" is intended. Everyone has a temperature, either normal or abnormal. A patient may have a *temperature* of 39.5°C (not "a fever of 39.5°C"). The following forms are also correct:

> The patient has a fever (temperature, 39.5°C).
>
> The patient is febrile (temperature, 39.5°C).
>
> The patient has an elevated temperature (39.5°C).

fewer, less—*Fewer* and *less* are not interchangeable. Use *fewer* for number (individual persons or things) and *less* for volume or mass (indicating degree or value).

> Fewer interventions may not always mean less care.
>
> The authors evaluated fewer than 100 studies yet still reported more support for the conventionally prescribed therapy.

Note: Spent less than $4000 (*not:* Spent fewer than $4000)

Reported fewer data (*not:* Reported less data)

One intervention fewer *or* One less intervention (*not:* One fewer intervention)

follow, follow up, observe—Cases are *followed.* Patients are not *followed* but *observed.* However, either cases or patients may be *followed up* (eg, the maintenance of contact with or reexamination of a person or patient, especially after treatment). Their clinical course may be *followed.* In a study, case or control subjects may be *lost to follow-up* (eg, the investigators were unable to locate them to complete documentation on subjects in the initial study groups) or *unavailable for follow-up* (eg, the investigators were unable to persuade them to complete the study).

> Patients with tuberculosis were followed up with home visits to ascertain compliance with the medication regimen.

gender, sex—*Sex* refers to the biological state of being male or female. *Gender* has been defined as a "grammatical term denoting whether words pertaining to a noun or pronoun are classed as masculine, feminine, or neuter." *Gender* has evolved to include not only a grammatical meaning but also social and cultural aspects: "Gender signifies an individual's personal, legal, and social status without reference to genetic sex; gender is a subjective cultural attitude while sex is an objective biological fact."[5]

In scientific and medical research, use the word *sex* when distinguishing men and women or boys and girls in an epidemiologic study, for example. If, in a given context, *sex* could be confused with the sex act, *gender* may be appropriate.

> The theory of gender and power is a social structural theory that examines the sexual division of labor, the sexual distribution of power and authority, affective influences, and gender-specified norms about what constitutes appropriate sexual conduct within heterosexual relationships, to guide intervention development.

health care, health care reform, health system, health system reform—Use these contemporary terms with care. *American Heritage Dictionary* defines *health care* as the "prevention, treatment, and management of illness and the preservation of mental and physical well-being through the services offered by the medical and allied health professions."[6] A *health system* is the infrastructure (hospitals, systems of reimbursement, and so on) that supports *health care.* Thus, the distinction between *health care reform* and *health system reform,* though subtle, is important. The care given to patients may be exemplary; the system that supports it may be in need of attention.

historic, historical—Although their meanings overlap and they are often used interchangeably, *historic* and *historical* have different usages. *Historic* means important or influential in history (a *historic* discovery). *Historical* is concerned with the events in history (a *historical* novel).

But: A historical novel may have historic impact.

-ic, -ical—*Merriam-Webster's Collegiate, Stedman's, Dorland's,* and *American Heritage* dictionaries are resources for determining the appropriate suffix form for adjectives. In some cases the "-ical" form is more remote from the word root and may have a meaning beyond that of the "-ic" form. Although "anatomic" may be used in the same sense as "anatomical," the latter is preferred as the adjectival form. The important guideline is that the use of terms must be consistent throughout an article or a chapter, preferably throughout the entire publication. Usually the "-al" may be omitted unless its absence changes the meaning of the word. Examples of such differences in meaning include *biologic, biological; classic, classical; economic, economical; empiric, empirical; historic, historical; pathologic, pathological; periodic, periodical; physiologic, physiological.*

identify: see **diagnose, evaluate, examine, identify**

ie: see **eg, ie**

immunity, immunize, inoculate, vaccinate—*Immunity* is the quality or state of being immune, ie, being able to resist a disease. *Immunize* means to induce or provide immunity by giving a vaccine, toxoids, or preformed antibodies. *Inoculate* means to introduce a serum, a vaccine, or an antigenic substance. *Vaccinate* refers to the act of administering a vaccine.

> To immunize the newborn infant of an HBsAg-positive woman against hepatitis B, the patient should be inoculated with both hepatitis B immunoglobulin and vaccine.
>
> The nurse vaccinated the infant with hepatitis B vaccine.

imply, infer—To *imply* is to suggest or to indicate or express indirectly. To *infer* is to conclude or to draw conclusions from facts, statements, or indications.

> These statistics imply a decrease in production, which the researchers inferred was the result of an increase in staff vacancies.

See also 17.4, Statistics, Glossary of Statistical Terms **(inference)**.

incidence, prevalence—See 17.4, Statistics, Glossary of Statistical Terms.

injecting, injection drug user; intravenous—The terms *injecting drug user* and *injection drug user* are not necessarily the same as *intravenous drug user.* Injecting or injection drug users can inject drugs intravenously, intramuscularly, or subcutaneously. Do not substitute one term for the other. If *intravenous* is used, ascertain that the route of administration is through a vein. If *injecting* or *injection drug user* is used, specify the type of injection (eg, intravenous, intradermal) at first mention, unless all types are meant.

injury: see **accident, injury**

inoculate: see **immunity, immunize, inoculate, vaccinate**

insure: see **assure, ensure, insure**

irregardless, regardless—*Irregardless,* a mistaken hybrid of *regardless* and *irrespective,* is incorrect, regardless of usage.

irritate: see **aggravate, irritate**

less: see **fewer, less**

liable: see **apt, liable, likely**

management, treatment—To avoid dehumanizing usage, it is generally preferable to say that cases are *managed* and patients are *cared for* or *treated.* However, constructions such as "the clinical management of the seriously ill patient" and "the management of patients with X" are acceptable when they refer to a general treatment protocol. *Management* is especially useful when the care of the patient does not involve specific "treatment" but may include, for example, watchful waiting (eg, for prostate cancer). *Management* may also be used to refer to the monitoring or periodic evaluations of the patient after a specific treatment.

manic: see **catatonic, manic, schizophrenic**

militate, mitigate—These 2 words are often confused, but they are not synonymous. *Militate* means to have weight or effect and is usually used with *against. Mitigate* means to moderate, abate, alleviate.

The leukocytosis militates against that diagnosis.

The cardiologist could not mitigate the effect of the unfavorable report of catheterization-related complications.

negative: see **abnormal, normal; negative, positive**

-ology—Derived from the Greek *logos,* the suffix *-ology* (also *-logia*) means "word," "idea," or "thought," denoting the *science of* or *study of*—a branch of learning. Nouns with this suffix, like *pathology* and *histology,* are general and abstract and should not be used to describe particular items.

Incorrect:	The pathology was located in the right upper lobe of the lung.
Correct:	The pathologic lesion was located in the right upper lobe of the lung.
Incorrect:	The histology was small cell carcinoma of the lung.
Correct:	The histologic diagnosis was small cell carcinoma of the lung.
Also correct:	Histologic examination disclosed small cell carcinoma of the lung.
But:	The quality of meta-analyses has improved as reports of their methodology have been published.

Exception: Etiology refers to all the possible *causes,* separate or related, of a condition or a disease.

Pyogenic granuloma is a common skin tumor of unknown etiology.

But: The cause of most cases of acute renal failure is either ischemia secondary to renal hypoperfusion or a reaction to toxins.

The etiology of aplastic anemia may involve dysfunction of a hematopoietic stem cell. Among the many reported causes are infections, toxic agents, and immune disorders.

operate, operate on—Surgeons *operate on* a patient or *perform an operation on* a patient. Similarly, patients are not *operated* but are *operated on.*

Incorrect:	The operated group recovered quickly.
Correct:	The surgical group recovered quickly.
Also correct:	The group that underwent surgery recovered quickly.

over, under—Correct usage of these words depends on context.

Time: Over may mean either *more than* or *for* (*a period of*). In cases in which ambiguity might arise, *over* should be avoided and *more than* used.

Ambiguous:	The cases were followed up over 4 years.
Preferred:	The cases were followed up for more than 4 years.
Also:	The cases were followed up for 4 years.

Age: When referring to age groups, *over* and *under* should be replaced by the more precise *older than* and *younger than* (see also **age, aged, school-age, school-aged, teenage, teenaged;** and **fewer, less**).

Avoid:	All members of the control and experimental groups were over 65 years old.
Preferred:	All members of the control and experimental groups were older than 65 years.

Note: It is unnecessary and redundant to add *of age* after the number of years. When the terms *younger* and *older* are used, age is implied. See also 9.2.1, Redundant Words.

Units: When numbers of persons, things, or groups are referred to, *over* and *under* should be replaced by *more than* and *less than.* Symbols such as < and > are appropriate to use in tables and figures but not in running text (exception: probability values, eg, $P < .05$), although these symbols may be used with numbers in parenthetical expressions.

Avoid: Over 300 people died during the epidemic.

Preferred: More than 300 people died during the epidemic.

Possible: The epidemic resulted in a high number of deaths (>300 as of January 1).

When replacing symbols such as ≤ in the text, observe the way the sentence reads. Do not replace the symbol or sign with its equivalent words without regard to elegance of expression. For example, do not rephrase "patients ≤60 years old" to "patients less than or equal to 60 years old." Instead, use "patients 60 years and younger."

Note: In some constructions, *over* may also mean *during:*

She was honored for her many contributions over the past decade.

pandemic: see **endemic, epidemic, hyperendemic, pandemic**

patient: see **case, client, consumer, patient, subject**

percent, percentage, percentage point, percentile—See 16.7.2, Numbers and Percentages, Percentages.

physician: see **doctor, physician**

place on, put on—The phrase "to put [or to place] a patient on a drug" is jargon and should be avoided. Medications are *prescribed* or patients are *given* medications; therapy or therapeutic regimens are started, administered, maintained, stopped, or discontinued.

Incorrect: The patient with depression was put on paroxetine.

Correct: Paroxetine was prescribed for the patient with depression.
Correct: The patient with depression was given paroxetine.
Correct: A therapeutic regimen of paroxetine, 20 mg/d, was begun.

"To put [or to place] on a ventilator" is more acceptable usage but should be avoided by using other expressions, eg, receive, undergo, continue, or discontinue.

Avoid: The patient was put on a respirator.
Preferred: The patient was given ventilatory assistance.
The patient underwent ventilatory assistance.

Avoid: The patient had been on a respirator for 2 months.
Preferred: The patient had been receiving mechanical ventilation [or ventilatory assistance] for 2 months.
The patient had been undergoing mechanical ventilation [or ventilatory assistance] for 2 months.

positive: see **abnormal, normal; negative, positive**

practitioner: see **clinician, practitioner**

prevalence: See 17.4, Statistics, Glossary of Statistical Terms **(incidence, prevalence)**.

provider—The term *provider* can mean a health care professional or a medical institution or organization. If the usage refers to 1 specific provider (eg, physician, hospital), use the specific name or alternative name for that provider (eg, pediatrician, tertiary care hospital, or managed care organization), rather than the general term *provider*. If the term connotes multiple providers, it can be used to avoid repeating lists of persons or institutions; however, the term should be defined at first mention.

> The task force comprised 7 health care providers (2 pediatricians, 1 psychiatrist, 2 nurse practitioners, and 2 social workers).

> The number of public health care providers (state-funded hospitals, clinics, and health departments) has decreased since 1990.

The phrase *nonphysician provider* is similarly imprecise and can refer to numerous health professionals licensed to provide a health care service. It is preferable to specify the provider (eg, nurse, pharmacist) and to use *nonphysician provider* only when speaking of all health professionals except physicians. If a phrase is needed to describe repeatedly and succinctly the many health professionals who are not physicians, then *nonphysician providers* is acceptable as long as the phrase is defined at first mention. This also applies to other professions (eg, nonnurses, nonpharmacists, nonastronauts).

See also **clinician, practitioner**.

radiograph, roentgen, x-ray—The term *roentgen* (R), meaning a unit of x- or γ-radiation, is now used only infrequently, having been replaced by the gray (Gy) as the international unit of measurement. An *x-ray* (formerly *roentgen ray*) is electromagnetic radiation about 10 keV that is capable of penetrating tissue. See also 15.7, Units of Measure, SI Units for Ionizing Radiation.

A *radiograph* is a film image made by means of x-rays, in a process known as *radiography* (formerly *roentgenography*). Specific terms such as *venogram* or *arthrogram* are more informative and preferred if available and appropriate for the article. *Radiograph* is synonymous with *x-ray film* but not with *x-ray*. In AMA journals, either *radiograph* or *x-ray film* may be used.

Radiograph may be used as a general term to describe all images produced by means of ionizing radiation; however, terms that indicate other specific imaging techniques, eg, *computed tomographic scan* and *radioactive isotope scan*, should not be changed. (Images made by ultrasound or magnetic resonance imaging, which do not involve ionizing radiation, are not radiographs.)

According to *Dorland's*, *radiogram* is synonymous with *radiograph*, but *radiogram* has a second meaning of "a message sent by wireless telegraphy." To avoid confusion, the term *radiograph* should be used.

regardless: see **irregardless, regardless**

regime, regimen—A *regime* is a form of government, a social system, or a period of rule. A *regimen* is a systematic schedule (involving diet, exercise, or medication, for example) designed to improve or maintain the health of a patient.

> His medical regimen for mild hypertension included hydrochlorothiazide, 25 mg once a day.

repeat, repeated—*Repeat* is a noun or a verb and should not be used in place of the adjective *repeated*. *Repeated* implies repetition. For the sake of precision and clarity, the exact number should be given.

Incorrect:	A repeat electrocardiogram was obtained.
Possible but misleading:	A repeated electrocardiogram was obtained.
Preferred:	A second electrocardiogram was obtained.
Preferred:	The electrocardiogram was repeated.
Preferred:	Two successive electrocardiograms showed no abnormalities.

report: see **describe, report**

respective, respectively—These words indicate a one-to-one correspondence that may not otherwise be obvious between members of 2 series. When only 1 series, or none at all, is listed, the distinction is meaningless and should not be used.

Incorrect:	The 2 patients were 12 and 14 years old, respectively.
Correct:	Kate and Jake were 12 and 14 years old, respectively.
Incorrect:	The 2 patients' respective ages were 12 and 14 years.
Correct:	The 2 patients were 12 and 14 years old.

Cumbersome and confusing sentence constructions containing *respectively* can often be simplified by rephrasing the sentence.

schizophrenic: see **catatonic, manic, schizophrenic**

sex: see **gender, sex**

side effect: see **adverse effect, adverse event, adverse reaction, side effect**

since: see **as, because, since**

subject: see **case, client, consumer, patient, subject**

suffer from, suffer with: See 9.10.4, Disabilities.

suggestive of, suspicious for, suspicious of—To be *suggestive of* is to give a suggestion of something or to evoke. To be *suspicious of* is to distrust. Thus, the 2 phrases are not synonymous, and care should be taken to avoid confusing them.

Incorrect:	The chest radiograph was suspicious for tuberculosis.
Correct:	The chest radiograph was suggestive of tuberculosis.
Also correct:	The chest radiograph showed abnormalities suggestive of tuberculosis.
Possible:	The physician was suspicious of the equivocal chest radiograph.

temperature: see **fever, temperature**

terminate: see **abort, terminate**

though: see **although, though**

toxic, toxicity—*Toxic* means pertaining to or caused by a poison or toxin. *Toxicity* is the quality, state, or degree of being poisonous. A patient is not toxic. A patient does not have toxicity.

Methotrexate is a toxic antineoplastic agent.

The drug had a toxic effect on the patient.

The patient had a toxic reaction to the drug.

The patient had a toxic appearance.

The toxicity of the drug must be considered.

transplant, transplantation—*Transplant* is both a noun (the organ or tissue that is transplanted) and a verb. *Transplantation* is a noun that describes the process of relocating the organ or tissue.

Incorrect: The patient was transplanted.
The surgeon transplanted the patient.

Correct: The patient received a transplant.
The patient underwent transplantation.
The researchers collected transplantation data.
A randomized trial in recipients of lung transplants yielded similar results.
Cyclosporine has been used successfully as monotherapy in pediatric liver transplantation.
The surgeon transplanted skin from the patient's back to her arm.
In emergencies, livers may be transplanted across the ABO blood type barrier.

treatment: see **management, treatment**

under: see **over, under**

uninterested: see **disinterested, uninterested**

use, usage, utility, utilize—*Use* is almost always preferable to *utilize,* which has the specific meaning "to find a profitable or practical use for," suggesting the discovery of a new use for something. However, even where this meaning is intended, *use* would be acceptable.

During an in-flight emergency, the surgeon utilized a coat hanger as a "trocar" during chest tube insertion.

Exception: Utilization review is acceptable terminology.

Usage refers to an acceptable, customary, or habitual practice or procedure, often linguistic in nature. For the broader sense in which there is no reference to a standard of practice, *use* is the correct noun form.

To say "between you and I" defies all rules of correct usage.

Some authors use the pretentious *usage* where *use* would be appropriate. As a rule of thumb, then, avoid *utilize* and be wary of *usage*. Use *use*.

Note: Utility—meaning fitness for some purpose, or usefulness—should never be changed to the noun *use*. Nor should the verb *employ* be routinely changed to *use*. Use *employ* to mean *hire*.

vaccinate: see **immunity, immunize, inoculate, vaccinate**

vision, visual acuity—*Vision* is a general term describing the overall ability of the eye and brain to perceive the environment. *Visual acuity* is a specific measurement of one aspect of the sensation of vision assessed by an examiner.

A patient describing symptoms of his or her visual sensation would be describing the overall visual performance of the eye(s) and would use the term *vision:* "My vision is improved [or worse]."

A practitioner reporting the examination findings at one specific time would describe *visual acuity* (20/30, 20/15, etc). However, the practitioner might also refer to the general visual function as *vision:* "As the vitreous hemorrhage cleared, the vision improved and visual acuity returned to 20/20." It is possible to have normal visual acuity despite marked vision impairment, eg, when the peripheral visual field is abnormal.

x-ray: see **radiograph, roentgen, x-ray**

9.2 ■ REDUNDANT, EXPENDABLE, AND INCOMPARABLE WORDS AND PHRASES.

9.2.1 ***Redundant Words.***—A redundancy is a term or phrase that unnecessarily repeats words or meanings. Below are some common redundancies that can usually be avoided (redundant words are *italicized*):

- adequate *enough*
- *advance* planning
- aggregate *together*
- brief *in duration*
- combine *together*
- *completely* full [empty]
- consensus *of opinion*
- contemporaneous *in age*
- count [divide] *up*
- distinguishing *the difference*
- each *individual* person
- eliminate *altogether*
- enter *into* [exception: enter into a contract]
- *equally* as well as
- estimated at *about*
- *fellow* colleagues
- fewer *in number*
- *skin* rash
- similar results were obtained *also* by
- soft [firm] *in consistency*
- sour [sweet, bitter] *tasting*
- *still* continues
- sum *total*
- tender *to the touch*
- filled *to capacity*
- fuse *together*
- *future* plans
- *general* rule
- *herein* we describe
- interval *of time*
- large [small, bulky] *in size*
- *major* breakthrough
- out *of* [*but:* out of bounds, out of the question, out of the jurisdiction]
- outside *of*
- oval [square, round, lenticular] *in shape*
- own *personal* view
- period *of time, time* period
- *personal* friend
- precedes *in time*
- red *in color*
- rough [smooth] *in texture*
- *true* fact
- *12* noon [midnight]
- *2* halves
- 2 *out* of 12
- *uniformly* consistent
- whether *or not* [unless the intent is to give equal emphasis to the alternative]
- younger [older] than 50 years *of age*

9.2.2 ***Expendable Words and Circumlocution.***—Some words and phrases can usually be omitted without affecting meaning, and omitting them often improves the readability of a sentence:

- as already stated
- in other words
- it goes without saying
- it is important [interesting] to note that

it may be said that

it stands to reason that

it was found that

it was demonstrated that

needless to say

take steps to

the fact that

the field of

to be sure

Quite, very, and *rather* are often overused and misused and can be deleted in many instances (see also 9.1, Commonly Misused Words and Phrases, **etc**).

Avoid roundabout and wordy expressions:

Change	*To*
in terms of	in, of, for
an increased [decreased] number of	more [fewer]
due to the fact that	since
as the result of	because
during the time that	while
at this [that] point in time	now [then]
in close proximity to	near
in regard to	about
the majority of	most
produce an inhibitory effect on	inhibit
commented to the effect that	said
draws to a close	ends
file a lawsuit against	sue
have an effect [impact] on	affect

9.2.3 ***Incomparable Words.***—Some words are regarded by grammarians as "absolute" adjectives, those not possessing a comparative or superlative form. Some words considered incomparable and needing no superlative or comparative modifier are listed below:

absolute

ambiguous

complete [*but:* almost or nearly complete]

comprehensive

entire

equal

omnipotent

original

perfect [*but:* almost or nearly perfect]

preferable

pregnant

supreme

total

eternal	ultimate
expert	unanimous [*but:* almost or nearly unanimous]
fatal [*but:* almost or nearly fatal]	unique
final	
full [*but:* half full; nearly full]	
infinite	

Note: In general, superlatives should be avoided in scientific writing.

9.3 ■ **BACK-FORMATIONS.**—The transformation of a noun into a verb is a back-formation, often seen in technical as well as informal writing. *Diagnose,* for example, is a mid-19th-century back-formation, from *diagnosis*. Back-formations now in use include *dialyze* (from *dialysis*) and *anesthetize* (from *anesthesia*). A back-formation that is not widely acceptable is *diurese* (from *diuresis*). Any use of back-formations should be checked in the dictionaries.

Back-formation:	The patient was diuresed.
Preferred:	The patient was given diuretics [or underwent diuresis].

9.4 ■ **JARGON.**—Words and phrases that are understandable in conversation but are vague, confusing, or depersonalizing are generally inappropriate in formal scientific writing (see also 9.1, Commonly Misused Words and Phrases, **-ology,** and 17.4, Statistics, Glossary of Statistical Terms).

Jargon	*Preferred Form*
4+ albuminuria	proteinuria (4+)
blood sugar	blood glucose [query author]
cardiac [diabetic] diet	diet for patients with cardiac disease [diabetes]
emergency room	emergency department
exam	examination
congenital heart	congenital heart disease; congenital cardiac anomaly
gastrointestinal infection	gastrointestinal tract infection *or* infection of the gastrointestinal tract
genitourinary infection	genitourinary tract infection *or* infection of the genitourinary tract
heart attack	myocardial infarction [query author]
hyperglycemia of 250 mg/dL	hyperglycemia (blood glucose level of 13.9 mmol/L [250 mg/dL])
jugular ligation	jugular vein ligation *or* ligation of the jugular vein
left heart failure	left ventricular failure [query author]; left-sided heart failure
normal range	reference range

Pap smear	Papanicolaou test
prepped	prepared
psychiatric floor	psychiatric department, service, unit, ward
respiratory infection	respiratory tract infection *or* infection of the respiratory tract
symptomatology	symptoms [query author]
therapy of [a disease or condition]	therapy for
treatment for [a disease or condition]	treatment of
urinary infection	urinary tract infection *or* infection of the urinary tract

When describing the administration of drugs, *intra-articular, intracardiac, intramuscular, intrathecal, intravenous, intraventricular, intravitreal, oral, parenteral, rectal, subconjunctival, subcutaneous, sublingual,* and *topical* are acceptable terms when these are the usual or intended routes of administration. Except for systemic chemotherapy, however, drugs are usually neither systemic nor local but are given for systemic or local effect.

Some topical steroid ointments produce systemic effects.

Oral penicillin is often preferred to parenteral penicillin.

Intravenously injected heroin may be contaminated.

Exceptions: Local anesthetics are a class of drug. Techniques for delivering anesthesia are general, local, and regional. Certain drugs may be inhaled.

The following terms and euphemisms should be changed to preferred forms:

Avoid	*Use*
expired, passed away, succumbed	died
sacrificed	killed; humanely killed [query author]

Note: Avoid trivializing or dehumanizing disciplines or specialties, for example:

Osteopathic physician and *osteopathic medicine,* not *osteopath* and *osteopathy*

Cardiologic consultant or *cardiology consultation,* not *cardiology*

Orthopedic surgeon, not *orthopod*

Colloquialisms, idioms, and vulgarisms should be avoided in formal scientific writing; exceptions may be made in editorials, informal articles, and the like.

9.5 ■ **AGE AND SEX REFERENTS.**—Use specific terminology to refer to age.

Neonates or *newborns* are persons from birth to 1 month of age.

Infants are children aged 1 month to 1 year (12 months).

Children are persons aged 1 to 12 years. Sometimes, *children* may be used more broadly to encompass persons from birth to 12 years of age. They may also be referred to as *boys* or *girls.*

Adolescents are persons aged 13 through 17 years. They may also be referred to as *teenagers* or as *adolescent boys* or *adolescent girls,* depending on the context.

Adults are persons 18 years and older and should be referred to as *men* or *women.*

Whenever possible, a patient should be identified as a man, woman, boy, girl, or infant, not as a male or female. Occasionally, however, a study group may comprise children and adults of both sexes. Then, the use of *male* and *female* as nouns is appropriate. *Male* and *female* are also appropriate adjectives.

See also 9.10.3, Age.

9.6 ■ **ANATOMY.**—Authors often err in referring to anatomic regions or structures as the "right heart," "left chest," "left neck," and "right brain." Generally, these terms can be corrected by inserting a phrase such as "part of the" or "side of the."

right side of the heart; right atrium; right ventricle

left side of the chest; left hemithorax

left aspect of the neck

right hemisphere [query author]

ascending [not right] and descending [not left] colon

Where appropriate, use specific anatomic descriptors:

proximal jejunum; distal esophagus; distal radius; distal ureter

The *upper extremity* comprises the arm (extending from the shoulder to the elbow), the forearm (from the elbow to the wrist), and the hand. The *lower extremity* comprises the thigh (extending from the hip to the knee), the leg (from the knee to the ankle), and the foot. Therefore, references to upper and lower arm and upper and lower leg are often redundant or ambiguous. When such references appear in a manuscript, the author should be queried.

9.7 ■ **CLOCK REFERENTS.**—Occasionally, reference to a locus of insertion, position, or attitude is given in terms of a clock-face orientation, as seen by the viewer (see also 16.1.3, Numbers and Percentages, Measures of Time).

Ambiguous: The foreign body was observed in the patient's left eye at 9 o'clock.
Use: The foreign body was observed in the patient's left eye at the 9-o'clock position.

Note: The terms *clockwise* and *counterclockwise* can also be misleading. The point of reference (eg, that of observer vs subject) should be specified if the usage is ambiguous.

9.8 ■ **LABORATORY VALUES.**—Usually, in reports of clinical or laboratory data, the substance per se is not reported; rather, a value is given that was obtained by measuring a substance or some function or constituent of it. For example, one does not report "blood" but rather blood pressure, blood cell count, or bleeding time. Some other correct forms are as follows:

differential white blood cell *count*

hemoglobin *level*

agglutination *titer*

prothrombin *time*

pulse *rate* (beats per minute)

sedimentation *rate* (per hour)

total serum cholesterol *value* or *level* or *concentration* increase in antibody *level*

creatinine *level* or *clearance*

serum phosphorus *concentration*

rise in bilirubin *level* or *increase* in bilirubin

In reports of findings from clinical examinations or laboratory studies, data may be enumerated without repeating *value, level,* etc, in accordance with the following example:

> Laboratory studies disclosed the following values: sodium, 128 mmol/L; potassium, 4.0 mmol/L; hematocrit, 0.28; serum urea nitrogen, 27 mmol/L (76 mg/dL) of urea; creatinine, 760 μmol/L (8.6 mg/dL); and total calcium, 2.54 mmol/L (10.2 mg/dL).

9.9 ■ **ARTICLES.**—The article *a* is used before aspirate *h* (eg, *a* historic occasion) and nonvocalic *y* (eg, *a* ubiquitous organism). Abbreviations and acronyms are preceded by *a* or *an* according to the *sound* following (eg, *a* UN resolution, *an* HMO plan). (See also 11.8, Abbreviations, Agencies and Organizations.)

a hypothesis [*h* sound]	an ultraviolet source [*u* sound]
a WMA report [*d* sound]	a UV source [*y* sound]
a hematocrit [*h* sound]	an honorarium [*o* sound]
an MD degree [*e* sound]	

9.10 ■ **INCLUSIVE LANGUAGE.**

> *To boldly go where no man has gone before.*
> Captain James T. Kirk
> "Star Trek" (1966-1969)

> *To boldly go where no one has gone before.*
> Captain Jean-Luc Picard
> "Star Trek: The Next Generation" (1987-1994)

(See also 5.8.5, Grammar, Split Infinitives.)

AMA journals avoid the use of language that imparts bias against persons or groups on the basis of sex, race or ethnicity, age, physical or mental disability, or sexual orientation. The careful writer avoids generalizations and stereotypes and is specific when choosing words to describe people.

9.10.1 ***Sex/Gender.***—*Sex* refers to the biological characteristics of males and females. *Gender* includes more than *sex* and serves as a cultural indicator of a person's personal and social status. An important consideration when referring to sex is the level of specificity required: specify sex when it is relevant. Choose sex-neutral terms that avoid bias, suit the material under discussion, and do not intrude on the reader's attention. See also 9.5, Age and Sex Referents.

Nouns

Avoid	*Preferred*
man, mankind	people, human beings, humans, humanity, humankind, human species [*but:* see note]
chairwoman, chairman	chair, chairperson [*but:* see note]

fireman	firefighter
layman	layperson
policeman, policewoman	police officer
steward, stewardess	flight attendant
mailman	letter carrier, mail carrier
mothering	parenting, nurturing, caregiving
spokesman, spokeswoman	spokesperson

Note: Use ***man*** or ***men*** when referring to a man or a group of men, ***woman*** or ***women*** when referring to a woman or a group of women. Similarly, ***chairman*** or ***spokesman*** might be used if the person under discussion is a man, and ***chairwoman*** or ***spokeswoman*** if she is a woman. Any of these might be used if it is an official title (verify with the author).

Do not attempt to change all words with ***man*** to ***person*** (eg, ***manmade, manhole, manpower***). If possible, choose a sex-neutral equivalent such as ***artificial*** (or ***synthetic*** or ***handmade***), ***sewer hole*** or ***utility access hole,*** and ***workforce.***

Many terms, such as ***physician, nurse,*** and ***scientist,*** are sex-neutral and do not require modification (eg, female physician, male nurse) unless the sex of the person or persons described is relevant to the discussion (eg, a study of only female physicians or male nurses).

When a specific person is being discussed, use appropriate sex-specific pronouns.

> The physician-astronaut underwent thorough preflight training. Her debriefing was equally rigorous.

Personal Pronouns

Avoid sex-specific pronouns in cases in which sex specificity is irrelevant. The creation of common-gender pronouns (eg, "s/he," "shem," "shim," "himorher," "he'er") unduly emphasizes the problem without really solving it. Reword the sentence to use a singular or plural non-sex-specific pronoun, neutral noun equivalent, or change of voice; or use "he or she" ("him or her," "his or her[s]," "they or their[s]").

Avoid	*Preferred*
The physician and his office staff can do much to alleviate a patient's nervousness.	Physicians and their office staff can do much to alleviate a patient's nervousness. [plural]
	The physician and the office staff can do much to alleviate a patient's nervousness. [neutral noun equivalent]
Everyone must allocate their time effectively.	One must allocate one's time effectively. [singular]
	People must allocate their time effectively. [plural]
	Time must be allocated effectively. [change of voice]

Note: In an effort to avoid both sex-specific pronouns and awkward sentence structure, some writers use plural pronouns with singular indefinite antecedents (eg, Everyone allocates their time [note singular verb and "their" instead of "his or her"]), particularly in informal writing. Editors of AMA journals recognize this trend but prefer that agreement in number be maintained in formal scientific writing (see 5.9, Grammar, Subject-Verb Agreement).

Avoid:	One must allocate their time.
	Everyone must allocate their time.
Preferred:	One must allocate one's time.
Or:	One must allocate time.
	Everyone must allocate time.

9.10.2 ***Race/Ethnicity.***—*Race* is defined as "possessing traits that are transmissible by descent and sufficient to characterize it as a distinct human type."[7] ***Ethnicity*** relates to "groups of people classed according to common racial, national, tribal, religious, linguistic, or cultural origin or background."[7]

Like gender, race and ethnicity are cultural constructs, but they can have biological implications. A person's genetic heritage can convey certain biological and therefore medically relevant predispositions (eg, sickle cell anemia for persons with African ancestry, lactose intolerance for persons with Chinese or Japanese ancestry, Tay-Sachs disease for Jewish persons with Eastern European ancestry).

Specifying subjects' race or ethnicity can provide information about the generalizability of a study. However, because many people in ethnically diverse countries such as the United States may have multiple racial and ethnic origins, a racial or ethnic distinction should not be considered absolute, and it is often based on a person's self-designation.

Racial categories should not be used automatically. Authors should explain and justify racial designators used, perhaps in the methods section of the manuscript. Any such terms should be used accurately.

When mention of race or ethnicity is relevant to an understanding of scientific information, be sensitive to the designations that individuals or groups prefer. Be aware also that preferences may change and that individuals within a group may disagree about the most appropriate designation.

For terms such as *white, black,* and *African American,* copy editors should follow author usage (*exception: Caucasian* is occasionally used to indicate *white* but is technically specific to people from the Caucasus region and thus should be avoided).

In the United States, the term *African American* may be preferred to *black* (note, however, that this term should be allowed only for US citizens of African descent). A hyphen is not used in either the noun or adjectival form (see also 6.3.1, Punctuation, Hyphen, When Not to Use Hyphens).

In references to persons (and their descendants) indigenous to North America, *American Indian* is generally preferred to the broader term *Native American,* which is also acceptable but includes (by US government designation) Hawaiian, Samoan, and Alaskan natives. Whenever possible, specify the nation or peoples (eg, Navajo, Nez Perce, Inuit) rather than use the more general term.

Hispanic and *Latino* are broad terms that may be used to designate Spanish-speaking persons as well as those descended from the Spanish-speaking people of Mexico, South and Central America, and the Caribbean. However, the terms are not interchangeable, since *Latino* is understood by some to exclude those of Mexican or Caribbean ancestry and may be preferred in certain geographic areas. In either case, these terms should not be used in noun form, and when possible, a more specific term (eg, Mexican, Mexican American, Latin American, Cuban, Cuban American, Puerto Rican) should be used.

Similarly, Asian persons may wish to be described according to their country or geographic area of origin, eg, Chinese, Indian, Japanese, Sri Lankan. Note that *Asian* and *Asian American* (*Chinese* and *Chinese American,* and so on) are not equivalent or interchangeable. Do not use *Oriental* or *Orientals*.

Note: Avoid using "non-" (eg, "white and nonwhite subjects"), which is a nonspecific "convenience" grouping and label. Such a "category" may be oversimplified and misleading, even incorrect. Occasionally, however, one sees these categorizations used for comparisons in data analysis. In such cases, the author should be queried. *People of color* and *multiracial* are sometimes used in part to address the heterogeneous ethnic background of many people.

9.10.3 ***Age.***—Discrimination based on age is *ageism,* usually relevant to older persons. Avoid using age descriptors as nouns because of the tendency to stereotype a particular group as having a common set of characteristics. While in general the phrase *the elderly* should be avoided, when referring to the entire population of elderly persons, use of *the elderly* may be appropriate (as in the impact of Medicare cuts on the elderly, for example). Otherwise, terms such as *older persons, older people, elderly patients, geriatric patients, older patients, aging adults,* or *the older population* are preferred.

Note: In studies that involve humans, age should always be given specifically. Researchers in geriatrics may use defined terms for older age groups, eg, young-old (usually defined as 60 or 65 to 70 or so years) and old-old (80 years and older).[8] (See also 9.5, Age and Sex Referents.)

9.10.4 ***Disabilities.***—According to the Americans With Disabilities Act, "a disability exists when an individual has any physical or psychological illness that 'substantially limits' a major life activity, such as walking, learning, breathing, working, or participating in community activities."[9]

Avoid labeling (and thus equating) people with their disabilities or diseases (eg, the blind, schizophrenics, epileptics). Instead, put the person first. Avoid describing persons as *victims* or with other emotional terms that suggest helplessness (*afflicted with, suffering from, stricken with*). Avoid euphemistic descriptors such as *physically challenged* or *special.*

Avoid	*Preferred*
the disabled, the handicapped	persons with disability
disabled child, mentally ill person, retarded adult	child with a disability, person with mental illness, adult with mental retardation
diabetics	persons with diabetes, subjects in the diabetes group [ie, in a study], diabetic patients
asthmatics	children with asthma, asthma group, asthmatic child
epileptic	person affected by epilepsy, person with epilepsy
AIDS victim, stroke victim	person with AIDS, person who has had a stroke
crippled, lame, deformed	physically disabled

Note: Some manuscripts use certain phrases many times, and changing, for example, "AIDS patient" to "person with AIDS" at every occurrence may result in awkward and stilted text. In such cases, the adjectival form may be used.

9.10.5 ***Sexual Orientation.***—Sexual orientation should be indicated in a manuscript only when scientifically relevant.

The nouns *lesbians* and *gay men* are preferred to the broader term *homosexuals* when referring to specific groups. Avoid using *gay* or *gays* as a noun. *Heterosexual* and *homosexual* may be used as adjectives (eg, *homosexual man*).

A member of a heterosexual or homosexual couple may be referred to as *spouse, companion, partner, life partner,* or *lover.*

ACKNOWLEDGMENTS

Principal author: Roxanne K. Young, ELS

Richard E. Appen, MD, University of Wisconsin-Madison Medical School; Thomas B. Cole, MD, MPH, 1995-1996 *JAMA* Fishbein Fellow in Medical Journalism; Ronald G. Evens, MD, Mallinckrodt Institute of Radiology, Washington University School of Medicine, St Louis, Mo; Phil Gunby, Division of Medical News and Humanities, American Medical Association, Chicago, Ill; Laura King, MA, Division of Editorial Processing, American Medical Association, Chicago; and Jody W. Zylke, MD, Contributing Editor, *JAMA,* Chicago.

REFERENCES

1. King LS. *Why Not Say It Clearly: A Guide to Expository Writing.* 2nd ed. Boston, Mass: Little Brown & Co Inc; 1991.
2. Kane RL, Kane RA. Long-term care. *JAMA.* 1995;273:1690-1691.
3. The Expert Committee on the Diagnosis and Classification of Diabetes Mellitus. Report of the Expert Committee on the Diagnosis and Classification of Diabetes Mellitus. *Diabetes Care.* 1997;20:1183-1197.
4. Publications Department, American College of Obstetricians and Gynecologists. *Publication Guidelines.* Washington, DC; American College of Obstetricians and Gynecologists; 1997:22-23.
5. Maggio R. *The Dictionary of Bias-Free Usage: A Guide to Nondiscriminatory Language.* Phoenix, Ariz: Oryx Press; 1991.
6. *The American Heritage Dictionary of the English Language.* 3rd ed. Boston, Mass: Houghton Mifflin Co; 1992.
7. *Merriam-Webster's Collegiate Dictionary.* 10th ed. Springfield, Mass: Merriam-Webster Inc; 1993.
8. Evans JG, Williams TF, eds. *Oxford Textbook of Geriatric Medicine.* New York, NY: Oxford University Press; 1992.
9. Orentlicher D. Rationing and the Americans With Disabilities Act. *JAMA.* 1994;271: 308-314.

ADDITIONAL READINGS AND GENERAL REFERENCES

American Psychological Association. *Publication Manual of the American Psychological Association.* 4th ed. Washington, DC: American Psychological Association; 1994.

Baron D. *Grammar and Gender.* New Haven, Conn: Yale University Press; 1986.

Baron D. *Grammar and Good Taste: Reforming the American Language.* New Haven, Conn: Yale University Press; 1982.

Brooks BS, Pinson JL. *Working With Words: A Concise Handbook for Media Writers and Editors.* 2nd ed. New York, NY: St Martins Press; 1993.

Caldwell SH, Popenoe R. Perceptions and misperceptions of skin color. *Ann Intern Med.* 1995;122:614-617.

The Chicago Manual of Style. 14th ed. Chicago, Ill: University of Chicago Press; 1993.

DeBakey L. Echolalia. *Int J Cardiol.* 1982;2:267-272.

DeBakey L, in collaboration with Cranefield PF, Gupta AP, Ingelfinger FJ, et al. *The Scientific Journal: Editorial Policies and Practices: Guidelines for Editors, Reviewers, and Authors.* St Louis, Mo: CV Mosby Co; 1976.

Editorial Policy Committee, Council of Biology Editors. *Ethics and Policy in Scientific Publication.* Bethesda, Md: Council of Biology Editors Inc; 1990.

Follett W; Barzun J, ed. *Modern American Usage: A Guide.* New York, NY: Hill & Wang; 1966:358.

Fowler HW; Gowers E, ed. *A Dictionary of Modern English Usage.* 2nd ed. Oxford, England: Clarendon Press; 1968.

Freudenheim E. *Healthspeak: A Complete Dictionary of America's Health Care System.* New York, NY: Facts on File Inc; 1996.

Goodwill Industries International Inc. *People With Disabilities Terminology Guide.* Bethesda, Md: Goodwill Industries International Inc; 1994. Publication 5032.10.

A Guide to Bias-Free Communications. Madison: University of Wisconsin, Office of University Publications; August 1992.

Huth EJ. Identifying ethnicity in medical papers. *Ann Intern Med.* 1995;122:619-621.

Huth EJ. *Medical Style & Format: An International Manual for Authors, Editors, and Publishers.* Philadelphia, Pa: ISI Press; 1987.

King RK. Race: an outdated concept. *AMWA J.* 1995;10:55-58.

Miller C, Swift K. *The Handbook of Nonsexist Writing.* New York, NY; Lippincott & Crowell; 1980.

Ontario Ministry of Health. *The SI Manual in Health Care.* 2nd ed. Toronto: Ontario Ministry of Health; 1982;appendix VI:36.

Osborne NG, Feit MD. The use of race in medical research. *JAMA.* 1992;267:275-279.

Schwartz M, and the Task Force on Bias-Free Language of the Association of American University Presses. *Guidelines for Bias-Free Writing.* Bloomington: Indiana University Press; 1995.

Council of Biology Editors Style Manual Committee. *Scientific Style and Format: The CBE Manual for Authors, Editors, and Publishers.* 6th ed. New York, NY: Cambridge University Press; 1994.

Sutcliffe AJ, ed. *The New York Public Library Writer's Guide to Style and Usage.* New York, NY: HarperCollins Publishers; 1994.

Tekwani NH, Sengupta AK. The importance of mentioning ethnicity in the clinical presentation [Pulse]. *JAMA.* 1996;275:733.

CHAPTER 10

10.0 NON-ENGLISH WORDS AND PHRASES; ACCENT MARKS (DIACRITICS)

10.1 ■ NON-ENGLISH WORDS AND PHRASES.

10.1.1 ***Use of Italics.***—Some words and phrases derived from other languages have become part of standard English usage (eg, in vivo, in vitro). Those that have not, ie, that do not appear in the most recent edition of *Merriam-Webster's Collegiate Dictionary* or in standard medical dictionaries, should be italicized (see 19.0, Typography).

> *Çao gio* (coin rolling) bruises have been reported as an example of apparent child abuse among Vietnamese refugees.
>
> Some 62% of the Dutch population—the lower-income groups—obtain health services through the *ziekenfonds,* or sickness funds.

Non-English names of streets (addresses), buildings, organizations, or government institutions should not be italicized or abbreviated (30, avenue de la Voie Romaine; Città del Vaticano; Museum für Volkerkunde) (see 11.4, Abbreviations, Local Addresses).

10.1.2. ***Translation.***—Non-English titles mentioned in text may be translated or not, at the author's discretion. If the original title is used, an English translation should be given parenthetically, except in cases in which the work is considered well known (eg, Pascal's *Pensées*).

This rule varies somewhat from that governing non-English titles in references (see 2.12.10, Manuscript Preparation, References, Non-English-Language Titles).

10.1.3 ***Capitalization and Punctuation.***—Non-English words should be capitalized and non-English phrases punctuated according to that language's standard of correctness. Follow language dictionaries and *The Chicago Manual of Style,* 14th edition, chapter 9 (see 2.12.10, Manuscript Preparation, References, Non-English-Language Titles, and 10.2, Accent Marks [Diacritics]).

10.2 **■ ACCENT MARKS (DIACRITICS).**—An accent mark (or *diacritic*), when added to a letter, confers a special phonetic value. English words once spelled with accent marks (eg, coöperation, rôle, naïve) now are written and printed without them. Recently published dictionaries provide alternate forms for words that have had accent marks at one time (eg, resume/resumé/résumé; facade/façade).

Accented letters are available in most word-processing software packages. Consult program and printer manuals for font information.

Accent marks should be retained in proper names. Otherwise, accent marks may be omitted, except in these instances:

- When correct spelling in the original language is shown (proper nouns in the original language are not italicized)

  Köln (Cologne)

Note: In general, the English-language version of city or country names is used in English-language publications. Consult the geographic names section of *Merriam-Webster's Collegiate Dictionary*—as well as the author—for preferred forms.

- In a person's name

  Behçet syndrome

- In quotations

  "On résiste à l'invasion des armées; on ne résiste pas à l'invasion des idées."—Victor Hugo [One can resist the invasion of armies, but not the invasion of ideas.]

- In terms in which accent marks are retained in current use (consult dictionary)

  garçon

  Möbius strip [alternative form: Moebius]

  tête-à-tête

Accent marks are also used to show pronunciation and syllabic emphasis (eg, for *lues,* lü-ez; for *endive,* ˈen-dīv, än-ˈdēv).

Accent marks should be clearly indicated on manuscript copy. Although for most typefaces the diaeresis and umlaut are indistinguishable, each should be marked specifically.

Diacritic	*Example of Usage*
acute	Ménétrier
breve	Omskiĭ
cedilla	Behçet
circumflex	Le Nôtre
diaeresis	dadaïsme
dot	faůst
grave	Akademiaì Kiadò
macron	gignōskein
ring	Ångstrom
slash	København
tilde	mañana
umlaut	für
wedge	Vrapče

ACKNOWLEDGMENT

Principal author: Roxanne K. Young, ELS

Terminology

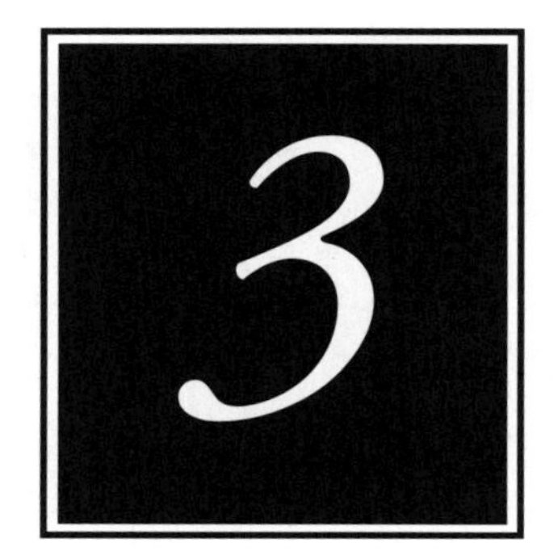

CHAPTER 11

The Greeks did not use abbreviations commonly; they had no instinct for abbreviating. When they did abbreviate, it was by simple suspension (or curtailment), usually self-intelligible. The purpose was often to save numerous repetitions in one document. . . . Greek abbreviations were not standardized, but depended on the whim of the scribe.

Herbert Weir Smyth[1]

11.0 ABBREVIATIONS

The Random House Dictionary of the English Language defines an abbreviation as "a shortened or contracted form of a word or phrase, used to represent the whole"[2] (eg, Dr for doctor, US for United States, mL for milliliter).

An acronym is "a word formed from the initial letters or groups of letters of words in a set phrase or series of words"[2] (eg, ELISA for enzyme-linked immunosorbent assay). Acronyms are pronounced as words.

An initialism is "a name or term formed from the initial letters of a group of words and pronounced as a separate word"[2] (eg, NATO for North Atlantic Treaty Organization) or "a set of initials representing a name, organization, or the like, with each letter pronounced separately"[2] (eg, DHHS for Department of Health and Human Services).

The editors of the AMA's scientific publications discourage the use of abbreviations, acronyms, and initialisms in their journals, with the exception of internationally approved and accepted units of measure and some well-recognized clinical, technical, and general terms and symbols. Overuse of abbreviations can be confusing and ambiguous for readers—especially those of another culture or those outside a specific specialty. However, since abbreviations save space, they may be acceptable to use when the original word or words are repeated numerous times.

Many instructions for authors published in medical and scientific journals include guidelines on the use of abbreviations, ranging from "limit of 4 per manuscript" to "use only approved abbreviations." Authors, editors, copy editors, and others involved in preparing manuscripts should use good judgment, flexibility, and common sense when considering the use of abbreviations. Abbreviations that some consider universally known may be obscure to others. Author-invented abbreviations should be avoided. See specific entries in this section and 12.0, Nomenclature, for further guidance in correct usage of abbreviations.

Note: The expanded form of an abbreviation is given in lowercase letters, unless the expansion contains a proper noun, is a formal name, or begins a sentence (capitalize first word only).

AMA style for abbreviations rarely calls for the use of periods. (*But:* see 11.6, Names and Titles of Persons.)

11.1 ■ **ACADEMIC DEGREES AND HONORS.**—The following academic degrees are abbreviated in bylines and in the text (see also 11.6, Names and Titles of Persons). These abbreviations are used only with the full name of a person. In some circumstances, however, use of the abbreviation alone is acceptable (eg, June is a doctor of medicine and also holds a PhD in biochemistry) (see also 7.1, Plurals, Abbreviations).

Generally, US fellowship designations (eg, FACP, FAAN) and honorary designations (eg, PhD[Hon]) are not used in bylines. In contrast, non-US designations such as the British FRCP and the Canadian FRCPC (attained through a series of qualifying examinations) should be listed.

Degrees below the master's level are generally not listed in bylines or elsewhere (BA and BS degrees from US institutions are so broad that little meaningful information about the authors is provided). However, if a bachelor's degree is the highest degree held, it may be listed. Exceptions are also made for specialized degrees, licenses, certifications, and credentials below the master's level in medical and health-related fields (included below). Any unusual degrees should be verified with the author.

ART	accredited record technician
BS, BCh, BC, CB, or ChB	bachelor of surgery
BSN	bachelor of science in nursing
CNM	certified nurse midwife
CNMT	certified nuclear medicine technologist
CO	certified orthoptist
COMT	certified ophthalmic medical technologist
CPFT	certified pulmonary function technologist
CRNA	certified registered nurse anesthetist
CRTT	certified respiratory therapy technician
DC	doctor of chiropractic
DCh or ChD	doctor of surgery
DDS	doctor of dental surgery
DMD	doctor of dental medicine
DME	doctor of medical education
DMSc	doctor of medical science
DNE	doctor of nursing education
DNS or DNSc	doctor of nursing science
DO or OD	doctor of optometry
DO	doctor of osteopathy
DPH or DrPH	doctor of public health; doctor of public hygiene
DPharm	doctor of pharmacy
DPM	doctor of podiatric medicine
DSW	doctor of social work
DTM&H	diploma in tropical medicine and hygiene

DTPH	diploma in tropical pediatric hygiene
DVM, DMV, or VMD	doctor of veterinary medicine
DVMS	doctor of veterinary medicine and surgery
DVS or DVSc	doctor of veterinary science
EdD	doctor of education
ELS	editor in the life sciences
EMT	emergency medical technician
EMT-P	emergency medical technician-paramedic
FCGP	fellow of the College of General Practitioners
FCPS	fellow of the College of Physicians and Surgeons
FFA	fellow of the Faculty of Anaesthetists
FFARCS	fellow of the Faculty of Anaesthetists of the Royal College of Surgeons
FNP	family nurse practitioner
FP	family practitioner
FRACP	fellow of the Royal Australian College of Physicians
FRCGP	fellow of the Royal College of General Practitioners
FRCOG	fellow of the Royal College of Obstetricians and Gynaecologists
FRCP	fellow of the Royal College of Physicians
FRCPath	fellow of the Royal College of Pathologists
FRCPC	fellow of the Royal College of Physicians of Canada
FRCPE or FRCP(Edin)	fellow of the Royal College of Physicians of Edinburgh
FRCP(Glasg)	fellow of the Royal College of Physicians and Surgeons of Glasgow *qua* Physician
FRCPI or FRCP(Ire)	fellow of the Royal College of Physicians of Ireland
FRCR	fellow of the Royal College of Radiologists
FRCS	fellow of the Royal College of Surgeons
FRCSC	fellow of the Royal College of Surgeons of Canada
FRCSE or FRCS(Edin)	fellow of the Royal College of Surgeons of Edinburgh
FRCS(Glasg)	fellow of the Royal College of Physicians and Surgeons of Glasgow *qua* Surgeon
FRCSI or FRCS(Ire)	fellow of the Royal College of Surgeons of Ireland
FRCVS	fellow of the Royal College of Veterinary Surgeons
FRS	fellow of the Royal Society
GNP	gerontologic or geriatric nurse practitioner
JD	doctor of jurisprudence
LLB	bachelor of laws
LLD	doctor of laws
LLM	master of laws
LPN	licensed practical nurse
LVN	licensed visiting nurse; licensed vocational nurse
MA or AM	master of arts
M(ASCP)	registered technologist in microbiology (American Society of Clinical Pathologists)
MB or BM	bachelor of medicine
MBA	master of business administration
MBBS or MB,BS	bachelor of medicine, bachelor of surgery
MD or DM	doctor of medicine
ME	medical examiner
MEd	master of education
MFA	master of fine arts
MHA	master of hospital administration
MLS	master of library science

MN	master of nursing
MPA	master of public administration
MPH	master of public health
MPharm	master of pharmacy
MRCP	member of the Royal College of Physicians
MRCS	member of the Royal College of Surgeons
MS, MSc, or SM	master of science
MS, SM, MCh, MSurg	master of surgery
MSN	master of science in nursing
MSPH	master of science in public health
MSW	master of social welfare; master of social work
MT	medical technologist
MTA	medical technical assistant
MT(ASCP)	registered medical technologist (American Society of Clinical Pathologists)
NP	nurse practitioner
OT	occupational therapist
OTR	occupational therapist, registered
PA	physician assistant
PA-C	physician assistant-certified
PharmD, DP, or PD	doctor of pharmacy
PharmG	graduate in pharmacy
PhD or DPhil	doctor of philosophy
PNP	pediatric nurse practitioner
PsyD	doctor of psychology
PT	physical therapist
RD	registered dietitian
RN	registered nurse
RNA	registered nurse anesthetist
RNC or RN,C	registered nurse, certified
RPFT	registered pulmonary function technologist
RPh	registered pharmacist
RPT	registered physical therapist
RRL	registered record librarian
RT	radiologic technologist; respiratory therapist
RTR	recreational therapist, registered
ScD, DSc, or DS	doctor of science

11.2 ■ **US MILITARY SERVICES AND TITLES.**—An abbreviation of a military service follows a name; an abbreviation of a military title (also called grade or rank) precedes a name (eg, 1LT Mary McNamara, AN, USAR). In most instances, the service and title replace the academic degree in bylines. Military titles and abbreviations should be verified with the author (see also 2.2, Manuscript Preparation, Bylines and End-of-Text Signatures, and 2.2.2, Manuscript Preparation, Degrees).

11.2.1 *US Military Services*

US Army

MC, USA	Medical Corps, US Army
AN, USA	Army Nurse Corps, US Army
SP, USA	Specialist Corps, US Army

MS, USA	Medical Service Corps, US Army
DC, USA	Dental Corps, US Army
VC, USA	Veterinary Corps, US Army

Note: All of the preceding designations also apply to the Army National Guard (ARNG) and US Army Reserve (USAR).

US Air Force

USAF, MC	Medical Corps, US Air Force
USAF, NC	Nurse Corps, US Air Force
USAF, MSC	Medical Service Corps, US Air Force
USAF, DC	Dental Corps, US Air Force
USAF, BSC	Bio-Sciences Corps, US Air Force

Note: All of the preceding designations also apply to the Air National Guard (ANG) and US Air Force Reserve (USAFR). The US Air Force has no veterinary corps; veterinarians are in the Bio-Sciences Corps.

US Navy

MC, USN	Medical Corps, US Navy
MSC, USN	Medical Service Corps, US Navy
NC, USN	Nurse Corps, US Navy
DC, USN	Dental Corps, US Navy

Note: All of the preceding designations also apply to the US Naval Reserve (USNR).

11.2.2 *US Military Officer Titles (Grades/Ranks).*

US Army

General	GEN
Lieutenant General	LTG
Major General	MG
Brigadier General	BG
Colonel	COL
Lieutenant Colonel	LTC
Major	MAJ
Captain	CPT
First Lieutenant	1LT
Second Lieutenant	2LT
Chief Warrant Officer	CWO
Warrant Officer	WO

US Navy and US Coast Guard

Admiral	ADM
Vice Admiral	VADM
Rear Admiral	RADM
Captain	CAPT
Commander	CDR
Lieutenant Commander	LCDR
Lieutenant	LT
Lieutenant (Junior Grade)	LTJG
Ensign	ENS
Chief Warrant Officer	CWO

Note: All medical professionals in the US Coast Guard (except physician assistants) are commissioned officers in the US Public Health Service (PHS). US Coast Guard chief warrant officers in medicine are designated CWO(Med). This also applies to the US Coast Guard Reserve.

US Air Force and US Marine Corps

General	Gen
Lieutenant General	Lt Gen
Major General	Maj Gen
Brigadier General	Brig Gen
Colonel	Col
Lieutenant Colonel	Lt Col
Major	Maj
Captain	Capt
First Lieutenant	1st Lt
Second Lieutenant	2nd Lt

Note: The US Marine Corps does not have a separate medical organization. The medical care of the US Marine Corps is provided by the US Navy.

11.3 ■ **DAYS OF THE WEEK, MONTHS, ERAS.**—Generally, days of the week and months are not abbreviated.

> The manuscript was received at *JAMA*'s offices in late December 1995 and accepted for publication on February 5, 1996, after expedited peer review, revision, and discussion among the editors. Because of the importance of its topic, the article was published 4 weeks later, on Wednesday, March 6.

In tables and figures, the following 3-letter abbreviations for days of the weeks and months may be used to conserve space (see 2.13, Manuscript Preparation, Tables, and 2.14, Manuscript Preparation, Figures):

Monday	Mon	January	Jan
Tuesday	Tue	February	Feb
Wednesday	Wed	March	Mar
Thursday	Thu	April	Apr
Friday	Fri	May	May
Saturday	Sat	June	Jun
Sunday	Sun	July	Jul
		August	Aug
		September	Sep
		October	Oct
		November	Nov
		December	Dec

Occasionally, scientific manuscripts may contain discussion of eras. Abbreviations for eras are set in small capitals with no punctuation. Numerals are used for years and words for the first through ninth centuries. The more commonly used era designations are AD (*anno Domini,* in the year of the Lord), BC (before Christ), CE (common era), and BCE (before the common era). CE and BCE are equivalent to AD and BC, respectively. In formal usage, the abbreviation AD precedes the year number, and BC, CE, and BCE follow it.

> William Withering was the first to report extensively, in the late 18th century, on the use of foxglove (*Digitalis purpurea*) for the treatment of dropsy (edema).
>
> Hippocrates, a prominent Greek medical practitioner and teacher of the fourth century BCE, has come to personify the ideal physician.
>
> The incidence of tuberculosis is thought to have increased greatly during the Middle Ages (roughly AD 500-1500), possibly because of the growth of towns across Europe.
>
> Cuneiform was invented probably by the Sumerians before 3000 BC.

11.4 ■ **LOCAL ADDRESSES.**—Use the following abbreviations when *complete* local addresses are given (eg, Front Street vs 13 Front St). In some cases, these designators may not be abbreviated, by convention (eg, Fort Collins, Mount Sinai, North Chicago):

Air Force Base	AFB
Army Post Office	APO
Avenue	Ave
Boulevard	Blvd
Building	Bldg
Circle	Cir
Court	Ct
Drive	Dr
East	E
Fleet Post Office	FPO
Fort	Ft
Highway	Hwy
Lane	Ln
Mount	Mt
North	N
Northeast	NE
Northwest	NW
Parkway	Pkwy
Place	Pl
Post Office	PO
Road	Rd
Route	Rte
Rural Free Delivery	RFD
Rural Route	RR
Saint	St or Ste (eg, Sault Ste Marie [verify])
South	S
Southeast	SE
Southwest	SW
Square	Sq
Street	St
Terrace	Terr
West	W

Do not abbreviate the non-English counterparts of the above designators (eg, boulevard, avenue, place, rue, via, Strasse, Platz) (see also *The Chicago Manual of Style,* 14th ed, chapter 9).

When the plural form is used, do not abbreviate (eg, Broad and Vine streets). When a street number is not given, do not abbreviate (eg, National Hospital for Neurology and Neurosurgery, Queen Square, London WC1N 3BG, England).

Do not abbreviate *room, suite, department* (except in references; see 2.12.38, Manuscript Preparation, References, Government Bulletins), or *division.*

Do not use periods or commas with *N, S, E, W,* or their combinations.

There may be exceptions to these rules. For example, "One IBM Plaza," "One Magnificent Mile," and "One Gustave L. Levy Place" are not only addresses but also proper names of buildings or office centers. In these cases it is appropriate to spell out address numbers that accompany designators such as "Place." In such cases, the editor or author should use common sense and verify unusual addresses.

Note: E-mail addresses should be used exactly as given (see also 2.3.8, Manuscript Preparation, Reprint or Correspondence Address).

11.5 ■ **US STATES, TERRITORIES, AND POSSESSIONS; PROVINCES; COUNTRIES.**—Names of US states, territories, and possessions should be spelled out in full when they stand alone. When the state name follows the name of a city, the abbreviation should be used, without periods. Use postal codes for states only when using ZIP codes. Do not abbreviate a state name after a county name.

Chicago, Ill
Chicago, IL 60610
Cook County, Illinois

US State, Territory, or Possession	*Abbreviation*	*Postal Code*
Alabama	Ala	AL
Alaska	Alaska	AK
American Samoa	American Samoa	AS
Arizona	Ariz	AZ
Arkansas	Ark	AR
California	Calif	CA
Canal Zone	Canal Zone	CZ
Colorado	Colo	CO
Connecticut	Conn	CT
Delaware	Del	DE
District of Columbia	DC	DC
Florida	Fla	FL
Georgia	Ga	GA
Guam	Guam	GU
Hawaii	Hawaii	HI
Idaho	Idaho	ID
Illinois	Ill	IL
Indiana	Ind	IN
Iowa	Iowa	IA
Kansas	Kan	KS
Kentucky	Ky	KY
Louisiana	La	LA
Maine	Me	ME
Maryland	Md	MD
Massachusetts	Mass	MA
Michigan	Mich	MI
Minnesota	Minn	MN
Mississippi	Miss	MS
Missouri	Mo	MO
Montana	Mont	MT
Nebraska	Neb	NE
Nevada	Nev	NV
New Hampshire	NH	NH
New Jersey	NJ	NJ
New Mexico	NM	NM
New York	NY	NY
North Carolina	NC	NC
North Dakota	ND	ND
Ohio	Ohio	OH
Oklahoma	Okla	OK
Oregon	Ore	OR
Pennsylvania	Pa	PA
Puerto Rico	Puerto Rico	PR
Rhode Island	RI	RI

US State, Territory, or Possession	*Abbreviation*	*Postal Code*
South Carolina	SC	SC
South Dakota	SD	SD
Tennessee	Tenn	TN
Texas	Tex	TX
Utah	Utah	UT
Vermont	Vt	VT
Virginia	Va	VA
Virgin Islands	Virgin Islands	VI
Washington	Wash	WA
West Virginia	WVa	WV
Wisconsin	Wis	WI
Wyoming	Wyo	WY

Note: The abbreviation "US" may be used as a modifier (ie, only when it directly precedes the word it modifies) but should be expanded to "United States" in all other contexts.

> The authors stratified all counties in the United States as urban or rural according to US census data.

Canadian city names should be followed by the province name (eg, London, Ontario, not London, Canada). Province names are not abbreviated. Whenever full addresses are given, both the province and "Canada" should be listed, in addition to the Canadian postal code: London, Ontario, Canada N6A 4L6.

At first mention in the text, the name of the appropriate state or country should follow the name of a city whenever clarification of location is thought to be important for the reader, as in the following examples:

> On August 24, 1992, Hurricane Andrew made landfall 56 km southwest of Miami, Fla, with sustained winds of 232 km/h.

> Hope was hard to find at the 10th International Conference on AIDS, which was held in Yokohama, Japan.

In addition to the city name, always provide the name of the state or country in the reprint request address, affiliation footnote, and signature block. (*But:* For the last 2, see below for how to handle situations in which the institution name contains the name of the state or country.) If the city, state, or country is clear from the context, as in the following examples, do not repeat it.

> Studies were carried out at the University of Michigan Medical School, Ann Arbor [unnecessary to add "Mich"].

> A cross-sectional survey assessing bicycle safety helmets was conducted in 3 Dutch primary schools in Breda, Maastricht, and Terneuzen.

> By 1995, scientists at Illinois' Argonne National Laboratory, located about 50 km west of Chicago, expected to switch on the brightest beams of light ever to shine on earth.

Do not provide the state or country name in cases in which the entity is well known and such clarification is excessive, eg, Chicago Bulls, Philadelphia chromosome, Uppsala virus, Lyme disease, *London Times*.

Do not provide the location of an institution if it is clear that the location is not important, eg, "Using the Centers for Disease Control and Prevention criteria for AIDS. . . ." or "Following the World Health Organization guidelines. . . ."

What does it matter that she was born in Boston, or that after her parents had instilled in her the guiding principles of life, Harvard University had its turn?

When giving the location of an institution or organization whose formal name includes a city, do not insert the state or country within the name:

Correct:	Stanford University School of Medicine in California
Also correct:	Stanford University School of Medicine, Stanford, Calif
Not:	Stanford University School of Medicine (Calif)
And not:	Stanford (Calif) University School of Medicine
And not:	Stanford University School of Medicine, California

The style used in the correct examples above may be applied in signature bylines:

Correct: Remy I. Smith, MD
Stanford University School of Medicine
Stanford, Calif

Not: Remy I. Smith, MD
Stanford (Calif) University School of Medicine

11.6 ■ **NAMES AND TITLES OF PERSONS.**—Given names should not be abbreviated in the text or in bylines except by using initials, when so indicated by the author. The editor should verify the use of initials with the author. (Some publishers prefer to use initials, instead of given names.)

Do not use Chas., Geo., Jas., Wm., etc, except when such abbreviations are part of the formal name of a company or organization that regularly uses such abbreviations (see 11.7, Business Firms). When an abbreviation is part of a person's name, retain the period after the abbreviation, eg, Oliver St. John Gogarty, MD.

Initials used in the text to indicate names of persons (eg, coauthors of an article) should be followed by periods and set close within parentheses. *Note:* This is one of the few instances in which periods are used with the abbreviation.

A method was devised to calculate familial risk (R.A.K., unpublished observations, 1996).

A person who is not an author may also be included in the text, in which case the full name and academic degree are used.

Although measurements of the various components were divided among 3 different examiners (K.Z., D.O.M., and Norris T. Friedlin, MD), each examiner measured the same components at each annual session.

Senior and *Junior* are abbreviated when they are part of a name. The abbreviations follow the surname and are set off by commas. (*But:* See 16.7.4, Numbers and Percentages, Roman Numerals, and 2.12.7, Manuscript Preparation, References, Authors.) *Note:* These abbreviations are used only with the full name (*never* Dr Forsythe Jr).

Peter M. Forsythe, Jr, MD, performed his landmark research in collaboration with James Philips, Sr, PhD, at the National Institutes of Health.

Names with roman numerals do not use a comma: John Paul II, Marshall Field IV.

Many titles of persons are abbreviated but only when they precede the full name (given name or initials and surname). Spell titles out when (1) used before a surname alone (except in some cases as described below), (2) used at the beginning of a sentence, and (3) used after a name (in this instance, the title should not be capitalized). (*But:* see also 11.2, US Military Services and Titles.)

Colonel Todd
COL Amelia Todd, MC, USA
Dr Todd, colonel in the army

Alderman Tillman
Ald Dorothy Tillman
Dorothy Tillman, alderman of the Third Ward of Chicago

Assistant Professor Ramirez
Asst Prof Maria Ramirez
Maria Ramirez, assistant professor, Department of Internal Medicine

Father Doyle
Fr Raymond G. Doyle
Raymond G. Doyle, SJ

Governor Edgar
Gov Jim Edgar
Jim Edgar, governor of Illinois

Representative McDermott
Rep Jim McDermott
Jim McDermott, MD, representative from the state of Washington

Senator Moseley-Braun
Sen Carol Moseley-Braun (D, Ill)
Carol Moseley-Braun, senator from Illinois

Sister Monica
Sr Monica Sobieski
Monica Sobieski, SJC, mother superior

Superintendent Smith
Supt H. B. Smith
Henry B. Smith, EdD, superintendent of schools

Exception, Heads of State: President is not abbreviated. It is capitalized when it precedes a name and set lowercase when following a name (see also 8.2, Capitalization, Titles and Degrees of Persons):

President John F. Kennedy
President and Mrs Kennedy
John F. Kennedy, president of the United States
the president

The following social titles are always abbreviated when preceding a surname, with or without first name or initials: *Dr, Mr, Messrs, Mrs, Mmes, Ms,* and *Mss.* In most instances, the title Dr should be used only after the specific academic degree has been mentioned and only with the surname.

Arthur L. Rudnick, MD, PhD, gave the opening address. At the close of the meeting, Dr Rudnick was named director of the committee on sports injuries.

The Reverend, Reverend, or *Rev* is used only when the first name or initials are given with the surname. When only the surname is given, use *the Reverend Mr* (or *Ms* or *Dr*), *Mr* (or *Ms* or *Dr*), or *Father* (Roman Catholic, sometimes Anglican). Never use *the Reverend Brown, Reverend Brown,* or *Rev Brown.*

the Reverend Katharine M. Burke

the Reverend Dr Burke

Rev Katharine M. Burke

11.7 ■ **BUSINESS FIRMS.**—In the text, use the name of a company exactly as the company uses it, but omit the period after any abbreviations used, such as *Co, Inc, Corp,* and *Ltd.* In the text, do not abbreviate these terms if the company spells them out, eg, Sandoz Pharmaceuticals Corporation. In the text, periods *are* used with a company namesake's initials.

However, to conserve space in *references,* abbreviate *Company, Corporation, Brothers, Incorporated, Limited,* and *and* (using an ampersand), without punctuation, even if the company expands them, and delete periods even with initials, in accordance with the following examples (see also 2.12.35, Manuscript Preparation, References, Publishers, and 12.5, Nomenclature, Equipment, Devices, and Reagents).

Text Style	*Reference Style*
Little, Brown & Co, Inc	Little Brown & Co Inc
J. B. Lippincott	JB Lippincott
American Mensa, Ltd	American Mensa Ltd
BasicBooks	BasicBooks
MEDSoft Corp	MEDSoft Corp

11.8 ■ **AGENCIES AND ORGANIZATIONS.**—Many organizations (eg, academies, associations, government agencies, research institutes) are known by abbreviations or acronyms rather than by their full names. Some of these organizations have identical abbreviations (eg, AHA for both American Heart Association and American Hospital Association). Therefore, to avoid confusion, the names of all organizations should be expanded at first mention in the text and other major elements of the manuscript, with the abbreviation following immediately in parentheses, in accordance with the guidelines offered in 11.11, Clinical and Technical Terms.

The article *the* is often used with abbreviated forms of agencies and organizations (eg, the UN, the AMA, the WHO); however, an article is not necessary with forms pronounced as words (eg, HCFA [hik-fuh], NASA [nas-ah], OSHA [oh-shuh]).

The following are associations and organizations commonly cited in AMA publications. This list is intended to show examples and is not all-inclusive. Because there are other expansions of some of the abbreviations, users should consider context before using them.

AAAAI
American Academy of Allergy, Asthma, and Immunology

AAAS
American Association for the Advancement of Science

AABB
American Association of Blood Banks

AACAP
American Academy of Child and Adolescent Psychiatry

AACC
American Association of Clinical Chemists

AACIA
American Association for Clinical Immunology and Allergy

AACCN
American Association of Critical Care Nurses

AACN
American Association of Colleges of Nursing

AAD
American Academy of Dermatology

AAFP
American Academy of Family Physicians

AAFPRS
American Academy of Facial Plastic and Reconstructive Surgery

AAHSLD
Association of Academic Health Science Library Directors

AAI
American Association of Immunologists

AAMC
Association of American Medical Colleges

AAMCH
American Association of Maternal and Child Health

AAN
American Academy of Neurology
American Academy of Neuropathologists
American Academy of Nursing

AANA
American Association of Nurse Anesthetists

AANP
American Academy of Nurse Practitioners

AANS
American Association of Neurological Surgeons

AAO
American Academy of Ophthalmology
American Association of Ophthalmology

AAOHNS
American Academy of Otolaryngology-Head and Neck Surgery

AAOS
American Academy of Orthopaedic Surgeons

AAP
American Academy of Pediatrics
American Association of Pathologists

AAPHP
American Association of Public Health Physicians

AAPM
American Academy of Pain Medicine
American Association of Physicists in Medicine

AAPMR
American Academy of Physical Medicine and Rehabilitation

AAPS
American Association of Plastic Surgeons

AARP
American Association of Retired Persons

AATM
American Academy of Tropical Medicine

AATS
American Association for Thoracic Surgery

AAUP
American Association of University Professors

AAWR
American Association for Women Radiologists

ABA
American Bar Association

ACA
American College of Allergists
American College of Anesthetists

ACAAI
American College of Allergy, Asthma, and Immunology

ACC
American College of Cardiology

ACCP
American College of Chest Physicians

ACEP
American College of Emergency Physicians

ACG
American College of Gastroenterology

ACHA
American College Health Association

ACHE
American College of Hospital Executives

ACIP
Advisory Committee on Immunization Practices

ACLM
American College of Legal Medicine

ACMQ
American College of Medical Quality

ACNM
American College of Nuclear Medicine
American College of Nurse-Midwives

ACNP
American College of Nuclear Physicians

ACOEM
American College of Occupational and Environmental Medicine

ACOG
American College of Obstetricians and Gynecologists

ACP
American College of Physicians

ACPE
American College of Physician Executives

ACPM
American College of Preventive Medicine

ACR
American College of Radiology
American College of Rheumatology

ACS
American Cancer Society
American College of Surgeons

ACSM
American College of Sports Medicine

ADA
American Dental Association
American Dermatological Association
American Diabetes Association
American Dietetic Association

ADRDA
Alzheimer's Disease and Related Disorders Association

AES
American Epilepsy Society

AFAR
American Federation for Aging Research

AFCR
American Federation for Clinical Research

AFIP
Armed Forces Institute of Pathology

AFS
American Fertility Society

AGA
American Gastroenterological Association

AGPA
American Group Practice Association

AGS
American Geriatrics Society

AHA
American Heart Association
American Hospital Association

AHCPR
Agency for Health Care Policy and Research

AHRA
American Healthcare Radiology Administrators

AJCC
American Joint Committee on Cancer

ALA
American Library Association
American Lung Association

ALROS
American Laryngological, Rhinological and Otological Society

AMA
Aerospace Medical Association
American Management Association
American Medical Association
Australian Medical Association

AMDA
American Medical Directors Association

AMPA
American Medical Publishers' Association

AMSA
American Medical Student Association

AMSUS
Association of Military Surgeons of the United States

AMWA
American Medical Women's Association
American Medical Writers Association

ANA
American Neurological Association
American Nurses Association

ANSI
American National Standards Institute

AOA
Alpha Omega Alpha
American Orthopedic Association
American Osteopathic Association

AOMA
American Occupational Medicine Association

AONE
American Organization of Nurse Executives

AORN
Association of Operating Room Nurses

AOS
American Otological Society

AOWHN
American Organization of Women's Health Nurses

APA
Ambulatory Pediatrics Association
American Pharmaceutical Association
American Psychiatric Association
American Psychological Association

APHA
American Public Health Association

APM
Academy of Physical Medicine

APS
American Psychological Society

ARA
American Rheumatism Association

ARC
American Red Cross

ARENA
Applied Research Ethics National Association

ARRS
American Roentgen Ray Society

ARVO
Association for Research in Vision and Ophthalmology

ASA
American Society of Anesthesiologists

ASAM
American Society of Addiction Medicine

ASCN
American Society of Clinical Nutrition

ASCO
American Society of Clinical Oncology
American Society of Clinical Ophthalmology

ASCP
American Society of Clinical Pathologists
American Society of Consultant Pharmacists

ASCPT
American Society of Clinical Pharmacology and Therapeutics

ASCRS
American Society of Cataract and Refractive Surgery
American Society of Colon and Rectal Surgeons

ASDR
American Society of Diagnostic Radiology

ASDS
American Society for Dermatologic Surgery

ASG
American Society for Genetics

ASGE
American Society for Gastrointestinal Endoscopy

ASHG
American Society of Human Genetics

ASIM
American Society of Internal Medicine

ASLME
American Society of Law, Medicine and Ethics

ASM
American Society for Microbiology

ASMT
American Society of Medical Technologists

ASPRS
American Society of Plastic and Reconstructive Surgeons

ASTHO
Association of State and Territorial Health Officers

ASTMH
American Society of Tropical Medicine and Hygiene

ASTRO
American Society for Therapeutic Radiology and Oncology

ASTS
American Society of Transplant Surgeons

ATA
American Thyroid Association

ATS
American Thoracic Society

AUA
American Urological Association

BELS
Board of Editors in the Life Sciences

BMA
British Medical Association

CAP
College of American Pathologists

CBE
Council of Biology Editors

CDC
Centers for Disease Control and Prevention

CMA
Canadian Medical Association

CNS
Child Neurology Society

DHHS
Department of Health and Human Services

EASE
European Association of Science Editors

EEOC
Equal Employment Opportunity Commission

EIS
Epidemic Intelligence Service
(Centers for Disease Control and Prevention)

EPA
Environmental Protection Agency

FASEB
Federation of American Societies for Experimental Biology

FCC
Federal Communications Commission

FDA
Food and Drug Administration

FTC
Federal Trade Commission

GLMA
Gay and Lesbian Medical Association

HCFA
Health Care Financing Administration

IARC
International Agency for Research on Cancer

ICMJE
International Committee of Medical Journal Editors

ICN
International Council of Nurses

ICRC
International Committee of the Red Cross

ICS
International College of Surgeons

IEEE
Institute of Electrical and Electronics Engineers

IOM
Institute of Medicine

IPPNW
International Physicians for the Prevention of Nuclear War

ISBT
International Society of Blood Transfusion

ISO
International Standards Organization

MLA
Medical Library Association

MRC
Medical Research Council (United Kingdom)

MSF
Médecins Sans Frontières

NAME
National Association of Medical Examiners

NAS
National Academy of Sciences

NASA
National Aeronautics and Space Administration

NCHS
National Center for Health Statistics

NCI
National Cancer Institute

NCRR
National Center for Research Resources

NEI
National Eye Institute

NHGRI
National Human Genome Research Institute

NHLBI
National Heart, Lung, and Blood Institute

NIA
National Institute on Aging

NIAAA
National Institute on Alcohol Abuse and Alcoholism

NIAID
National Institute of Allergy and Infectious Diseases

NIAMSD
National Institute of Arthritis and Musculoskeletal and Skin Diseases

NICHD
National Institute of Child Health and Human Development

NIDA
National Institute on Drug Abuse

NIDCD
National Institute on Deafness and Other Communication Disorders

NIDDK
National Institute of Diabetes and Digestive and Kidney Diseases

NIDR
National Institute of Dental Research

NIEHS
National Institute of Environmental Health Sciences

NIGMS
National Institute of General Medical Sciences

NIH
National Institutes of Health

NIMH
National Institute of Mental Health

NINDS
National Institute of Neurological Disorders and Stroke

NINR
National Institute of Nursing Research

NIOSH
National Institute for Occupational Safety and Health

NISO
National Information Standards Organization

NLM
National Library of Medicine

NLN
National League for Nursing

NMA
National Medical Association

NMHA
National Mental Health Association

NRC
National Research Council
Nuclear Regulatory Commission

NSF
National Science Foundation

NSPB
National Society for the Prevention of Blindness

OMAR
Office of Medical Applications of Research

ONS
Oncology Nursing Society

OPRR
Office for Protection From Research Risks

ORI
Office of Research Integrity

ORWH
Office of Research on Women's Health

OSHA
Occupational Safety and Health Administration

PAHO
Pan American Health Organization

PHR
Physicians for Human Rights

PHS
Public Health Service

PMA
Pharmaceutical Research and Manufacturers of America

PPRC
Physician Payment Review Commission

PSR
Physicians for Social Responsibility

PSRO
Professional Standards Review Organization

RERF
Radiation Effects Research Foundation

RPB
Research to Prevent Blindness

RSNA
Radiological Society of North America
Rehabilitation Society of North America

SAMBA
Society for Ambulatory Anesthesia

SAMHSA
Substance Abuse and Mental Health Services Administration

SCCM
Society of Critical Care Medicine

SID
Society for Investigative Dermatology

SMA
Southern Medical Association

SMCAF
Society of Medical Consultants to the Armed Forces

SNM
Society of Nuclear Medicine

SSA
Social Security Administration

SSO
Society of Surgical Oncology

SSP
Society for Scholarly Publishing

STS
Society of Thoracic Surgeons

UICC
Union Internationale Contre le Cancer

UN
United Nations

UNHCR
United Nations High Commissioner for Refugees

UNICEF
United Nations Children's Fund

UNOS
United Network for Organ Sharing

USAN
United States Adopted Names [Council]

VA
Department of Veterans Affairs

WAME
World Association of Medical Editors

WFP
World Food Program

WHO
World Health Organization

WMA
World Medical Association

For more detailed listings of US and international agencies and associations, consult the current editions of *The Official American Board of Medical Specialties (ABMS) Directory of Board Certified Medical Specialists, The United States Government Manual, Federal Yellow Book, Congressional Yellow Book, Encyclopedia of Associations, Directory of European Medical Organisations, Directory of European Professional & Learned Societies, Civil Service Yearbook, The Medical Registry,* and *The World of Learning.*

11.9 ■ **COLLABORATIVE GROUPS.**—Collaborative groups usually include study groups, multicenter trials, task forces, expert and ad hoc consensus groups, and periodic national and international health surveys. Such an entity's full name should be provided in addition to its abbreviation, even if it appears only once in a manuscript. Because some of these groups are often better recognized by their acronyms than by their full names, the acronym can be placed first, with the *expansion* in parentheses, contrary to the order usually recommended.

To save space in titles, however, the acronym may be used alone if its expansion is provided early in the manuscript, for example, in the abstract and in the text. Alternatively, the acronym might be given in the manuscript's title and the expansion in its subtitle; or, if space permits and both the expansion and the acronym convey separate and essential concepts, both could be given in the title or subtitle. The collaborative group name may be used as the byline (see also 3.1.6, Ethical and Legal Considerations, Group and Collaborative Authorship, 2.2, Manuscript Preparation, Bylines and End-of-Text Signatures, and 2.10, Manuscript Preparation, Acknowledgments).

Example:

(Title) Value of the Ventilation/Perfusion Scan
in Acute Pulmonary Embolism

(Subtitle) Results of the Prospective Investigation
of Pulmonary Embolism Diagnosis (PIOPED)

(Byline) The PIOPED Investigators

Consider the manuscript's context and audience, database searches, and ease of comprehension when choosing the form in which collaborative group information is presented. Remember that many literature databases contain only the title and article citation; some, but not all, also provide the abstract.

11.10 ■ **NAMES OF JOURNALS.**—In reference listings, abbreviate names of journals according to the US National Library of Medicine's current *Index Medicus.* Journal names are italicized. In references, the abbreviations are followed by a period, which denotes the close of the title group of bibliographic elements (see also 2.12.13, Manuscript Preparation, Names of Journals).

The following commonly referenced journals and their abbreviations are indexed in *Abridged Index Medicus* (in this list, the article *The* has been omitted in the expanded journal titles, as in *The Journal of . . .*). Single-word journal titles are not abbreviated.[3,4]

Academic Medicine (formerly *Journal of Medical Education,* abbreviated *J Med Educ*)
Acad Med

AJR: American Journal of Roentgenology
AJR Am J Roentgenol

American Family Physician
Am Fam Physician

American Heart Journal
Am Heart J

American Journal of Cardiology
Am J Cardiol

American Journal of Clinical Nutrition
Am J Clin Nutr

American Journal of Clinical Pathology
Am J Clin Pathol

American Journal of the Medical Sciences
Am J Med Sci

American Journal of Medicine
Am J Med

American Journal of Nursing
Am J Nurs

American Journal of Obstetrics and Gynecology
Am J Obstet Gynecol

American Journal of Ophthalmology
Am J Ophthalmol

American Journal of Pathology
Am J Pathol

American Journal of Physical Medicine and Rehabilitation
Am J Phys Med Rehabil

American Journal of Psychiatry
Am J Psychiatry

American Journal of Public Health
Am J Public Health

American Journal of Respiratory and Critical Care Medicine
Am J Respir Crit Care Med

American Journal of Surgery
Am J Surg

American Journal of Tropical Medicine and Hygiene
Am J Trop Med Hyg

Anaesthesia
Anaesthesia

Anesthesia and Analgesia
Anesth Analg

Anesthesiology
Anesthesiology

Annals of Emergency Medicine
Ann Emerg Med

Annals of Internal Medicine
Ann Intern Med

Annals of Otology, Rhinology, and Laryngology
Ann Otol Rhinol Laryngol

Annals of Surgery
Ann Surg

Annals of Thoracic Surgery
Ann Thorac Surg

Archives of Dermatology
Arch Dermatol

Archives of Disease in Childhood
Arch Dis Child

Archives of Disease in Childhood. Fetal and Neonatal Edition
Arch Dis Child Fetal Neonatal Ed

Archives of Environmental Health
Arch Environ Health

Archives of Family Medicine
Arch Fam Med

Archives of General Psychiatry
Arch Gen Psychiatry

Archives of Internal Medicine
Arch Intern Med

Archives of Neurology
Arch Neurol

Archives of Ophthalmology
Arch Ophthalmol

Archives of Otolaryngology-Head & Neck Surgery
Arch Otolaryngol Head Neck Surg

Archives of Pathology & Laboratory Medicine
Arch Pathol Lab Med

Archives of Pediatrics & Adolescent Medicine (formerly *American Journal of Diseases of Children*, abbreviated *Am J Dis Child* [abbreviated *AJDC* in AMA journals])
Arch Pediatr Adolesc Med

Archives of Physical Medicine and Rehabilitation
Arch Phys Med Rehabil

Archives of Surgery
Arch Surg

Arthritis and Rheumatism
Arthritis Rheum

Blood
Blood

BMJ (formerly *British Medical Journal*, abbreviated *Br Med J*)
BMJ

Brain
Brain

British Journal of Obstetrics and Gynaecology
Br J Obstet Gynaecol

British Journal of Radiology
Br J Radiol

British Journal of Rheumatology
Br J Rheumatol

British Journal of Surgery
Br J Surg

CA: A Cancer Journal for Clinicians
CA Cancer J Clin

Canadian Medical Association Journal
Can Med Assoc J

Cancer
Cancer

Chest
Chest

Circulation-Journal of the American Heart Association (formerly *Circulation*)
Circ J Am Heart Assoc

Clinical Orthopaedics and Related Research
Clin Orthop

Clinical Pediatrics
Clin Pediatr (Phila)

Clinical Pharmacology and Therapeutics
Clin Pharmacol Ther

Critical Care Medicine
Crit Care Med

Current Problems in Surgery
Curr Probl Surg

Diabetes
Diabetes

Digestive Diseases and Sciences
Dig Dis Sci

Disease-a-Month
Dis Mon

Endocrinology
Endocrinology

Gastroenterology
Gastroenterology

Geriatrics
Geriatrics

Gut
Gut

Heart (formerly *British Heart Journal,* abbreviated *Br Heart J*)
Heart

Heart and Lung
Heart Lung

Hospital Practice (Office Edition)
Hosp Pract (Off Ed)

Hospitals and Health Networks (formerly *Hospitals*)
Hosp Health Netw

Journal of Allergy and Clinical Immunology
J Allergy Clin Immunol

Journal of the American College of Cardiology
J Am Coll Cardiol

Journal of the American College of Surgeons (formerly *Surgery, Gynecology & Obstetrics,* abbreviated *Surg Gynecol Obstet*)
J Am Coll Surg

Journal of the American Dental Association
J Am Dent Assoc

Journal of the American Dietetic Association
J Am Diet Assoc

Journal of the American Medical Association
JAMA

Journal of Bone and Joint Surgery. American Volume
J Bone Joint Surg Am

Journal of Bone and Joint Surgery. British Volume
J Bone Joint Surg Br

Journal of Clinical Endocrinology and Metabolism
J Clin Endocrinol Metab

Journal of Clinical Investigation
J Clin Invest

Journal of Clinical Pathology
J Clin Pathol

Journal of Family Practice
J Fam Pract

Journals of Gerontology. Series A, Biological Sciences and Medical Sciences
J Gerontol A Biol Sci Med Sci

Journals of Gerontology. Series B, Psychological Sciences and Social Sciences
J Gerontol B Psychol Sci Soc Sci

Journal of Immunology
J Immunol

Journal of Infectious Diseases
J Infect Dis

Journal of Laboratory and Clinical Medicine
J Lab Clin Med

Journal of Laryngology and Otology
J Laryngol Otol

Journal of the National Cancer Institute
J Natl Cancer Inst

Journal of Nervous and Mental Disease
J Nerv Ment Dis

Journal of Neurosurgery
J Neurosurg

Journal of Nursing Administration
J Nurs Adm

Journal of Oral and Maxillofacial Surgery
J Oral Maxillofac Surg

Journal of Pediatrics
J Pediatr

Journal of Thoracic and Cardiovascular Surgery
J Thorac Cardiovasc Surg

Journal of Toxicology. Clinical Toxicology
J Toxicol Clin Toxicol

Journal of Trauma
J Trauma

Journal of Urology
J Urol

Lancet
Lancet

Mayo Clinic Proceedings
Mayo Clin Proc

Medical Clinics of North America
Med Clin North Am

Medical Letter on Drugs and Therapeutics
Med Lett Drugs Ther

Medicine
Medicine (Baltimore)

MMWR Morbidity and Mortality Weekly Report
MMWR Morb Mortal Wkly Rep

Neurology
Neurology

New England Journal of Medicine
N Engl J Med

Nursing Clinics of North America
Nurs Clin North Am

Nursing Outlook
Nurs Outlook

Nursing Research
Nurs Res

Obstetrics & Gynecology
Obstet Gynecol

Orthopedic Clinics of North America
Orthop Clin North Am

Pediatric Clinics of North America
Pediatr Clin North Am

Pediatrics
Pediatrics

Physical Therapy
Phys Ther

Plastic and Reconstructive Surgery
Plast Reconstr Surg

Postgraduate Medicine
Postgrad Med

Proceedings of the National Academy of Sciences of the United States of America
Proc Natl Acad Sci U S A

Progress in Cardiovascular Diseases
Prog Cardiovasc Dis

Public Health Reports
Public Health Rep

Radiologic Clinics of North America
Radiol Clin North Am

Radiology
Radiology

Southern Medical Journal
South Med J

Surgery
Surgery

Surgical Clinics of North America
Surg Clin North Am

Urologic Clinics of North America
Urol Clin North Am

Western Journal of Medicine
West J Med

The National Library of Medicine's abbreviations used in *Index Medicus* are based on the *American National Standard for Information Sciences—Abbreviation of Titles of Publications* (ANSI Z39.5) (1985), as well as abbreviations formulated under earlier ANSI guidelines. Use the following guide to abbreviate or not abbreviate words that may appear in journal titles. (Single-word journal titles are not abbreviated.) These words are capitalized, and articles, conjunctions, prepositions, punctuation, and diacritical marks are omitted in the abbreviated title form.

The correct abbreviations of journal titles indexed in MEDLINE can also be located through Grateful Med access (see also 22.3, Resources, Online Resources).

Word	*Abbreviation or Word Used*
Abnormal	Abnorm
Abuse	Abuse
Academia	Acad
Academy	Acad

Word	*Abbreviation or Word Used*
Acoustical	Acoust
Actions	Actions
Acupuncture	Acupunct
Acute	Acute
Addiction	Addict
Addictions	Addict
Additives	Addit
Administration	Adm
Adolescence	Adolescence
Adolescent	Adolesc
Advanced	Adv
Advancement	Adv
Advances	Adv
Adverse	Adverse
Aesthetic	Aesthetic
Affairs	Aff
Affective	Affective
African	Afr
Age	Age
Ageing	Ageing
Agents	Agents
Aging	Aging
Air	Air
Alabama	Ala
Alaska	Alaska
Alcohol	Alcohol
Alcoholism	Alcohol
Allergy	Allergy
Allied	Allied
America	Am
American	Am
Anaesthesia	Anaesth
Anaesthetists	Anaesth
Analgesia	Analg
Anatomical	Anat
Anatomy	Anat
Andrology	Androl
Anesthesia	Anesth
Anesthesiology	Anesthesiol
Angiology	Angiol
Angle	Angle
Animal	Anim
Ankle	Ankle
Annals	Ann
Annual	Annu
Anthropology	Anthropol
Antibiotics	Antibiot
Anticancer	Anticancer
Antigens	Antigens
Antimicrobial	Antimicrob
Antiviral	Antiviral
Apheresis	Apheresis
Appetite	Appetite
Applied	Appl
Archives	Arch

Word	*Abbreviation or Word Used*
Argentina	Argent
Arizona	Ariz
Arkansas	Ark
Army	Army
Arteriosclerosis	Arterioscl
Artery	Artery
Arthritis	Arthritis
Artificial	Artif
Asian	Asian
Assessment	Assess
Association	Assoc
Asthma	Asthma
Audiovisual	Audiov
Auditory	Aud
Australia	Aust
Australian	Aust
Autism	Autism
Autonomic	Auton
Avian	Avian
Aviation	Aviat
Bacteriology	Bacteriol
Bangladesh	Bangladesh
Basic	Basic
Behavior	Behav
Behavioral	Behav
Behaviors	Behav
Biochemical	Biochem
Biochemistry	Biochem
Biocommunications	Biocomm
Biofeedback	Biofeedback
Biological	Biol
Biology	Biol
Biomaterials	Biomater
Biomechanical	Biomech
Biomedical	Biomed
Biometrics	Biometrics
Biophysical	Biophys
Biophysics	Biophys
Bioscience	Biosci
Biosocial	Biosoc
Biosystems	Biosystems
Biotechnological	Biotechnol
Biotechnology	Biotechnol
Birth	Birth
Blood	Blood
Bone	Bone
Brain	Brain
Brazilian	Braz
Breast	Breast
British	Br
Bulletin	Bull
Burns	Burns
Calcified	Calcif
Calcium	Calcium
Canadian	Can

Word	*Abbreviation or Word Used*
Cancer	Cancer
Carbohydrate	Carbohydr
Carcinogenesis	Carcinog
Carcinogenic	Carcinog
Cardiography	Cardiogr
Cardiology	Cardiol
Cardiovascular	Cardiovasc
Care	Care
Caries	Caries
Catheterization	Cathet
Cell	Cell
Cells	Cells
Cellular	Cell
Central	Cent
Cephalalgia	Cephalalgia
Cerebral	Cereb
Ceylon	Ceylon
Chemical	Chem
Chemicals	Chem
Chemistry	Chem
Chemists	Chem
Chemotherapy	Chemother
Chest	Chest
Child	Child
Childhood	Child
Children	Child
Childs	Childs
Chinese	Chin
Chromatographic	Chromatogr
Chromatography	Chromatogr
Chronic	Chronic
Chronicle	Chron
Circulation	Circ
Circulatory	Circ
Cleft	Cleft
Cleveland	Cleve
Clinic	Clin
Clinical	Clin
Clinics	Clin
Cognition	Cogn
Collagen	Coll
College	Coll
Colon	Colon
Colorado	Colo
Communicable	Commun
Communication	Commun
Communications	Commun
Community	Community
Comparative	Comp
Complement	Complement
Comprehensive	Compr
Computerized	Comput
Computers	Comput
Connecticut	Conn
Connective	Connect

Word	*Abbreviation or Word Used*
Consulting	Consult
Contact	Contact
Contaminants	Contam
Contamination	Contam
Contemporary	Contemp
Contributions	Contrib
Control	Control
Controlled	Control
Copenhagen	Copenh
Cornea	Cornea
Cornell	Cornell
Corps	Corps
Cortex	Cortex
Council	Counc
Craniofacial	Craniofac
Critical	Crit
Cryobiology	Cryobiol
Culture	Cult
Current	Curr
Currents	Curr
Cutaneous	Cutan
Cutis	Cutis
Cybernetics	Cybern
Cyclic	Cyclic
Cytogenetics	Cytogenet
Cytology	Cytol
Cytometry	Cytometry
Dairy	Dairy
Danish	Dan
Deaf	Deaf
Decision	Decis
Defects	Defects
Deficiency	Defic
Delivery	Deliv
Demography	Demogr
Dental	Dent
Dentistry	Dent
Dependencies	Dependencies
Dermatitis	Dermatitis
Dermatological	Dermatol
Dermatology	Dermatol
Dermatopathology	Dermatopathol
Detection	Detect
Development	Dev
Devices	Devices
Diabetes	Diabetes
Diagnosis	Diagn
Diagnostic	Diagn
Dialysis	Dial
Diarrhoeal	Diarrhoeal
Dietetic	Diet
Differentiation	Differ
Digestion	Digestion
Digestive	Dig
Dimensions	Dimens

Word	*Abbreviation or Word Used*
Directions	Dir
Directors	Dir
Discussions	Discuss
Disease	Dis
Diseases	Dis
Disorders	Disord
Disposition	Dispos
DNA	DNA
Drug	Drug
Drugs	Drugs
Ear	Ear
Early	Early
East African	East Afr
Economic	Econ
Ecotoxicology	Ecotoxicol
Educational	Educ
Egyptian	Egypt
Electrocardiology	Electrocardiol
Electroencephalography	Electroencephalogr
Electromyography	Electromyogr
Electron	Electron
Electrotherapeutics	Electrother
Embryo	Embryo
Embryology	Embryol
Emergency	Emerg
Endocrine	Endocr
Endocrinological	Endocrinol
Endocrinology	Endocrinol
Endoscopy	Endosc
Engineering	Eng
Enteral	Enteral
Entomology	Entomol
Environmental	Environ
Enzyme	Enzyme
Enzymology	Enzymol
Epidemiologic	Epidemiol
Epidemiology	Epidemiol
Ergology	Ergol
Ergonomics	Ergonomics
Essays	Essays
Ethics	Ethics
Eugenics	Eugen
European	Eur
Evaluation	Eval
Exceptional	Except
Exercise	Exerc
Experimental	Exp
Eye	Eye
Factors	Factors
Family	Fam
Federation	Fed
Fertility	Fertil
Finnish	Finn
Fitness	Fitness
Florida	Fla

Word	*Abbreviation or Word Used*
Food	Food
Foot	Foot
Forensic	Forensic
Foundation	Found
Function	Funct
Fundamental	Fundam
Gastroenterology	Gastroenterol
Gastrointestinal	Gastrointest
Gene	Gene
General	Gen
Genetic	Genet
Genetics	Genetics
Genitourinary	Genitourin
Geographical	Geogr
Georgia	Ga
Geriatric	Geriatr
Geriatrics	Geriatr
Gerontologist	Gerontologist
Gerontology	Gerontol
Group	Group
Groups	Groups
Growth	Growth
Gut	Gut
Gynaecological	Gynaecol
Gynaecology	Gynaecol
Gynecologic	Gynecol
Gynecology	Gynecol
Haematology	Haematol
Haemostasis	Haemost
Hastings Center	Hastings Cent
Hawaii	Hawaii
Head	Head
Headache	Headache
Health	Health
Hearing	Hear
Heart	Heart
Hematological	Hematol
Hematology	Hematol
Hemoglobin	Hemoglobin
Hemostasis	Hemost
Hepatology	Hepatol
Heredity	Hered
Hip	Hip
Histochemical	Histochem
Histochemistry	Histochem
Histology	Histol
Histopathology	Histopathol
History	Hist
Homosexuality	Homosex
Horizons	Horiz
Hormone	Horm
Hormones	Horm
Hospital	Hosp
Hospitals	Hospitals
Human	Hum

Word	*Abbreviation or Word Used*
Humans	Hum
Hybridoma	Hybridoma
Hygiene	Hyg
Hypertension	Hypertens
Hypnosis	Hypn
Hypotheses	Hypotheses
Imaging	Imaging
Immunity	Immun
Immunoassay	Immunoassay
Immunobiology	Immunobiol
Immunogenetics	Immunogenet
Immunological	Immunol
Immunology	Immunol
Immunopharmacology	Immunopharmacol
Immunotherapy	Immunother
Implant	Implant
Including	Incl
India	India
Indian	Indian
Indiana	Indiana
Industrial	Ind
Infection	Infect
Infectious	Infect
Inflammation	Inflamm
Informatics	Inf
Inherited	Inherited
Injury	Inj
Inorganic	Inorg
Inquiry	Inquiry
Institutes	Inst
Instrumentation	Instrum
Insurance	Insur
Intellectual	Intellect
Intelligence	Intell
Intensive	Intensive
Interactions	Interact
Interferon	Interferon
Internal	Intern
International	Int
Internist	Internist
Interventional	Intervent
Intervirology	Intervirol
Intraocular	Intraocul
Invasion	Invasion
Invertebrate	Invertebr
Investigation	Invest
Investigational	Investig
Investigations	Invest
Investigative	Invest
Iowa	Iowa
Irish	Ir
Isotopes	Isot
Isozymes	Isozymes
Israel	Isr
Issues	Issues

Word	*Abbreviation or Word Used*
Istanbul	Istanbul
Japanese	Jpn
Joint	Joint
Journal	J
Kansas	Kans
Kentucky	Ky
Kidney	Kidney
Kinetics	Kinet
Laboratory	Lab
Language	Lang
Laparoendoscopic	Laparoendosc
Laryngology	Laryngol
Larynx	Larynx
Lasers	Lasers
Law	Law
Lectures	Lect
Legal	Leg
Leprosy	Lepr
Letters	Lett
Leukocyte	Leukoc
Leukotriene	Leukotriene
Leukotrienes	Leukotrienes
Library	Libr
Life	Life
Life-threatening	Life Threat
Lipid	Lipid
Lipids	Lipids
Literature	Lit
Louisiana	La
Lung	Lung
Lymphokine	Lymphokine
Lymphology	Lymphol
Madagascar	Madagascar
Magnesium	Magnesium
Magnetic	Magn
Main	Main
Making	Making
Malaysia	Malaysia
Management	Manage
Manipulative	Manipulative
Marital	Marital
Maritime	Marit
Maryland	Md
Mass	Mass
Mathematical	Math
Maxillofacial	Maxillofac
Measurement	Meas
Mechanisms	Mech
Media	Media
Medical	Med
Medicinal	Med
Medicine	Med
Membrane	Membr
Mental	Ment
Metabolic	Metab

Word	*Abbreviation or Word Used*
Metabolism	Metab
Metastasis	Metastasis
Methods	Methods
Mexico	Mex
Michigan	Mich
Microbial	Microb
Microbiological	Microbiol
Microbiology	Microbiol
Microcirculation	Microcirc
Microscopy	Microsc
Microvascular	Microvasc
Microwave	Microw
Military	Milit
Mineral	Miner
Minnesota	Minn
Mississippi	Miss
Missouri	Mo
Modification	Modif
Molecular	Mol
Monographs	Monogr
Morphology	Morphol
Motility	Motil
Muscle	Muscle
Mutagenesis	Mutagen
Mutation	Mutat
Mycobacterial	Mycobact
Narcotics	Narc
National	Natl
Natural	Nat
Nature	Nat
Naval	Nav
Nebraska	Nebr
Neck	Neck
Neglect	Negl
Neonate	Neonate
Nephrology	Nephrol
Nephron	Nephron
Nervosa	Nerv
Nervous	Nerv
Netherlands	Neth
Neural	Neural
Neurobehavioral	Neurobehav
Neurobiology	Neurobiol
Neurochemistry	Neurochem
Neurocytology	Neurocytol
Neuroendocrinology	Neuroendocrinol
Neurogenetics	Neurogenet
Neuroimmunology	Neuroimmunol
Neurologic	Neurol
Neurological	Neurol
Neurology	Neurol
Neuropathology	Neuropathol
Neuropediatrics	Neuropediatr
Neuropeptides	Neuropeptides
Neuropharmacology	Neuropharmacol

Word	*Abbreviation or Word Used*
Neurophysiology	Neurophysiol
Neuropsychobiology	Neuropsychobiol
Neuropsychology	Neuropsychol
Neuropsychopharmacology	Neuropsychopharmacol
Neuroradiology	Neuroradiol
Neuroscience	Neurosci
Neurosurgery	Neurosurg
Neurosurgical	Neurosurg
Neurotoxicology	Neurotoxicol
Neurotrauma	Neurotrauma
New	N
New England	N Engl
New Jersey	N J
New Orleans	New Orleans
New York	N Y
New Zealand	N Z
North America	North Am
North Carolina	N C
Nose	Nose
Nuclear	Nucl
Nucleotide	Nucleotide
Nurse	Nurse
Nursing	Nurs
Nutrition	Nutr
Nutritional	Nutr
Obesity	Obes
Obstetric	Obstet
Obstetrics	Obstet
Occupational	Occup
Ocular	Ocul
Official	Off
Ohio	Ohio
Oklahoma	Okla
Oncology	Oncol
Ophthalmic	Ophthalmic
Ophthalmological	Ophthalmol
Ophthalmology	Ophthalmol
Optical	Opt
Optics	Opt
Optometric	Optom
Optometry	Optom
Oral	Oral
Organization	Organ
Organs	Organs
Orthodontics	Orthod
Orthodontist	Orthod
Orthopaedic	Orthop
Orthopsychiatry	Orthopsychiatry
Orthotics	Orthot
Osaka	Osaka
Oslo	Oslo
Osteopathic	Osteopath
Otolaryngology	Otolaryngol
Otology	Otol
Otorhinolaryngology	Otorhinolaryngol

Word	*Abbreviation or Word Used*
Pace	Pace
Paediatric	Paediatr
Paediatrics	Paediatr
Palate	Palate
Panama	Panama
Pan American	Pan Am
Paper	Pap
Papua New Guinea	Papua New Guinea
Parasite	Parasite
Parasitology	Parasitol
Parenteral	Parenter
Pathology	Pathol
Pediatrician	Pediatrician
Pediatrics	Pediatr
Pennsylvania	Pa
Peptide	Pept
Peptides	Pept
Perception	Perception
Perceptual	Percept
Perinatal	Perinat
Perinatology	Perinatol
Periodontal	Periodont
Periodontology	Periodontol
Personality	Pers
Perspectives	Perspect
Pharmaceutical	Pharm
Pharmacokinetics	Pharmacokinet
Pharmacology	Pharmacol
Pharmacopsychiatry	Pharmacopsychiatry
Pharmacotherapy	Pharmacother
Pharmacy	Pharm
Philosophical	Philos
Phosphorylation	Phosphorylation
Photobiology	Photobiol
Photochemistry	Photochem
Photodermatology	Photodermatol
Photography	Photogr
Physical	Phys
Physician	Physician
Physicians	Physicians
Physics	Phys
Physiological	Physiol
Physiology	Physiol
Placenta	Placenta
Planning	Plann
Plastic	Plast
Podiatric	Podiatr
Podiatry	Podiatry
Poisoning	Poisoning
Policy	Policy
Politics	Polit
Pollution	Pollut
Population	Popul
Postgraduate	Postgrad
Poultry	Poult

Word	*Abbreviation or Word Used*
Practice	Pract
Practitioners	Pract
Pregnancy	Pregnancy
Prenatal	Prenat
Preparative	Prep
Prevention	Prev
Preventive	Prev
Primary	Primary
Primatology	Primatol
Proceedings	Proc
Process	Process
Processes	Processes
Products	Prod
Programs	Programs
Progress	Prog
Prostaglandin	Prostaglandin
Prostaglandins	Prostaglandins
Prostate	Prostate
Prosthetic	Prosthet
Prosthetics	Prosthet
Protein	Protein
Protozoology	Protozool
Psyche	Psyche
Psychiatric	Psychiatr
Psychiatry	Psychiatry
Psychoactive	Psychoactive
Psychoanalysis	Psychoanal
Psychoanalytic	Psychoanal
Psycholinguistic	Psycholinguist
Psychologist	Psychol
Psychology	Psychol
Psychoneuroendocrinology	Psychoneuroendocrinol
Psychopathology	Psychopathol
Psychopharmacology	Psychopharmacol
Psychophysiology	Psychophysiol
Psychosocial	Psychosoc
Psychosomatic	Psychosom
Psychosomatics	Psychosom
Psychotherapy	Psychother
Public	Public
Puerto Rico	P R
Quantitative	Quant
Quarterly	Q
Radiation	Radiat
Radiography	Radiogr
Radioisotopes	Radioisotopes
Radiologists	Radiol
Radiology	Radiol
Rational	Ration
Reactions	React
Recombinant	Recomb
Reconstructive	Reconstr
Record	Rec
Rectum	Rectum
Regional	Reg

Word	*Abbreviation or Word Used*
Regulation	Regul
Regulatory	Regul
Rehabilitation	Rehabil
Renal	Renal
Report	Rep
Reports	Rep
Reproduction	Reprod
Reproductive	Reprod
Research	Res
Residue	Residue
Resonance	Reson
Respiration	Respir
Respiratory	Respir
Response	Response
Resuscitation	Resuscitation
Retardation	Retard
Retina	Retina
Review	Rev
Reviews	Rev
Rheumatic	Rheum
Rheumatism	Rheum
Rheumatology	Rheumatol
Rhinology	Rhinol
Rhode Island	R I
Safety	Safety
Scandinavian	Scand
Scanning	Scan
Schizophrenia	Schizophr
School	Sch
Science	Sci
Sciences	Sci
Scientific	Sci
Scottish	Scott
Security	Secur
Seminars	Semin
Series	Ser
Service	Serv
Sex	Sex
Sexual	Sex
Sexually	Sex
Shock	Shock
Singapore	Singapore
Skeletal	Skeletal
Sleep	Sleep
Social	Soc
Societies	Soc
Society	Soc
Sociological	Sociol
Sociology	Sociol
Somatic	Somatic
Somatosensory	Somatosens
South African	S Afr
South Carolina	S C
South Dakota	S D
Southeast	Southeast

Word	*Abbreviation or Word Used*
Southern	South
Space	Space
Spectrometry	Spectrom
Speech	Speech
Spine	Spine
Sports	Sports
Stain	Stain
Standardization	Stand
Standards	Stand
Statistical	Stat
Steroid	Steroid
Steroids	Steroids
Stockholm	Stockh
Strabismus	Strabismus
Stress	Stress
Stroke	Stroke
Structure	Struct
Studies	Stud
Subcellular	Subcell
Submicroscopic	Submicrosc
Substance	Subst
Suicide	Suicide
Superior	Super
Support	Support
Surgeon	Surg
Surgeons	Surg
Surgery	Surg
Surgical	Surg
Swedish	Swed
Symposia	Symp
Symposium	Symp
System	Syst
Systems	Syst
Technical	Tech
Technology	Technol
Tennessee	Tenn
Teratogenesis	Teratogenesis
Teratology	Teratol
Thailand	Thai
Theoretical	Theor
Therapeutics	Ther
Therapies	Ther
Therapy	Ther
Thermal	Therm
Thoracic	Thorac
Thorax	Thorax
Throat	Throat
Thrombosis	Thromb
Thromboxane	Thromboxane
Thymus	Thymus
Tissue	Tissue
Today	Today
Tokyo	Tokyo
Tomography	Tomogr
Topics	Top

Word	*Abbreviation or Word Used*
Total	Total
Toxicologic	Toxicol
Toxicological	Toxicol
Toxicology	Toxicol
Traditional	Tradit
Transactions	Trans
Transfer	Transfer
Transfusion	Transfusion
Transmission	Transm
Transmitted	Transm
Transplant	Transplant
Transplantation	Transplantation
Traumatic	Trauma
Tropical	Trop
Tuberculosis	Tuberc
Tumour	Tumour
Tunis	Tunis
Turkish	Turk
Ulster	Ulster
Ultramicroscopy	Ultramicrosc
Ultrasonic	Ultrason
Ultrasonics	Ultrasonics
Ultrasound	Ultrasound
Ultrastructural	Ultrastruct
Ultrastructure	Ultrastruct
Undersea	Undersea
Union	Union
Uremia	Uremia
Vision	Vis
Visual	Vis
Vital	Vital
Vitamin	Vitam
Vitaminology	Vitaminol
Vitamins	Vitam
Vitro	Vitro
Welfare	Welfare
Western	West
West Indian	West Indian
West Virginia	W Va
Wildlife	Wildl
Wisconsin	Wis
Women	Women
Women's	Womens
Yale	Yale
Zoology	Zool
Zoonoses	Zoonoses

11.11 ■ **CLINICAL AND TECHNICAL TERMS.**—This compilation of common clinical and technical terms and their abbreviations is not intended to be all-encompassing but is provided as an aid to the stylebook user. There are many published listings of abbreviations, acronyms, and initialisms[5-7]; see also 22.1, Resources, Readings.

Many terms share the same abbreviation (eg, EMS for emergency medical services, eosinophilia-myalgia syndrome, European Medical Society, electrical muscle stimulation, and Elvis Presley Memorial Society of Syracuse). Thus, context is an important consideration. In addition, some abbreviations encompass more than one grammatical variant (eg, noun, adjective) of a term. For example, *CT* represents both *computed tomography* and *computed tomographic*. Therefore, it is unnecessary to redefine the abbreviation for each variation in usage within a body of work. Similarly, terms that have singular and plural forms (eg, *RBC* and *RBCs*) are defined once for whichever form is mentioned first.

In cases in which the expanded form is possessive at first mention, the parenthetical abbreviation is also possessive at first mention (and vice versa):

> The American Medical Association's (AMA's) Council on Ethical and Judicial Affairs prepared a report that was later adopted as AMA policy.

The following terms should be expanded at first mention. (*But:* see note below.) Use common sense in deciding whether to abbreviate these and other terms. For example, if "toxic shock syndrome" appears only once or twice in an article, spell it out; if the article concerns toxic shock syndrome and the term is used several times (perhaps 5 or more times), expand the term at first mention with the abbreviation immediately following in parentheses. Abbreviate it thereafter.

Avoid using abbreviations at the beginning of a sentence unless the expansion is cumbersome, eg, a collaborative group name or other acronym pronounced as a word (PIOPED, AIDS, CLIA, HCFA) (see also 11.8, Agencies and Organizations, and 11.9, Collaborative Groups). Do not use an abbreviation as the sole term in a subheading. Also avoid introducing an abbreviation in a subheading:

> *Avoid*
> **Provider Reimbursement Review Board (PRRB)**
> In 1972, Congress established the PRRB to furnish providers with an impartial forum for resolving Medicare payment disputes arising from cost reports.
>
> *Preferred*
> **Provider Reimbursement Review Board**
> In 1972, Congress established the Provider Reimbursement Review Board (PRRB) to furnish providers with an impartial forum . . .

Apply the foregoing concepts to each element of the manuscript. See also 11.0, Abbreviations, and 2.0, Manuscript Preparation, as well as specific nomenclature sections (eg, 17.5, Statistics, Statistical Symbols and Abbreviations) for additional guidelines for correct use of specialized terms and their abbreviations. (See also 2.14, Manuscript Preparation, Figures, and 2.13, Manuscript Preparation, Tables.)

Note: Considerations for which this general rule might be set aside include comprehensibility, recognition, and space, as well as avoidance of cumbersome expressions. Exceptions include using the abbreviation instead of the expansion in a long title or subtitle, a letter to the editor, or an informal essay.

Some technical and subspecialty publications—with readers who are familiar with unusual abbreviations—by policy never expand certain abbreviations. Examples of these abbreviations are indicated with an asterisk in the following list.

Abbreviation	*Expanded Form*
ABC	avidin-biotin complex
AC	alternating current
ACE	angiotensin-converting enzyme
ACTH	Use *corticotropin* (previously adrenocorticotropic hormone).

*This abbreviation may be used without expansion.

Abbreviation	*Expanded Form*
ADHD	attention-deficit/hyperactivity disorder
ADH	antidiuretic hormone
ADL	activities of daily living (*but:* 1 ADL, 6 ADLs)
aDNA	ancient DNA
ADP	adenosine diphosphate
ADPase	adenosine diphosphatase
AFP	α-fetoprotein
AIDS	acquired immunodeficiency syndrome
ALL	acute lymphoblastic leukemia; acute lymphocytic leukemia
ALT	alanine aminotransferase (previously SGPT)
AML	acute monocytic leukemia; acute myeloblastic leukemia; acute myelocytic leukemia
AMP	adenosine monophosphate
ANA	antinuclear antibody
ANCOVA	analysis of covariance
ANLL	acute nonlymphocytic leukemia
ANOVA	analysis of variance
APACHE	Acute Physiology and Chronic Health Evaluation
APB	atrial premature beat
ARC	AIDS-related complex (use *symptomatic HIV infection*)
ARDS	acute respiratory distress syndrome; adult respiratory distress syndrome
AST	aspartate aminotransferase (previously SGOT)
ATP	adenosine triphosphate
ATPase	adenosine triphosphatase
AUC	area under the curve
BCG	bacille Calmette-Guérin (*but:* do not expand as a drug: BCG vaccine)
BDI	Beck Depression Inventory
BMD	bone mineral density
BMI	body mass index
BMT	bone marrow transplantation
BP	blood pressure
BPD	bronchopulmonary dysplasia
BPH	benign prostatic hyperplasia
BPRS	Brief Psychiatric Rating Scale
BSA	body surface area
BSE	breast self-examination
BTPS	body temperature, pressure, saturated
BUN	blood urea nitrogen (use *serum urea nitrogen*)
C	complement (use with a number, eg, C1, C2, . . . C9; see 12.8.1, Nomenclature, Complement)
CA	contrast angiography
CABG	coronary artery bypass graft
CAD	coronary artery disease
cAMP	cyclic adenosine monophosphate
CARS	compensatory anti-inflammatory response syndrome
CBC	complete blood cell (add *count*)
CCU	cardiac care unit
CD*	clusters of differentiation (use with a number, eg, CD4 cell; see 12.8.4, Nomenclature, Lymphocytes)

**This abbreviation may be used without expansion.*

Abbreviation	*Expanded Form*
CD*	compact disc
cDNA	complementary DNA
CD-ROM*	compact disc read-only memory
CEA	carcinoembryonic antigen
CEU	continuing education unit
CFT	complement fixation test
CFU	colony-forming unit
cGMP	cyclic guanosine monophosphate
CHD	coronary heart disease
CHF	congestive heart failure
CI	confidence interval
CIN	cervical intraepithelial neoplasia
CL	confidence limit
CK	creatine kinase
CK-BB	creatine kinase-BB (BB designates the isozyme)
CK-MB	creatine kinase-MB
CK-MM	creatine kinase-MM
CME	continuing medical education (often used without expansion when describing credit hours, eg, category 1 CME credit)
CMV	cytomegalovirus
CNS	central nervous system
COPD	chronic obstructive pulmonary disease
CPK	Use *creatine kinase*.
CPR	cardiopulmonary resuscitation
CPT	*Current Procedural Terminology*
CQI	continuous quality improvement
CRF	corticotropin-releasing factor
cRNA	complementary RNA
CSF	cerebrospinal fluid; colony-stimulating factor
CT	computed tomographic; computed tomography
CVS	chorionic villus sampling
DALY	disability-adjusted life-year
dAMP	deoxyadenosine monophosphate (deoxyadenylate)
DCIS	ductal carcinoma in situ
D&C	dilation and curettage
DC	direct current
DDT*	dichlorodiphenyltrichloroethane (chlorophenothane)
DE	dose equivalent
DEV	duck embryo vaccine
dGMP	deoxyguanosine monophosphate (deoxyguanylate)
DIC	disseminated intravascular coagulation
DIF	direct immunofluorescence
DNA*	deoxyribonucleic acid
DNAR	do not attempt resuscitation
DNase	deoxyribonuclease
DNR	do not resuscitate
DOS*	disk operating system
DOT	directly observed therapy
DRD2	D_2 dopamine receptor [gene]
DRE	digital rectal examination
DRG	diagnosis related group
DS	duplex sonography

This abbreviation may be used without expansion.

Abbreviation	*Expanded Form*
DSM-III	*Diagnostic and Statistical Manual of Mental Disorders, Third Edition*
DSM-III-R	*Diagnostic and Statistical Manual of Mental Disorders, Revised Third Edition*
DSM-IV	*Diagnostic and Statistical Manual of Mental Disorders, Fourth Edition*
DTP	diphtheria and tetanus toxoids and pertussis [vaccine]
DXA	dual-energy x-ray absorptiometry
EBV	Epstein-Barr virus
EC	ejection click
ECA	epidemiologic catchment area
ECG	electrocardiogram; electrocardiographic
ECT	electroconvulsive therapy
ED	effective dose; emergency department
ED_{50}	median effective dose
EDTA*	ethylenediaminetetraacetic acid
EEE	eastern equine encephalomyelitis
EEG	electroencephalogram; electroencephalographic
EIA	enzyme immunoassay
ELISA	enzyme-linked immunosorbent assay
EM	electron microscope; electron microscopic; electron microscopy
EMG	electromyogram; electromyographic
EMIT	enzyme-multiplied immunoassay technique
EMS	electrical muscle stimulation; emergency medical services; eosinophilia-myalgia syndrome
ENG	electronystagmogram; electronystagmographic
EOG	electro-oculogram; electro-oculographic
ERCP	endoscopic retrograde cholangiopancreatography
ERG	electroretinogram; electroretinographic
ESR	erythrocyte sedimentation rate
ESRD	end-stage renal disease
ESWL	extracorporeal shock wave lithotripsy
EVR	evoked visual response
F*	French (add *catheter;* use only with a number, eg, 12F catheter)
$FEF_{25\%-75\%}$	forced expiratory flow, midexpiratory phase
FEV	forced expiratory volume
FEV_1	forced expiratory volume in 1 second; forced expiratory volume in the first second
F_{IO_2}	fraction of inspired oxygen
FISH	fluorescence in situ hybridization
FSH	follicle-stimulating hormone
FTA	fluorescent treponemal antibody
FTA-ABS	fluorescent treponemal antibody absorption (add *test*)
FUO	fever of unknown origin
FVC	forced vital capacity
GABA	γ-aminobutyric acid
GCS	Glasgow Coma Scale
GDP	guanosine diphosphate
GDS	Geriatric Depression Scale
GERD	gastroesophageal reflux disease
GFR	glomerular filtration rate

**This abbreviation may be used without expansion.*

Abbreviation	*Expanded Form*
GH	growth hormone
GI	gastrointestinal
GIFT	gamete intrafallopian transfer
GLC	gas-liquid chromatography
GMP	guanosine monophosphate (guanylate, guanylic acid)
GMT	geometric mean titer
GnRH	gonadotropin-releasing hormone (*gonadorelin* as diagnostic agent)
GUI	graphical user interface
HALE	health-adjusted life expectancy
Hb_{CO}	carboxyhemoglobin
HBO	hyperbaric oxygen
Hb_{O_2}	oxyhemoglobin; oxygenated hemoglobin
HbS	sickle cell hemoglobin
HBsAg	hepatitis B surface antigen (see 12.12.2, Nomenclature, Viruses)
HBV	hepatitis B virus
hCG	human chorionic gonadotropin (do not abbreviate when used as drug)
HCV	hepatitis C virus (see 12.12.2, Nomenclature, Viruses)
HDL	high-density lipoprotein
HDL-C	high-density lipoprotein cholesterol
HDRS	Hamilton Depression Rating Scale
hGH	human growth hormone
Hib	*Haemophilus influenzae* type b [vaccine or disease]
HIV	human immunodeficiency virus
HLA*	human leukocyte antigen (say "HLA antigen"; see 12.8.2, Nomenclature, The Human Leukocyte Antigen [HLA] System)
HMG-CoA	3-hydroxy-3-methylglutaryl coenzyme A
HMO	health maintenance organization
HPF	high-power field
HPLC	high-performance liquid chromatography; high-pressure liquid chromatography
HPV	human papillomavirus (add hyphen to abbreviation when indicating type, eg, HPV-6)
HRQOL	health-related quality of life
HSV	herpes simplex virus
5-HT	Use *serotonin* (also 5-hydroxytryptamine).
HTLV	human T-lymphotropic virus
IADL	instrumental activities of daily living (*but:* 1 IADL, 6 IADLs)
ICD-9	*International Classification of Diseases, Ninth Revision*
ICD-9-CM	*International Classification of Diseases, Ninth Revision, Clinical Modification*
ICD-10	*International Statistical Classification of Diseases, 10th Revision*
ICU	intensive care unit
ID	infective dose
IDDM	insulin-dependent diabetes mellitus
IDU	injecting drug user; injection drug user
Ig	immunoglobulin (abbreviate only with specification of class, eg, IgA, IgG, IgM; see 12.8.3, Nomenclature, Immunoglobulins)
IL	interleukin (abbreviate only when indicating a specific protein factor, eg, IL-2) (see 12.4.10, Nomenclature, Special Drug Categories, and 12.8.5, Nomenclature, Cytokines)

**This abbreviation may be used without expansion.*

Abbreviation	*Expanded Form*
IM	intramuscular; intramuscularly
IND	Investigational New Drug
INF	interferon (do not abbreviate as drug; see 12.4.10, Nomenclature, Special Drug Categories)
INR	international normalized ratio
IOP	intraocular pressure
IQ*	intelligence quotient
IRB	institutional review board
IRMA	immunoradiometric assay
ISBN*	International Standard Book Number
ISG	immune serum globulin
ISSN*	International Standard Serial Number
ITI	intratubal insemination
ITP	idiopathic thrombocytopenic purpura
IUD	intrauterine device
IUGR	intrauterine growth retardation
IUI	intrauterine insemination
IV	intravenous; intravenously
IVF	in vitro fertilization
IVP	intravenous pyelogram
KUB	kidneys, ureter, bladder [plain abdominal radiograph]
LA	left atrium
LAD	left anterior descending coronary artery
LAO	left anterior oblique coronary artery
LAV	lymphadenopathy-associated virus
LBW	low birth weight
LCA	left coronary artery
LCX, CX	left circumflex coronary artery
LD	lethal dose
LD_{50}	median lethal dose
LDH	lactate dehydrogenase
LDL	low-density lipoprotein
LDL-C	low-density lipoprotein cholesterol
LH	luteinizing hormone
LHRH	luteinizing hormone-releasing hormone (*gonadorelin* as diagnostic agent)
Lp(a)	lipoprotein(a)
LSD	lysergic acid diethylamide
LV	left ventricle; left ventricular
LVEDV	left ventricular end-diastolic volume
LVEF	left ventricular ejection fraction
LVOT	left ventricular outflow tract
*m-**	meta- (use only in chemical formulas or names)
MAOI	monoamine oxidase inhibitor
MBC	minimum bactericidal concentration
MCH	mean corpuscular hemoglobin
MCHC	mean corpuscular hemoglobin concentration
MCO	managed care organization
MCV	mean corpuscular volume
MD	muscular dystrophy
MDR	multidrug-resistant

**This abbreviation may be used without expansion.*

Abbreviation	*Expanded Form*
MEC	mean effective concentration
MEN	multiple endocrine neoplasia (do not add hyphen when specifying type, eg, multiple endocrine neoplasia type 2A [MEN 2A])
MeSH	Medical Subject Headings [vocabulary, terms, etc]
MET	metabolic equivalent
MHC	major histocompatibility complex
MI	myocardial infarction
MIC	minimum inhibitory concentration
MICU	medical intensive care unit
MMPI	Minnesota Multiphasic Personality Inventory
MMR	measles-mumps-rubella [vaccine]
MMSE	Mini-Mental State Examination
MODS	multiple-organ dysfunction syndrome
MPS	Mortality Probability Score
MRA	magnetic resonance angiography
MRI	magnetic resonance imaging
mRNA	messenger RNA
MS	multiple sclerosis
MSA	metropolitan statistical area
MSET	multistage exercise test
MVC	motor vehicle crash
NDA	New Drug Application
Nd:YAG*	neodymium:yttrium-aluminum-garnet [laser]
NEC	necrotizing enterocolitis
NF	*National Formulary*
NICU	neonatal intensive care unit
NIDDM	non-insulin-dependent diabetes mellitus (*but:* see 9.1, Correct and Preferred Usage, Commonly Misused Words and Phrases [diabetes mellitus])
NK	natural killer (add *cells*)
NNT	number needed to treat
NS	not significant
NSAID	nonsteroidal anti-inflammatory drug
o-*	ortho- (use only in chemical formulas)
OC	oral contraceptive
OD*	oculus dexter (right eye) (use only with a number)
OGTT	oral glucose tolerance test
OR	odds ratio
OS*	oculus sinister (left eye) (use only with a number)
OS	opening snap
OU*	oculus unitas (both eyes) or oculus uterque (each eye) (use only with a number)
p-*	para- (use only in chemical formulas or names)
PA	pulmonary artery
$Pa\textsc{co}_2$*	partial pressure of carbon dioxide, arterial
$Pa\textsc{o}_2$*	partial pressure of oxygen, arterial
$P\textsc{ao}_2$	partial pressure of oxygen in the alveoli
PAS	periodic acid-Schiff
$P\textsc{co}_2$*	partial pressure of carbon dioxide
PCP	*Pneumocystis carinii* pneumonia

This abbreviation may be used without expansion.

Abbreviation	*Expanded Form*
PCR	polymerase chain reaction
PCW	pulmonary capillary wedge [pressure]
PDA	patent ductus arteriosus
PEEP	positive end-expiratory pressure
PEG	percutaneous endoscopic gastrostomy; pneumoencephalographic; pneumoencephalography
PET	positron emission tomographic; positron emission tomography
pH*	hydrogen ion concentration; negative logarithm of hydrogen ion activity
PHO	physician hospital organization
PICC	peripherally inserted central catheter
PID	pelvic inflammatory disease
PKU	phenylketonuria
PMS	premenstrual syndrome
Po_2*	partial pressure of oxygen
PPD	purified protein derivative (tuberculin)
PPO	preferred provider organization
PRO	peer review organization; professional review organization
PSA	prostate-specific antigen
PSRO	professional standards review organization
PSVT	paroxysmal supraventricular tachycardia
PT	prothrombin time
PTCA	percutaneous transluminal coronary angioplasty
PTSD	posttraumatic stress disorder
PTT	partial thromboplastin time
PUVA	psoralen-UV-A
PVC	premature ventricular contraction
PVR	pulmonary vascular resistance
PVS	permanent vegetative state; persistent vegetative state
QA	quality assurance
QALY	quality-adjusted life-year
QC	quality control
QOL	quality of life
RA	rheumatoid arthritis
RAM*	random access memory
RAST	radioallergosorbent test
RBC	red blood cell
RBRVS	resource-based relative value scale
RCA	right coronary artery
RCT	randomized controlled trial
RDA	recommended daily allowance; recommended dietary allowance
RDC	Research Diagnostic Criteria
rDNA	recombinant DNA; ribosomal DNA
RDS	respiratory distress syndrome
REM	rapid eye movement
RFLP	restriction fragment length polymorphism
RIA	radioimmunoassay
RNA*	ribonucleic acid
ROC	receiver operating characteristic [curve]
ROM*	read-only memory
RPR	rapid plasma reagin

**This abbreviation may be used without expansion.*

Abbreviation	*Expanded Form*
RR	relative risk; risk ratio
RSV	respiratory syncytial virus
RV	right ventricle; right ventricular
RVEF	right ventricular ejection fraction
RVOT	right ventricular outflow tract
SAD	seasonal affective disorder
SADS	Schedule for Affective Disorders and Schizophrenia
SAPS	Simplified Acute Physiology Score
SCID	severe combined immunodeficiency
SD*	standard deviation
SE*	standard error
SEM*	standard error of the mean
SEM	scanning electron microscope; systolic ejection murmur
SGA	small for gestational age
SGOT	serum glutamic-oxaloacetic transaminase (use *aspartate aminotransferase*)
SGPT	serum glutamic-pyruvic transaminase (use *alanine aminotransferase*)
SIADH	syndrome of inappropriate secretion of antidiuretic hormone
SICU	surgical intensive care unit
SIDS	sudden infant death syndrome
SIP	Sickness Impact Profile
SIRS	systemic inflammatory response syndrome
SLE	St Louis encephalitis; systemic lupus erythematosus
sp g	specific gravity (use with a number, eg, sp g 13.6)
SSC*	standard saline citrate
SSPE*	sodium chloride, sodium phosphate, EDTA [buffer]
SSPE	subacute sclerosing panencephalitis
SSRI	selective serotonin reuptake inhibitor
STD	sexually transmitted disease
SUN	serum urea nitrogen
SVR	systemic vascular resistance
$t_{1/2}$	half-life
T_3	triiodothyronine
T_4	thyroxine
TAHBSO	total abdominal hysterectomy with bilateral salpingo-oophorectomy
TAT	Thematic Apperception Test
TB	tuberculosis
TCA	tricyclic antidepressant
TCD_{50}	median tissue culture dose
THA	total-hip arthroplasty
TIA	transient ischemic attack
TIBC	total iron-binding capacity
TLC	thin-layer chromatography; total lung capacity
TNF-α	tumor necrosis factor α
TNM*	tumor, node, metastasis (see 12.2.2, Nomenclature, The TNM Staging System)
tPA	tissue-type plasminogen activator
TPN	total parenteral nutrition
TQM	total quality management

**This abbreviation may be used without expansion.*

Abbreviation	*Expanded Form*
TRH	thyrotropin-releasing hormone (*protirelin* as diagnostic agent)
tRNA	transfer ribonucleic acid
TRUS	transrectal ultrasound
TSH	Use *thyrotropin* (previously thyroid-stimulating hormone).
TSS	toxic shock syndrome
TTP	thrombotic thrombocytopenic purpura
UHF	ultrahigh frequency
ul*	uniformly labeled (used within parentheses; see 12.9.5, Nomenclature, Uniform Labeling)
US	ultrasonography, ultrasound
USAN	*United States Adopted Names*
USP	*United States Pharmacopeia*
UV*	ultraviolet
UV-A*	ultraviolet A
UV-B*	ultraviolet B
UV-C*	ultraviolet C
VAIN	vaginal intraepithelial neoplasia
VDRL*	Venereal Disease Research Laboratory (add *test*)
VEP	visual evoked potential
VER	visual evoked response
VHDL	very high-density lipoprotein
VHF	very high frequency
VLBW	very low birth weight (*but:* very low-birth-weight infant)
VLDL	very low-density lipoprotein
VO_2	oxygen consumption per unit time
VO_{2max}	maximum oxygen consumption
VPB	ventricular premature beat
$\dot{V}/\dot{Q}$	ventilation-perfusion ratio
VT	tidal volume
WAIS	Wechsler Adult Intelligence Scale
WBC	white blood cell
WEE	western equine encephalomyelitis

**This abbreviation may be used without expansion.*

11.12 ■ **UNITS OF MEASURE.**—The AMA journals report quantitative values in the International System of Units (SI units, Système International d'Unités) and require SI measurements for submitted manuscripts (see also 15.5.2, Units of Measure, Dual Reporting).

Use the following abbreviations and symbols with a numerical quantity in accordance with guidelines in 15.0, Units of Measure. See especially 15.6, Non-SI Reporting of Common Measurements, 15.5.1, SI Conversion Tables, and 6.4, Punctuation, Virgule (Solidus).

Note: Do not capitalize abbreviated units of measure (unless the abbreviation itself is always capitalized or contains capital letters) in titles, subtitles, table heads, centerheads, sideheads, or line art.

acre	acre
ampere	A
angstrom	Convert to nanometers (1 Å = 0.1 nm).
atmosphere, standard	atm
bar	bar
barn	b*
base pair	bp*
becquerel	Bq
Bessey-Lowry unit	Bessey-Lowry unit
billion electron volts	GeV*
Bodansky unit	BU*
British thermal unit	BTU
calorie	cal (Convert to joule; 1 cal = 4.184 J.)
candela	cd*
Celsius	C (Close up to degree symbol, eg, 40°C.)
centigram	cg
centimeter	cm
centimeters of water	cm H_2O
centipoise	cP
coulomb	C*
counts per minute	cpm
counts per second	cps
cubic centimeter	cm^3 (Use milliliter for liquids and gases.)
cubic foot	cu ft
cubic inch	cu in
cubic meter	m^3
cubic micrometer	μm^3
cubic millimeter	mm^3 (Use microliter for liquids and gases.)
cubic yard	cu yd
curie	Ci (Convert to becquerel; 1 Ci = 3.7×10^{10} Bq.)
cycles per second	Use hertz.
dalton	d
day	d†
decibel	dB
decigram	Convert to grams.
deciliter	dL
decimeter	Convert to meters.
diopter	D*
disintegrations per minute	dpm*
disintegrations per second	dps*
dram	dram
dyne	dyne
electron volt	eV
electrostatic unit	ESU*
equivalent	Eq
equivalent roentgen	equivalent roentgen
Fahrenheit	F (Close up to degree symbol, eg, 99°F.)
farad (electric capacitance)	F

**Expand at first mention, with the abbreviation following immediately in parentheses. Abbreviate thereafter, except at the beginning of a sentence (see also 15.3.4, Units of Measure, Beginning of Sentence, Title, Subtitle).*

†Use the abbreviation only in a virgule construction and in tables and line art. Note: Do not abbreviate (except in a virgule construction) in table footnotes or figure legends.

femtogram	fg
femtoliter	fL
femtomole	fmol
fluid ounce	fl oz
foot	ft
foot-candle	ft-c*
foot-lambert	foot-lambert
foot-pound	ft-lb
gallon	gal
gas volume	gas volume
gauss	G
grain	grain
gram	g
gravity (acceleration due to)	*g* (Use closed up to preceding number, eg, 200*g*.)
gray	Gy
henry	H*
hertz	Hz
horsepower	hp
hour	h†
immunizing unit	ImmU*
inch	in
international benzoate unit	IBU*
international unit	IU
joule	J
katal	kat*
kelvin	K
kilobase	kb*
kilocalorie	kcal (Convert to kilojoule; 1 kcal = 4.2 kJ.)
kilocurie	kCi
kilodalton	kd
kiloelectron volt	keV
kilogram	kg
kilohertz	kHz
kilojoule	kJ
kilometer	km
kilovolt	kV
kilovolt-ampere	kVA
kilovolt (constant potential)	kV(cp)*
kilovolt (peak)	kV(p)*
kilowatt	kW
King-Armstrong unit	King-Armstrong unit
knot	knot
liter	L
lumen	lumen
lux	lux
megacurie	MCi
megacycle	Mc
megahertz	MHz

**Expand at first mention, with the abbreviation following immediately in parentheses. Abbreviate thereafter, except at the beginning of a sentence (see also 15.3.4, Units of Measure, Beginning of Sentence, Title, Subtitle).*

†Use the abbreviation only in a virgule construction and in tables and line art. Note: Do not abbreviate (except in a virgule construction) in table footnotes or figure legends.

megaunit	megaunit
megawatt	MW
meter	m
metric ton	metric ton
microampere	μA
microcurie	μCi
microfarad	μF*
microgram	μg
microliter	μL
micrometer	μm
micromicrocurie	Use picocurie.
micromicrogram	Use picogram.
micromicrometer	Use picometer.
micromolar	Use μmol/L.
micromole	μmol
micron	Use micrometer.
micronormal	μN
micro-osmole	μOsm
microunit	μU
microvolt	μV
microwatt	μW
mile	mile
miles per hour	mph
milliampere	mA
millicurie	mCi
millicuries destroyed	mCid*
milliequivalent	mEq
millifarad	mF*
milligram	mg
milligram-element	mg-el*
milli-International Unit	mIU
milliliter	mL
millimeter	mm
millimeters of mercury	mm Hg
millimeters of water	mm H_2O
millimolar	Use mmol/L.
millimole	mmol
million electron volts	MeV
milliosmole	mOsm
millirem	mrem
milliroentgen	mR
millisecond†	ms
milliunit	mU
millivolt	mV
milliwatt	mW
minute (time)	min†
molar	Use mol/L.
mole	mol
month	mo†
mouse unit	MU*
nanocurie	nCi
nanogram	ng

**Expand at first mention, with the abbreviation following immediately in parentheses. Abbreviate thereafter, except at the beginning of a sentence (see also 15.3.4, Units of Measure, Beginning of Sentence, Title, Subtitle).*

†Use the abbreviation only in a virgule construction and in tables and line art. Note: Do not abbreviate (except in a virgule construction) in table footnotes or figure legends.

nanometer	nm
nanomolar	Use nmol/L.
nanomole	nmol
newton	N
normal (solution)	N
ohm	Ω
osmole	osm
ounce	oz
outflow (weight)	C*
parts per million	ppm
pascal	Pa
picocurie	pCi
picogram	pg
picometer	pm
picomolar	Use pmol/L.
picomole	pmol
pint	pt
pound	lb
pounds per square inch	psi
pounds per square inch absolute	psia*
pounds per square inch gauge	psig*
prism diopter	PD, Δ*
quart	qt
rad	rad (Convert to gray; 1 rad = 0.01 Gy.)
radian	radian
rat unit	RU*
revolutions per minute	rpm
roentgen	R
roentgen equivalents man (or mammal)	rem
roentgen equivalents physical	rep
Saybolt seconds universal	SSU*
second	s†
siemens	siemens
sievert	Sv
square centimeter	cm^2
square foot	sq ft
square inch	sq in
square meter	m^2
square millimeter	mm^2
Svedberg flotation unit	Sf*
tesla	T
tonne (metric ton)	tonne
torr	Use millimeters of mercury.
tuberculin unit	TU
turbidity-reducing unit	TRU*
unit	U
volt	V
volume	vol
volume per volume	vol/vol

**Expand at first mention, with the abbreviation following immediately in parentheses. Abbreviate thereafter, except at the beginning of a sentence (see also 15.3.4, Units of Measure, Beginning of Sentence, Title, Subtitle).*

†Use the abbreviation only in a virgule construction and in tables and line art. Note: Do not abbreviate (except in a virgule construction) in table footnotes or figure legends.

volume percent	vol%
watt	W
week	wk†
weight	wt
weight per volume	wt/vol
weight per weight	wt/wt
yard	yd
year	y†

**Expand at first mention, with the abbreviation following immediately in parentheses. Abbreviate thereafter, except at the beginning of a sentence (see also 15.3.4, Units of Measure, Beginning of Sentence, Title, Subtitle).*

†Use the abbreviation only in a virgule construction and in tables and line art. Note: Do not abbreviate (except in a virgule construction) in table footnotes or figure legends.

11.13 ■ **ELEMENTS AND CHEMICALS.**—In general, the names of chemical elements and compounds may be expanded in the text at first mention and elsewhere in accordance with the guidelines for clinical and technical terms (see also 12.4.4, Nomenclature, Chemical Names, and 12.9, Nomenclature, Isotopes). However, in some circumstances it may be helpful or necessary to provide the chemical symbols or formulas in addition to the expansion if the compound under discussion is new or relatively unknown or if no nonproprietary term exists. For example:

> 2,3,7,8-Tetrachlorodibenzo-p-dioxin (TCDD, or dioxin) is often referred to as the most toxic synthetic chemical known. [Use "TCDD" or "dioxin" thereafter; TCDD is more specific, because there is more than one form of dioxin.]

> 3,4-Methylenedioxymethamphetamine (MDMA, ecstasy, XTC), a synthetic analog of 3,4-methylenedioxyamphetamine, has been the center of controversy over its potential for abuse vs its use as a psychotherapeutic agent. [Use "MDMA," "ecstasy," or "XTC" thereafter, depending on the article's context.]

The following format may also be used:

> Isorhodeose (chemical name, 6-deoxy-D-glucose [$CH_3(CHOH)_4CHO$]) is a sugar derived from cinchona bark. [Use "isorhodeose" thereafter.]

Names such as "sodium lauryl sulfate" are easier to express and understand (and typeset) than "$CH_3(CH_2)_{10}CH_2OSO_3Na$." Similarly, "oxygen" and "water" do not take up much more space than "O_2" and "H_2O" and hence should remain expanded throughout a manuscript, unless specific measurements (eg, gas exchange) are under discussion.

> The venous CO_2 pressure is always greater than arterial CO_2 pressure; specifically, $P\textsc{v}CO_2/P\textsc{a}CO_2$ is greater than 1.0 except when PO_2 plus PCO_2 is measured. Nevertheless, the CO_2 levels should be carefully measured.

> Near the earth's surface, the atmosphere has a well-defined chemical composition, consisting of molecular nitrogen, molecular oxygen, and argon. It also contains small amounts of carbon dioxide and water vapor, along with trace quantities of methane, ammonia, nitrous oxide, hydrogen sulfide, helium, neon, krypton, xenon, and various other gases.

In the following example, sodium and potassium are not abbreviated.

> Repeated serum chemistry studies confirmed a serum sodium level of 131 mmol/L and a serum potassium level of 4.8 mmol/L.

In the text and elsewhere, the expansion of such symbols as Na^+ or Ca^{2+} can be cumbersome, since these symbols have a specific meaning for the reader. Usage should follow the context. For example, in nontechnical pieces, the flavor of the writing might be lost if, for example, the editor arbitrarily changed "CO_2" to "carbon dioxide" ("What's the patient's CO_2?").

When chemical symbols and formulas are used, they must be carefully marked for the printer, especially when chemical bonds are expressed (see also 18.1, Mathematical Composition, Copy Marking). Three types of chemical bonds commonly seen in organic and biochemical compounds are single, double, and triple:

$$H_3{-}CH_3 \qquad H_2C{=}CH_2 \qquad HC{\equiv}CH$$

When deciding whether to expand or abbreviate element and chemical names, the editor and the author should consider guidelines for established terminology, the manuscript's subject matter, technical level, and audience, and the context in which the term appears.

11.14 ■ **RADIOACTIVE ISOTOPES.**—In general, the expanded terms for radioactive isotopes are used in AMA journals, as described in 12.9, Nomenclature, Isotopes, with exceptions noted, for example, in radioactive pharmaceuticals and certain chemical notations. The following table lists radioactive isotopes (and their symbols) used in medical diagnosis and therapy (see also 12.9.2, Nomenclature, Radiopharmaceuticals, and 12.9.3, Nomenclature, Radiopharmaceutical Compounds Without Approved Names) (adapted from *The Merck Index*[8]).

Name	*Symbol*	*Name*	*Symbol*
americium	Am	mercury	Hg
calcium	Ca	phosphorus	P
cesium	Cs	potassium	K
chromium	Cr	radium	Ra
cobalt	Co	radon	Rn
copper	Cu	ruthenium	Ru
fluorine	F	selenium	Se
gadolinium	Gd	sodium	Na
gallium	Ga	strontium	Sr
gold	Au	sulfur	S
indium	In	technetium	Tc
iodine	I	thallium	Tl
iridium	Ir	xenon	Xe
iron	Fe	ytterbium	Yb
krypton	Kr		

ACKNOWLEDGMENT

Principal author: Roxanne K. Young, ELS

REFERENCES

1. Smyth HW; Messing GM, rev ed. *Greek Grammar.* Cambridge, Mass: Harvard University Press; 1984:104.

2. Flexner SB, ed. *The Random House Dictionary of the English Language.* 2nd ed, unabridged. New York, NY: Random House; 1987.

3. Patrias K. *National Library of Medicine Recommended Formats for Bibliographic Citation.* Bethesda, Md: National Library of Medicine, Reference Service; 1991.

4. National Library of Medicine, National Institutes of Health. *List of Journals Indexed in Index Medicus.* Bethesda, Md: National Library of Medicine; 1997. NIH publication 97-267.

5. Jablonski S, ed. *Dictionary of Medical Acronyms & Abbreviations.* 2nd ed. Philadelphia, Pa: Hanley & Belfus Inc; 1993.

6. Logan CM, Rice MK. *Logan's Medical and Scientific Abbreviations.* Philadelphia, Pa: JB Lippincott Co; 1987.

7. Mossman J, Dear P, Longe JL, Sisung KS, Skirpan RH. *Acronyms, Initialisms & Abbreviations Dictionary.* 18th ed. Detroit, Mich: Gale Research Inc; 1994.

8. Budavari S, ed. *The Merck Index.* 11th ed. Rahway, NJ: Merck & Co Inc; 1989.

Chapter 12

12.0 Nomenclature

A generally accepted and universally used system of nomenclature is an essential tool in any area of study.

Julia G. Bodmer[1(p2)]

This chapter is devoted to nomenclature: the systematic formulation of names for specific entities. During the last half century, many medical disciplines have set up committees to develop and promulgate official systems of nomenclature, which are described in the subsections of this chapter.

Accelerating knowledge, particularly from molecular biology, necessitated the official nomenclature systems, sometimes with dramatic results. In coagulation, 1 factor alone was referred to by 14 different names.[2] An investigator deemed the official coagulation nomenclature "one of the most significant, even if only semantic, recent advances in the field."[3(p16)] The results, probably true in other disciplines as well, were that "[a]n impenetrable confusion was cleared away, apparent disagreements were often shown to be conflicts of terminology, not of fact, and a much freer exchange of information was made possible."[3(p16)]

In microbiology, with publication of the approved list of bacterial names in 1980, "[t]he number of names of bacteria decreased dramatically, from approximately 29,000 to just over 1,700."[4(p250)] The CD (clusters of differentiation) nomenclature is thought to have prevented mistakes in laboratory and clinical research.[5]

Such are some examples of the compelling need for systematic nomenclature, which requires the exhaustive and ongoing work of international groups. The development of nomenclature, however, faces challenges besides the confusion of multiple names. There is tradition—"the ruins of previous systems"[6(p7)]—which investigators are reluctant to give up. When disciplines converge—for instance, when the genetics of a physiologic system are delineated—preexisting systems of nomenclature may operate in parallel.

Sometimes the resulting differences in names are only typographic. However, a phenomenon like interspecies homology, as described in the human HLA system and the mouse H-2 system, can pose a seemingly insurmountable nomenclatural challenge:

> The situation is perhaps similar to what one might have encountered in the field of immunoglobulins had researchers working with immunoglobulins in different species not realized relatively early that the classes of heavy chains and light chains they were working with were homologous and been willing to adopt a common nomenclature. We might then have separate names in each species for IgM, IgG, IgA, kappa, lambda, and so on. It is obvious that a common nomenclature is preferable, but once work has progressed very far in each field independently, it becomes increasingly difficult to achieve this goal. The opportunity for a common MHC [major histocompatibility complex] nomenclature has recently presented itself, since the molecular biology of the MHC has identified interspecies homologs. However, for the present, one must learn both sets of nomenclature if one is to be able to make use of information in both species.[7(p578)]

A system of nomenclature may face the test of sheer numbers. The count of symbols in the catalog of human gene nomenclature has risen from a few hundred into the thousands, and human genes numbering 50 000 to 100 000 can be anticipated. Other systems may face name changes when entities discovered in pathological contexts, such as blood group and tissue antigens, have their physiologic functions revealed.

Another challenge is to remain flexible. Those who deal with nomenclature accept it as a construct[8-11] and have noted the need to reflect new knowledge[9,12] and "evolve with new technology rather than be restrictive as sometimes occurs when historical . . . systems are applied."[13(p12)]

Such flexibility, however, places a burden on clinicians, who must replace familiar names with new ones.[14] Often, "colorful or descriptive names,"[5(p1245)] which are more easily retained,[15] give way to more efficient terms, such as the alphanumeric epithets of many systems.

Official systems of nomenclature are not universally observed to the letter, but, because of their contribution to scientific communication, they deserve, and in this chapter receive, cognizance.

Our purpose in the nomenclature section is not to explain how entities should be named. We cite the sources of such rules, for readers who need them. Editors have the task of mediating between official systems and authors' actual usage. To that end, the goals of this chapter are 2-fold: to present style used for various terms in order to reduce ambiguities and achieve typographic consistency; and to explain terms in hopes that they are then more easily dealt with.

In medical nomenclature the stylistic trend has been toward typographic simplicity, driven by computers. Terms lose hyphens, superscripts, subscripts, and spaces. However, such features have not been eliminated completely, either within or beyond these pages. In 1950 standardized terms in pulmonary-respiratory medicine and physiology were put forth, and typographic features impossible on a typewriter were expressly retained, seen as indispensable components of a systematic and enlightening nomenclature.[12] Computers are increasingly capable of generating unusual characters, and typographic simplification and electronic sophistication may cross paths before medical nomenclature loses its last defining flourishes.

ACKNOWLEDGMENTS

Principal authors: Harriet S. Meyer, MD, for sections 12.0 through 12.3, 12.6 through 12.8, and 12.10 through 12.13; Margaret A. Winker, MD, for sections 12.4, 12.5, and 12.9.

The assistance of the following is gratefully acknowledged; any errors belong exclusively to the authors of the sections:

The following reviewed drafts and provided invaluable suggestions:

Blood Groups and Platelet Antigens: Geoff L. Daniels, PhD, Peter D. Issitt, PhD, Albert E. G. von dem Borne, MD, PhD; Cancer: Donald Earl Henson, MD, Robert V. P. Hutter, MD, Charis Eng, MD, PhD; Cardiology: Alan D. Bernstein, EngScD, Harvey Feigenbaum, MD, J. Willis Hurst, MD (electrocardiography and auscultation), Jonathan Langberg, MD (electrophysiology, pacemakers), Randolph P. Martin, MD (echocardiography), Galen S. Wagner, MD; Drugs: Donald R. Bennett, MD, PhD, Ruta Freimanis, PharmD, RPh; Genetics: Dr Charles Cantor, Dr Athel Cornish-Bowden (nucleic acids and amino acids), R. G. H. Cotton, DSc, Phyllis J. McAlpine, PhD (human gene nomenclature), Bert Vogelstein, MD, PhD (oncogenes and tumor suppressor genes), Janet Rowley, MD, Diane Roulston, MD, PhD (chromosomes), Muriel T. Davisson, PhD (animal genes); Hemostasis: Leon W. Hoyer, MD, Karen L. Kaplan, MD; Immunology: John P. Atkinson, MD (complement), Steven G. E. Marsh (HLA), Tristram G. Parslow, MD, PhD (immunoglobulins and lymphocytes), Dr Joost J. Oppenheim (cytokines); Isotopes: Donald R. Bennett, MD, PhD, Ruta Freimanis, PharmD, RPh; Neurology: Michael J. Aminoff, MD, Robert J. Joynt, MD, PhD, Donald W. Kass, MD; Organisms: Kevin C. Hazen, PhD, Frank L. Iber, MD (hepatitis), Bernard Roizman, PhD (viruses); Pulmonary and Respiratory Terminology: John B. West, MD.

Charl Richey adapted the illustrations.

Bruce B. Dan, MD, Dee Egger, Leo Manack, MD, Ronald M. Meyer, MD, Carin M. Olson, MD, and Don Riesenberg, MD, provided helpful suggestions.

Karen Lindau (Karger), Douglas Macbeth (The Jackson Library, Bar Harbor, Me), and Carol Rozmiarek (Institute of Laboratory Animal Resources, Washington, DC) provided helpful information.

Maurice Bell, Yolanda Davis-Ellis, and Sandra Schefris, AMA Library and Information Services, Toni Reed, University of Illinois, Chicago, InfoQuic, and the Evanston, Ill, Webster Library provided assistance in obtaining references.

REFERENCES

1. Bodmer JG. Nomenclature 1991 foreword. *Hum Immunol.* 1991;34:2-3.

2. Abe T, Alexander B, Astrup T, et al, and the International Committee for the Nomencla-

ture of Blood Clotting Factors; Wright IS, chair. The nomenclature of blood clotting factors. *JAMA*. 1962;180:733-735.

3. Biggs R, ed. *Human Blood Coagulation, Hemostasis and Thrombosis.* 2nd ed. Oxford, England: Blackwell Scientific Publications; 1976:15-16.
4. Baron EJ, Weissfeld AS, Fuselier PA, Brenner DJ. Classification and identification of bacteria. In: Murray PR, ed. *Manual of Clinical Microbiology.* 6th ed. Washington, DC: ASM [American Society for Microbiology] Press; 1995:249-264.
5. Singer NG, Todd RF, Fox DA. Structures on the cell surface: update from the Fifth International Workshop on Human Leukocyte Differentiation Antigens. *Arthritis Rheum.* 1994;37:1245-1248.
6. Wildy P. *Classification and Nomenclature of Viruses: First Report of the International Committee on Nomenclature of Viruses.* New York, NY: S Karger AG; 1971;5:7. Melnick JL, ed. Monographs in Virology.
7. Hansen TH, Carreno BM, Sachs DH. The major histocompatibility complex. In: Paul WE, ed. *Fundamental Immunology.* 3rd ed. New York, NY: Raven Press; 1993:577-628.
8. Staley JT, Krieg NR. Bacterial classification, I: classification of procaryotic organisms: an overview. In: Krieg NR, Holt JF, eds. *Bergey's Manual of Systematic Bacteriology.* Baltimore, Md: Williams & Wilkins; 1984;1:1-4.
9. Erzinclioglu YZ, Unwin DM. The stability of zoological nomenclature [letter]. *Nature.* 1986;320:687.
10. Lublin DM, Telen MJ. What is a blood group antigen [letter]? *Transfusion.* 1992;32:493.
11. Lublin DM, Telen MJ. More about use of the term Drb [letter]. *Transfusion.* 1993;33:182.
12. Pappenheimer JR, chairman; Comroe JH, Cournand A, Ferguson JKW, et al. Standardization of definitions and symbols in respiratory physiology. *Fed Proc.* 1950;9:602-605.
13. Shows TB, McAlpine PJ, Boucheix C, et al. Guidelines for human gene nomenclature: an international system for human gene nomenclature (ISGN, HGM9). *Cytogenet Cell Genet.* 1987;46:11-28.
14. Patterson PY, Sommers HM. A proposed change in bacterial nomenclature: a rose by any other name. *J Infect Dis.* 1981;144:85-86.
15. Flexner CW. In praise of descriptive nomenclature [letter]. *Lancet.* 1996;347:68.

12.1 ■ BLOOD GROUPS AND PLATELET ANTIGENS.

12.1.1 ***Blood Groups.***—*Blood groups* are characterized by erythrocyte (red blood cell) antigens with common immunologic properties. *Blood group systems* are series of antigens with a common inheritance.[1(p77)]

The principal entities of a blood group are the antigenic phenotype or specificity (eg, A), the alleles (specific genes for each phenotype, eg, *A*), and the antibodies to the antigen (eg, anti-B).

Historically, as with many systems of medical nomenclature, the approach to blood group terminology changed as more entities were discovered. The names of the 22 currently identified blood group systems have varied origins. For instance, the earliest systems were named with single letters. In the MNSs system, *M* was taken from "immune" ("'I' was avoided because of confusion with the numeral 1"[1(p78)]). Rhesus monkey cells led to the name of the Rh system, although the experiments using them actually uncovered the related LW antigen, named for the investigators Landsteiner and Wiener. Later systems are usually named for the patient in whom antibodies of that system were discovered (eg, Duffy, Kell[eher]).[2]

The Xg and Xk systems take their names from their genetic loci on the X chromosome.

Nomenclature of blood group systems is inconsistent as to whether specific antigen products of different alleles are designated using uppercase or lowercase letters (eg, K, k), superscripts or subscripts (A_1, Jk^a, Jk^b), plus and minus signs, or other forms (see examples that follow).[1(p79)]

Other aspects of blood group nomenclature, however, are consistent[2]:

- About half the systems have a conventional name and all have standard abbreviations (eg, "Lewis system," "Le system").
- As in classical genetics, genetic terms are italicized, phenotypic terms are not.
- Erythrocyte antigen and phenotype terminology uses single letters (eg, A) or dual letters (eg, AB, Le), often with a letter or number as a superscript or subscript.
- If a subscript letter or number is part of an antigen symbol, *it becomes a superscript* in the symbol for the allele (eg, A_1 antigen; A^1 allele).
- If a superscript letter is part of an antigen symbol, *it remains a superscript* in the symbol for the allele (eg, Fy^a antigen; Fy^a allele).

In general, editors should question deviations from the abovementioned conventions. Table 1 shows sample terms from some of the more commonly encountered blood group systems (see also 12.6.2, Human Gene Nomenclature). In some cases, alternative forms for the same antigen are in use, and author preference is acceptable.

Terms such as O+ ("O positive"), A+, and AB− are in common parlance but are misleading and absolutely proscribed in scientific articles. Although such terms are shorthand for blood of the ABO system and its Rh specificity, use instead standard terms that specifically indicate Rh status, eg:

O Rh-positive

O Rh+

or more specific designations of phenotype, eg:

group B, D-negative

group A, Rh D-positive

Individual elements of a blood group profile may be separated by commas, as above, or, for more complex specificities, with semicolons:

The patient's blood was group B, D+ C+ c+ E− e+; M+ N+ S− s+; P_1+; Le(a−b−); K− k+; Fy(a−b+); Jk(a+b−).[3(p85)]

12.1.2 ***ISBT Name and Number.***[1(p79),4-8]—In the 1980s the Working Party on Terminology for Red Cell Surface Antigens of the International Society of Blood Transfusion (ISBT) developed an alphanumeric system of blood group notation. The system's use of all capitals and characters set on the line was intended to facilitate and standardize electronic processing of blood group data, superseding individual notations devised to circumvent computer character limitations. The system was proposed as and remains an alternative to the classical blood group nomenclature described above. In AMA journals, at the author's discretion, the alphanumeric ISBT term may appear within parentheses following the classical term.

In the ISBT terminology, each blood group system has a symbol, usually of 1 to 3 capital letters, and a system number of 3 digits. Each antigen within the system also has a 3-digit number. The partial table on page 343 is excerpted from Lewis et al[6]:

TABLE 1. SAMPLE BLOOD GROUP TERMS

System or Group	Phenotypes	Antigens	Antibodies	Genotypes
ABO system*	Groups: O, A, B, AB, O_h, O_h^A Subgroups: A_1, A_2, A_1B, A_2B	A, A_1, A_2, A_x, B	Anti-A, anti-A_1, anti-A,B	A^1O, A^1A^1, A^1B, *OO*
Lewis (Le) system	Le(a−b+), Le(a+b−), Le(a−b−)	Le^a, Le^b	Anti-Le^b, anti-Le^{bH}, anti-Le^{bL}	*Lele, LeLe, lele*
Ii group	I, i	I, i, i_1, i_2, i_{cord}, I^T	Anti-I, anti-HI, anti-BI, anti-Hi, Anti-Bi, anti-P_1I, anti-HILe^b	
MNSs system	M+N+, M+N−, M−N+, S+s+, S+s−, S−s+	M, N, S, s, U, M^g	Anti-M, anti-M-like, anti-M_1, anti-N, anti-s	*MN, MM, NN, MSNs*
P system and related groups	P_1, P_2, P_1^k, P_2^k, p	P_1, P, P^k	Anti-P_1, anti-P, anti-PP_1P^k	
Rh system†	D-positive (Rh positive) D-negative (Rh negative) DCcE, DCce Rh: −1, −2, −3 Rh_{null}	D, C, E, c, e Rh1, Rh2, Rh3, Rh4, Rh5 f, Ce, . . . JAL Rh6, Rh7, . . . Rh48	Anti-D Anti-Rh1 Epitopes of D: epD1, epD2, . . . epD6/7, epD8	*DCe/DCe* (R^1R^1) *DcE/dce* (R^2r) *dce/dce* (*rr*) *D−−/D−−*
Kell (K) system	K+k−, Kp(a−b+), Js(a−b+) K: 1, −2, −3, 4, −6, 7	K, k, Kp^a, Kp^b, Ku, Js^a, Js^b K1, K2, K3, K4, K5, K6, K7	Anti-K, anti-k, anti-Js^a, anti-Js^b	*Kk*, Kp^bKp^b, Js^bJs^b K^1, K^2, K^{-3}, K^4, K^{-5}, K^6
Lutheran (Lu) system	Lu(a−b+), Lu(a+b−), Lu(a+b+)	Lu^a, Lu^b	Anti-Lu^a, anti-Lu^b, anti-Lu3 or anti-Lu^{ab}	Lu^aLu^a, Lu^bLu^b, Lu^aLu^b
Duffy (Fy) system	Fy(a−b+), Fy(a+b−), Fy(a−b−)	Fy^a, Fy^b	Anti-Fy^a, anti-Fy^b	Fy^aFy^a, Fy^bFy^b, *FyFy*
Kidd (Jk) system	Jk(a−b+), Jk(a+b−), Jk(a+b+)	Jk^a, Jk^b	Anti-Jk^a, anti-Jk^b	Jk^aJk^a, Jk^bJk^b, Jk^aJk^b
Xg system	Xg(a+), Xg(a−)	Xg^a	Anti-Xg^a	Female: Xg^aXg^a, Xg^aXg, *XgXg* Male: Xg^aY, *XgY*

* *Sample expressions for ABO, typical for all blood group systems: ABO antigens, A cell, type AB recipient, type O donor. Secretors of ABH antigens have a secretor* (Se) *gene. Their genotype may be* SeSe *or* Sese. *The nonsecretor genotype is* sese.

† *Historically Rh nomenclature has used 3 alternative schemes: The Rh-Hr nomenclature, the CDE nomenclature, and the numerical nomenclature (for a discussion see Mollison et al*[205-207]*). Terms from the first, eg, rh′, hr″, rh^x, Rh^A, are appropriate in historical discussions, but otherwise, the CDE and numerical nomenclatures are favored.*

System			*Antigen No. Within System*			
Name	*Symbol*	*No.*	*001*	*002*	*003*	*004*
ABO	ABO	001	A	B	A,B	Al
MNS	MNS	002	M	N	S	s
Rh	RH	004	D	C	E	c

Sinistral (left-hand) zeros can be dropped from system and antigen terms, and system letter symbols can be used as part of the alphanumeric term. The following, for instance, are all acceptable for blood type AB:

001003

1003

1,3

ABO3

In systems that use pluses and minuses to express presence and absence of particular antigens, phenotypic expressions in the numerical notation employ a colon and use numbers in place of letters, as in this example:

LE:−1,2 [for Le(a−b+)]

FY:1,−2 [for Fy(a+b−)]

Genotypic expressions are italicized, eg:

FY 1/2 or *FY*1/2* (for Fy^aFy^b)

To find further conventions for phenotypic and genotypic designations, consult Issitt and Moulds[8] and Lewis et al.[6]

12.1.3 ***Platelet Antigens.***—(This section is based largely on a report by von dem Borne and Décary[9] and a written communication from A. E. G. von dem Borne, MD, PhD, October 1994.) All platelet-specific antigen systems discovered so far are biallelic systems. Molecular studies have shown that they are the result of single

TABLE 2. PLATELET ANTIGEN SYSTEMS

Antigen System	Other Names	Antigens	Other Names
HPA-1	Zw, P1A	HPA-1a	Zw^a, $P1^{A1}$
		HPA-1b	Zw^b, $P1^{A2}$
HPA-2	Ko, Sib	HPA-2a	Ko^b
		HPA-2b	Ko^a, Sib^a
HPA-3	Bak, Lek	HPA-3a	Bak^b
		HPA-3b	Bak^a, Lek^a
HPA-4	Pen, Yuk	HPA-4a	Pen^a, Yuk^b
		HPA-4b	Pen^b, Yuk^a
HPA-5	Br, Zav, Hc	HPA-5a	Br^b, Zav^b
		HPA-5b	Br^a, Zav^a, Hc^a
HPA-6	Ca, Tu	HPA-6b	Ca, Tu
HPA-7	Mo	HPA-7b	Mo^a
HPA-8	Sr	HPA-8b	Sr^a
HPA-9W	Max	HPA-9Wb	Max^a

base substitutions, resulting in single amino acid substitutions, in the genes of platelet membrane glycoproteins (GPIIIa, GPIIIb, GPIa, GPIbα).

Platelet antigen and antigen system nomenclature is the responsibility of the Platelet Serology Working Party of the International Society of Blood Transfusion and the International Society of Hematology. New systems that are still under evaluation are designated with a W (from Workshop), eg, HPA-9W, a recently discovered new system. Names of antigens will be issued only when specific antisera are available.

To date 9 systems have been defined; they are summarized in Table 2. The most recently described antigens (HPA-6b to HPA-9Wb) are all low-frequency antigens.

REFERENCES

1. Mollison PL, Engelfriet CP, Contreras M. *Blood Transfusion in Clinical Medicine.* 9th ed. Boston, Mass: Blackwell Scientific Publications; 1993.
2. Issitt PD, Crookston MC. Blood group terminology: current conventions. *Transfusion.* 1984;24:2-7.
3. Whitsett CF, Hare VW, Oxendine SM, Pierce JA. Autologous and allogeneic red cell survival studies in the presence of autoanti-AnWj. *Transfusion.* 1993;33:845-847.
4. Daniels GL, Moulds JJ, Anstee DJ, et al. ISBT Working Party on Terminology for Red Cell Surface Antigens: Sao Paulo Report. *Vox Sang.* 1993;65:77-80.
5. Lewis M, Allen FH, Anstee DJ, et al. ISBT Working Party on Terminology for Red Cell Surface Antigens: Munich Report. *Vox Sang.* 1985;49:171-175.
6. Lewis M, Anstee DJ, Bird GWG, et al. Blood group terminology 1990. *Vox Sang.* 1990;58:152-169.
7. Lewis M, Anstee DJ, Bird GWG, et al. ISBT Working Party on Terminology for Red Cell Surface Antigens: Los Angeles Report. *Vox Sang.* 1991;61:158-160.
8. Issitt PD, Moulds JJ. Blood group terminology suitable for use in electronic data processing equipment. *Transfusion.* 1992;32:677-682.
9. von dem Borne AEG, Décary F. ICSH/ISBT Working Party on Platelet Serology: nomenclature of platelet-specific antigens. *Vox Sang.* 1990;58:176.

ADDITIONAL READINGS AND GENERAL REFERENCES

Calhoun L, Petz LD. Erythrocyte antigens and antibodies. In: Beutler E, Lichtman MA, Coller BS, Kipps TJ, eds. *Williams Hematology.* 5th ed. New York, NY: McGraw-Hill; 1995:1595-1610.

Mueller-Eckhardt C, Kiefel V, Santoso S. Review and update of platelet alloantigen systems. *Transfus Med Rev.* 1990;4:98-109.

Schroeder ML, Rayner HL. Red cell, platelet, and white cell antigens. In: Lee GR, Bithell TC, Foerster J, Athens JW, Lukens JN, eds. *Wintrobe's Clinical Hematology.* 9th ed. Philadelphia, Pa: Lea & Febiger; 1993:616-650.

12.2 ■ CANCER.

12.2.1 ***Cancer Stage.***—Cancer stages commonly are expressed using capital roman numerals:

stage I	stage III
stage II	stage IV

The term *stage 0* indicates carcinoma in situ.

Histologic grades are expressed using arabic numerals, eg, grade 2.

Letter and numerical suffixes, usually set on the line, may be added to subdivide individual cancer stages, as in the following examples:

stage 0a	stage III_{E+S}
stage 0is	stage II_3
stage IA	stage IVA
stage I_E	stage IVB

Note: Subscripts are used with lymphomas; for instance, the subscript E refers to extralymphatic spread, the subscript S to splenic involvement, and subscript numerals to the number of involved lymph node regions; "is" indicates "in situ."

12.2.2 ***The TNM Staging System.***—Authors will frequently use and editors frequently encounter the TNM staging system,[1,2] an internationally standardized system in its fifth decade of continuing formulation used for the staging of cancer. The TNM classification is put forth by the American Joint Committee on Cancer (AJCC) and the Union Internationale Contre le Cancer (UICC). The AJCC *Cancer Staging Manual*[1] and the UICC *TNM Classification of Malignant Tumours*[2] present the stages of cancer as defined by TNM classifications. The TNM definitions and stage groupings are based on outcome. The TNM symbols follow.

- T: tumor (indicates size, extent, or depth of penetration of the primary tumor)
  T is followed by numerical suffixes or other suffixes set on the line, eg:
  - TX: primary tumor cannot be assessed
  - T0: no evidence of a primary tumor
  - Tis: in situ carcinoma
  - T1, T2, T3, T4: increasing size, extent, or other characteristics of the primary tumor

  (*Note:* The number following T does not refer to a specific size for all tumors. For example, for one type of tumor, T1 may indicate size of 2 cm or less, for another, size of 0.75 mm or less, and for another, confinement within the underlying mucosa.)
- N: node (indicates the absence or presence and extent of regional lymph node involvement)
  - NX: regional lymph nodes cannot be assessed
  - N0: no regional lymph node metastasis
  - N1, N2, N3: increasing metastatic involvement of regional lymph nodes according to criteria that vary for the different anatomic sites
- M: metastasis (indicates absence or presence of distant metastasis)
  - MX: extent of metastasis cannot be determined
  - M0: no metastasis
  - M1: distant metastasis

  Site of metastasis may be indicated by such 3-letter abbreviations as PUL (pulmonary), OSS (osseous), or HEP (hepatic).

The TNM System and Cancer Staging: Various combinations of the T, N, and M categories are used to define cancer stages. For example, stage I is defined as T1 N0 M0 for many types of cancer.

The combinations that define individual stages differ among the anatomic sites. In laryngeal cancer, for example, stage II is defined as T2 N0 M0, while in pancreatic cancer, stage II is defined as T3 N0 M0.

More than one combination of the T, N, and M categories may constitute the definition of a single stage: eg, in a given cancer, stage III may be defined as T1 N1 M0 *or* T2 N1 M0 *or* T3 N0 M0 *or* T3 N1 M0.

Optional Descriptors: Additional descriptors, although not part of the TNM staging system, may be used as adjuncts to the T, N, and M categories for defining the extent of disease; these are indicated by capital letters as follows:

lymphatic vessel invasion	LX, L0, L1
venous invasion	VX, V0, V1, V2
residual tumor	RX, R0, R1, R2
histopathological grading	GX, G1, G2, G3, G4
scleral invasion or serum marker(s)	SX, S0, S1, S2

Lowercase prefixes to the T, N, M, and other symbols may be used to indicate the mode of determining criteria for tumor description and staging; these are as follows:

c	clinical T, N, or M classification or stage
p	pathologic T, N, or M classification or stage
r	recurrent tumor T, N, or M classification or stage
a	autopsy T, N, or M classification or stage
y	classification during or following multimodality treatment

Examples: cTNM, pT3

(For further explanation, see the AJCC *Cancer Staging Manual*[1] or the UICC *TNM Classification of Malignant Tumours.*[2])

The T, N, M, and other symbols used in cancer staging may be followed by suffixes in addition to the common X, 0, and numerals, which further specify qualities such as size, invasiveness, and extent of metastasis, eg:

Ta	T2a	N1a	pN1a
T1b	T2(m)	N2a	pN1biv
T1c	T2(5)	N2b	M1a
T1a1	T3a	N2c	M1b
	Tis		

The parenthetical suffix "m" indicates multiple primary tumors at a single site.

Usage: Terms such as "stage I cancer," "TNM staging system," and "T1 N1 M0" are widely recognized and may be used in articles. However, authors should also specify the clinical and/or pathologic criteria that define any stage and should reference the staging system of the AJCC or UICC manuals.

Stage and TNM designations are acceptable modifiers for nouns such as *tumor, lesion,* and *cancer,* as in "stage III cancer," "T1 N0 M0 tumor," and "N1 lesions." Expressions such as "TX N0 M0 classification" and "T1 N0 M0 cases" are acceptable. Improper would be "stage III patient" or "T1 N0 patients"; instead use "patient assigned [or with] stage III cancer," "patients with T1 N0 M0 tumors," and the like (see also 9.1, Correct and Preferred Usage, Commonly Misused Words and Phrases [case, client, consumer, patient, subject]).

For some sites, the histologic grade has been integrated into the staging system.

Other Staging Systems and the TNM System: The AJCC/UICC TNM classification and stage grouping is not the only system used for staging cancer, and equivalency of the same stage number among different systems cannot be assumed. However, 2 cancer staging systems, the FIGO (International Federation of Gynecologists and Obstetricians) staging system for gynecologic cancers and the Dukes stage system for colon and rectal cancers, have total equivalence with the AJCC/UICC stage. The AJCC/UICC system contains subsets of TNM classifications within stage groups that provide greater prognostic precision within each stage for colorectal cancer than does the Dukes system. For example, colorectal carcinoma AJCC/UICC stage I (the equivalent of Dukes A) has 2 subsets: T1 N0 M0, with 5-year survival of 100%; T2 N0 M0, with 5-year survival of 85%.[3]

12.2.3 ***Multiple Endocrine Neoplasia.***—Abbreviations for types of multiple endocrine neoplasia (MEN) feature arabic numerals and a space, as follows[4]:

MEN 1

MEN 2

MEN 2A

MEN 2B

MEN 3

Gene terms close up the space (see 12.6.2, Human Gene Nomenclature), eg:

MEN1

REFERENCES

1. Fleming ID, Cooper JS, Henson DE, et al (American Joint Committee on Cancer), eds. *Cancer Staging Manual.* 5th ed. Philadelphia, Pa: Lippincott-Raven; 1997.
2. Sobin LH, Wittekind C (International Union Against Cancer [UICC]), eds. *TNM Classification of Malignant Tumours.* 5th ed. Baltimore, Md: Wiley-Liss; 1997.
3. Hutter RVP, Sobin LH. A universal staging system for cancer of the colon and rectum: let there be light. *Arch Pathol Lab Med.* 1986;110:367-368.
4. Glossary: Second International Workshop on MEN-2. *Henry Ford Hosp Med J.* 1987;35:93.

12.3 ■ **CARDIOLOGY.**—Several areas of cardiology use typographically atypical terms that need not be expanded at first mention.

12.3.1 ***Electrocardiographic Terms.***—Note the use of capitals, lowercase letters, subscripts, and hyphens in the following examples of electrocardiographic (ECG) terms.

Leads: Leads (recording electrodes) are designated as follows:

standard (bipolar) leads	I, II, III
augmented limb leads (unipolar extremity leads)	aVR, aVL, aVF (a stands for augmented, V for voltage, R for right arm, L for left arm, and F for foot)
inverted aVR lead	−aVR
(unipolar) precordial (chest) leads	V_1, V_2, V_3, V_4, V_5, V_6, V_7, V_8, V_9
right precordial leads	V_2R, V_3R, V_4R, V_5R, V_6R
modified chest lead using V_1	MCL_1

Example: The abnormality appeared in leads V_3 through V_6 [not V_3-V_6 or V_{3-6}].

Deflections: The main deflections of the ECG are named in an alphabetical sequence (P, Q, R, S, T, U); other deflections use initial letters of the entity being described.

The following are examples of terms descriptive of deflections and patterns in ECG tracings:

delta wave (preferred over Δ wave)

F wave (atrial flutter wave)

f wave (atrial fibrillation wave)

J point, J junction

P wave, axis, etc

PR interval, segment, etc (*not* P-R)

Q wave, q wave

QRS complex, configuration, axis, etc

QS wave, qs wave

QT interval, prolongation, etc (*not* Q-T)

QTc (corrected QT interval)

R wave, r wave, R′ wave, r′ wave

R-on-T

R-R interval

rSR′ pattern

S wave, s wave

S′ wave, s′ wave

ST segment, depression, axis, etc (*not* S-T segment)

ST-segment abnormality

ST-T segment, elevation, axis, etc (*not* S-T-T)

T wave, axis, etc

U wave

Symbols used in connection with paced ECGs:

A atrial stimulus

V ventricular stimulus

AV interval from atrial stimulus to succeeding ventricular stimulus

AR interval from atrial stimulus to conducted spontaneous ventricular depolarization

PV interval from spontaneous atrial depolarization to succeeding "atrial-synchronous" ventricular stimulus

Capital letters are used to describe ECG deflections in general. For example:

Improper paper speed will spuriously alter the QRS configuration [*not* qrs configuration].

In reference to an individual ECG tracing, or in descriptions of some specific ECG patterns, capitals may indicate larger waves and lowercase letters smaller waves; in practice, this most often applies to the Q, R, and S waves:

> Pathologic Q waves occur in myocardial infarction.
>
> The q wave in aVF and the Rr′ pattern in lead V_3 in this patient's ECG were considered normal findings.
>
> An rSR′ complex in the anterior chest leads and qRs in the left chest leads may indicate right bundle-branch block.

Lead and tracing terms may be combined to describe pattern and location together, eg:

R_I	R wave in lead I
RaVL	R wave in aVL
S_{III}	S wave in lead III
${}_RV_3$	R in V_3
$S_1Q_3T_3$ pattern	prominence of S wave in lead I, Q wave in lead III, and T-wave inversion in lead III
$SV_1 + RV_5$	sum of voltages of S wave in V_1 and R wave in V_5

P Axis, QRS Axis, ST Axis, T Axis: These axes are specified with a plus or minus sign followed by the number of degrees in arabic numerals, eg, +60°, −30°. Should the interpreter use Grant's method, he or she should state how many degrees the axis (or vector) is directed anteriorly or posteriorly.

12.3.2 ***Heart Sounds.***—Four heart sounds and 4 components are commonly abbreviated in discussions of cardiac auscultatory findings; numerical subscripts are used:

S_1 first heart sound
  M_1 mitral valve component
  T_1 tricuspid valve component

S_2 second heart sound
  A_2 aortic valve component
  P_2 pulmonic valve component

S_3 third heart sound (helpful to indicate if the S_3 is left ventricular or right ventricular)

S_4 fourth heart sound (helpful to indicate if the S_4 is left ventricular or right ventricular)

> The presence of an audible S_3 was consistent with the patient's left ventricular aneurysm.
>
> An audible S_4 may be due to a variety of cardiac and systemic conditions.

Sound names may be written out in full, especially at the beginning of a sentence:

> Third heart sounds are suggestive of congestive heart failure, but an S_3 gallop may be a normal finding in children and young adults.

12.3.3 ***Murmurs.***—Murmurs are graded from soft (lower grade) to loud (higher grade). Murmur grades are written in arabic numerals. Systolic murmurs may be graded from 1 to 6, diastolic from 1 to 4. Murmurs may also be presented using ratios, eg, grade 4/6 systolic murmur, grade 2/4 diastolic murmur.

> The patient had a grade 3 systolic murmur radiating to the axilla consistent with the diagnosis of mitral valve regurgitation.

12.3.4 ***Jugular Venous Pulse.***—The jugular venous pulse contours are expressed with italic single letters and roman words:

a wave (atrial)	*x* descent
z point	*y* descent
c wave	*h* wave
v wave (ventricular)	

12.3.5 ***Echocardiography.***—The names of major echocardiographic methods are listed. Expand any abbreviations at first mention, unless otherwise indicated:

Name	*Common Abbreviation*
2-dimensional echocardiography	2DE
motion mode echocardiography	M-mode echocardiography (expansion not necessary)
Doppler echocardiography	
spectral Doppler echocardiography	
continuous wave Doppler echocardiography	CW Doppler
color flow Doppler, Doppler flow imaging, color Doppler echocardiography	
contrast echocardiography	
transesophageal echocardiography	TEE
stress or exercise or pharmacologic or dobutamine echocardiography	
intravascular ultrasound	IVUS
amplitude modulation echocardiography	A-mode echocardiography (expansion not necessary)
brightness modulation echocardiography	B-mode echocardiography (expansion not necessary)

The following commonly used echocardiographic entities should also be expanded at first mention but are included for reference and to indicate typical use of subscripts:

FS	fractional shortening
FAC	fractional area change
EF	ejection fraction
EPSS	E point septal separation
SAM	systolic anterior motion of the mitral valve
PHT	pressure half-time
MVA	mitral valve area

Table 3. Pacemaker Code*

Position I (Chamber Paced)	Position II (Chamber Sensed)	Position III (Responding to Sensing)	Position IV (Programmability, Rate Modulation)	Position V (Antitachyarrhythmia Functions)
O = none	O = none	O = none	O = none	O = none
A = atrium	A = atrium	T = triggered	P = simple programmable	P = pacing (antitachyarrhythmia)
V = ventricle	V = ventricle	I = inhibited	M = multiprogrammable	S = shock
D = dual (A + V)	D = dual (A + V)	D = dual (T + I)	C = communicating	D = dual (P + S)
			R = rate modulation	

Reprinted from Bernstein et al[1] by permission of Futura Publishing Co.

Table 4. Defibrillator Code*

Position I (Shock Chamber)	Position II (Antitachycardia Pacing Chamber)	Position III (Tachycardia Detection)	Position IV (Antibradycardia Pacing Chamber)
O = none	O = none	E = electrogram	O = none
A = atrium	A = atrium	H = hemodynamic	A = atrium
V = ventricle	V = ventricle		V = ventricle
D = dual (A + V)	D = dual (A + V)		D = dual (A + V)

Reprinted from Bernstein et al[3] by permission of Futura Publishing Co.

AVA	aortic valve area
LVID	left ventricular internal dimension
IVS, IVST	interventricular septal thickness
PW, PWT	posterior wall thickness
d or ed	end diastole (subscript, eg, $LVID_d$)
s or es	end systole (subscript)

Ejection Fraction: Ejection fraction is expressed as a number (eg, 0.60), not as a percentage (not 60%) (see also 15.0, Units of Measure, and 16.0, Numbers and Percentages).

12.3.6 ***Pacemaker Codes.***—The capabilities and operation of cardiac pacemakers are described by 3- to 5-letter codes,[1,2] as in "VVI pacemaker" or "DDIR pacing." The code system for antibradycardia pacemakers and antitachyarrhythmia devices endorsed by the North American Society of Pacing and Electrophysiology and the British Pacing and Electrophysiology Group is known as the NASPE/BPEG Generic Code or NBG Code. Although when mentioned in passing the code need not be expanded, it is good practice to describe pacing modes in prose at first mention, eg, "DDDR (dual-chamber, adaptive-rate) pacing."

In Table 3, positions I through V refer to the first through fifth letters of the NBG Code. The character for "None" is the letter O, not the numeral 0. In practice, the first 3 positions are always given; the fourth and fifth are added when necessary to provide additional information.

12.3.7 ***Implanted Cardioverter/Defibrillators (ICDs).***—A similar code, known as the NASPE/BPEG Defibrillator Code or NBD Code,[3] exists for implanted cardioverter/defibrillators, as defined in Table 4. Examples are "VOEO defibrillator" and "DDH defibrillator."

There is also a Short Form of the NBD code intended only for use in conversation:

ICD-S	ICD with shock capability only
ICD-B	ICD with antibradycardia pacing as well as shock
ICD-T	ICD with antitachycardia pacing as well as shock and antibradycardia pacing

Because ICD-S, ICD-B, and ICD-T can each represent a variety of devices, only the Long Form is used in writing. As in the case of the NBG Code, at first mention of an ICD it is good practice to include a prose description as well as the NBD Code designation.

For maximal conciseness and completeness in ICD labeling and record keeping, the first 3 positions of the NBD Code are given, followed after a hyphen by the first 4 positions of the NBG Code. Thus, "VAE-DDDR" refers to an ICD providing ventricular shock, atrial antitachycardia pacing, electrogram sensing for tachycardia detection, and dual-chamber, adaptive-rate antibradycardia pacing.

REFERENCES

1. Bernstein AD, Camm AJ, Fletcher RD, et al. The NASPE/BPEG Pacemaker Code for antibradyarrhythmia and adaptive-rate pacing and antitachyarrhythmia devices. *Pacing Clin Electrophysiol.* 1987;10:794-799.

2. Bernstein AD, Parsonnet V. Pacemaker and defibrillator codes. In: Ellenbogen K, Kay GN, Wilkoff B, eds. *Textbook of Cardiac Pacing,* Philadelphia, Pa: WB Saunders Co; 1995:279-283.

3. Bernstein AD, Camm AJ, Fisher JD, et al. North American Society of Pacing and Electrophysiology Policy Statement: the NASPE/BPEG Defibrillator Code. *Pacing Clin Electrophysiol.* 1993;16:1776-1780.

ADDITIONAL READINGS AND GENERAL REFERENCES

Freed M, Grines C, eds. *Essentials of Cardiovascular Medicine.* Birmingham, Mich: Physician's Press; 1994.

Isselbacher KJ, Braunwald E, Wilson JD, Martin JB, Fauci AS, Kasper DL, eds. *Harrison's Principles of Internal Medicine.* 13th ed. New York, NY: McGraw-Hill; 1994.

Parsonnet V, Furman S, Smyth NPD. Implantable cardiac pacemakers status report and resource guideline: Pacemaker Study Group. *Circulation.* 1974;50:A21-A35 (of historical interest).

Schlant RC, Alexander RW, eds. *Hurst's The Heart.* 8th ed. New York, NY: McGraw-Hill; 1994.

Swanton RH. *Cardiology Pocket Consultant.* 3rd ed. Boston, Mass: Blackwell Scientific Publications; 1994.

Wagner GS. *Marriott's Practical Electrocardiography.* 9th ed. Baltimore, Md: Williams & Wilkins; 1994.

12.4 ■ **DRUGS.**—Physicians and other health professionals, researchers, manufacturers, and the public may refer to drugs by several names, including the nonproprietary (often referred to as *generic*) name and at least 1 proprietary (brand) or trademark name selected by the manufacturer of the drug. Other drug identifiers include chemical names, trivial (unofficial) names, and code designations.[1(pp6-11)] During the drug development process, different names are used to identify the same substance. The multiplicity of drug identifiers necessitates a consistent and uniform policy when drugs are referred to in biomedical publications, to ensure that the drugs intended are clear and the dosages and forms of administration accurate. To ensure that accurate information is conveyed in biomedical publications, the nonproprietary name should be used whenever possible[1(p6)] (see 12.4.2, Nonproprietary Names). A brief summary of the drug development process is provided here to help readers understand the origins of different drug identifiers.

12.4.1 ***The US Drug Development and Approval Process.***—Drugs approved for human use in the United States must first complete preclinical studies in vitro and in animals for 1 to 5 years (average, 2.6 years), followed by 3 phases of clinical testing. Animal studies are usually continued during clinical testing to monitor long-term toxic effects, teratogenicity, carcinogenicity, and effects on reproduction.[2(p56)] During preclinical studies, a drug is referred to by its chemical name or code designation.

If the drug appears promising for use in humans and the developer of the drug or a sponsoring manufacturer wants to initiate clinical trials, an Investigational New Drug (IND) application must be filed with the US Food and Drug Administration (FDA).[2(p55)] The sponsoring manufacturer must also obtain approval for a nonproprietary name. In the United States, the US Adopted Names (USAN) Council approves the nonproprietary or US adopted name. Until a nonproprietary name has been approved, the developers of a drug may refer to it by a code designation. The code designation is often alphanumeric, with letters to refer to the institution or manufacturer that assigns the code designation for the drug and numbers to refer to the chemical compound.[1(p11)] (For example, the code designation assigned to zidovudine by its manufacturer, Burroughs Wellcome, was BW A509U.)

Phase 1 Studies: Once an IND application has been approved by the FDA, the developers of the drug can begin testing the drug in humans. First, phase 1 studies are conducted in 20 to 80[3(p113)] healthy volunteers, or occasionally special populations such as those with impaired drug metabolism, to establish safety and pharmacologic effects of the drug at escalating doses and to determine detailed pharmacokinetics and drug interactions.[2(p56)]

Phase 2 Studies: Phase 2 studies are conducted to establish the therapeutic efficacy of a drug for its proposed indication and to study dose range, kinetics, adverse effects, and metabolism. The trial usually includes 80 to 100 patients who have the condition under investigation and compares in a randomized manner the new drug with a placebo or active drug already approved for the indication.[3(p113)]

Phase 3 Studies: A phase 3 trial is a randomized controlled trial that tests a drug's efficacy and adverse effects in 500 to 3000 carefully selected patients.[2(p57)] The trial tests the drug under conditions of anticipated usage that will be included in product labeling. Occasionally, if the disease being treated is life-threatening and no effective treatment is available, and results of phase 1 testing are promising, phases 2 and 3 may be omitted as part of the expedited drug approval process. The 3 phases of clinical testing take from 2 to 10 years (average, 5.6 years).[2(p56)]

Preapproval Use: Occasionally, drugs may be used clinically while still in testing. Compassionate use may be justified in a desperate situation when there is no response to available treatment or no recognized treatment is available. However, in the past this use was applied in some cases for thousands of patients, so in 1982 the FDA introduced formally a new category of investigations called *treatment protocols* or *Treatment INDs*.[4(p1661)] Treatment INDs may be used for patients with serious or life-threatening conditions for which no comparable or satisfactory treatment is available, if a drug appears promising and is being studied in ongoing controlled trials.[4(p1661)] (Zidovudine first became available for patients with human immunodeficiency virus infection under a Treatment IND.) In 1992, another form of preapproval use, the Parallel Track drug availability program, became available for drugs used to treat acquired immunodeficiency syndrome (AIDS).[4(p1661)] Although formal assessment of efficacy is not conducted, all preapproval uses require that patients be monitored for adverse events.

New Drug Application: When the sponsor of an IND believes that sufficient information has been generated to support a drug's safety and efficacy, often in consultation with the FDA, the sponsor submits a New Drug Application (NDA) to the FDA. The NDA includes all research data and information regarding development accumulated in the study of a new drug. The NDAs received by the FDA are prioritized according to the potential benefits of the drug, with drugs intended to treat life-threatening conditions being given the highest priority. Time from submission to approval of an NDA ranges from 2 months to 7 years (average, 2.6 years).[2(p56)]

FDA Approval: When a drug is approved by the FDA, the FDA approves labeling for the drug that defines the indications for which the drug can be marketed. The

FDA does not approve indications for which a drug may be prescribed. The package insert is intended for use by physicians and includes pharmacologic information, approved indications, contraindications, precautions, warnings, adverse reactions, usual dosage, and available preparations.[2(pp56-57)] Changes in labeling to include new indications must be requested by the pharmaceutical company through a Supplemental New Drug Application. The *Physicians' Desk Reference*[5] provides verbatim the approved labeling for a drug.

Postmarketing Surveillance: After a drug has been approved and marketed, the pharmaceutical company marketing the drug must report adverse drug reactions and drug toxic effects to the FDA. Although pharmaceutical companies may conduct postmarketing surveillance or phase 4 testing, formal analysis is usually conducted only if reports of adverse events suggest the possibility of harm. All physicians in the United States participate in phase 4 testing through the voluntary reporting system MEDWATCH.[6] Physicians in the United Kingdom, Canada, New Zealand, Denmark, and Sweden participate in legally mandated adverse event reporting systems.[2(p58)]

Orphan Drugs: Orphan drug products are a category of drugs that are unlikely to be profitable commercially but may be useful for rare diseases. To encourage development of such drugs, the FDA, under the Orphan Drug Act of 1983,[7] may give a drug a special orphan product classification. Orphan drugs are listed in the *USP Dictionary of USAN and International Drug Names (USP Dictionary).*[1(pp817-844)]

12.4.2 ***Nonproprietary Names.***—The nonproprietary or generic name is the established, official name of a drug. The nonproprietary name is in the public domain and therefore may be used without restrictions. In the United States and other countries, the drug manufacturer is required by law to use the nonproprietary name in labels, advertising, and brochures. In the United States, nonproprietary names for new chemical entities of potential medicinal use are approved by the USAN Council. The USAN Council follows established rules and guidelines for creating new nonproprietary names.[1(pp6-7)] Suffixes common to a particular drug class ("stems") are incorporated into new drug names to indicate a chemical and/or pharmacological relationship to older drugs,[1(p846)] for example:

cimetidine, ranitidine, famotidine

diazepam, lorazepam, clonazepam

saquinavir, ritonavir, telinavir

A table of "stems" is provided in the *USP Dictionary.*[1(pp849-852)]

Drug nomenclature councils also exist (as of 1996) in Great Britain, France, Italy, Japan, the Scandinavian countries, Spain, and Switzerland. The World Health Organization (WHO) International Nonproprietary Name (INN) Committee makes recommendations to each of the drug nomenclature councils to maintain consistent nomenclature and to attempt to identify a single INN that will be used by all countries and will not be confused with other drug names already in use. However, because drugs are marketed under different proprietary names in different countries, proprietary and proposed nonproprietary names may conflict in one country but not in another. When this occurs, the nomenclature agency of the country with the potential conflict may choose to approve a nonproprietary name different from the name approved as the INN.[1(p8)] The INN, USAN, and other nonproprietary names are provided in the *USP Dictionary.*[1]

Nonproprietary names may also differ among countries if the substance was in existence before the coordination of nomenclature by the WHO. The drug named acetaminophen in the United States is one example; its INN, British Approved Name (BAN), and Dénomination Commune Français (DCF, French approved nonproprietary name) is paracetamol. Similarly, the USAN albuterol has an INN and a BAN of salbutamol.[1(p29)] For AMA publications, the USAN should be used preferentially, although for international audiences providing both the USAN and the INN at first mention would be appropriate.

> Acetaminophen (paracetamol) was recommended as an initial treatment for pain in the practice guidelines.

Databases: Unfortunately, databases used for searching the medical literature about a specific topic do not link all nonproprietary names as search terms (although other nonproprietary names may be listed as synonyms). If more than one nonproprietary name exists internationally, all nonproprietary names listed in the *USP Dictionary*[1] should be used as search terms to ensure that the relevant material is identified.

Changes in Nonproprietary Names: Nonproprietary names may be changed if they are believed to be potentially confusing. For example, one antineoplastic compound was originally named *mithramycin*, but the name was changed to *plicamycin* to avoid confusing mithramycin with the similar-sounding antineoplastic mitomycin and its proprietary name Mutamycin.

12.4.3 ***Proprietary Names.***—The manufacturer's name for a drug (or other product) is called a *proprietary name, trademark,* or *brand name*.[1(p10)] Proprietary names for drugs often differ between countries (for example, nifedipine initially was marketed as Procardia in the United States and Adalat in Europe). Most US proprietary names are listed in the *USP Dictionary*[1] and cross-referenced to their USAN name.

Proprietary names use initial capitals, with a few exceptions (eg, pHisoHex). AMA publications do not use the trademark symbol (TM) because capitalization indicates the proprietary nature of the name (see also 3.6, Ethical and Legal Considerations, Intellectual Property: Ownership, Rights, and Management). The International Trademark Association has information about specific trademarks and may be reached at http://plaza.interport.net/inta/tmchklst.htm or INTA, 1133 Avenue of the Americas, New York, NY 10036-6710.[8]

Use of Proprietary Names in Scientific Articles: Proprietary names should not be used in scientific articles except in specific instances in which the proprietary name is essential to reproduce or interpret the study. For example, the proprietary name should be provided if a study reports an adverse event that might be unique to a specific product formulation or if a study compares a generic formulation of a drug with the drug that was first approved. When both the nonproprietary and proprietary names are listed in text, the nonproprietary name should be listed first, with the proprietary name capitalized and in parentheses.

> The lot of penicillin G potassium (Pentids) was inspected and found to meet the industry production standards.

Proprietary names may be used in questionnaires when the individuals being questioned may be unfamiliar with the nonproprietary name or if the specific proprietary product is important; in that case the exact wording of the question should be maintained but the nonproprietary name should still be provided.

Parents were asked, "Have you ever given your child Tylenol [acetaminophen], products containing Tylenol, or any other Tylenol-containing products?"

12.4.4 ***Chemical Names.***—The chemical name describes a drug in terms of its chemical structure.[1(p9)] Chemical names are rarely used in medical publications, and the nonproprietary name is preferred.

zidovudine (3′-azido-3′-deoxythymidine)

triamterene (2,4,7-triamino-6-phenylpteridine)

12.4.5 ***Code Designations.***—A code designation is a temporary designation assigned to a product by the institution or manufacturer and may be used to refer to a drug under development before a nonproprietary name has been assigned. Codes may be numeric, alphabetic, or alphanumeric; alphanumeric codes often include letters to designate the institution or manufacturer assigning the code designation of the drug, followed by numbers to designate the chemical compound.[1(p11)] In contrast to proprietary names, the code designations for compounds are usually identical regardless of the country in which they are studied.

Because code designations become obsolete in the literature once a nonproprietary name has been assigned, code designations are rarely seen in medical publications. If both the code and nonproprietary name are provided, such as in an article discussing the history of a drug, the nonproprietary name should be used preferentially.

Zidovudine was originally assigned the code BW A509U. It became known as azidothymidine (AZT) during testing and eventually was marketed as Retrovir by its manufacturer, Burroughs Wellcome.

Semustine was developed under the code NSC-95441, but was referred to in scientific literature by its trivial name, methyl-CCNU, a contraction of its chemical name 1-(2-chloroethyl)-3-(4-methylcyclohexyl)-1-nitrosourea.

12.4.6 ***Trivial Names.***—Drugs occasionally become known by an unofficial trivial name (*trivial* in this case refers to the unofficial status of the name). The trivial name should be used in biomedical publications only when the name was used specifically as part of a study (eg, in a questionnaire) or on rare occasions when readers may be unfamiliar with the nonproprietary name. In either case, the nonproprietary name should be used preferentially and the trivial name provided in parentheses at first mention.

The subjects were asked, "Have you ever taken AZT [zidovudine] or ddI [didanosine]?" Subjects who said they had taken zidovudine or didanosine were classified as having had prior exposure to antiretroviral agents.

12.4.7 ***Drugs With Nonbase Moieties.***—Drugs often contain a component that, although not directly responsible for the drug's mechanism of action, lends chemical stability or increases bioavailability.[1(pp846-847)] Since different formulations of a drug may require different dosages for an equivalent effect and may have a different spectrum of effects, the complete nonproprietary name should be provided at first mention in both the abstract and the text (for exceptions to this rule, see Circumstances in Which the Nonbase Moiety May Not Require Mention). If editors encounter a nonproprietary name in text that may also exist with a nonbase moiety (eg, tetracycline is mentioned, which could also be tetracycline hydrochloride or tetracycline phosphate complex), the editor should clarify with the author which drug compound is meant.

The inactive moieties include salts, esters, and complexes. Salts may contain, for example, sodium, potassium, chloride, hydrochloride, sulfate, mesylate, or fumarate.

acyclovir sodium

midazolam hydrochloride

benztropine mesylate

morphine sulfate

Quaternary ammonium salts usually are designated by a 2-part name and have the suffix *-ium* on the first word of the name.

atracurium besylate

alcuronium chloride

octonium bromide

Salts and esters are frequently designated by the ending *-ate*. Salts and esters can have a 1- or 2-word nonproprietary name. Three-word names are used for compounds that are both salts and esters.

clomegestone acetate [ester]

hydrocortisone valerate [ester]

testosterone cypionate [ester]

methylprednisolone sodium phosphate [salt and ester]

roxatidine acetate hydrochloride [ester and salt]

Complexes may contain the word *complex* or a second word ending in *-ex*.

bisacodyl tannex

nicotine polacrilex

tetracycline phosphate complex

Nonbase Moieties Used With Proprietary Names: The nonbase substance may also be used with the proprietary name.

Apresoline Hydrochloride is a proprietary name for hydralazine hydrochloride.

If both the nonproprietary name and the proprietary name are provided, the inactive moiety is given only once.

The patient had been taking hydralazine (Apresoline) hydrochloride for a week before developing an urticarial papular rash.

Circumstances in Which the Nonbase Moiety Should Not Be Used: When a drug is mentioned in the context of testing a microorganism's susceptibility to the drug, the concentration of the drug measured in body fluids, or a patient's allergy to the drug, only the base substance of the drug should be named. (Since the nonbase substance is no longer part of the drug once it has been absorbed [ie, a drug that has dissolved will be dissociated from its salt], a microorganism will be susceptible or not susceptible to the base substance only, and the concentration of a drug in the bloodstream reflects only the concentration of the base substance. A person allergic to a drug with a base substance and nonbase substance likely will be allergic to any drug with the same base substance.)

> The strain of *Streptococcus pneumoniae* isolated by the laboratory was highly resistant to penicillin.

> The patient's plasma lithium level at 8 AM was 2.0 mmol/L.

Circumstances in Which the Nonbase Moiety May Not Require Mention: In some circumstances in which brevity is important, such as titles or headings in the text, providing only the active portion of the drug name may be sufficient. In these cases the complete name should be given in the text. Referring to the base substance alone may also be appropriate for brevity when drugs are referred to in general, such as in editorials or other text that does not refer to specific dosages. However, if an article refers to 2 different formulations of the same drug and the distinction is important, the nonbase moiety should be mentioned along with the base substance in the title and throughout the text.

> The β-blockers most selective for β_1 activity are bisoprolol and metoprolol; acebutolol, carvedilol, and nebivolol are somewhat selective. All lose their selectivity when given at higher doses.

> Long-acting calcium channel blockers were not available at the time; only nifedipine, diltiazem, and verapamil had been approved by the Food and Drug Administration.

12.4.8 ***Combination Products.***—For combination products (mixtures), the names of the active ingredients should be provided. The proprietary name of the combination may be given in parentheses, if necessary to clarify the product to which the article refers.

> pseudoephedrine hydrochloride and triprolidine hydrochloride (Actifed)

> povidone and hydroxyethylcellulose (Adsorbotear)

If the list of active ingredients is too long to use when referring to the combination product, the active ingredients should be listed at first mention along with the proprietary name and either an abbreviation or, if necessary, the proprietary name used thereafter.

> The patient reported having taken several doses of Vanex-HD (a liquid suspension of hydrocodone bitartrate, 10 mg, phenylephrine hydrochloride, 30 mg, and chlorpheniramine maleate, 12 mg, per 30 mL) the previous day.

> The patient had been administered an artificial tear product (Adsorbotear, a sterile solution containing 0.42% hydroxyethylcellulose and 1.67% povidone).

Only the active ingredients must be listed. However, in some circumstances it may be necessary to include all ingredients, including preservatives, if sensitivity to an ingredient may be important.

> The patient had complained of red, itching eyes after using an artificial tear product (Adsorbotear, a sterile solution containing hydroxyethylcellulose and povidone with edetate disodium and thimerosal as preservatives).

The prefix *co-* is sometimes used for combination products. The USP may provide a Pharmacy Equivalent Name (PEN)[1(pp8-9)] to refer to a combination product, such as co-triamterzide for the combination of triamterene and hydrochlorothiazide. However, PEN terms should be used only if they are familiar and clear to readers.

Since co-triamterzide is unlikely to be familiar to most readers, the following approach can be used:

> Subjects were given a capsule containing a combination of 25 mg of hydrochlorothiazide and 50 mg of triamterene each day at 8 AM. If subjects were not able to tolerate hydrochlorothiazide-triamterene, they were given 50 mg of metoprolol at 8 AM.
>
> Trimethoprim-sulfamethoxazole (80 mg of trimethoprim and 400 mg of sulfamethoxazole) administered once daily effectively prevented reinfection in 93% of patients.

12.4.9 ***Multiple-Drug Regimens.***—Regimens that include multiple drugs may be referred to by an abbreviation after the nonproprietary names of the drugs have been provided at first mention (and dosages have been provided if appropriate) (see also 11.11, Abbreviations, Clinical and Technical Terms). Drug regimens used in oncology frequently use abbreviations to refer to the combinations of antineoplastic agents, but often the abbreviations are not derived from the USAN names. For example, the letter *O* in MOPP is derived from Oncovin, the proprietary name for vincristine sulfate, and the *A* in ABVD is derived from Adriamycin, the proprietary name for doxorubicin hydrochloride. The proprietary name may be provided in parentheses after the nonproprietary name to clarify the origin of the abbreviation.

> The MOPP (methotrexate, vincristine sulfate [Oncovin], prednisone, and procarbazine hydrochloride) regimen for advanced Hodgkin disease was compared with MOPP alternating with ABVD (doxorubicin hydrochloride [Adriamycin], bleomycin sulfate, vinblastine sulfate, and dacarbazine).

12.4.10 ***Special Drug Categories.***—Special drug categories, such as hormones given as drugs, other endogenous substances, and vitamins, require special mention since the drug name differs from the name used for the endogenous substance. Using the appropriate name can help clarify that the substance referred to is a drug, although for less familiar drug names it may be necessary to include the endogenous hormone name in parentheses to clarify the action of the drug for readers. (For more information on appropriate abbreviations for hormones, see 11.11, Abbreviations, Clinical and Technical Terms.)

Hypothalamic Hormones: The USAN Council in conjunction with the WHO Committee has chosen the suffix *-relin* to denote hypothalamic peptide hormones that stimulate release of pituitary hormones and the suffix *-relix* for hormones that inhibit release.

Native Substance	*Diagnostic/Therapeutic Agent*
thyrotropin-releasing hormone (TRH)	protirelin
luteinizing hormone-releasing hormone (LHRH) (or gonadotropin-releasing hormone [GnRH])	buserelin acetate, gonadorelin acetate (or hydrochloride), histrelin, lutrelin acetate, nafarelin acetate
growth hormone-releasing factor (GHRF)	somatorelin
growth hormone release-inhibiting factor (somatostatin, GHRIF)	detirelix acetate

Example:

> After venipuncture, protirelin (synthetic thyrotropin-releasing hormone) was injected.

Pituitary Hormones: Nonproprietary names for synthetic corticotropins use suffixes such as *-actide, -tropin,* and *-pressin*.

Native Substance	*Diagnostic/Therapeutic Agent*
corticotropin (ACTH)	seractide acetate, cosyntropin, corticotropin
growth hormone (GH)	somatrem, somatropin
follicle-stimulating hormone (FSH), luteinizing hormone (LH)	urofollitropin (FSH only); follitropin alfa, follitropin beta (FSH manufactured from recombinant DNA); menotropins (both LH and FSH)
thyroid-stimulating hormone (TSH)	thyrotropin
arginine vasopressin (AVP)	vasopressin

Thyroid Hormones: Abbreviations for thyroxine and triiodothyronine are provided in parentheses and may be used after the name is expanded at first mention.

Description	*Therapeutic Agent*
levorotatory thyroxine (T_4)	levothyroxine sodium
triiodothyronine (T_3)	liothyronine sodium
dextrorotatory triiodothyronine	dextrothyroxine sodium
mixture of liothyronine and levothyroxine sodium	liotrix sodium
thyroid gland extract	thyroglobulin

Other Hormones Administered as Drugs: Hormones normally released by the placenta may also be used as drugs.

gonadotropin, chorionic (human chorionic gonadotropin)

Insulin: Insulin terminology can be a source of clinically important confusion, particularly with regard to insulin concentrations and types. Insulin concentrations are as follows (not necessary to expand at first mention):

U100	contains 100 U/mL (the most commonly used concentration)
U40	contains 40 U/mL
U80	contains 80 U/mL (no longer available in the United States)
U500	contains 500 U/mL (for use in severe insulin resistance)

Insulin types include those that may be administered intravenously, subcutaneously, or intramuscularly (termed *injections*), and those that may be administered only subcutaneously or intramuscularly (termed *suspensions*). Insulin is prepared with the use of recombinant DNA technology (referred to as *insulin, human,* since the source is human DNA) or as a synthetic modification of porcine insulin.

Injections

Preferred Term	*Other Terms*
insulin injection	regular insulin
insulin injection, human	regular insulin, human

Suspensions

Preferred Term	*Proprietary Name*
insulin zinc [suspension], prompt	Semilente (proprietary)
insulin zinc [suspension]	Lente (proprietary)
insulin zinc [suspension], extended	Ultralente
insulin [suspension], isophane	NPH
insulin [suspension], protamine zinc	

Note: The following section on nomenclature for biological products was adapted from the *USP Dictionary,*[1(pp847-848)] with permission (Copyright 1996, USP Convention Inc).

Interferons: Use the nonproprietary names and trademarks given in the *USP Dictionary,*[1] which also provides the following nomenclature system[1(p847-848)] (see also 12.8.5, Cytokines):

interferon alfa (formerly leukocyte or lymphoblastoid interferon)

The *f* is used rather than *ph* to avoid the confusing *ph* in international usage. When referring to interferon outside the therapeutic context, ie, when the nonproprietary name is not being used, then "alpha" is acceptable, eg, "the alpha interferons."

interferon beta (formerly fibroblast interferon)

interferon gamma (formerly immune interferon)

Subcategories are designated by a numeral and lowercase letter. The numbers conform to the recommendation of the International Nomenclature Committee; the lowercase letter after the number is assigned by the drug nomenclature committee to differentiate one manufacturer's interferon from another's. Examples of pure interferons are as follows:

interferon alfa-2a

interferon alfa-2b

interferon beta-1a

interferon beta-1b

interferon gamma-la

The following are names of mixtures of interferons from natural sources (designated by "n" preceding the arabic numeral):

interferon alfa-n1

interferon alfa-n2

Interleukins: The suffix ***-leukin*** is used for naming interleukin 2 type substances (see also 12.8.5, Cytokines).

aldesleukin

celmoleukin

teceleukin

Colony-Stimulating Factors: Recombinant colony-stimulating factors are named according to the following guidelines[1(p848)] (see also 12.8.5, Cytokines):

The suffix ***-grastim*** is used for granulocyte colony-stimulating factors (G-CSF):

lenograstim

filgrastim

The suffix ***-gramostim*** is used for granulocyte macrophage colony-stimulating factors (GM-CSF):

molgramostim

regramostim

sargramostim

The suffix ***-mostim*** is used for macrophage colony-stimulating factors (M-CSF):

mirimostim

The suffix ***-plestim*** is under consideration for interleukin 3 (IL-3) and derivatives.

Erythropoietins: The word *epoetin* is used to describe erythropoietin preparations that have an amino acid sequence identical to the endogenous cytokine. The words *alfa, beta,* and *gamma* are added to designate differences in composition and carbohydrate moieties on the compound.[1(p848)]

epoetin alfa

epoetin beta

epoetin gamma

Monoclonal Antibodies: The suffix ***-mab*** is used for monoclonal antibodies and fragments. Monoclonal antibodies are derived from animals as well as from humans and the nomenclature is based on the source of the antibody (mouse, rat, hamster, primate, or human) and the disease target or antibody subclass. More details regarding nomenclature are available from the *USP Dictionary.*[1(p848)] Some examples of monoclonal antibodies follow:

abciximab

dacliximab

satumomab

If the monoclonal antibody is radiolabeled or conjugated to a chemical such as a toxin, additional designations are used. When a toxin is used, *-tox* is used in a second word to name the conjugate:

zolimomab aritox

For radiolabeled products, the isotope, element symbol, and isotope number precede the monoclonal antibody:

technetium Tc 99m biciromab

indium In 111 altumomab pentetate

Vitamins and Related Compounds: The familiar letter names of most vitamins are reserved for referring to the substances as found in food and in vivo. The same vitamins given therapeutically have other nonproprietary USAN names listed in the *USP Dictionary.*[1] The following are some examples:

Native Vitamin	*Drug Name*
vitamin A	beta carotene
vitamin B_1	thiamine hydrochloride
vitamin B_1 mononitrate	thiamine mononitrate
vitamin B_2	riboflavin
vitamin B_6	pyridoxine hydrochloride
vitamin B_8	adenosine phosphate
vitamin B_{12}	cyanocobalamin
vitamin C	ascorbic acid
vitamin D	cholecalciferol
vitamin D_1	dihydrotachysterol
vitamin D_2	ergocalciferol
vitamin E	vitamin E
vitamin G	riboflavin
vitamin K_1	phytonadione
folate	folic acid
niacin	nicotinic acid
niacinamide	nicotinamide

REFERENCES

1. Fleeger CA, ed. *USP Dictionary of USAN and International Drug Names.* 34th ed. Rockville, Md: US Pharmacopoeial Convention Inc; 1996.

2. Nies AS, Spielberg SP. Principles of therapeutics. In: Hardman JG, Limbird LE, eds. *Goodman & Gilman's The Pharmacological Basis of Therapeutics.* 9th ed. New York, NY: McGraw-Hill Book Co; 1996.

3. McPhillips JJ. Drug testing in humans. In: Craig CR, Stitzel RE, eds. *Modern Pharmacology.* 3rd ed. Boston, Mass: Little Brown & Co Inc; 1990:108-113.

4. Temple R. Development of drug law, regulations, and guidance in the United States. In: Munson PL, ed. *Principles of Pharmacology: Basic Concepts and Clinical Applications.* New York, NY: International Thomson Publishing; 1996.

5. *Physicians' Desk Reference.* 50th ed. Montvale, NJ: Medical Economics; 1996.

6. Kessler DA. Introducing MEDWATCH, a new approach to reporting medication and device adverse effects and product problems. *JAMA.* 1993;269:2765-2768.

7. Orphan Drug Act, Pub L No. 97-414.

8. Kruh S. Trademark checklist. *Editorial Eye.* May 1997:10.

Additional Readings and General References

Billups NF, Billups SM, eds. *American Drug Index.* 40th ed. St Louis, Mo: Facts and Comparisons; 1996.

Olin BR, ed. *Drug Facts and Comparisons.* St Louis, Mo: Facts and Comparisons; 1995.

Reynolds JEF, ed. *Martindale: The Extra Pharmacopoeia.* 30th ed. London, England: The Pharmaceutical Press; 1993.

12.5 ■ **EQUIPMENT, DEVICES, AND REAGENTS.**—As with drugs and isotopes, nonproprietary names or descriptive phrasing is preferred to proprietary names for devices, equipment, and reagents. However, if several brands of the same product are being compared or if the use of proprietary names would enhance clarity, proprietary names should be given at first mention along with the nonproprietary name. Occasionally information regarding the manufacturer or supplier and location is important and authors should include this information in parentheses after the nonproprietary name or description. Authors should provide this information for any reagents, antibodies, enzymes, or probes used in investigations.

> Currently, treatment by Nd:YAG laser is the accepted method to surgically open the opacified posterior capsule. [This general statement does not require specific product information.]
>
> The positron emission tomography (PET) unit (4096 Plus; General Electric Systems, Milwaukee, Wis) comprised 8 detector rings positioned in a cylindrical array. Image processing and reconstruction were performed with a VAX 4000-300 computer system and a VAX 3100 workstation (Digital Equipment, Marlboro, Mass). [For the methods section of a study, specific equipment information is important to enable another researcher to attempt to replicate the study.]
>
> All magnetic resonance angiography examinations were performed with a 1.5-T whole-body imager (General Electric Medical Systems, Milwaukee, Wis).

As with drugs and isotopes, proprietary names should be capitalized; the registered trademark symbol is not used.

> Some hearing loss may result from use of a portable radio or cassette player equipped with headphones (Walkman-style) played at high decibel levels. [More specific information is not needed since the brand name is used as a generic description of a product.]

If a device is described as "modified," the modification should be explained or an explanatory reference cited. If equipment or apparatus is provided free of charge by the manufacturer, this fact should be included in the acknowledgments (see 2.10.2, Manuscript Preparation, Acknowledgments, Other Assistance).

If a study evaluates a medical device that has not been approved by the Food and Drug Administration, the author of the study should specify whether the device is considered a significant or nonsignificant risk device (as defined under the Medical Device Amendments of 1976[1]) and provide information regarding institutional review board approval and patient informed consent, just as with a drug study.

REFERENCE

1. Medical Device Amendments, Pub L No. 94-295.

12.6 ■ GENETICS.

12.6.1 *Nucleic Acids and Amino Acids.*—The recommendations in this section are based on conventions put forth by the IUPAC-IUB Commission on Biochemical Nomenclature.[1]

DNA: The 2 nucleic acids, DNA and RNA, are nucleotide polymers whose function in living systems is to transmit genetic information.

Deoxyribonucleic acid, or DNA, is the embodiment of the genetic code and is contained in the chromosomes. It is made up of molecules called *bases,* the sugar 2-deoxyribose, and phosphate groups. The bases fall into 2 classes: *pyrimidine* and *purine*.

Structurally, DNA is a helical polymer of deoxyribose linked by phosphate groups; 1 of its 4 bases projects from each sugar molecule of the sugar-phosphate chain.

A base-sugar unit is a *nucleoside.* A base-sugar-phosphate unit is a *nucleotide.*

Each nucleotide has a 1-letter designation, corresponding to the base in that nucleotide. These letters are commonly used without expansion:

Base	*Nucleoside*	*Nucleotide Abbreviation*	*Molecular Class*
thymine	thymidine	T	pyrimidine
cytosine	cytidine	C	pyrimidine
adenine	adenosine	A	purine
guanine	guanosine	G	purine

When a nucleotide in a sequence is not specified as T, C, A, or G, additional single-letter designators are used; because these are not as well known, it is best to define them as shown below (adapted from Liébecq[1(p123)] by permission of Portland Press and The Biochemical Society):

Symbol	*Stands for*	*Explanation*
R	G or A	puRine
Y	T or C	pYrimidine
M	A or C	aMino
K	G or T	Keto
S	G or C	Strong interaction (3 H bonds)
W	A or T	Weak interaction (2 H bonds)
H	A or C or T	not G (H follows G in alphabet)
B	G or T or C	not A (B follows A)
V	G or C or A	not T (not U [see RNA]; V follows U)
D	G or A or T	not C (D follows C)
N	G or A or T or C	aNy base

Several forms of DNA are commonly abbreviated as follows; expand at first use:

bDNA	branched DNA
cDNA	complementary DNA
dsDNA	double-stranded DNA
hn-cDNA	heteronuclear cDNA (heterogeneous nuclear cDNA)
mtDNA	mitochondrial DNA
nDNA	nuclear DNA
rDNA	recombinant DNA
rDNA	ribosomal DNA
scDNA	single-copy DNA
ssDNA	single-stranded DNA

There are 4 known classes of DNA helices, which differ in the direction of rotation and the tightness of the spiral (number of base pairs per turn):

A-DNA

B-DNA

C-DNA

Z-DNA

In eukaryotic cells, DNA is bound with protein in a complex known as chromatin. DNA in chromatin is organized into nucleosomes by proteins known as histones. The 5 classes of histones are as follows:

H1

H2A

H2B

H3

H4

Almost all DNA exists in the form of a double helix, in which 2 DNA polymers are paired, linked by hydrogen bonds between individual bases on each chain. Because of the biochemical structure of the nucleotides, A always pairs with T and C with G. Such pairs individually may be indicated as follows:

A · T   C · G

In the event of a mispairing (eg, as a consequence of a mutation), a mismatch may be indicated as follows:

C · T

Base pairs are often quantified and then are abbreviated as bp (base pairs), kbp (thousand base pairs), or Mbp (million base pairs):

a 235-bp repeat sequence

a 47-kbp vector genome

1 Mbp of DNA

The size of the human haploid genome is $3.3 \cdot 10^9$ bp.[2]

Sometimes length of nucleotide molecules is qualified using the suffix *-mer,* eg:

20mer 20 nucleotides

24mer 24 nucleotides

(This formation is based on the terms *dimer, trimer, tetramer,* etc.)
A DNA sequence might be depicted as follows:

GTCGACTG

A double-stranded sequence consisting of the above strand and its complement would be:

GTCGACTG
CAGCTGAC

To show correct pairing between the bases in the 2 strands, sequences need to be aligned properly. In the sequence above, the first base pair is G · C, the next is T · A, etc. The first G is above the first C, the first T above the first A, etc.

A codon is a sequence of 3 nucleotides in a DNA molecule that codes for an amino acid or biosynthetic message. Codons are also referred to as codon triplets. Examples are shown below:

CAT ATC ATT

The genetic code—the complete list of each codon and its specific product—is widely reproduced, eg, in medical dictionaries and textbooks.

Sequences of repeating single nucleotides are named as follows:

polyA polyT polyC polyG

or, optionally, with lowercase d for deoxyribose:

poly(dT)

The phosphate groups are sometimes indicated with a lowercase p, and methylated bases with a superscript lowercase m, eg:

pGpApApTpTpC

$GAT^{m}CC$

The m applies to the next base to the right, as does the p when it is within an expression (ie, not referring to the 3′ or 5′ terminal phosphate).

Sequences of repeating nucleotides, also known as tandem repeats, are indicated as follows (n represents the number of repeats):

$(TTAGGG)_n$

$(GT)_n$

$(CGG)_n$

The carbons and nitrogens of the bases are numbered 1 through 6 (pyrimidines) or 1 through 9 (purines), and the carbons of deoxyribose are numbered 1′ through 5′.

The phosphates that join the DNA nucleotides link the 5′-carbon of 1 deoxyribose to the 3′ carbon of the next deoxyribose. For single strands, the 5′ end is at the left and the 3′ end at the right; thus, a sequence such as the following:

CCCATCTCACTTAGCTCCAATG

would be assumed to have this directionality:

5′-CCCATCTCACTTAGCTCCAATG-3′

The complementary strands of dsDNA have opposite directionality; by convention, the top strand reads from the 5′ end to the 3′ end, while its complementary strand appears below it with the 3′ end on the left. The example

CCCATCTCACTTAGCTCCAATG
GGGTAGAGTGAATCGAGGTTAC

would imply this directionality:

5′-CCCATCTCACTTAGCTCCAATG-3′
3′-GGGTAGAGTGAATCGAGGTTAC-5′

Long sequences pose special typesetting problems. Such sequences should be depicted as separate figures, rather than within text or tables, whenever possible.

For DNA, first and foremost it must be made clear whether the sequence is single-stranded or double-stranded. Double-stranded sequences such as:

CCCATCTCACTTAGCTCCAATG
GGGTAGAGTGAATCGAGGTTAC

have been mistaken for single-stranded sequences and set as such, eg:

CCCATCTCACTTAGCTCCAATGGGGTAGAGTGAATCGAGGTTAC

Of course, conversely, mistaking a single-stranded sequence for a double-stranded sequence and typesetting accordingly would also be an error.

Always maintain alignment in 2-stranded sequences—take care not to have this:

CCCATCTCACTTAGCTCCAATG
GGGTAGAGTGAATCGAGGTTAC

become this:

 CCCATCTCACTTAGCTCCAATG
GGGTAGAGTGAATCGAGGTTAC

Numbering and spacing may be used as visual aids in presenting sequences. A space every 3 bases indicates the codon triplets:

. . . GCA GAG GAC CTG CAG GTG GGG . . .

In a sequence that consists of exons and introns, more than 1 type of spacing is used. An intron that actually occurs within the above sequence is designated by the 5-base groups on either side of the middle ellipsis (examples from Cooper[3(p273)]):

. . . GCA GAG GAC CTG CAG G GTGAG . . . GGCAG TG GGG . . .

In longer sequences, spaces every 5 or 10 bases are customary visual aids, eg:

GAATT CCTGAC CTCAG GTGAT CTGCC CGCCT CGGCC TCCCA AAGTG CTGG

GAATTCCTGA CCTCAGGTGA TCTGCCCGCC TCGGCCTCCC AAAGTGCTGG

Several types of numbering are further aids. In the following example (from Cooper[3(p133)]), numbers on the left specify the number of the first base on that line and "lowercase letters indicate uncertainty in the base call":

1	5′-GAATTCCTGA	CCTCAGGTGA	TCTGCCCGCC	TCGGCCTCCC	AAAGTGCTGG
51	GATTTACAGG	CATGAGGCAC	CACACCTGGC	CAGTTGCTTA	GCTCTCTAAG
101	TCTTATTTGC	TTTACTTACA	AAATGGAGAT	ACAACCTTAT	AGAACATTCG
151	ACATATACTA	GGTTTCCATG	AACAGCAGCC	AGATCTCAAC	TATATAGGGA
201	CCAGTGAGAA	ACCAATCTCA	GGTAGCTGAT	GATGGGCAAa	GGgATGGGgA
251	CTGATATGCC	cNNNNNGACG	ATTCGAGTGA	CAAGCTACTA	TGTACCTCAG
301	CTTTtCATCT	tGATCTTCAC	CACCCATGGg	TAGGTGTCAC	TGAAaTT-3′

Alternatively, numbers may appear above bases of special interest:

     6   39
GAATTCCTGA CCTCAGGTGA TCTGCCCGCC TCGGCCTCCC AAAGTGCTGG

When a long sequence is run within text, use a hyphen at the right-hand end of the line to indicate the bond linking successive bases:

GATTTACAGGCATGAGGCACCACACCTGGCCAGTTGCTTAGCTCTCTAAGTCTTAT-
TGCTTTACTTACAAAATGGAGATACAACCTTATAGACATTCG

A hyphen is not necessary if spacing is used, as long as the break between groups occurs at the end of the line, eg:

. . . 5′CCT GGG

CAA AGC AAG GTA GG-3′

Recognition sequences are sections of a sequence recognized by proteins such as restriction enzymes that cleave DNA in specific locations (see below, Nucleic Acid Analysis and Modification). To indicate sites of cleavage, virgules may be used, eg:

GT/MKAC

GG/CGCGCC

C/TCGTG

Mutations—Nucleotides (see also Mutations—Amino Acids): Various shorthand forms using the single-letter nucleotide abbreviations can be used to designate mutations. In general medical publications, textual explanations should accompany the shorthand terms at first mention:

G1691A	G-to-A substitution at nucleotide 1691
977insA	A inserted at base 977
186/insC/187	frameshift mutation with insertion of C between nucleotides 186 and 187
Y253N	missense mutation with a pyrimidine at position 253 replaced by another base
185delAG	deletion of A and G at position 185
617delT	deletion of T at position 617
926ins11	insertion of 11 bases at position 926
188del11	11-bp deletion at nucleotide 188
1294del40	40-bp deletion at nucleotide 1294

RNA: Functionally associated with DNA is ribonucleic acid (RNA). It contains the 3 bases cytosine (C), adenine (A), and guanine (G) but differs from DNA in having the base uracil (U; nucleoside: uridine) instead of thymine (T) and the sugar ribose rather than deoxyribose.

An example of an RNA sequence is:

5′-UUAGCACGUGCUAA-3′

Examples of RNA codons are:

CAU UUG AUU

Expand these commonly described types of RNA at first use:

cRNA	complementary RNA
hnRNA	heterogeneous nuclear RNA
mRNA	messenger RNA
mtRNA	mitochondrial RNA
nRNA	nuclear RNA
rRNA	ribosomal RNA
snRNA	small nuclear RNA
tRNA	transfer RNA

Types of tRNA may be further specified; follow typographic style closely (these need not be expanded):

$tRNA^{fMet}$	tRNA specific for formylmethionine
$fMet\text{-}tRNA^{fMet}$ *or* $fMet\text{-}tRNA_f$	*N*-formylmethionyl-tRNA
$tRNA^{Met}$	tRNA specific for methionine
$Met\text{-}tRNA^{Met}$	methionyl-tRNA

aminoacyl-tRNAs (see also Amino Acids):

$tRNA^{Ala}$	tRNA specific for alanine
$tRNA^{Val}$	tRNA specific for valine

The 3-dimensional structure of tRNA has several different arms: the amino acid arm, the DHU (dihydrouridine) arm, and the anticodon arm. The fourth arm of tRNA contains the unusual base pseudouridine and is named for that base as follows (ψ for *pseudo-*):

TψC arm

Other Nucleotides: The nucleosides of DNA and RNA are also important individually as the precursors of DNA and RNA and as energy molecules. They may bind 1, 2, or 3 phosphate molecules, giving rise to nucleotides with the following abbreviations (see also 11.11, Abbreviations, Clinical and Technical Terms) or alternative shorthand, eg:

Term	*Abbreviation*	*Alternative Shorthand*
adenosine monophosphate	AMP	pA
adenosine diphosphate	ADP	ppA
adenosine triphosphate	ATP	pppA
thymosine monophosphate	dTMP	pT
thymosine diphosphate	dTDP	ppT
thymosine triphosphate	dTTP	pppT

Nucleic Acid Analysis and Modification: Laboratory methods of analyzing DNA make use of properties of its nucleotide sequences, such as VNTRs (variable number of tandem repeats), STRs (short tandem repeats), STSs (sequence tagged sites), and RFLPs (restriction fragment length polymorphisms). Polymerase chain reaction (PCR) is a well-known method of amplifying particular DNA segments.

Recombinant DNA is DNA created by combining isolated DNA sequences of interest. Among the tools used in this process are cloning vectors, such as plasmids, phages (see 12.12.2, Viruses), and hybrids of these, cosmids and phagemids. Another tool is the yeast artificial chromosome, or YAC.

Basic explanations of these entities are available in medical dictionaries and textbooks. A few that present special nomenclatural problems are described here.

BLOTTING. Southern blotting is a technique for identifying previously isolated DNA. It was named for its originator, E. Southern. When a similar technique was applied to RNA, it was drolly named Northern blotting, and for proteins, Western blotting.[4]

CLONING VECTORS. Plasmids are typically named with a lowercase p followed by a letter or alphanumeric designation; spacing may vary, eg:

pBR322 pJS97 pUC pUC18 pSPORT pSPORT 2

Phage cloning vectors are named for the phages, for example:

phage λ: λgt22A λgt11 λgt10

M13 phage: M13KO7 M13mp

RESTRICTION ENZYMES. Restriction enzymes (or restriction endonucleases) are special enzymes that cleave DNA at specific sites. They are named for the organism from which they are isolated, usually a bacterial species or strain. As originally proposed,[5] their names consist of a 3-letter term, italicized and beginning with a capital letter, taken from the organism of origin, eg:

Hpa for *Haemophilus parainfluenzae*

followed by a roman numeral, which is a series number, eg:

*Hpa*I *Hpa*II

In some cases, the series number is preceded by a roman letter (lowercase or capital) and/or an arabic numeral, which refers to the strain of bacterium, eg:

*Eco*RI *Hin*fI *Sau*96I *Sau*3AI

Many variations in the form of the names of these enzymes have appeared, eg, *Hin* d III, *Hin* dIII, *Hind* III, *Hind* III. It is currently recommended that the style displayed herein be followed. The following list gives examples:

Enzyme Name	*Organism of Origin*
*Acc*I	*Acinetobacter calcoaceticus*
*Alu*I	*Arthrobacter luteus*
*Alw*NI	*Acinetobacter lwoffii* N
*Bam*HI	*Bacillus amyloliquefaciens* H
*Bst*EII	*Bacillus stearothermophilus* ET

Enzyme Name	*Organism of Origin*
*Bst*XI	*Bacillus stearothermophilus* X
*Dpn*I	*Streptococcus* (diplococcus) *pneumoniae* M
*Eco*RI	*Escherichia coli* RY13
*Eco*RII	*Escherichia coli* R245
*Hae*II	*Haemophilus aegyptius*
*Hinc*II	*Haemophilus influenzae* Rc
*Hind*III	*Haemophilus influenzae* Rd
*Hinf*I	*Haemophilus influenzae* Rf
*Msp*I	*Moraxella* species
*Sau*3AI	*Staphylococcus aureus* 3A
*Sau*96I	*Staphylococcus aureus* PS96
*Sst*I	*Streptomyces stanford*
*Taq*I	*Thermus aquaticus* YT-1
*Xba*I	*Xanthomonas badrii*
*Xho*I	*Xanthomonas holicola*

These enzyme names are often seen as modifiers, eg:

a *Taq*I RFLP

a *Bam*HI fragment

MODIFYING ENZYMES. Enzymes exist that synthesize DNA and RNA (polymerases), cleave DNA (nucleases), join nucleic acid fragments (ligases), methylate nucleotides (methylases), and synthesize DNA from RNA (reverse transcriptases). Those in laboratory use come from living systems, often from the same organisms that furnish restriction enzymes. Because the names may be similar, it is essential to specify the type of enzyme, eg:

*Alu*I methylase   *Pfu* DNA polymerase

*Taq*I methylase   *Taq* DNA ligase

(*Pfu: Pyrococcus furiosus*)

In the following enzyme terms, T plus numeral refers to the related phage (see 12.12.2, Viruses):

T7 DNA polymerase

T4 DNA polymerase

T4 polynucleotide kinase

T4 RNA ligase

Amino Acids: Twenty amino acids are products of the genetic code (see above, DNA) and constituents of proteins. Each has 1 or more distinct codons in DNA, eg, GCU, GCC, GCA, and GCG code for alanine.

The following table gives the amino acids of proteins and their preferred 3- and single-letter symbols. Although these amino acids have systematic names (eg, alanine is 2-aminopropanoic acid), the trivial names given are the most widely recognized and used. The single-letter symbols are intended for longer sequences, and a key should always define the letters. In shorter sequences, the 3-letter symbols are preferred, and it is helpful in general publications to expand them as well:

Amino Acid	*3-Letter Symbol*	*Single-Letter Symbol*
alanine	Ala	A
arginine	Arg	R
asparagine	Asn	N
aspartic acid	Asp	D
asparagine or aspartic acid	Asx	B
cysteine	Cys	C
glutamine	Gln	Q
glutamic acid	Glu	E
glutamic acid or glutamine	Glx	Z
glycine	Gly	G
histidine	His	H
isoleucine	Ile	I
leucine	Leu	L
lysine	Lys	K
methionine	Met	M
phenylalanine	Phe	F
proline	Pro	P
serine	Ser	S
threonine	Thr	T
tryptophan	Trp	W
tyrosine	Tyr	Y
valine	Val	V
unspecified amino acid	Xaa	X

(The symbols Asp and Glu apply equally to the anions aspartate and glutamate, respectively, the forms that exist under most physiologic conditions.)

Do not mix the symbol X and 3-letter symbols, but use Xaa with other 3-letter symbols for amino acids. Do not mix single-letter and 3-letter amino acid symbols.

Other amino acids are also well known by their trivial names and have 3-letter codes. These, however, should always be expanded, as the example of cystine, whose 3-letter code is the same as that of cysteine, bears out:

citrulline	Cit
cystine	Cys
homocysteine	Hcy
hydroxyproline	Hyp

ornithine	Orn
thyroxine	Thx

The side chains of amino acids are known as R groups, and the letter R is used in molecular formulas when indicating a nonspecified side chain, as in this general formula for an amino acid:

```
      COOH
       |
NH2—C—H
       |
       R
```

Do not confuse the R with the single-letter abbreviation for arginine (see amino acid list).

The carboxyl (COOH) group is referred to as the α-carboxyl group, which contains the C-1 carbon. The amino (NH_2) group is referred to as the α-amino group, which contains the N-2 nitrogen.

(The true structure is not neutral, as above, but rather contains NH_3^+ and COO^-. However, the structure above is often used, as it is herein, for purposes of discussion.)

Peptide bonds are bonds between the α-carboxyl group of 1 amino acid and the α-amino group of the next. Long peptide sequences are the backbones of proteins. A peptide sequence might be indicated as follows, with hyphens representing peptide bonds:

Gly-Ile-Val-Glu-Gln-Cys-Cys-Ala-Ser-Val-Cys-Ser-Leu-Tyr

In such a sequence, the amino end (amino acid with the free amino group, also known as the N terminal) is on the left and the carboxyl end (amino acid with the free carboxyl group, also known as the C terminal) is on the right. The NH_2 and COOH can be included in the representation of the peptide sequence, as follows:

NH_2-Gly-Ile-Val-Glu-Gln-Cys-Cys-Ala-Ser-Val-Cys-Ser-Leu-Tyr-COOH

The same left-to-right convention applies to sequences using single letters. The above sequence using single letters would be:

GIVEQCCASVCSLY

When the NH_2 group appears on the right of a sequence, it has a meaning other than amino end. For instance, in the following sequence, Val-NH_2 indicates the amide derivative of valine:

His-Phe-Arg-Lys-Pro-Val-NH_2

To indicate bonds other than the peptide bonds previously described, lines, rather than hyphens, are used:

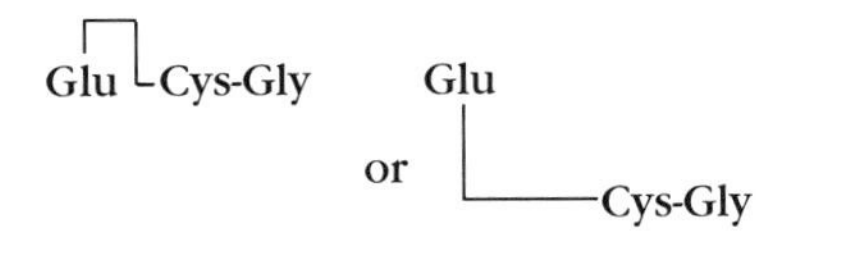

Cys-Tyr-Ile-Gln-Asn-Cys-Pro-Leu-Gly-NH_2 (oxytocin)

(From Liébecq.[1(pp57,59)])

For a multiline peptide sequence in running text, use a hyphen at the right end of one line to indicate a break and at the start of the next line to indicate the peptide bond, eg:

Ala-Ser-Tyr-Phe-Ser-
-Gly-Pro-Gly-Trp-Arg

or, in figures, use a line, eg:

```
     Ala-Ser-Tyr-Phe-Ser ─┐
┌─────────────────────────┘
└─Gly-Pro-Gly-Trp-Arg
```

(From Liébecq.[1(p58)])

In special cases, such as cyclic compounds, the bond from C-2 to N-2 can be shown with arrows, as in

```
┌→Val→Orn→Leu→DPhe→Pro─┐
│                       │
└─Pro←DPhe←Leu←Orn←Val←─┘
```

(From Liébecq.[1(p59)])

As with nucleic acid sequences, alignment can be most important with protein sequences. In the following examples, the amino acid residues must remain aligned with the nucleic acid triplets:

```
   Me t S e r I l eG l nH i s              Me t-S e r-I l e-G l n-H i s
AGTATGAGTATTCAACAT        or        AGT ATG AGT ATT CAA CAT
TCATACTCATAAGTTGTA                  TCA TAC TCA TAA GTT GTA
```

(From Liébecq.[1(p60)])

An amino acid term plus number refers to the amino acid by codon number (when known) or by protein residue, eg:

Arg506

Mutations—Amino Acids (see also Mutations—Nucleotides): As with mutations described by the altered nucleotides, shorthand forms are used for mutations described according to altered amino acids, eg:

Arg506→Gln

or

Arg506Gln

or, in 1-letter notation:

R506Q

(This amino acid substitution is the result of the G1691A mutation.[6])

Explanation of such terms at first mention is recommended.

Note: The same single letters that designate the nucleotides also designate many amino acids (see earlier), eg, A for alanine, C for cysteine, R for arginine. It has been proposed, but not uniformly observed, that mutation terms beginning with a letter refer to amino acids and mutation terms beginning with a number refer to nucleotides.[7] This has not been honored in the observance, however, as of this writing. Therefore, it is usually best in general medical publications to (1) reserve the single-letter form for nucleotide substitutions and use the 3-letter amino acid abbreviation when indicating amino acid substitutions, and (2) define such terms at first mention.

For more examples and conventions on codon/residue numbering, see Beaudet and Tsui.[7]

REFERENCES

1. Liébecq C. *Biochemical Nomenclature and Related Documents: A Compendium.* London, England: International Union of Biochemistry and Molecular Biology/Portland Press Ltd; 1992. Available from: Portland Press Inc, PO Box 2191, Chapel Hill, NC 27515-2191. (Note: recommendations originally appeared in *Biochem J.* 1984;219:345-373, *Eur J Biochem.* 1984;138:9-37, *J Biol Chem.* 1985;260:14-42, *Pure Appl Chem.* 1984;56:595-624, and others.)
2. Lewin B. *Genes V.* New York, NY: Oxford University Press; 1994.
3. Cooper NG. *The Human Genome Project: Deciphering the Blueprint of Heredity.* Mill Valley, Calif: University Science Books; 1994.
4. Steel CM. DNA in medicine: the tools: part I. *Lancet.* 1984;2:908-911.
5. Smith HO, Nathans D. A suggested nomenclature for bacterial host modification and restriction systems and their enzymes. *J Mol Biol.* 1973;81:419-423.
6. Online Mendelian Inheritance in Man (OMIM). National Center for Biotechnology Information. Available at: http://www3.ncbi.nlm.nih.gov/Omim/. Accessed February 20, 1997.
7. Beaudet AL, Tsui L-C. A suggested nomenclature for designating mutations. *Hum Mutat.* 1993;2:245-248.

ADDITIONAL READINGS AND GENERAL REFERENCES

GibcoBRL Product Catalogue and Reference Guide 1995-1996. Gaithersburg, Md: Life Technologies; 1995.

Instructions for authors. *J Biol Chem.* 1994;269:777-785.

Lehninger AL, Nelson DL, Cox MM. *Principles of Biochemistry.* 2nd ed. New York, NY: Worth Publishers; 1993.

New England BioLabs 1996/7 Catalog. Beverly, Mass: New England BioLabs Inc; 1996.

Shattuck-Eidens D, McClure M, Simard J, et al. A collaborative study of 80 mutations in the *BRCA1* breast and ovarian cancer susceptibility gene: implications for presymptomatic testing and screening. *JAMA.* 1995;273:535-541.

Weber BL. Genetic testing for breast cancer. *Sci Am Sci Med.* 1996;3:12-21.

12.6.2 ***Human Gene Nomenclature.***—The International System for Human Gene Nomenclature (ISGN), a system for gene symbols, was inaugurated in 1979.[1,2] The Human Gene Mapping Nomenclature Committee, which developed the ISGN, has put forth a "one human genome-one gene language" principle:

> Certainly there exists a genetic and molecular basis for a single human gene language without dialects. All human nuclear genes as we know them follow the same genetic, molecular, and evolutionary principles. . . . Thus it is reasonable and logical to develop a standard and consolidated gene nomenclature system rather than have a human gene language based on different gene systems. . . .[3(p12)]

The typographic simplicity of the ISGN—all-capital letters, no superscripts or subscripts—has been well suited to digital text, which became widespread soon after the ISGN was formulated. The ISGN has accommodated new methods of gene identification that have arisen in the decades since its formulation. Thus, genes defined in a multitude of ways, from inferential pedigree analysis through direct study of human DNA, and genes named for diseases, enzymes, or DNA segments have a consistent place in the system. Consistency is bound to be further ensured by the practice of reserving gene names with the Human Gene Mapping Nomenclature Committee.[4,5]

The annual *Human Gene Mapping* compendia, which contain all assigned gene names, are published by The Johns Hopkins University Press (Baltimore, Md). Computerization and linkage of genetics databases have been under way since 1983.[6-8] The Genome Data Base (GDB), the major repository of human genome data and an up-to-date source of gene markers and symbols, is accessible through accounts at GDB nodes (in the United States: The Johns Hopkins University School of Medicine, 2024 E Monument St, Baltimore, MD 21205-2100) or via the World Wide Web (http://gdbwww.gdb.org). The international Chromosome Coordinating Meetings issue annual catalogs of approved genes and updates on nomenclature (published by S Karger AG, Basel, Switzerland, and New York, NY). Authors should consult the GDB regarding the existence of an approved symbol.

Genetic diseases are catalogued in *Mendelian Inheritance in Man* (*MIM*),[9] a publication available from The Johns Hopkins University Press and in an online form known as OMIM. OMIM is now distributed by the National Center for Biotechnology Information on the World Wide Web at http://www3.ncbi.nlm.nih.gov /omim/. Further information on access is obtainable at GDB User Support, 2024 E Monument St, Baltimore, MD 21205, or by e-mail at help@gdb.org. When referring to genetic disease phenotypes, authors are strongly encouraged to include the MIM number. Many diseases have multiple names, and the use of the MIM number greatly facilitates identification of the precise disorder and gives multiple links to other citations (Phyllis J. McAlpine, PhD, written communications, March 1996 and May 1996).

The purpose of this section is not to explain *how* to name a gene; ISGN deals fully with this, and interested readers are referred to the above sources and those in the bibliography. Rather, the style recommendations that follow are meant to convey the *form* of gene and allele symbols (ie, the typographic recommendations of ISGN) and to explain some conventions, to allow readers and editors to decode terms frequently encountered.

Examples of gene symbols in this section are taken from the aforementioned catalogs, which include "only marker assignments and linkages that are supported by factual genetic evidence."[10(p7)] This section is not meant to be a source of information on the human genome, knowledge of which is ever in flux and subject to revision. Some gene symbols used as examples were "reserved" but unassigned to a map location at time of publication. The reader should not infer that a gene, if mentioned, has been isolated or is the gene responsible for all occurrences of a condition (eg, *HPT* is not the source of all instances of hypoparathyroidism) or that all human traits and diseases are due to single genes.

An excellent recent summary of gene nomenclature guidelines with information on genomic databases, including bacteria, plants, and animals, has been compiled by the journal *Trends in Genetics:* the *TIG Genetic Nomenclature Guide* (see Additional Readings and General References, this section).

Typography—Basic Rules for Genes

GENE AND LOCUS SYMBOLS. Genes are the molecular units of heredity. The locus is the location of the gene, eg, on the chromosome. (For instance, one might refer to the gene for renin, *REN*, or the *REN* locus. In this section, the term *gene symbol* is used synonymously with *locus symbol*.) Alleles are alternative forms of a gene, and their nomenclature is described later in this section.

A gene may be named for a hereditary disease, an inherited characteristic, a biochemical constituent—enzyme, structural protein, antigen, etc—or the DNA sequence that makes up the gene. The gene symbol is often recognizable as an abbreviation for the gene name or a quality of the gene. "The first character of a gene symbol must be the first letter of the gene name."[11(p39)] Expanding the gene term at first mention of the gene symbol is helpful, unless context otherwise clarifies the gene's identity, eg:

the D_2 dopamine receptor gene (*DRD2*)
or
DRD2 (the D_2 dopamine receptor gene)

Human gene symbols consist of all-letter or alphanumeric expressions from 2 to 9 characters long (usually 3-7 characters long; the ISGN prefers that the letter component be 3-5 characters long). All letters in human gene terms are capitalized (in contrast to animal genes—see 12.6.5, Animal Genetic Terms). The entire term is italicized (or underlined in typescript; see also Writing About Genes; Italics in Gene Symbols):

MB	myoglobin
CMH1	cardiomyopathy, hypertrophic 1
HMS1	homosexuality 1
HPR	haptoglobin-related protein

The first character is always a capital letter and is never a number:

RN5S1@ [not *5SRN1@*]	5S RNA, cluster 1

Within gene symbols, roman numerals are changed to arabic numerals and Greek letters are changed to English letters, eg:

AFP	α-fetoprotein
AT3	antithrombin III
B2M [traditionally $\beta_2 m$]	β_2-microglobulin
TCRA	TCRα (T-cell receptor, alpha)

In keeping with ISGN recommendations, numerals and (nearly always) Greek letter equivalents do not begin a gene term, but instead appear at or near the end of the gene term, to facilitate location of the gene name in alphabetical listings, eg:

GLA	α-galactosidase
GLB1	β_1-galactosidase
NT5	5′ nucleotidase

There are no superscripts or subscripts—all characters of the term are typeset on the line:

CA1 [formerly CA^1]	carbonic anhydrase I
TBXA2R	thromboxane A_2 receptor

Likewise, there are no punctuation marks or spaces within the symbol:

HNRPA2B1	heterogeneous nuclear ribonucleoprotein A2/B1
IL1A	interleukin 1α
MCF2	MCF.2 cell line-derived transforming sequence

Important exceptions, however, include the genes for the molecules of the HLA system (see 12.8.2, The Human Leukocyte Antigen [HLA] System), which include hyphens within the gene term, eg:

HLA-A	HLA-A
HLA-B	HLA-B
HLA-C	HLA-C
HLA-K	HLA-K
HLA-L	HLA-L

Gene expressions used in the study of human blood group systems long used a capital-lowercase format that antedated the all-capital ISGN style. The Human Gene Nomenclature Committee with the International Society of Blood Transfusion (ISBT) has recommended an all-capital style for blood group genes "in the genetic context . . . not intended to replace blood bank usages."[3(p18)] Therefore, both types of gene term as seen in the examples below are acceptable (see also 12.1, Blood Groups and Platelet Antigens):

Traditional	*ISGN*	*Blood Group*
Do	*DO*	Dombrock blood group
Fy	*FY*	Duffy blood group
Ii	*II*	Ii blood group
Jk	*SLC14A1* (formerly *JK*)	solute carrier family 14 (urea transport), member 1 (Kidd blood group)
Lu	*LU*	Lutheran blood group
Rd	*RD*	Radin blood group
Sc	*SC*	Scianna blood group
Sf	*SF*	Stoltzfus blood group
Xg	*XG*	Xg blood group
Xk	*XK*	Kell blood group precursor

WRITING ABOUT GENES; ITALICS IN GENE SYMBOLS. Discussions of genes often do not use or necessarily require the use of gene symbols:

Acceptable Expression	*Gene Symbol Equivalent*
the MHC region of the genome	various genes
the gene for parathyroid hormone	*PTH*
the cystic fibrosis locus	*CFTR*
the gene for synapsin I	*SYN1*

Acceptable Expression	*Gene Symbol Equivalent*
the hemophilia A locus	*F8C*
gene for the tumor protein p53	*TP53*

Authors sometimes object to the recommendation to italicize gene names, and the ISGN allows for roman typeface in compendia of gene symbols, such as *Human Gene Mapping.*[10,12] Originally, the gene symbol was italicized because the gene was only inferred to exist; molecular technology has rendered this reason for italics moot, and a number of genetics journals now feature gene symbols in roman typeface (Phyllis J. McAlpine, PhD, oral communication, March 1996). However, the value of italics also lies in distinguishing those genes and gene products that have identical names, and, for now, AMA journals will continue to observe this convention.

Some well-known gene names are readily distinguishable from their gene product or phenotype (and appear widely throughout the literature in roman typeface), eg:

BRCA1, breast and ovarian cancer susceptibility gene

Yet a great many other gene symbols, if not italicized, are easily confused with terms for the products of those genes, or with other terms, for instance:

Gene	*Potentially Confusing Nongene Term*
ABO	ABO blood group system (see also 12.1, Blood Groups and Platelet Antigens)
APOE	apoE (apolipoprotein E)
CEA	carcinoembryonic antigen (commonly abbreviated CEA)
EPO	erythropoietin, the physiologic entity, is commonly abbreviated EPO; the therapeutic agent, recombinant human erythropoietin, is also sometimes abbreviated EPO
ESR	estrogen receptor; but ESR is also a common abbreviation of erythrocyte sedimentation rate
GIF	GIF (gastric intrinsic factor)
GIP	GIP (gastric inhibitory polypeptide)
HLA-A, HLA-B, etc	HLA-A, HLA-B, etc (see also 12.8.2, The Human Leukocyte Antigen [HLA] System)
MAD	MAD protein (MAX-binding protein)
MS	multiple sclerosis
many hormone genes, eg, *CRH, GHRH, GNRH, GNRHR, PTH, TRH*	CRH, GHRH, GNRH, GNRH receptor, PTH, TRH

An article on Huntington disease that abbreviated the condition as *HD* and used the gene symbol HD might contain expressions like the following:

HD, *HD*	the first is the abbreviation for Huntington disease; the second is the gene symbol; the 2 are distinguishable only with italics

patient with HD	patient with the disease (or patient with the *HD* gene in an article that does not italicize gene symbols)
HD gene	equivalent to *HD* gene
HD gene product, *HD* gene product	huntingtin, the protein product of the gene for HD: either expression is acceptable
expression of *HD*	expression of the *HD* gene
expression of HD	by inference, expression of the *HD* gene; italics would greatly clarify this phrase
prevalence of HD	prevalence of Huntington disease
prevalence of *HD*	prevalence of the *HD* gene; not necessarily equal to prevalence of HD

With more than 5000 genes in the GDB and an estimated 50 000 to 100 000 in the human genome, researchers might recognize through context or familiarity every abbreviation as a gene or gene product, but even the well-informed nongeneticist reader seeking information in an unfamiliar field would have few clues. It is up to authors to make unambiguously clear when a specific gene, rather than some other entity, is under discussion. Because the choice of italics involves some nuance, editors must ultimately defer to author preference, but only after vigorously prompting authors to italicize any gene symbols in their articles.

In some expressions, italics may be moot, such as a gene named for its biochemical product. For instance, the gene symbol for the enzyme tyrosine hydroxylase gene is *TH*. The enzyme is commonly abbreviated TH. The following table shows equivalent expressions:

Expression	*Meaning*
TH gene or *TH* gene	gene for tyrosine hydroxylase
TH gene product or *TH* gene product	tyrosine hydroxylase, the product of the TH gene

Note, however, that when quantity is involved, the gene and its product must be distinguished, eg:

TH deficiency	deficiency of the enzyme TH
TH deficiency	deletion of the *TH* gene

GENE SYMBOL CONVENTIONS. Genes are named for the condition associated with the gene, the biochemical product of the gene, or the function of the gene, if known, eg:

CFTR	cystic fibrosis transmembrane conductance regulator (formerly *CF*)
DFNA1	deafness, autosomal dominant 1
HCL1	hair color 1 (brown)
HCL2	hair color 2 (red)
HPT	hypoparathyroidism
IDDM2	insulin-dependent diabetes mellitus 2
MAGE2	melanoma antigen 2
PDCD1	programmed cell death 1
REN	renin

RENBP renin-binding protein

TUBA1 tubulin, α1 (testis specific)

The letter L at the end of a gene symbol often signifies a "like" sequence:

G6PD glucose-6-phosphate dehydrogenase

G6PDL glucose-6-phosphate dehydrogenase-like

INS insulin

INSL1 insulinlike 1

INSL2 insulinlike 2

INSR insulin receptor

INSRL insulin receptor-like

Not all near-terminal Ls, however, stand for "like," eg:

CDL1 Cornelia de Lange syndrome 1

A terminal LG stands for ligand:

CD40LG CD40 antigen ligand (hyper-IgM syndrome)

Pseudogenes are "nontranscribed sequences that bear striking homologies to structural gene sequences."[3(p16)] The letter P at or near the end of a gene symbol often signifies "pseudogene":

HBA1 hemoglobin-α_1

HBAP1 hemoglobin-α_1 pseudogene

However, not every final *P* stands for pseudogene, eg:

C4B complement component 4B (C4B)

C4BPA complement component 4-binding protein (C4bp) α

GARP glycoprotein A repetitions predominant

HIVE1 human immunodeficiency virus 1 (HIV-1) expression (elevated) 1

HIVEP2 human immunodeficiency virus 1 enhancer-binding protein 2

MHP1 migraine, hemiplegic 1

The *MT* prefix often signifies mitochondrial:

MT7SDNA 7S mitochondrial DNA

Zinc finger proteins are proteins with zinc-binding loops or "fingers" that interact with DNA. The gene symbols for those proteins consist of *ZNF* followed by a number, eg:

ZNF1

ZNF162

Homeobox genes are genes first discovered in the fruitfly *Drosophila melanogaster* but found throughout the animal kingdom, which are involved in embryological development. Such genes begin with the sequence *HOX*,[13] eg:

HOXA7 (homeobox A7)

The symbol @ is used at the end of terms to signify a gene family or cluster,[14] eg:

PGA@ pepsinogen A gene cluster

Anonymous DNA segments have been mapped to chromosomes but await the discovery of defined products. "The D-number nomenclature . . . has been developed to distinguish the loci (genomic segments) from the probes used to recognize them."[15] Terms for anonymous DNA segments contain these elements: the letter *D*; the chromosome number or letter (*0* for unassigned); the letter *S* (unique sequence), *Z* (repetitive sequence), or *F* (member of a family of sequences found on more than 1 chromosome); and the sequence number. A site number (*S* plus number) and the suffix *E* (expressed segment)[5] sometimes follow, eg:

Symbol	*Explanation*	
D4S57	**D***4S57*	**D** for DNA
D17S9	*D***17***S9*	**17** for chromosome 17
DXS580	*D***X***S580*	**X** for X chromosome
DYS29	*D***Y***S29*	**Y** for Y chromosome
DXYS14	*D***XY***S14*	**XY** for sequence present at homologous sites on chromosomes X and Y
D19S394	*D19***S***394*	**S** for unique sequence
D13Z9	*D13***Z***9*	**Z** for repetitive sequence
D19F11S1	*D19***F***11S1*	**F** for family sequence
DXYF36S1	*DXYF36***S***1*	**S** for site
D9F173S1E	*D9F173S1***E**	**E** for expressed segment

A number of sites on chromosomes defined as "fragile" are heritable and may be associated with various human syndromes. Locus designations for such fragile site genes begin with *FRA*, contain the number of the chromosome on which they are located, and end with a sequential letter, eg:

FRA1E

FRA13C

FRAXB

The cytogenetic designation of *FRAXB* is fra(X)(p22.31). (See also 12.6.4, Human Chromosomes.)

The following list gives gene families associated with disciplines covered elsewhere in this chapter.

ECG-related terms (see 12.3, Cardiology)	*LQT1*	long QT syndrome, Ward-Romano syndrome 1
	LQT2	long QT syndrome 2
	LQT4	long QT syndrome 4
	SCN5A (formerly *LQT3*)	sodium channel, voltage-gated, type V, α-polypeptide (long QT syndrome 3)
coagulation (see 12.7, Hemostasis)	*A2M*	α_2-macroglobulin
	AT3	antithrombin III
	F2	factor II
	F2L	factor II-like
	F2R	factor II receptor
	F3	factor III

	F5	factor V
	F7	factor VII
	F7R	factor VII regulator
	F8C	factor VIIIc, procoagulant component (hemophilia A)
	F9	factor IX (Christmas disease, hemophilia B)
	F10	factor X
	F11	factor XI
	F12	factor XII (Hageman factor)
	F13A1	factor XIII, A1 polypeptide
	F13A2	factor XIII, A2 polypeptide
	F13A3	factor XIII, A3 polypeptide
	F13B	factor XIII, B polypeptide
	FGA	fibrinogen A α polypeptide
	FGB	fibrinogen B β polypeptide
	FGG	fibrinogen γ polypeptide
	HCF2	heparin cofactor II
	PAI1	plasminogen activator inhibitor, type I
	PCI	protein C inhibitor
	PI	protease inhibitor 1, α_1-antitrypsin
	PLAT	plasminogen activator, tissue (tPA)
	PLAU	plasminogen activator, urokinase (uPA)
	PLAUR	uPA receptor
	PLG	plasminogen
	PLI	α_2-plasmin inhibitor
	PROC	protein C
	PROC-PEN	protein C receptor (endothelial)
	TFPI	tissue factor pathway inhibitor
	TFPI2-PEN	tissue factor pathway inhibitor 2
	VWF	von Willebrand factor
	VWFP	von Willebrand factor pseudogene
nucleic acids, amino acids, and histones (see 12.6.1, Nucleic Acids and Amino Acids)	*H1F1*	H1 histone, family 1
	H1F2	H1 histone, family 2
	H1F3	H1 histone, family 3
	H1F4	H1 histone, family 4
	H1FV	H1° histone
	H2A	H2A histone
	H2AX	H2AX histone
	H2AZ	H2AZ histone
	H2B	H2B histone
	H3F2	H3 histone, family 2
	H3F3A	H3 histone, family 3A
	H3F3B	H3 histone, family 3B (H3.3B)
	H4F2	H4 histone, family 2
	H4F3	H4 histone, family 3
	HNRPA1	heterogeneous nuclear ribonucleoprotein A1
	HNRPA1L	heterogeneous nuclear ribonucleoprotein A1-like
	HNRPG	heterogeneous nuclear ribonucleoprotein G
	MTTA	tRNA alanine (mitochondrial)
	MTTC	tRNA cysteine (mitochondrial)

	MTTH	tRNA histidine (mitochondrial)
	MTTV	tRNA valine (mitochondrial)
	RN7SK	RNA, 7SK, nuclear
	RN7SL	RNA, 7SL, cytoplasmic
	RN7SLP1	RNA, 7SL, cytoplasmic, pseudogene 1
	RNE1	RNA, small nucleolar E1
	RNR1	RNA, ribosomal 1
	RNU1A	RNA, U1A small nuclear
	RNY1	RNA, Y1 small cytoplasmic
	TRC	tRNA cysteine
	TRN	tRNA asparagine
	TRG1	tRNA glycine (CCC) 1
	TRR1	tRNA arginine 1
	TRV2	tRNA valine 2
complement (see 12.8.1, Complement)	*BF*	B factor, properdin
	C1NH	C1 inhibitor (hereditary angioedema)
	C1QA	C1q α
	C1QB	C1q β
	C1QBP	C1q binding protein
	C1QG	C1q γ
	C1R	C1r
	C1S	C1s
	C2	C2
	C3	C3
	C4A	C4a
	C4B	C4b
	C4BPA	C4bp α
	C4BPAL1	C4bp α-like 1
	C4BPAL2	C4bp α-like 2
	C4BPB	C4bp β
	C5	C5
	C5R1	C5 receptor 1 (C5a ligand)
	C6	C6
	C7	C7
	C8A	C8A
	C8B	C8B
	C8G	C8G
	C9	C9
	CRARF	C4/C2 activating component of Ra-reactive factor
	DF	factor D
	HF1	factor H 1
	HF2	factor H 2
	HFL1	factor H-like 1
	HFL2	factor H-like 2
	HFL3	factor H-like 3
	IF	factor I
	PFC	P (properdin) factor
	PFD	P factor deficiency
HLA (see above and also 12.8.2, The Human Leukocyte Antigen [HLA] System)	*HLA-DMA*	HLA-DM α chain
	HLA-DMB	HLA-DM β chain
	HLA-DNA	HLA-DN α chain
	HLA-DOB	HLA-DO β chain
	HLA-DPA1	HLA-DP α chain 1
	HLA-BPB1	HLA-DP β chain 1

	HLA-DQA1	HLA-DQ α chain 1
	HLA-DRA	HLA-DR α chain
	HLA-DRB1	HLA-DR β chain 1
	HLA-DRB6	MHC class II β 6 (pseudogene)
	HLA-E	HLA-E
	HLA-F	HLA-F
	HLA-G	HLA-G
	HLA-H	MHC class II, H (pseudogene)
	HLA-J	MHC class II, J (pseudogene)
Fc receptors and Ig components (see 12.8.3, Immunoglobulins	*FCAR*	FcαR
	FCER1A	FcεRI, α
	FCGR1A	FcγRIa (CD64)
	FCGR1B	FcγRIb (CD64)
	IGA	Ig-α membrane-associated protein
	IGB	Ig-β membrane-associated protein (B29)
	IGER	IgE responsiveness (atopic)
	IGH@	immunoglobulin heavy-chain gene cluster (V, D, J, C)
	IGHA1	α1 heavy chain
	IGHA2	α2 heavy chain (A2M marker)
	IGHD	δ heavy chain
	IGHDY2	immunoglobulin heavy polypeptide diversity region 2
	IGHE	ε heavy chain
	IGHEP1	ε pseudogene 1
	IGHG1	γ1 heavy chain
	IGHGP	γ1 pseudogene
	IGHJ	H joining region
	IGHM	μ heavy chain
	IGHMBP2	μ binding protein 2
	IGHV2@	immunoglobulin heavy polypeptide, variable region 2 cluster
	IGHV@	immunoglobulin heavy polypeptide, variable region cluster
	IGJ	J chain
	IGJP1	J chain pseudogene 1
	IGKC	κ constant region
	IGKJRB1	κ J region recombination signal binding protein 1
	IGKV	κ variable region
	IGKV1	κ variable region 1
	IGKV268	κ variable region 268
	IGKV3	κ variable region 3
	IGKVP1	κ variable region pseudogene 1
	IGKVP@	κ variable region pseudogene cluster
	IGKVPZ1	κ variable region pseudogene Z1
	IGL@	λ gene cluster
	IGLC1	λ constant region 1 (Mcg marker)
	IGLL1	λ-like polypeptide 1, pre-B-cell specific
	IGLV@	λ variable region gene cluster
CD cell markers (see 12.8.4, Lymphocytes)	*CD1A*	CD1A antigen, α polypeptide
	CD4	CD4 antigen (p55)
	CD8A	CD8 antigen, α polypeptide (p32)
	CD40	CD40 antigen

T-cell receptors (see 12.8.4, Lymphocytes)	*TCRA*	T-cell receptor α chain (TCRα) (V, D, J, C)
	TCRB	TCRβ cluster
	TCRD	TCRδ (V, D, J, C)
	TCRG	TCRγ cluster
	TCRGJ1	TCRγ joining segment J1
	TCRGV1	TCRγ variable region V1 (pseudogene)
	TCRGV2	TCRγ variable region V2
interferons, interleukins, and tumor necrosis factor (see 12.8.5, Cytokines)	*IFN1@*	interferon, type 1, cluster
	IFNA1	IFN-α1
	IFNA10	IFN-α10
	IFNAP22	IFN-α pseudogene 22
	IFNAR1	IFN-α, IFN-β, and IFN-ω receptor 1
	IFNG	IFN-γ
	IFNW1	IFN-ω1
	IL1A	interleukin 1α
	IL1B	IL-1β
	IL1RA	IL-1RI
	IL1RB	IL-1RII
	IL1RN	IL-1RA
	IL2	IL-2
	IL2RA	IL-2Rα
	IL2RB	IL-2Rβ
	IL3	IL-3 (colony-stimulating factor, multiple)
	IL4	IL-4
	IL4R	IL-4R
	IL13	IL-13
	TNF	tumor necrosis factor (TNF)
viruses (see also 12.6.5, Animal Genetic Terms and 12.12.2, Viruses)	*A12M1*	adenovirus 12 chromosome modification site 1C
	AAVS1	adenoassociated virus integration site 1
	CXB3S	coxsackie virus B3 sensitivity
	E11S	echovirus (serotypes 4, 6, 11, 19) sensitivity
	EBI1	Epstein-Barr virus-induced gene 1
	HCVS	human coronavirus sensitivity
	HIVEP1	HIV-1 enhancer-binding protein 1
	HPV6AI1	human papillomavirus 6a integration site 1
	HPV18I1	human papillomavirus 18 integration site 1
	HPV18I2	human papillomavirus 18 integration site 2
	HVBS1	hepatitis B virus integration site 1
	HVBS4	hepatitis B virus integration site 4
	HVBS6	hepatitis B virus integration site 6
	HVBS7	hepatitis B virus integration site 7
	HVBS8	hepatitis B virus integration site 8
	MX1	myxovirus (influenza) resistance 1
	PE5L-LSB	papillomavirus 18 E5-like protein
	PVR	poliovirus receptor
	VDI	vesicular stomatitis virus defective interfering particle suppression

ALLELES. Alleles are alternative forms of a particular gene. Thus, they are expressed using both the gene name and an appendage that indicates the specific allele.

According to ISGN, allele symbols consist of the gene symbol plus an asterisk plus the allele designation, eg:

*HBB*S* allele of the *HBB* gene

As with gene terms, Greek letters are changed to roman in allele terms:

*APOE*E4* allele producing the ε4 type of apolipoprotein E

If clear in context, the allele symbol may be used in a shorthand form that omits the gene symbol and includes only the asterisk and the allele designation that follows, eg:

**S*

**E4*

In the case of alleles of the major histocompatibility locus (see 12.8.2, The Human Leukocyte Antigen [HLA] System), a portion of the gene name is usually included in the shortened form and the term appears in roman, eg:

Full Name	*Shortened Form*
HLA-DRB1*0301	DRB1*0301

In practice, the same allele is often expressed in different ways that diverge from the recommended nomenclature. Taking *APOE*E4* as an example, consider the many expressions for the same term now in use:

APOE ε4

ε4 allele

epsilon 4 allele

E4 allele

*APOE*4*

apo e4

APOE4

For now, it is sufficient to follow author preference.

Names for mutant alleles are currently evolving to a molecularly based nomenclature, with designations that indicate the amino acid or nucleic acid substitution (see 12.6.1, Nucleic Acids and Amino Acids)[16,17] (Phyllis J. McAlpine, PhD, oral and written communications, March 1996).

Genotype Terminology: The genotype comprises the collection of alleles in an individual. Because most individuals have 2 copies of most chromosomes (see 12.6.4, Human Chromosomes), individuals have 2 alleles (which may be the same alleles or 2 different alleles) for most genes.

The simplest genotype term for an individual would describe 1 gene and consist of the names of 2 alleles. Larger genotypes would contain 2 or more allele symbol pairs.

According to ISGN, allele groupings may be indicated by placement above and below a horizontal line or on the line. As seen in the following examples (from Shows et al[2,3]), such placement as well as *order, spacing,* and *punctuation marks* (virgules [/], semicolons, spaces, and commas) have specific meanings.

Alleles of the same gene are indicated by placement above and below a *horizontal line* or with a *virgule*:

$$\frac{ADA*1}{ADA*2} \quad or \quad ADA*1/ADA*2 \quad or \quad ADA*1/*2$$

Semicolons separate pairs of alleles at *unlinked* loci:

$$\frac{ADA*1}{ADA*2};\frac{ADH1*1}{ADH1*1};\frac{AMY1*A}{AMY1*B}$$

or

*ADA*1/ADA*2; ADH1*1/ADH1*1; AMY1*A/AMY1*B*

or

*ADA*1/*2; ADH*1/*1; AMY1*A/*B*

A single *space* represents alleles together on the *same chromosome* from alleles together on another chromosome (*phase known*):

$$\frac{AMY1*A\ PGM1*2}{AMY1*B\ PGM1*1}$$

or

*AMY1*A PGM1*2/AMY1*B PGM1*1*

Commas indicate that alleles above and below the line (or on either side of the virgule) are on the *same chromosome* pair, but not on which chromosome of the pair specifically (*phase unknown*):

$$\frac{PGM1*1}{PGM1*2},\frac{AMY1*A}{AMY1*B}$$

or

*PGM1*1/PGM1*2, AMY1*A/AMY1*B*

A special form for hemizygous males is:

*G6PD*A/Y*

When the *order* of genes along the chromosome is *known,* the genes are listed from short-arm end (pter) to the centromere (cen) or long-arm end (qter) (see 12.6.4, Human Chromosomes):

pter-*ENO1-PGM1-AMY1*-cen

When the *order* of genes along the chromosome is *not known,* the genes are listed *alphabetically* and *parentheses* are used:

pter-*PGD-AK2-(ACTA,APOA2,REN)*-qter

Phenotype Terminology: The phenotype is the collection of actual traits in an individual resulting from the individual's genotype. Phenotypes can be expressed in terms of the specific genes of genotypes such as those in the examples above. The *phenotype term* derives from the genotype term, but no italics are used, and, instead of asterisks, spaces are used. Genotypes usually contain pairs of symbols, while phenotypes contain single symbols. The following examples are from Shows et al[3]:

Genotype	*Phenotype*
*ADA*1/ADA*1*	ADA 1
*ADA*1/ADA*2*	ADA 1-2
*C2*C/C2*QO*	C2 C,QO
*HBB*A/HBB*6V*	HBB A,S [traditional, Hb A/S]
*ABO*A1/ABO*O*	ABO A1
*CFTR*N/CFTR*R*	CFTR N
*G6PD*A/Y*	G6PD A

REFERENCES

1. Klinger HP. Progress in nomenclature and symbols for cytogenetics and somatic-cell genetics. *Ann Intern Med.* 1979;91:487-488.
2. Shows TB, Alper CA, Bootsma D, et al. International system for human gene nomenclature (1979). *Cytogenet Cell Genet.* 1979;25:96-116.
3. Shows TB, McAlpine PJ, Boucheix C, et al. Guidelines for human gene nomenclature: an international system for human gene nomenclature (ISGN, HGM9). *Cytogenet Cell Genet.* 1987;46:11-28.
4. McAlpine PJ, Shows TB, Boucheix C, et al. Report of the Nomenclature Committee and the 1989 Catalog of Mapped Genes. In: Human Gene Mapping 10 (1989): Tenth International Workshop on Human Gene Mapping. *Cytogenet Cell Genet.* 1989; 51:13-66.
5. McAlpine PJ, Shows TB, Boucheix C, Huebner M, Anderson WA. The 1991 Catalog of Mapped Genes and Report of the Nomenclature Committee. In: Human Gene Mapping 11 (1991). *Cytogenet Cell Genet.* 1991;58:1.
6. Bodmer WF. Introduction. In: Human Gene Mapping 10.5 (1990): Update to the Tenth International Workshop on Human Gene Mapping. *Cytogenet Cell Genet.* 1990;55:1.
7. Craig I, Rawlings C. Overview of HGM10.5. In: Human Gene Mapping 10.5 (1990): Update to the Tenth International Workshop on Human Gene Mapping. *Cytogenet Cell Genet.* 1990;55:2.
8. Rawlings CJ, Lucier RE. Report of the Informatics Committee. In: Human Gene Mapping 10.5. *Cytogenet Cell Genet.* 1990;55:779-782.
9. McKusick VA. *Mendelian Inheritance in Man: A Catalog of Human Genes and Genetic Disorders.* 11th ed. Baltimore, Md: The Johns Hopkins University Press; 1994.
10. Cuticchia AJ, ed. *Human Gene Mapping 1994: A Compendium.* Baltimore, Md: The Johns Hopkins University Press; 1995.
11. McAlpine P. Vetebrates. In: Stewart A, ed. Trends in Genetics *Genetic Nomenclature Guide.* Tarrytown, NY: Elsevier Science; 1995:39-41.
12. Cuttichia AJ, Chipperfield MA, Foster PA. *Human Gene Mapping 1995: A Compendium.* Baltimore, Md: The Johns Hopkins University Press; 1996.
13. McAlpine PJ, Stranc LC, Boucheix C, Shows TB. The 1990 Catalog of Mapped Genes and Report of the Nomenclature Committee. In: Human Gene Mapping 10.5. *Cytogenet Cell Genet.* 1990;55:5-76.
14. McAlpine PJ, Boucheix C, Pakstis AJ, Stranc LC, Berent TG, Shows TB. The 1988 Catalog of Mapped Genes and Report of the Nomenclature Committee. In: Human

Gene Mapping 9.5 (1988): Update to the Ninth International Workshop on Human Gene Mapping. *Cytogenet Cell Genet.* 1988;49:4-38.

15. Kidd KK, Bowcock AM, Pearson PL, et al. Report of the Committee on Human Gene Mapping by Recombinant DNA Techniques. In: Human Gene Mapping 9.5 (1988): Update to the Ninth International Workshop on Human Gene Mapping. Cytogenet Cell Genet. 1988;49:132-218.
16. Beaudet AL, Tsui L-C. A suggested nomenclature for designating mutations. *Hum Mutat.* 1993;2:245-248.
17. McAlpine PJ, Shows TB, Boucheix C, Pericak-Vance MA, Anderson WA. The 1992 catalog of mapped genes and report of the nomenclature committee. In: Cuticchia AJ, Pearson PL, Klinger HP, eds. *Chromosome Coordinating Meeting (1992): Genome Priority Reports.* Vol 1. Basel, Switzerland: S Karger AG; 1993:11-142.

ADDITIONAL READINGS AND GENERAL REFERENCES

Cuticchia AJ, Pearson PL, Klinger HP, eds. *Chromosome Coordinating Meeting (1992): Genome Priority Reports.* Vol 1. Basel, Switzerland: S Karger AG; 1993.

The Genome Database: An International Collaboration in Support of the Human Genome Project. Hosted by: Johns Hopkins University School of Medicine, Baltimore, Md. Available at: http://gdbwww.gdb.org/.

Human Gene Mapping 9.5 (1988): Update to the Ninth International Workshop on Human Gene Mapping. *Cytogenet Cell Genet.* 1988;49:1-258.

Human Gene Mapping 10 (1989): Tenth International Workshop on Human Gene Mapping. *Cytogenet Cell Genet.* 1989;51:1-1148.

Human Gene Mapping 10.5 (1990): Update to the Tenth International Workshop on Human Gene Mapping. *Cytogenet Cell Genet.* 1990;55:1-785.

Human Gene Mapping 11 (1991). *Cytogenet Cell Genet.* 1991;58:1-2200.

Stewart A. *TIG Genetic Nomenclature Guide.* Cambridge, England: Elsevier Trends Journals; 1995.

12.6.3 *Oncogenes and Tumor Suppressor Genes.*

Oncogenes: Oncogenes, genes that can induce cancer, were discovered and characterized in viruses and animal experimental systems. These genes exist widely outside the systems in which they were discovered, and their normal cellular homologues are important in cell division and differentiation. Their nomenclature, however, remains rooted in the virus or tumor of discovery.

A style typical of that for microbial genes characterizes oncogenes, namely, 3 letters, italicized and in lowercase. The terms are usually taken from the names of the associated viruses (eg, *abl,* Abelson murine leukemia virus; *mos,* Moloney sarcoma virus; *myb,* avian myeloblastosis; *sis,* simian sarcoma virus; *src,* Rous sarcoma virus):

abl *mos* *fes* *myb* *myc* *erb* *ras* *sis* *src*

"Determining which genes in the tumor DNA could transform the normal cells identified a form of *ras* that had been mutated in the process of tumorigenesis."[1(p146)]

The protein products of the oncogenes use the same 3-letter term in roman type with an initial capital letter:

Abl Mos Fes Myb Myc Erb Ras Sis Src

"Thus, the activation and inactivation of Ras are carefully orchestrated."[2(p304)]

Commonly, the oncogene term contains 1 of 2 prefixes, which indicate the source or location of the gene: v- for virus or c- for the oncogene's cellular or chromosomal counterpart. The c- form is also known as a proto-oncogene and in the International Standard Gene Nomenclature (ISGN; see 12.6.2, Human Gene Nomenclature) is given in all capitals:

c-*abl* (*ABL1*) c-*mos* (*MOS*)

v-*abl* v-*mos*

Editors should follow author usage and not substitute one type of term for another.

The protein product may be similarly prefixed:

c-Abl c-Mos

v-Abl v-Mos

Additional prefixes occur to further identify oncogenes, eg, to identify members of the *ras* family. Expansions of some prefixes are given below, but it should not be inferred that the gene in question is associated only with the tumor it is named for:

Oncogene	*Prefix Expansion*
H-*ras* c-H-*ras* v-H-*ras*	Harvey rat sarcoma
K-*ras* c-K-*ras* v-K-*ras*	Kirsten rat sarcoma
N-*ras*, N-*myc*	neuroblastoma
B-*lym*	B-cell lymphoma
L-*myc*	small cell lung carcinoma

Numbers or letters designate genes in a series, eg:

K-*ras*-2

H-*ras*-1

erb-b2

Tumor Suppressor Genes: Follow author style for tumor suppressor genes (also known as recessive oncogenes), as in the examples below (expansions in the third column are for information only and need not be included by editors):

Gene	*Gene Product*	*Explanation*
TP53	p53	a 53-kd protein
RB	Rb protein (also p105-RB)	retinoblastoma (a 105-kd protein)
WT1	a zinc finger protein	Wilms tumor locus
NFI	nuclear factor I	nuclear factor I/neurofibromatosis
DCC		deleted in colorectal cancer

REFERENCES

1. Carbone DP. Oncogenes and tumor suppressor genes. *Hosp Pract.* 1993;28:145-148, 153-154, 156, 161.

2. Krontiris TG. Oncogenes. *N Engl J Med.* 1995;333:303-306.

ADDITIONAL READINGS AND GENERAL REFERENCES

Cuticchia AJ, ed. *Human Gene Mapping 1994: A Compendium.* Baltimore, Md: The Johns Hopkins University Press; 1995.

Hall E. The gene as theme in the paradigm of cancer. *Br J Radiol.* 1993;66:1-11.

Levy JA, Fraenkel-Conrat H, Owens RA. *Virology.* 3rd ed. Englewood Cliffs, NJ: Prentice-Hall; 1994:125-141.

Perkins AS, Vande Woude GF. Principles of molecular cell biology of cancer: oncogenes. In: DeVita VT, Hellman S, Rosenberg SA, eds: *Cancer: Principles and Practice of Oncology.* 4th ed. Philadelphia, Pa: JB Lippincott; 1993:35-59.

Varmus HE, Lowell CA. Cancer genes and hematopoiesis. *Blood.* 1994;83:5-9.

12.6.4 ***Human Chromosomes.***—Formalized standard nomenclature of human chromosomes dates from 1960 and since 1978 has been known as the International System for Human Cytogenetic Nomenclature (ISCN).

Material in this section is based on recommendations in *ISCN 1995,*[1] which includes cancer cytogenetic nomenclature. *ISCN 1991*[2] and *ISCN 1985*[3] have also been consulted. Examples and clarifications are from these 3 sources and from written communications (Janet Rowley, MD, and Diane Rouslton, MD, PhD, December 15, 1995, January 11, 1996, and February 13, 1996).

Human chromosomes are numbered from 1 to 22. There are 2 additional chromosomes, X and Y. The numbered chromosomes are known as autosomes, X and Y as the sex chromosomes. Before the introduction of chromosome banding techniques, many chromosomes were indistinguishable from those with similar size and shape. Similar sized chromosomes were grouped together, and the groups were identified by capital letters:

Group	*Chromosomes*
A	1-3
B	4, 5
C	6-12, X
D	13-15
E	16-18
F	19, 20
G	21, 22, Y

One may refer to a chromosome by number or by group, eg:

chromosome 14

a D group chromosome

(Most usage of group designation has been obviated by banding techniques.)

Chromosome Bands: Chromosome bands are elicited by special staining methods; terms in the left-hand column need not be expanded:

Banding Pattern	*Technique*
Q-banding, Q bands	quinacrine
G-banding, G bands	Giemsa
R-banding, R bands	reverse Giemsa

Banding Pattern	*Technique*
C-banding, C bands	constitutive heterochromatin
T-banding, T bands	telomeric
NOR-staining	nucleolar organizing region

Two- and 3-letter banding technique codes provide more information about the banding method. These abbreviations must be expanded, but the letters in the examples above (Q, G, R, C, T, NOR) within those terms need not be expanded, eg:

Abbreviation	*Expansion*
QF	Q-bands by fluorescence
QFQ	Q-bands by fluorescence using quinacrine
CBG	C-bands by barium hydroxide using Giemsa stain

Chromosomes contain short and long arms, which are joined at the centromere (Figure 1). The long arm is designated by q and the short arm by p. Arm designations follow the chromosome number:

17p	short arm of chromosome 17
3q	long arm of chromosome 3
Xq	long arm of the X chromosome

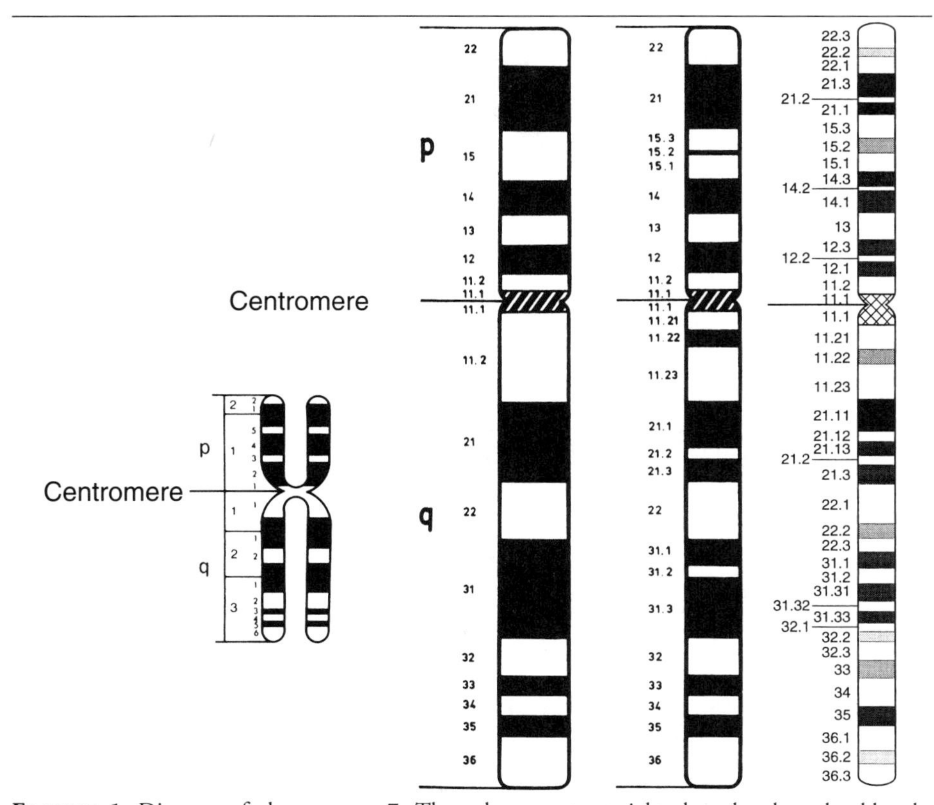

FIGURE 1 Diagram of chromosome 7. The enlargements at right show bands and subbands. Reproduced with permission from Mitelman.[1(pp17,109)]

Such expressions as 17p, 3q, and Xq need not be expanded. It is incorrect to refer to chromosome arms as chromosomes, eg, "chromosome 17p" should be "chromosome arm 17p" or simply "17p."

Regions are determined by major chromosome band landmarks. Chromosome arms contain 1 to 4 regions, numbered outward from the centromere. The region number follows the p or the q:

4q3	region 3 of long arm of chromosome 4

The regions are divided into bands, also numbered outward from the centromere. Bands have subdivisions or subbands (these are seen only when the chromosomes are extended). The band number follows the region number, and the subband number follows a period after the band number. When a subband is further subdivided, the sub-subband number follows the subband number without a period or other intervening punctuation:

11q23	chromosome 11, long arm, band 23 (region 2, band 3)
11q23.3	band in above subdivided, resulting in subband 23.3
20p11.23	chromosome 20, short arm, sub-subband 11.23 (region 1, band 1, subband 2, sub-subband 3)

It is correct usage to refer to the above expressions as "band 11q23," "band 11q23.3," and "band 20p11.23."

The centromere is indicated by p or q plus 10, as follows:

p10	region from middle of centromere to band p11
q10	region from middle of centromere to band q11

Karyotype: Karyotype is the chromosome complement, often expressed as the number of chromosomes per cell including the sex chromosomes with the sex chromosomes also specified, as in the following examples:

46,XX	46 chromosomes including 2 X chromosomes (2 each of chromosomes 1-22 and 2 X chromosomes in human female karyotype)
46,XY	46 chromosomes (2 each of chromosomes 1-22, 1 X and 1 Y in human male karyotype)
45,X	45 chromosomes, 1 X chromosome (Turner syndrome)
47,XXY	47 chromosomes, 2 X chromosomes, 1 Y (Klinefelter syndrome)
47,XYY	47 chromosomes, 1 X, 2 Y chromosomes
69,XXX	3 each of chromosomes 1-22 and X

A virgule is used to indicate more than 1 karyotype in an individual, tumor, cell line, etc:

45,X/46,XX

A karyotype description may contain both constitutional and acquired elements. For instance, the karyotype of a tumor cell from a person with constitutional trisomy 21 (Down syndrome) could show both the constitutional anomaly and an acquired neoplastic anomaly, eg, an acquired extra chromosome 8, and would be expressed as:

48,XX,+8,+21c

The lowercase c specifies that the trisomy 21 is constitutional, as distinguished from the acquired trisomy 8.

An individual with more than 1 karyotypic clone may be a *mosaic* (single-cell origin) or a *chimera* (multicell origin), which should be specified in the text and, with a 3-letter abbreviation, at first mention of the karyotype, eg:

mos 45,X/46,XY

chi 46,XX/46,XY

Brackets indicate the number of cells observed in a clone, eg:

chi 46,XX[25]/46,XY[10]

Chromosome Rearrangements: The following abbreviations and symbols are used in descriptions of chromosomes, including chromosome rearrangements. The list below is adapted from *ISCN 1995*.[1] Former designations based on *ISCN 1985*[3] appear in parentheses.

AI	first meiotic anaphase
AII	second meiotic anaphase
ace	acentric fragment
add	additional material of unknown origin
b	break
c	constitutional anomaly
cen	centromere
chi	chimera
chr (formerly cs)	chromosome
cht (formerly ct)	chromatid
cp	composite karyotype
cx	complex chromatid interchanges
del	deletion
de novo	chromosome abnormality not inherited
der	derivative
dia	diakinesis
dic	dicentric
dip	diplotene
dir	direct
dis	distal
dit	dictyotene
dmin	double minute
dup	duplication
e	exchange
end	endoreplication
fem	female
fis	fission
fra	fragile site

g	gap
h	heterochromatin
hsr	homogeneously staining region
i	isochromosome
idem	stemline karyotype in subclones
ider	isoderivative
idic	isodicentric
inc	incomplete karyotype
ins	insertion
inv	inversion or inverted
mar	marker chromosome
mat	maternal origin
med	medial
min	minute acentric fragment
ml	mainline
mn	modal number
mos	mosaic
oom	oogonial metaphase
p	short arm
PI	first meiotic prophase
pac	pachytene
pat	paternal origin
pcc	premature chromosome condensation
pcd	premature centromere division
prx	proximal
psu	pseudo-
pvz	pulverization
q	long arm
qdp	quadruplication
qr	quadriradial
r	ring form
rcp	reciprocal
rea	rearrangement
rec	recombinant chromosome
rob	robertsonian translocation
roman numerals	
I	univalent
II	bivalent

III	trivalent
IV	quadrivalent
s	satellite
sce	sister chromatid exchange
sct	secondary constriction
sdl	sideline
sl	stemline
spm	spermatogonial metaphase
stk	satellite stalk
t	translocation
tan	tandem
tas	telomeric association
tel	telomere
ter	terminal
tr	triradial
trc (formerly tri)	tricentric
trp	triplication
upd	uniparental disomy
v (formerly var)	variant or variable region
xma	chiasma(ta)
zyg	zygotene
:	break
::	break and reunion
;	separates chromosomes and chromosome bands in structural rearrangements involving 2 or more chromosomes
→	from-to
+	gain
−	loss
~	intervals in a chromosome segment where breakpoint is uncertain
<>	brackets for ploidy
[]	brackets for number of cells
=	number of chiasmata
× [multiplication sign]	multiple copies
?	questionable identification
/	separates clones

Single-letter abbreviations combined with other abbreviations are set closed up, eg:

chte	chromatid exchange
qter	long arm terminal

Three-letter symbols combined are set with a space, eg:

cht del	chromatid deletion
psu dic	pseudodicentric

The symbols in the list of chromosomes from *ISCN 1995* are part of an efficient shorthand, which describes the exact changes in a karyotype containing rearranged chromosomes. In publications that range beyond the field of cytogenetics, the symbols should always be defined.

Chromosome rearrangement terms can be written using a "short system" or short form. Complex abnormalities are designated by the more specific "detailed system" or long form. The detailed form uses symbols such as arrows to describe individual derivative chromosomes resulting from complex rearrangements (even the short system can result in a complex expression), eg:

short:
46,XY,t(2;5)(q21;q31)

long:
46,XY,t(2;5)(2pter→2q21::5q31→5qter;5pter→5q31::2q21→2qter)

The complete nomenclature, formulated for consistency in the description of chromosomal rearrangements, is detailed in *ISCN 1995.*[1] The following sections contain terms that illustrate some basic principles of the ISCN. Terms such as these may stand alone or may be part of longer expressions such as those above.

Order: In aberrations involving more than 1 chromosome, the sex chromosome appears first, then other chromosomes in numerical order (or, less commonly, in group order if only group is specified).

t(X;13)(q27;q12)	translocation involving bands Xq27 and 13q12

For 2 breaks in the same chromosome, the short arm precedes the long arm, and there is no internal punctuation, eg:

inv(2)(p21q31)	inversion of chromosome 2

Exceptions to numerical order convey special conditions, eg, when a piece of 1 chromosome is inserted into another, the recipient chromosome precedes the donor:

ins(5;2)(p14;q21q31)	insertion of portion of long arm of chromosome 2 into short arm of chromosome 5

PLUS AND MINUS SIGNS. A plus sign preceding a chromosome indicates a gain, eg:

+14	entire chromosome 14 gained

Recommendations have changed for additions involving chromosome regions or bands (terms with p or q). As of *ISCN 1995,* descriptions of karyotypes should use more specific terms incorporating symbols such as add, der, and ins (depending on the type of rearrangement); older terminology may still be appropriate for discussions. For instance, in the example below, the older notation on the left is appropriate for discussions (text) while the notation on the right is to be used in descriptions of karyotypes, eg:

Text	*Karyotype*
14p+ (addition to 14p)	add(14)(p13)

A minus sign preceding a chromosome signifies loss of the entire chromosome, eg:

−5	all of chromosome 5 missing

Similarly, a minus sign following a chromosome arm signifies loss *from* that arm, but this should be reserved for discussions, while more specific notation is used in karyotype descriptions, eg:

Text	*Karyotype*
5q− (part of 5q missing)	del(5)(q13q31)

A deletion of the long arm of a chromosome should be expressed not with a minus sign, but as:

del(5q)

PUNCTUATION

- Parentheses. The number of the affected chromosome follows the rearrangement symbol in parentheses:

inv(2)	inversion in chromosome 2

Details of the aberration follow in a second set of parentheses:

inv(2)(p13p24)	inversion in chromosome 2 involving bands 13 and 24 of the short arm

- Semicolon. Rearrangements involving a single chromosome do not take a semicolon. In rearrangements involving 2 or more chromosomes, a semicolon is used, eg:

1 Chromosome—no semicolon	
inv(2)(p21q31)	inversion within chromosome 2 with breaks at p21 and q31
dup(1)(q32q44)	duplication of segment from 1q32 to 1q44
del(9)(q22q33)	deletion of segment from 9q22 to 9q33

More than 1 chromosome—semicolon is used	
t(2;5)(q21;q31)	translocation involving breaks at 2q21 and 5q31

- Comma. Commas separate the chromosome number, sex chromosomes, and each term describing an abnormality:

46,XX,r(18)(p11q22)	female karyotype with ring chromosome 18

UNDERLINING. Underlining distinguishes different clones with "homologous chromosomes . . . involved in identical aberrations,"[1(pp56-57)] eg:

46,XX,der(1)t(1;3)(p34;q21)/46,XX,der(1)t(1;3)(p34;q21)

In unpublished text, authors should indicate that the underline is intended, so that it will not be set as italics, per typographic convention, in the published version.

OR. This word indicates "alternative interpretations of an aberration,"[1(p40)] eg:

add(19)(p13 or q13)

SPACING. As seen in previous examples, there is no spacing between the elements of a karyotype description except following "mos" and "chi," between 3-letter abbreviations, and before and after "or."

Derivative Chromosomes, Marker Chromosomes, and the Philadelphia Chromosome: The definitions of derivative and marker chromosomes have been recast in *ISCN 1995:* "A derivative chromosome is a structurally rearranged chromosome generated by (1) more than one rearrangement within a single chromosome . . . or (2) rearrangements involving two or more chromosomes. . . . An abnormal chromosome *in which no part can be identified* is referred to as a marker chromosome [italics added for emphasis]."[1(p35)]

Philadelphia chromosome is the name given to a particular derivative chromosome found in chronic myelogenous leukemia and some types of acute leukemia. It is the result of a rearrangement that juxtaposes the oncogene *ABL* with the breakpoint cluster region gene *BCR*[4] (see 12.6.2, Human Gene Nomenclature, and 12.6.3, Oncogenes and Tumor Suppressor Genes). The Philadelphia chromosome can be abbreviated as "Ph chromosome" or, if clear in context, "Ph." Although it is still seen with appendages, eg, Ph^1, Ph1, Ph_1, or Ph′, they are not necessary, and Ph is the current acceptable form. The Ph chromosome is the derivative chromosome 22 resulting from the translocation t(9;22)(q34;q11) and may be described as follows:

der(22)t(9;22)(q34;q11)

Long Karyotypes: Multiline karyotypes carry over from 1 line to the next with no punctuation other than that of the original expression (eg, no hyphen at the end of the first line), as in the following tumor karyotype:

46,XX,t(8;21)(q22;q22)[12]/45,idem,−X[19]/46,idem,
−X,+8[5]/47,idem,−X,+8,+9[8]

REFERENCES

1. Mitelman F, ed. *ISCN 1995: An International System for Human Cytogenetic Nomenclature 1995.* Basel, Switzerland: S Karger AG; 1995.

2. Mitelman F, ed. *ISCN (1991): Guidelines for Cancer Cytogenetics: Supplement to an International System for Human Cytogenetic Nomenclature.* Basel, Switzerland: S Karger AG; 1991.

3. Harnden DG, Klinger HP, eds. *ISCN (1985): An International System for Human Cytogenetic Nomenclature.* Basel, Switzerland: S Karger AG; 1985.

4. Rowley JD, Mitelman F. Principles of molecular cell biology of cancer: chromosome abnormalities in human cancer and leukemia. In: DeVita VT Jr, Hellman S, Rosenberg SA, eds. *Cancer: Principles and Practice of Oncology.* 4th ed. Philadelphia, Pa: JB Lippincott; 1993:68-69.

12.6.5 *Animal Genetic Terms.*

> *[T]he word* mouse . . . *comes originally from the Sanskrit* mush *derived from a verb meaning* to steal. . . . *Mice and rats, through their voracious activities in grain larders and as carriers of disease, inflicted considerable losses in food and lives upon ancient civilizations. . . .*
>
> H. C. Morse III[1(p6)]

> *A very obvious gap in our understanding of human genome evolution lies in the complete absence of any mapping data from the eutherian orders most distantly related to man, particularly the edentates. We would urge anyone with an interest in the genetics of the aardvark and the armadillo to consider a unique mapping project which will be at the forefront (alphabetically, at least) of the comparative mapping effort.*
>
> J. A. Marshall Graves et al[2(p964)]

As comparative mapping of human and animal genomes has intensified,[2] consistency of nomenclature has become a central goal, with similar or identical names designating the same gene across species whenever possible.

Traditionally, nonprimate animal gene terms have differed stylistically from human gene terms in some respects. The most notable difference is the use of lowercase letters. Mouse gene nomenclature may be considered prototypic of such terms.

Mouse Gene Nomenclature: The preponderance of mapped animal genes homologous to human genes have been identified in the mouse *Mus musculus*. The Mouse Genome Informatics Project and the Human Genome Database (GDB) cooperate closely.[3,4] Nomenclature of laboratory mouse genes is determined by the International Committee on Standardized Genetic Nomenclature for Mice.[3,5]

Mouse gene symbols resemble human symbols in several respects (see 12.6.2, Human Gene Nomenclature). They are descriptive, preferably short (2-4 characters), and italicized. They commence with letters, not numbers, and convert Greek letters to roman and roman numerals to arabic.

Mouse gene symbols differ from human symbols in using lowercase letters. Symbols usually contain an initial capital. A symbol with all lowercase letters (ie, no initial capital) conveys the meaning that the locus was "first discovered because of a recessive mutation."[6(p158)] Animal gene symbols also use hyphens (although only where hyphenation is required for clarity).

The following examples feature mouse genes with the related human gene term according to the International System for Human Gene Nomenclature (ISGN) when available[4,5]:

Mouse Gene Symbol	*Gene or Product*	*ISGN Term (When Available)*
a	nonagouti	
B2m	β_2-microglobulin	*B2M*
Car	carbonic anhydrase	*CA*
Cas	catalase	*CAT*
Cd5	(formerly *Ly1*) CD5 antigen	*CD5*

Mouse Gene Symbol	*Gene or Product*	*ISGN Term (When Available)*
C3	complement component 3	*C3*
Es1	esterase	
G6pd	glucose-6-phosphate dehydrogenase	*G6PD*
Gus	β-glucuronidase	
gus^{mps}	mutation in *Gus* gene causing mucopolysaccharidosis VII	
H2	major histocompatibility complex	*HLA*
Hbb	hemoglobin β-chain	*HBB*
Hras1	c-H-*ras* homologue (the prefix c is not used in animal genetic terms; see 12.6.3, Oncogenes and Tumor Suppressor Genes)	*HRAS*
Lamb1-1	β-laminin 1 gene, subunit 1	*LAMB1*
nmd	neuromuscular degeneration	
Pcx	pyruvate decarboxylase	*PC*
Pgk1-ps2	second pseudogene, phosphoglycerate kinase 1	*PGK1P2*
Tcra	T-cell receptor α-chain	*TCRA*

DNA segment nomenclature contains the elements of ISGN for humans plus interpolated information about the mouse chromosome, eg:

D16S259	ISGN symbol for segment on chromosome 16 in humans
D17H16S259	same segment is on mouse chromosome 17, with "H16" indicating that it resides on human chromosome 16

Symbols for DNA loci identified only in the mouse include laboratory codes (see Laboratory Codes), eg:

D1Mit1

Alleles: Whereas in ISGN human alleles are indicated by the gene term plus asterisk plus allele term, all set on the line, alleles in mice are represented by the gene symbol plus the allele designation as an italicized superscript. For use on computers, the Committee on Standardized Genetic Nomenclature for Mice recommends asterisks or angular brackets as alternatives to superscripts. Editors should convert the digital forms seen in the examples in the second column below to the forms in the first column for printed text. Authors should use the print text form on hard copy or indicate it by marking the hard copy (see 20.1, Copyediting and Proofreading Marks, Copyediting Marks).

Print Text	*Digital Text*	*Explanation*
$Gpi1^{a}$	*Gpi1*a* or *Gpi1<a>*	glucose phosphate isomerase 1a
c^{cb}	*c*cb* or *c<cb>*	chinchilla allele of albino coat color gene
d^{+2J}	*d*+2J* or *d<+2J>*	(+ signifies wild type; here, dilute locus, second reversion to wild type at The Jackson Laboratory)

When a mutant gene is cloned, its symbol becomes an allelic superscript of the cloned gene; for instance, *ob* (obese) is now

Lep^{ob}

(*Lep* is the gene symbol for leptin.)

Alleles do not always have superscripts (eg, *B, Ca* [caracul], *ob* [obese]) and the context in addition to the term itself must clarify whether the gene, locus, or allele is under discussion.

Mouse phenotype symbols are capitalized and appear in roman type, eg:

Gene/Locus	*Phenotype*
Gpi1	GPI1A, GPI1B, GPIAB
Pgm2	PGMB
$Ldh1^a/Ldh1^a$	$LDHA^a_4$

Mouse Chromosomes: Chromosomal nomenclature is similar for animals and humans (see 12.6.4, Human Chromosomes). However, rearrangement terms are capitalized. The following listing and subsequent examples are from the Committee on Standardized Genetic Nomenclature for Mice[5(pxxiv)]:

Cen	centromere
Del	deletion
Df	deficiency
Dp	duplication
Hc	pericentric heterochromatin
Hsr	homogeneous staining region
In	inversion
Is	insertion
Ms	monosomy
Ns	nullisomy
Rb	robertsonian translocation
Sp	supernumerary chromosome
T	translocation
Tel	telomere
Tet	tetrasomy
Tg	transgenic insertion
Tp	transposition
Ts	trisomy

As with human chromosomes, lowercase p represents the short arm and lowercase q the long arm.

Chromosome anomaly symbols usually include a unique laboratory code (see Laboratory Codes, below) and a series number, eg:

T37H	37th translocation found at Harwell
In5Rk	fifth inversion found by Roderick

Chromosome number appears in parentheses, eg:

In(2)5Rk   inversion in chromosome 2

Semicolons separate chromosomes involved in translocations, eg:

T(4;X)37H

Periods indicate the centromere in robertsonian translocations:

Rb(9.19)163H

Laboratory Codes: Laboratory registration codes appear as 1- to 4-letter symbols in animal genetic terminology, including chromosomal, DNA locus, and mouse strain nomenclature (see below). Such codes help identify specific colonies, useful in genetic studies that can extend over many generations. Laboratory codes are registered with the Institute of Laboratory Animal Resources at the National Academy of Sciences in Washington, DC, and are used to "uniquely identif[y] an investigator, laboratory, or institution that breeds rodents or rabbits." Laboratory codes appear without expansion. Examples are as follows:

Rpw   Richard P. Woychik, Oak Ridge National Laboratory

Arb   Arthritis and Rheumatism Branch, National Institute of Arthritis and Musculoskeletal and Skin Diseases

Mouse Strains: Names of inbred strains of mice are frequently encountered in discussions of genetics. Such names consist of capital letters or combinations of letters and numbers, which may be followed by a virgule and then by a substrain symbol, which may be a number, letter, or number-letter combination. Initial letters indicating substrains are usually Laboratory Registration codes and begin with a capital letter, eg:

CBA/J

in which J signifies The Jackson Laboratory. Exceptions exist in the case of 2 well-known strains of mouse:

BALB/c

C57BR/cd

Strain symbols may be abbreviated when used to designate new strains derived from them. For instance, C designates BALB/cJ-like and B designates C57BL/6J-like in a recombinant inbred strain, as follows:

CXB

For standard abbreviations, see the Rules for Mouse Genetic Nomenclature (Mouse Genome Database or The Jackson Laboratory's *Handbook on Genetically Standardized JAX Mice*[7]).

Many standard laboratory mouse strains are derived from crosses dating back to the early 20th century or even older lines, and the names reflect abbreviations for characteristics, for instance, BALB/c for *B*gg, *alb*ino, and DBA for *d*ilute, *b*rown, non*a*gouti.

Examples of mouse strain designations are

DBA/1   DBA/2   A/He   C57BL/6J   CBA/HN

Standardized abbreviations of strain-isolating methods used formerly (eg, e, egg transfer; f, foster nursing) have been discontinued from strain designations, except for some traditional strain names.

Capital F followed by a number in parentheses may appear after a strain designation to indicate the number of inbred generations, eg:

F(20)	20 inbred generations

No expansion of such terms is necessary.

Particular colonies are indicated by the symbol @ followed by the laboratory registration code, eg:

C57BL/6J@Arc	J substrain of substrain 6 of C57BL bred at Arc (Animal Resources Center, Australia)

The complete Nomenclature Guidelines for Mouse are available online from the Mouse Genome Database at The Jackson Laboratory (http://www.informatics.jax.org/).

Bacterial Gene Nomenclature: Bacterial gene and allele terms need not be expanded. Gene terms typically consist of an italicized lowercase 3-letter abbreviation plus a roman uppercase locus designator. The phenotype or encoded entity (eg, enzyme) is expressed with an initial capital and roman letters.[8,9]

Gene	*Phenotype (Explanation)*
inhA	InhA (protein involved in isoniazid action in mycobacteria)
katE	KatE (catalase)
sodA	SodA (superoxide dismutase)
sodB	SodB (superoxide dismutase)
wapA	WapA (wall-associated protein)

Alleles are designated with a number after the uppercase letter or following a hyphen, when not assigned to a locus, eg (the first 2 examples from Chater et al[8]):

araA1

ara-23

kat-19 (now *katA*)

Retroviral Genes[10-13]*:* (see also 12.6.3, Oncogenes and Tumor Suppressor Genes).

Viruses of the family Retroviridae, or retroviruses, contain these 3 main genes in common:

gag	group-specific core antigen gene
pol	polymerase gene
env	envelope gene

Compare typographic style of gene names and their products (p stands for protein, gp for glycoprotein):

Gene	*Gene Product (Protein or Polypeptide)*	*Subunits of Gene Products (Examples—Vary With Virus)*
gag	Gag	p18 p24 p53
pol	Pol	p31 p32 p66
env	Env	gp21 gp61/68 gp120

Additional human immunodeficiency virus genes include:

nef *rev* *tat* *vif* *vpr* *vpu*

REFERENCES

1. Morse HC III. The laboratory mouse—a historical perspective. In: Foster HL, Fox F, eds. *The Mouse in Biomedical Research.* Vol 1. Orlando, Fla: Academic Press Inc; 1981:6-10.

2. Marshall Graves JA, Wakefield MJ, Peters J, Searle AG, Womack JE, O'Brien SJ. Report of the Committee on Comparative Gene Mapping. In: Cuticchia AJ, ed. *Human Gene Mapping 1994: A Compendium.* Baltimore, Md: The Johns Hopkins University Press; 1995:962-1016.

3. Eppig JT, Maltais LJ. Locus nomenclature updates by e-mail. *Mamm Genome.* 1993;4:301-302.

4. McAlpine PJ, Shows TB, Povey S, et al. The 1994 Catalog of Approved Genes and Report of the Nomenclature Committee. In: Cuticchia AJ, ed. *Human Gene Mapping 1994: A Compendium.* Baltimore, Md: The Johns Hopkins University Press; 1995:6-147.

5. Committee on Standardized Genetic Nomenclature for Mice; Davisson MT, chair. Rules and guidelines for genetic nomenclature in mice. *Mouse Genome.* 1994;92:vii-xxxii.

6. Davisson MT. Rules and guidelines for nomenclature of mouse genes. *Gene.* 1994;147:157-160.

7. Green MC, Witham BA, eds. *Handbook on Gentically Standardized JAX Mice.* 4th ed. Bar Harbor, Me: The Jackson Laboratory; 1991.

8. Chater K, Berlyn M, Bachmann B. Bacteria. In: Stewart A, ed. Trends in Genetics *Genetic Nomenclature Guide.* Tarrytown, NY: Elsevier Science Publishers; 1995:5-8.

9. Demerec M, Adelberg EA, Clark AJ, Hartman PE. A proposal for a uniform nomenclature in bacterial genetics. *Genetics.* 1966;54:61-76.

10. Cullen BR, ed. *Human Retroviruses.* New York, NY: Oxford University Press; 1993:1-11.

11. Hsiung GD. Retroviridae. In: Hsiung GD, Fond CKY, Landry ML, eds. *Hsiung's Diagnostic Virology: As Illustrated by Light and Electron Microscopy.* 4th ed. New Haven, Conn: Yale University Press; 1994:201-217.

12. Levy JA, Fraenkel-Conrat H, Owens RA. *Virology.* 3rd ed. Englewood Cliffs, NJ: Prentice-Hall; 1994:125-141.

13. Collier L, Oxford J. *Human Virology: A Text for Students of Medicine, Dentistry and Microbiology.* New York, NY: Oxford University Press; 1993:281-295.

ADDITIONAL READING AND GENERAL REFERENCE

Silver M. Encyclopedia of the mouse genome III: October 1993: master list. *Mamm Genome.* 1993;4:S2-S9.

12.7 ■ **HEMOSTASIS.**—Hemostasis consists of platelet plug formation (primary hemostasis) and blood coagulation (secondary hemostasis, coagulation, clotting). Hemostasis and its control involve complex interactions of more than 50 procoagulants and anticoagulants. Description of hemostatic processes depends on consistent use of terms.

12.7.1 ***Primary Hemostasis.***—Note the typography of the following terms, which are found in descriptions of platelet hemostasis (use parenthetical abbreviated terms in accordance with 11.11, Abbreviations, Clinical and Technical Terms):

prostaglandin endoperoxides PGG_2 and PGH_2

thromboxanes A_2 (TXA_2) and B_2 (TXB_2, stable metabolite of TXA_2)

prostacyclin (PGI_2)

6-keto $PGF_{1\alpha}$ (a prostaglandin F, a stable metabolite of PGI_2)

von Willebrand factor (vWF; see below)

platelet factor 4 (PF4; see below)

β-thromboglobulin (βTG or BTG)

phospholipase C

phospholipase A_2

phosphatidylinositol 4,5-biphosphate (PIP_2)

inositol triphosphate (IP_3)

platelet glycoprotein Ia/IIa complex (GpIa-IIa)

platelet glycoprotein Ib/IX complex (GpIb-IX)

platelet glycoprotein IIb/IIIa complex (GpIIb-IIIa)

Platelet Factors: Arabic numerals are used to designate platelet factors, eg, platelet factor 3 (PF3), platelet factor 4 (PF4).

12.7.2 ***Secondary Hemostasis.***—Blood coagulation is the phase of clot formation dependent on plasma coagulation factors, or clotting factors.

Pathways: Plasma factor-dependent coagulation has been divided into 2 pathways (systems, phases). The following terms and synonyms are used for these:

Term	*Synonym*
intrinsic pathway	contact system-initiated pathway
extrinsic pathway	tissue factor-mediated or tissue factor-dependent pathway

Clotting Factors: An international system of nomenclature, completed in the early 1960s, clarified clotting factor terminology and, as Biggs[1] has observed, scientific findings in coagulation.

Roman numerals are used to designate plasma coagulation factors.

The following gives roman numeral designations, descriptive names, and synonyms for the plasma coagulation factors. Asterisks indicate preferred names. Synonyms that are rarely used are enclosed in parentheses. If a term other than the preferred term is used, the preferred term should be given in parentheses at the first mention of a factor. Common abbreviations appear here, but their use should conform to guidelines in 11.11, Abbreviations, Clinical and Technical Terms. (The term *factor VI,* originally designating activated factor V, is not used.)

Factor No.	*Descriptive Name*	*Synonym(s)*
(factor I)	fibrinogen*	. . .
factor II	prothrombin*	prethrombin

Factor No.	*Descriptive Name*	*Synonym(s)*
(factor III)	tissue factor	thromboplastin tissue thromboplastin tissue extract
(factor IV)	calcium*	calcium ion Ca^{2+}
factor V*	proaccelerin	(labile factor) (accelerator globulin [AcG]) (Ac globulin) (thrombogen)
factor VII*	proconvertin	(stable factor) (serum prothrombin conversion accelerator [SPCA]) (autoprothrombin I)
factor VIII*	antihemophilic factor (AHF)	antihemophilic globulin (AHG) antihemophilic factor A (platelet cofactor 1) (thromboplastinogen)
factor IX*	plasma thromboplastin component (PTC)	Christmas factor antihemophilic factor B (autoprothrombin II) (platelet cofactor 2)
factor X*	Stuart factor	Prower factor Stuart-Prower factor (autoprothrombin III) (thrombokinase)
factor XI*	plasma thromboplastin antecedent (PTA)	(antihemophilic factor C)
factor XII*	Hageman factor	contact factor (glass factor)
factor XIII	fibrin stabilizing factor (FSF)	plasma transglutaminase fibrinoligase (Laki-Lorand factor [LLF]) (fibrinase)
. . .	prekallikrein*	Fletcher factor
. . .	high-molecular-weight kininogen,* HMW kininogen (HMWK)	Fitzgerald factor Williams factor Flaujeac factor (contact activation cofactor) (Reid factor) (Washington factor)

A lowercase a designates the activated form of a factor, eg, IXa.

In diagrams of coagulation pathways, activation is indicated with a solid arrow:

X———→Xa

and action on another factor, with a dashed arrow:

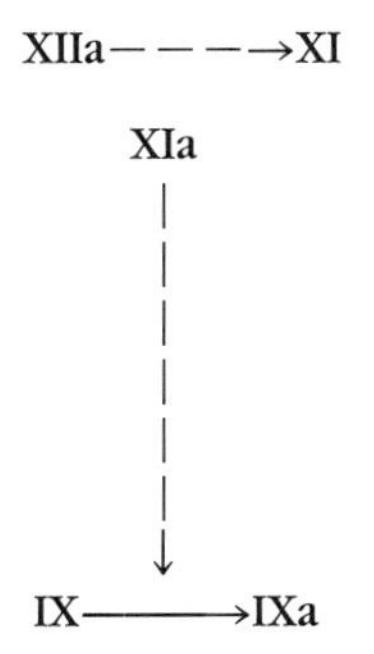

Clotting Factor Variants: Specific variants or abnormal forms may be named for locations, as follows (the first 3 examples are from Lee et al[2]):

fibrinogen Paris

prothrombin Barcelona

factor X Friuli

factor V Leiden

There is increasing use of molecular characterizations of abnormal forms as recommended by the International Society of Thrombosis and Haemostasis Scientific and Standardization Subcommittee on Factor VIII and Factor IX (Leon W. Hoyer, MD, written communication, June 13, 1995). For instance, variants such as factor VIII East Hartford and factor VIII Hiroshima are abnormal factors that contain an arginine-to-cysteine substitution at residue 1689[3-5] (see also 12.6.1 Nucleic Acids and Amino Acids), which can be designated as:

factor VIII Arg 1689 Cys

The abbreviations ins (insertion), del (deletion), In (intron), Ex (exon), and ter (termination codon) are also used within such terms as needed, as part of the subcommittee recommendations. See Peake and Tuddenham[6] for the complete recommendations.

Hemophilia: The terms ***hemophilia A*** and ***hemophilia B*** are used for factor VIII deficiency and factor IX deficiency (Christmas disease), respectively. Variants may be named ***hemophilia A Leiden, hemophilia A, CRM(+) variant, hemophilia B Leyden*** [*sic*], ***hemophilia Bm,*** etc (CRM: cross-reacting material). See Clotting Factor Variants for molecularly based nomenclature, which is increasingly preferred.

von Willebrand Factor: Because factor VIII, involved in coagulation, and von Willebrand factor (vWF), involved in platelet adhesion, form a noncovalent bimolecular complex, they were originally difficult to distinguish biochemically and immunologically. Nomenclature reflected this difficulty; for instance, what was first referred to as ***factor VIII-related antigen*** (abbreviated VIIIR:Ag) was found to be the factor that is deficient in von Willebrand disease.

Factor VIII and vWF, although functionally associated, are physiologically, genetically, and clinically distinct. In 1985 the International Committee on Coagulation and Thrombosis put forth preferred terminology that was meant to (1) distinguish VIII from vWF and (2) clarify exactly which entity was being specified. The committee noted that it is acceptable to use the term VIII-vWF for the biomolecular complex but not for either single component.[7,8]

TABLE 5. FACTOR VIII AND VON WILLEBRAND FACTOR

Preferred	Synonym	Old (Avoid)	Meaning
factor VIII	antihemophilic factor (AHF)	VIII:C	factor VIII protein
VIII:Ag	factor VIII antigen	VIII:CAg	factor VIII antigen
VIII:c	...	...	factor VIII coagulant activity
vWF	von Willebrand factor	VIIIR:Ag VIII/vWF AHF-like protein	von Willebrand factor protein
vWF:Ag	...	VIIIR:Ag	von Willebrand factor antigen
ristocetin cofactor (RCoF)	...	VIIIR:RCoF VIII:R:RCo VIIIR:vWF	von Willebrand factor function, ie, platelet adhesion–promoting property of vWF in the presence of the drug ristocetin

In Table 5, the terms in column 1 are not only preferred but also familiar exactly as shown to those conversant with the field. However, for most audiences, authors should clarify the preferred term by including the synonym or an explanation (eg, column 4, "Meaning") at first mention.

von Willebrand Disease: Variants of von Willebrand disease are designated as follows:

type I

type IIA

type IIB

type III

platelet type

Clot Degradation (Fibrinolysis, Thrombolysis): The following sample terms are included for reference. Expand at first mention in accordance with 11.11, Abbreviations, Clinical and Technical Terms:

tPA	tissue-type plasminogen activator *or* tissue plasminogen activator (When a specific therapeutic formulation of tPA is intended, use the USAN term; see 12.4, Drugs.)
PAI-1	a plasminogen activator inhibitor
uPA	urokinase or urinary-type plasminogen activator
α_2PI	α_2-plasmin inhibitor, α_2-antiplasmin
FDP or FSP	fibrin degradation products or fibrin split products
D-dimer	dimerized plasmin fragment D

PLASMA ANTICOAGULANT PROTEINS. The following sample terms are included for reference:

antithrombin III (ATIII)

heparin cofactor 2

protein C

activated protein C (APC)

protein S

tissue factor pathway inhibitor (TFPI); old terms: extrinsic pathway inhibitor (EPI), lipoprotein-associated coagulation inhibitor (LACI)

PLASMA PROTEINASE INHIBITORS. The following inhibit coagulation proteases as well as other plasma proteases:

α_2-macroglobulin

α_1-antitrypsin

C_1-esterase inhibitor

LUPUS ANTICOAGULANTS AND ANTIPHOSPHOLIPID ANTIBODIES. Lupus anticoagulants are immunoglobulins identified by their inhibitory activity in clotting assays, whereas antiphospholipid antibodies are identified by immunologic tests. Patients with one may or may not also have the other, and they have similar clinical implications.

Tests of Coagulation: Two among several tests of coagulation are the prothrombin time (PT) and the partial thromboplastin time (PTT). When the more common activated partial thromboplastin time (aPTT) is used, this should be specified.

Traditionally, the PT has been reported as a ratio of the patient's PT to the mean laboratory control PT, the PT ratio, or PTR. Reporting the PTR has been refined by use of a modified PTR, the international normalized ratio (INR).[9-11] In accordance with a 1985 policy statement of the International Committee for Thrombosis and Hemostasis and the International Committee for Standardization in Hematology,[9] authors are encouraged to report the INR if at all possible. Unlike conversions between conventional and SI units (see 15.1, Units of Measure, SI Units), there is no simple conversion factor from the PTR to the INR because the international sensitivity index (ISI) of the thromboplastin used in the actual assay performed must be known. The INR is calculated as shown:

$$INR = PTR^{ISI}$$

Authors should specify the exact method by which their results were initially reported by the laboratory performing the assay and the method of conversion, if any, used on the original results.

REFERENCES

1. Biggs R. *Human Blood Coagulation, Haemostasis, and Thrombosis.* 2nd ed. Oxford, England: Blackwell Scientific Publications; 1976:15-16. (A third edition of this work came out in 1984.)
2. Lee GR, Bithell TC, Foerster J, Athens JW, Lukens JN. *Wintrobe's Clinical Hematology.* 9th ed. Philadelphia, Pa: Lea & Febiger; 1993.
3. Arai M, Higuchi M, Antonarakis SE, et al. Characterization of a thrombin cleavage site mutation (Arg 1689 to Cys) in the factor VIII gene of two unrelated patients with cross-reacting material-positive hemophilia A. *Blood.* 1990;75:384-389.
4. Kamisue S, Shima M, Nishimura T, et al. Abnormal factor VIII Hiroshima: defect in crucial proteolytic cleavage by thrombin at Arg^{1689} detected by a novel ELISA. *Br J Haematol.* 1994;86:106-111.
5. O'Brien DP, Tuddenham EGD. Purification and characterization of factor VIII 1,689-Cys: a nonfunctional cofactor occurring in a patient with severe hemophilia A. *Blood.* 1989;73:2117-2122.

6. Peake I, Tuddenham E. A standard nomenclature for factor VIII and factor IX gene mutations and associated amino acid alterations: on behalf of the ISTH SSC Subcommittee on Factor VIII and Factor IX. *Thromb Haemost.* 1994;72:475-476.

7. Marder VJ, Mannucci PM, Firkin BG, Hoyer LW, Meyer D. Standard nomenclature for factor VIII and von Willebrand factor: a recommendation by the International Committee on Thrombosis and Haemostasis. *Thromb Haemost.* 1985;54:871-872.

8. Marder VJ, Roberts HR. Proposed symbols for factor VIII and von Willebrand factor [letter]. *Ann Intern Med.* 1986;105:627.

9. Loeliger EA. ICSH/ICTH recommendations for reporting prothrombin time in oral anticoagulant control. *Thromb Haemost.* 1985;53:155-156.

10. Hirsch J, Dalen JE, Deykin D, Poller L. Oral anticoagulants: mechanism of action, clinical effectiveness, and optimal therapeutic range. *Chest.* 1992;102:312S-324S.

11. Hirsch J, Poller L. The international normalized ratio: a guide to understanding and correcting its problems. *Arch Intern Med.* 1994;154:282-288.

Additional Readings and General References

Bloom AL, Forbes CD, Thomas DP, Tuddenham EGD, eds. *Haemostasis and Thrombosis.* 3rd ed. London, England: Churchill Livingstone; 1994.

Eckman MH, Levine HJ, Pauker SG. Effect of laboratory variation in the prothrombin-time ratio on the results of oral anticoagulant therapy. *N Engl J Med.* 1993;329:696-702.

Isselbacher KJ, Braunwald E, Wilson JD, Martin JB, Fauci AS, Kasper DL, eds. *Harrison's Principles of Internal Medicine.* 13th ed. New York, NY: McGraw-Hill; 1994.

12.8 ■ IMMUNOLOGY.

> *In many cases the host lives in symbiosis with potentially infectious microorganisms. Until very recent times, one's survival was entirely dependent on the immune system. . . . The student of immunity needs to remember that the immune system evolved to allow one to live at least until the age of reproduction. Autoimmune diseases that primarily develop in older individuals do not exert evolutionary pressure on a population.*
>
> M. K. Liszewski, J. P. Atkinson[1(p934)]

12.8.1 *Complement.*

> *It is estimated that one C3b deposited on an organism can become four million in about 4 min.*
>
> M. K. Liszewski, J. P. Atkinson[1(p922)]

The term *complement* refers to a group of proteins involved as a system in providing resistance to pathogens. The resistance is both direct (alternative pathway, also properdin system) and through antigen-antibody reactions (classical pathway), converging in a final common pathway (terminal pathway or the membrane attack complex). The complement system was so named because it was originally discovered to be complementary to humoral immunity.

Current nomenclature derives largely from the 1968 World Health Organization bulletin "Nomenclature of Complement"[2] with some subsequent de facto modifications having been brought about by changes in understanding of the mechanisms of action. Components of complement are designated with C and a number (reflective of order of discovery of the component rather than the reaction sequence, as evident below) or with another capital letter. (The prime, as in C′, has been discontinued.)

Classical pathway:	C1, C4, C2, C3
Alternative pathway:	D, B, P (properdin), C3
Membrane attack complex (MAC):	C5, C6, C7, C8, C9

For fragments of complement components, *lowercase* letters, often a or b, are added, eg:

C3b C3c C3d C3dg C3f

C4a C5b Bb

Usually, a lowercase b indicates the larger, membrane-binding fragment and lowercase a the smaller, released fragment. One inconsistency is the use of C2a as the binding fragment (with C2b as the release fragment). To correct this, some sources have reversed these designations to fit with the rest of the scheme.[3]

A lowercase letter i no longer necessarily specifies inactive complement fragments but rather simply a complement subfragment, eg:

C3bi or iC3b

Isoforms of C4 have *capital* letters appended, eg:

C4A C4B

The subunits of C1 are as follows:

C1q C1r C1s

Various notations combining these subunits convey the stoichiometry of the complex, and all are acceptable, eg:

$(C1r)_2$

$C1r^2{:}C1s^2$

$C1qC1r_2C1s_2$

$C1qr_2s_2$

C1s-C1r-C1r-C1s

Functionally associated elements of a complement complex are written in a series without spaces, eg:

C4b2a3b

C4bC2

Sometimes a hyphen is used:

C5b67 *or* C5b-7

C5-9

An asterisk shows nascent or metastable state:

C4b*

C3b*

C5b*

C5b-7*

Convertase complexes are linked complement fragments that activate other complement components. For example, the convertase that activates C3 is known as the C3 convertase. As in the following example, the convertases consist of different subunits, depending on which complement pathway generated them:

	Classical Pathway Fragments	*Alternative Pathway Fragments*
C3 convertase:	C4b2a	C3bBb
	C4b2b	C3bBbP
		C3(H_2O)Bb(Mg^{2+})
C5 convertase:	C4b2a3b	C3bBbC3bP
	C4b2b3b	(C3b)2Bb

A bar over the suffix(es) was proposed in 1968 to designate activated complement (eg, C$\overline{4}$, C$\overline{423}$, C$\overline{4b2a}$), but this convention is increasingly not observed.

Complement Receptors: Complement receptors are found on a variety of cells that participate in the effects of complement activation. A complement receptor may be named by number, by the complement component with which it binds (ligand), or by 1 or more CD (cluster of differentiation) designations, as shown in the list below, modified from Liszewski and Atkinson,[1(p926)] Table 3, with permission (see also 12.8.4, Lymphocytes).

Numbering System	*Ligand*	*CD*
CR1	C3b/C4b receptor	CD35
CR2	C3d/C3bi receptor C3dg	CD21
CR3	C3bi receptor	CD11b/18
CR4	C3bi receptor	CD11c/18
C3aR	C3a receptor	. . .
C5aR	C5a receptor	. . .
C1qR	C1q receptor	. . .

Complement Regulators: Complement regulators include the following:

delay accelerating factor (DAF) = CD55

membrane cofactor protein (MCP) = CD46

C1 inhibitor (C1-INH or C1-esterase INH)

MAC inhibitor = CD59

factor B

factor I

factor H (formerly β_1H)

C4 binding protein (C4bp)

S protein (vitronectin)

CH_{50}: The term "CH_{50}" denotes an assay for total complement, the *CH* referring to hemolytic complement and the subscript *50* to 50% lysis, an end point of the assay.

Official Nomenclature for Allotypes and Variants of Human Complement: Recommendations for these from the WHO-IUIS Nomenclature Sub-Committee appear regularly in the *Bulletin of the World Health Organization* and the *Journal of Immunological Methods,* and other journals.[4-6]

REFERENCES

1. Liszewski MK, Atkinson JP. The complement system. In: Paul WE, ed. *Fundamental Immunology.* 3rd ed. New York, NY: Raven Press; 1993:917-939.
2. World Health Organization. Nomenclature of complement. *Bull World Health Organ.* 1968;39:935-938.
3. Letendre P. Complement: to be or not to be? *Transfusion.* 1990;30:478-479.
4. WHO-IUIS Nomenclature Sub-Committee. Nomenclature for human complement factor B. *Bull World Health Organ.* 1992;70:541-546. *J Immunol Methods.* 1993;163:9-11.
5. WHO-IUIS Nomenclature Sub-Committee. Nomenclature for human complement component C2. *Bull World Health Organ.* 1992;70:527-530. *J Immunol Methods.* 1992;163:1-2.
6. WHO-IUIS Nomenclature Sub-Committee. Revised nomenclature for complement component C4. *Bull World Health Organ.* 1992;70:531-540.

ADDITIONAL READINGS AND GENERAL REFERENCES

Isselbacher KJ, Braunwald E, Wilson JD, Martin JB, Fauci AS, Kasper DL. *Harrison's Principles of Internal Medicine.* 13th ed. New York, NY: McGraw-Hill, 1994:1554-1555, 1636-1637.

Mollison PL, Engelfried CP, Contreras M. *Blood Transfusion in Clinical Medicine.* 9th ed. Boston, Mass: Blackwell Scientific Publications; 1993:134, 138-147.

Paraskevas F, Foerster J. Cell interactions in the immune response: complement. In: Lee GR, Bithell TC, Foerster J, Athens JW, Lukens JN, eds. *Wintrobe's Clinical Hematology.* 9th ed. Philadelphia, Pa: Lea & Febiger; 1993:458-467.

12.8.2 *The Human Leukocyte Antigen (HLA) System.*

> *[I]n transplantation, **H**istocompatibility **L**eads to **A**cceptance; in anthropology, **H**uman populations are **L**ocated by **A**llelic variation; in disease, **HLA** alleles in **L**inkage disequilibrium **A**ccount for disease. . . .*
>
> Julia G. Bodmer[1(p7)]

Nomenclature: Nomenclature of the HLA system, first formalized in 1967, is determined by the World Health Organization Nomenclature Committee for Factors of the HLA System.[2] Reports on HLA nomenclature, which present officially recognized antigens and alleles, appear annually in the journals *Human Immunology, European Journal of Immunogenetics, Tissue Antigens,* and *Vox Sanguinis;* the first 3 also publish monthly updates.[3]

HLA antigens appear not only on leukocytes but on virtually all nucleated cells of human tissues and on platelets. Just as red blood cell antigens determine blood type (see 12.1, Blood Groups and Platelet Antigens), HLA antigens determine tissue type.

HLA antigens were discovered to be determinants of the success of tissue transplantation (histocompatibility, *histo-* meaning "relating to tissue"), and certain specific HLA antigens are associated with particular diseases. Because these antigens are highly polymorphic, they are also used in forensic identification of individuals.

Latterly, but more fundamentally, the HLA antigens have been shown to have an important role in immunity, functioning as antigen-presenting molecules on the surface of antigen-presenting cells.[1] The antigen-presenting cells bind with T-lymphocyte receptors (T-cell receptors; see 12.8.4, Lymphocytes), activating cytotoxic or helper T cells, depending on the class of HLA antigen.

The molecules of the HLA system are encoded by at least 35 contiguous genes on the short arm of chromosome 6, a site known as the major histocompatibility complex (MHC). The at least 158 different antigens of the HLA system were originally identified serologically, and the nomenclature directly reflected this. As the molecular biology of the system began to be explored via nucleotide and amino acid sequencing techniques, it was found that single antigen specificities as defined serologically might represent multiple alleles as defined biochemically, ie, a single antigen could be expressed by multiple alleles. Accordingly, in 1987, new nomenclature for these alleles (which now number at least 560) consistent with the International System for Human Gene Nomenclature (see 12.6.2, Human Gene Nomenclature) was built onto the original serologically defined nomenclature. A prime goal was that the nomenclature would reflect the relationship between recognized serological antigen specificities and molecularly defined alleles.[2]

Because, in keeping with this goal, the genetic nomenclature follows from the earlier conventions for serological specificities,[4] the latter terminology is presented first.

HLA: This abbreviation has come to signify *human leukocyte antigen(s)*. However, it is proper, and not redundant, to refer to "HLA antigens" (the "A" originally was a simple letter designation and did not stand for "antigen"). The term HLA refers both to the antigens on cells and to the loci on the human genome responsible for those antigens.

Class I MHC Antigens: The 3 class I HLA antigens are present on all nucleated cells, bind short (9-amino acid) peptides from self or viral antigens, and interact with cytotoxic T cells. These antigens are:

HLA-A HLA-B HLA-C

The components of a class I MHC molecule include

an α chain (coded in the MHC)
α_1, α_2, α_3: subregions or subdomains of the α chain

β_2-microglobulin (not coded in the MHC)

Class II MHC Antigens: The class II antigens are found on monocytes, macrophages, some lymphocytes, epithelial cells, and dendritic cells; bind longer (10- to 14-amino acid) peptides from exogenous antigens; and interact with helper T cells. They are:

HLA-DP HLA-DQ HLA-DR

(DR originally signified "D-related"; DP and DQ were then named alphabetically.)

The components of a class II MHC molecule, which are all coded on the MHC, include:

an α chain with α_1 and α_2 domains

a β chain with β_1 and β_2 domains

(The terms *MB, DC, MT, DS,* and *SB,* formerly used for class II loci, should no longer be used.)

Note: α and β chains are also components of the homologous but not identical T-cell receptors—do not confuse with those chains or with the heavy chain of the IgA molecule; see 12.8.3, Immunoglobulins, and 12.8.4, Lymphocytes.

Antigenic Specificities: Antigen specificities of the major HLA loci are indicated with numbers following the major locus letter(s), eg:

HLA-A1 HLA-B27 HLA-DR1

With DNA sequencing now necessary for official recognition of most HLA antigens, the "w" (for "workshop," indicating provisional status, as determined serologically) is now used for only 3 specificity groups:

- HLA-C (to distinguish the C antigens from complement), eg, HLA-Cw1
- Dw and DPw specificities, which are still defined by 2 cellular assays, mixed lymphocyte culture (MLC) and primed lymphocyte typing (PLT), eg, Dw12
- Bw4 and Bw6

Parenthetical numbers may be part of the term for an HLA antigen; these indicate subspecificities or "splits" of the antigen (and its gene), such that 2 antigens (or alleles) are recognized instead of 1.[2]

HLA-A23(9) HLA-A24(9) HLA-B49(21) HLA-Dw18(w6)

These examples indicate, respectively, that A23 and A24 are splits of HLA-A9, that B49 is a split of B21, and that Dw18 is a split of Dw6.

Haplotypes: The HLA haplotype is the set of HLA alleles on 1 chromosome. Each person possesses 2 such haplotypes, 1 from each parent, and thus has 2 HLA antigens determined by each major locus, ie, 2 HLA-A antigens, 2 HLA-B antigens, etc. HLA typing is used clinically, eg, before tissue and bone marrow transplantation and platelet transfusion. When HLA typing is done, the HLA antigens are determined without respect to haplotype and are given as the phenotype, eg:

A1, A3, B5, B8, Cw1, Cw3, Dw1, Dw3

If the HLA types of the parents or siblings are known, it may be possible to determine the 2 HLA haplotypes, in which case an alternate form of expression, known as the genotype, can be given. In this form, the 2 haplotypes are expressed as 2 series of HLA specificities, separated by a virgule:

A1, B8, Cw1, Dw3/A3, B5, Cw3, Dw1

On occasion, it may be possible to type only 1 antigen from a given locus. In the next example, only Dw3 can be typed at the Dw locus, and a hyphen indicates the undetermined Dw antigen:

A1, A2, B8, B27, Cw4, Cw5, Dw3,–

The individual either may have an untypeable Dw antigen or may have 2 identical Dw3 antigens. In the former case, the genotype would be given as:

A1, B8, Cw4, Dw3/A2, B27, Cw5,–

In the latter case, the genotype is expressed as:

A1, B8, Cw4, Dw3/A2, B27, Cw5, Dw3

Other Histocompatibility Antigens: HLA antigens represent only some of the products of the MHC. Others, also important in immunity, are:

class III loci (loci for 4 components of complement; see also 12.8.1, Complement)

C2

C4a

C4b

Bf (properdin factor B)

LMP (large multifunctional protease)

TAP (transporter associated with antigen processing)

A haplotype of complement types is called a *complotype,* eg:

BfS, C2C, C4AQO, C4B1

(QO designates a deficiency; see also below, Class III Alleles.)

Additional HLA-Related Terminology: The following terms are provided as a reference. When writing for a general medical audience, expanded forms should be used.

The HLA-DR antigens are also referred to as "Ia-like" antigens.

CREG stands for cross-reactive group, as in A1-CREG, A2-CREG, B15-CREG.

Genetic Nomenclature (see also 12.6.2, Human Gene Nomenclature): Genetic methods (nucleotide sequencing) are now the preeminent means of defining new genes and alleles of the HLA system.

Use italics to distinguish HLA genes, eg, HLA-A1, *HLA-A1.* As HLA alleles are usually not italicized (in contrast to other alleles), authors should make clear through context whether genotype or phenotype is being discussed.

The components of the genetic name for an HLA allele begin with the gene:

HLA-A or *HLA-A* or *A*

For the HLA-D region, the gene name includes the name of the chain that the gene codes (A for α, B for β), often followed by a number for the chain gene (*not* the domain number as described in the previous sections on class I and class II molecules). For instance, the gene for the first DRβ chain is:

DRB1

The allele is then identified by an asterisk followed by 4 digits, eg:

DRB1*1201

DQA1*0302

A final N indicates a nonexpressed allele, eg:

DRB4*01012N

An occasional fifth digit indicates a "noncoding substitution" ("a mutation that is unlikely to cause any immunologic response"[2]), eg:

DRB*11042

Shorthand for a group of alleles at the same locus uses a hyphen, eg, the alleles at the HLA-B27 locus:

HLA-B*2701, *2702, *2703, *2704, *2705, *2706, *2707

which may also be expressed as:

HLA-B*2701-7

As mentioned in the introduction to this section, a single HLA specificity may coincide with multiple alleles; for instance, HLA-A1 corresponds to both A*0101 and A*0102. Since 1991, new serologically defined antigens have been named for the known DNA sequences with which they are associated,[1] sometimes resulting in numerically similar allele and specificity names, eg:

Specificity	*Allele Name*
HLA-A203	HLA-A*2303
B7801	B*7801

However, because most known specificities were defined before 1991, most do not have 4-digit designations. Also, some loci have been found to produce molecules of differently numbered specificities, so the specificity and allele numbering may often correspond only in part or not at all, eg:

Specificity	*Allele Name*
B64(14)	B*1401
DR53	DRB4*01

HLA pseudogenes (see also 12.6.2, Human Gene Nomenclature) resemble and are located near the class I loci but are not transcribed to produce functional products[5]:

HLA-H *HLA-J* *HLA-K* *HLA-L*

These class II gene loci were discovered before their products (if any) and the roles of those products had been elucidated:

HLA-DM *HLA-DN* *HLA-DO*

Class III Alleles: The following are examples of alleles of this region of the MHC (QO designates a deficiency allele):

BF*F BF*S BF*F1 BF*S1

C2*C C2*A C2*QO

C4A (formerly "Rogers")
C4A*1
C4A*QO

C4B (formerly "Chido")
C4B*1
C4B*QO

Animals: The names for the histocompatibility locus in other animals[6] usually correspond to the expression HLA for humans (but not always, eg, the prototypical mouse locus, H-2). In this convention, the name is based on a common name or species name, combined with "LA" for "leukocyte antigen," for example:

cat	FLA
dog	DLA
domestic cattle	BoLA

domestic fowl	B
guinea pig	GPLA
horse	EqLA
mole rat	Smh
mouse	H-2
pig	SLA
rabbit	RLA
rat	RT1

A new style has been adopted by primate researchers in the Mhc field (in nonhuman animals, this abbreviation mixes an initial capital and lowercase letters; see also 12.6.5, Animal Genetic Terms). The primate terminology is based on the genus and species name (see 12.12, Organisms) and substitutes Mhc for LA, as more representative of the true distribution of these antigens, for example:

Animal Name	*Recommended Term*	*Former Term*
chimpanzee (*Pan troglodytes*)	MhcPatr	ChLA
gorilla (*Gorilla gorilla*)	MhcGogo	GoLA
orangutan (*Pongo pygmaeus*)	MhcPopy	OrLA
rhesus macaque (*Macaca mulatta*)	MhcMamu	RhLA

After first use, the Mhc prefix may be dropped:

MhcMamu-A26	Mamu-A26
MhcGogo-DRB	Gogo-DRBY*01

REFERENCES

1. Bodmer WF. HLA 1991. In: Tsuji K, Aizawa M, Sasazuki S, eds. *HLA 1991: Proceedings of the Eleventh International Histocompatibility Workshop and Conference Held in Yokohama, Japan, 6-13 November, 1991.* New York, NY: Oxford University Press; 1992:7-16.

2. Bodmer JG. Nomenclature 1991 foreword. *Hum Immunol.* 1991;34:2-3.

3. Bodmer JG, Marsh SGE, Albert ED, et al. Nomenclature for factors of the HLA system, 1995. *Tissue Antigens.* 1995;46:1-18.

4. Wordsworth P. HLA nomenclature: a user-friendly system? *Ann Rheum Dis.* 1994;53:153-154.

5. Bodmer JG, Marsh SGE, Albert ED, et al. Nomenclature for factors of the HLA system, 1994. *Tissue Antigens.* 1994;44:1-18.

6. Klein J, Bontrop RE, Dawkins RL, et al. Nomenclature for the major histocompatibility complexes of different species: a proposal. *Immunogenetics.* 1990;31:217-219.

ADDITIONAL READINGS AND GENERAL REFERENCES

Carpenter CB. The major histocompatibility gene complex. In: Isselbacher KJ, Braunwald E, Wilson JD, Martin JB, Fauci AS, Kasper DL, eds. *Harrison's Principles of Internal Medicine.* 13th ed. New York, NY: McGraw-Hill; 1994:380-386.

Hansen TH, Carreno BM, Sachs DH. The major histocompatibility complex. In: Paul WE, ed. *Fundamental Immunology.* 3rd ed. New York, NY: Raven Press; 1993:577, 578, 586, 606-628.

Paraskevas F, Foerster J. Cell interactions in the immune response. In: Lee GR, Bithell TC, Foerster J, Athens JW, Lukens JN, eds. *Wintrobe's Clinical Hematology.* 9th ed. Philadelphia, Pa: Lea & Febiger; 1993:431-437.

Reisner EG. Human leukocyte and platelet antigens. In: Beutler E, Lichtman MA, Coller BS, Kipps TJ, eds. *Williams Hematology.* 5th ed. New York, NY: McGraw-Hill; 1995:1611-1617.

12.8.3 ***Immunoglobulins.***—Immunoglobulins are the glycoproteins that constitute antibodies. They were first recognized by serum electrophoresis and, because they were localized to the electrophoretic gamma zone, were originally referred to as γ-globulins,[1] a term that is still in use.

The term *immunoglobulin* and terminology for immunoglobulin classes were put forth in the early 1960s.[2-6] The most abundant class of immunoglobulin (Ig) molecules was named IgG, the G deriving from the electrophoretic gamma mobility. The M in IgM originates in an earlier designation as a macroglobulin.

The 5 classes of immunoglobulins, in decreasing order of abundance, are

IgG IgA IgM IgD IgE

Each can be found either on a cell surface (where it serves as an antigen receptor) or in tissue fluids such as blood (where it serves as a protective antibody).

Figure 2 shows schematically the basic structural unit of all immunoglobulin molecules, including many components defined herein. An immunoglobulin can be composed of 1 or more such units, often called monomers.

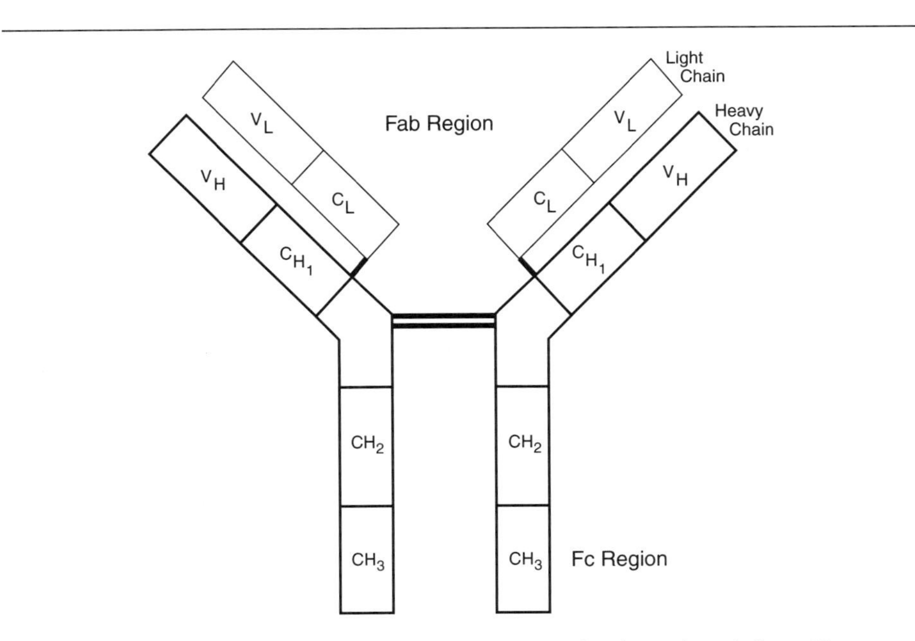

FIGURE 2 Basic structural unit of immunoglobulin molecules. Adapted from Haynes and Fauci,[7(p1553)] reprinted by permission.

Enzymes cleave the immunoglobulin molecule into fragments with specific names. Expansion of these terms is not necessary:

Fab (antigen-binding fragment)

Fab′

$F(ab')_2$ (2 linked Fab′ fragments)

Fb

Fc (crystallizable fragment)

pFc′

Fd

Fv (variable part of Fab)

Each immunoglobulin monomer contains 2 heavy chains and 2 light chains, commonly signified simply as follows:

H L

Each H chain and L chain protein in turn contains both variable and constant regions:

C V

It is useful to define H, L, C, and V for most audiences and to use their expansions in general discussions.

Heavy Chains: The type of heavy chain identifies the class (isotype) of immunoglobulin. Heavy chains are named with the Greek letter that corresponds to the class of the immunoglobulin:

Heavy-Chain Name	*Immunoglobulin Class*
γ	IgG
α	IgA
μ	IgM
δ	IgD
ε	IgE

IgG and IgA have subclasses with corresponding heavy chains:

Heavy-Chain Name	*Immunoglobulin Subclass*
$\gamma 1$	IgG1
$\gamma 2$	IgG2
$\gamma 3$	IgG3
$\gamma 4$	IgG4
$\alpha 1$	IgA1
$\alpha 2$	IgA2

Light Chains: There are 2 types of light chain:

κ λ

Both types are associated with all 5 immunoglobulin classes; that is, an immunoglobulin molecule of any type might have κ or λ light chains (but not both types in the same molecule). In humans, there are 6 classes (isotypes) of λ chain:

$\lambda 1$ $\lambda 2$ $\lambda 3$ $\lambda 4$ $\lambda 5$ $\lambda 6$

Variable and Constant Regions: Different nonallelic forms of the light- or heavy-chain variable regions can be designated by numbers as follows (these numbers are not subscript):

V_H: variable region of the heavy chain

specific forms of the heavy-chain variable region:

V_H1 V_H2 V_H3 V_H4

V_L: variable region of the light chain

specific forms of the κ and λ light-chain variable regions:

$V_\kappa 1$ $V_\kappa 2$ $V_\kappa 3$ $V_\kappa 4$

$V_\lambda 1$ $V_\lambda 2$ $V_\lambda 3$ $V_\lambda 4$

Constant regions of the various H-chain or L-chain proteins are denoted by subscript letters and numbers as follows:

C_L: constant region of the light chain
C_L regions specified for light-chain type:

C_κ $C_\lambda 1$ $C_\lambda 2$

C_H: constant region of the heavy chain
C_H domains of the Ig molecule:

C_H1 C_H2 C_H3

C_H regions specified for heavy-chain class:

C_μ $C_\gamma 1$ $C_\gamma 3$ C_ε

Specific hypervariable regions within the variable regions of the immunoglobulin are known as complementarity-determining regions (CDRs) and are named as follows:

CDR1 CDR2 CDR3

(Do not confuse CDRs with the CD cell markers, eg, CD3; see 12.8.4, Lymphocytes.) Heavy- or light-chain CDRs are termed HCDR1, etc, or LCDR1, etc, respectively.

Framework regions (relatively invariable regions between hypervariable regions) are designated

FR1 FR2 FR3 FR4

Ig Prefixes: The following are examples of terms combining Ig and a single-letter prefix. It is best to expand these terms at first mention (especially those with the letter s, which has more than one meaning in this context):

sIg	surface immunoglobulin
sIgM	surface IgM
mIgM	monomeric IgM (equivalent to sIgM)
sIgA	secretory IgA

pIg	polymerized immunoglobulin
pIgA	polymerized IgA
pIgR	receptor to polymerized immunoglobulin

Other Immunoglobulin Components: The secretory forms of IgM and IgA contain an additional polypeptide, the

J chain

(not to be confused with the joining or J segments of the immunoglobulin gene loci; see Additional Selected Immunoglobulin Genetic Terms below).

Secreted IgA also contains a secretory component, SC.

Molecular Formulas: These indicate how many of each polypeptide chain constitute an immunoglobulin molecule:

γ_2L_2	IgG monomer with 2 γ chains and 2 light chains
α_2L_2	IgA monomer with 2 α chains and 2 light chains
$(\alpha_2L_2)_2SCJ$	IgA dimer with 4 α chains, 4 light chains, an SC, and a J chain
$(\mu_2L_2)_5$	IgM pentamer with 10 μ chains and 10 light chains
$(\mu_2L_2)_5J$	IgM pentamer with 10 μ chains, 10 light chains, and a J chain
$\delta_2\kappa_2$	IgD monomer with 2 δ chains and 2 κ light chains
$\varepsilon_2\lambda_2$	IgE monomer with 2 ε chains and 2 λ light chains

Fc Fragments and Fc Receptors[8]*:* Fc fragments may be specified by heavy-chain class:

Fcγ1 Fcγ2 Fcγ3 Fcγ4

Fcα1 Fcuα2

Fcμ

Fcδ

Fcε

Many cells bear receptors for the Fc portion of immunoglobulin molecules. Those currently characterized are named as follows (cell surface marker identities, if applicable, are shown in parentheses; see 12.8.4, Lymphocytes):

IgG receptors:	FcγRI (CD64) FcγRII (CD32) FcγRIII (CD16)
IgA receptor:	FcαR
IgM receptor:	FcμR
IgE receptors:	FcεRI FcεRII (CD23)

Potentially Confusing Terms: These membrane proteins associated with immunoglobulins and immune cells should not be confused with terms for immunoglobulin classes or heavy chains:

Ig-α (This is not IgA or the α heavy chain.)

Ig-β

Although, as noted above in the context of immunoglobulins, a subscript H indicates the immunoglobulin heavy chain, T_H is shorthand for the helper T cell (see 12.8.4, Lymphocytes).

Immunoglobulin Genes: Each immunoglobulin L- or H-chain gene is made up of 1 variable (V), 1 joining (J), and 1 constant (C) gene segment. Each H-chain gene also has 1 diversity (D) segment. These segments (also called regions) can be referred to as:

V_L J_L C_L V_H D_H J_H C_H

or more specifically as:

V_κ V_λ $C_{\lambda 2}$ C_μ $C_{\alpha 2}$

Various nonallelic forms of the V, D, or J gene segments are specified numerically (the *numbers* are *not* subscript):

V_K1 $V_\lambda 3$ J_H1 J_K2

Not all cells express all segments. A B cell expressing a particular segment, or an immunoglobulin protein containing that segment, might be referred to with the name of that segment and a plus sign, eg:

V_K3^+

The V, D, and J gene segments must be brought together by DNA rearrangement to form a single exon that codes for the variable region of a heavy- or light-chain protein. This is called a

V/J exon	in L-chain genes
V/D/J exon	in H-chain genes
V/(D)/J exon	when referring to L and/or H chain genes; also VDJ, V/D/J, V/(D)/J, V-D-J (variable-diversity-joining)

A potential source of confusion is that the V, D, and J segments together code for the variable (V) region (or V domain) of the immunoglobulin protein. Since gene segments are sometimes called "regions," context must make clear whether the term "V region" refers to a gene segment or to a protein domain. It is unusual to refer to D or J regions of an immunoglobulin protein.

Each C-region (C_μ, $C_\gamma 1$, etc) protein domain is encoded by 5 or more exons. The individual exons are denoted as follows:

$C_\mu 1$ $C_\mu 3$ $C_{\gamma 1}1$ $C_{\gamma 1}2$ $C_{\alpha 2}5$

(For alternative expressions of some of these terms using official human gene terminology, consult 12.6.2, Human Gene Nomenclature. Both types of terminology are acceptable, and editors should follow author usage.)

Additional Selected Immunoglobulin Genetic Terms: Many such terms relate to the components of the immunoglobulin molecule as previously described. (When the convention of italicizing gene terms is not observed, context must differentiate identical gene and gene-product terminology.)

C segment, C exon

D_H segment (diversity segment)

J segment (not the same entity as the J chain of IgA and IgM—see above, Other Immunoglobulin Components)

J_κ, J_λ

J_H segment

J_1 J_2 J_3 J_4 J_5 J_6

N region (non-germline-encoded region inserted into an immunoglobulin gene)

RAG-1, RAG-2 (products of recombination-activating genes)

S (switch region)

S_μ, S_ε

V segment

REFERENCES

1. Bennington JL, ed. *Saunders Dictionary and Encyclopedia of Laboratory Medicine and Technology.* Philadelphia, Pa: WB Saunders Co; 1984:623.
2. Kao NL. How immunoglobulins were named. *Ann Intern Med.* 1992;117:445.
3. Ceppellini R, Dray S, Edelman G, et al. Nomenclature for human immunoglobulins. *Bull World Health Organ.* 1964;30:447-449.
4. Ishizaka K, Ishizaka T, Hornbook MM. Physico-chemical properties of human reaginic antibody, IV: presence of a unique immunoglobulin as a carrier of reaginic activity. *J Immunol.* 1966;97:75-85.
5. Rowe DS, Fahey JL. A new class of human immunoglobulins, I: a unique myeloma protein. *J Exp Med.* 1965;121:171-184.
6. Rowe DS, Fahey JL. A new class of human immunoglobulins, II: normal serum IgD. *J Exp Med.* 1965;121:185-199.
7. Haynes BF, Fauci AS. Cellular and molecular basis of immunity. In: Isselbacher KJ, Braunwald E, Wilson JD, Martin JB, Fauci AS, Kasper DL, eds. In: *Harrison's Principles of Internal Medicine.* 13th ed. New York, NY: McGraw-Hill; 1994.
8. IUIS Subcommittee on Nomenclature. Nomenclature of the Fc receptors. *Bull World Health Organ.* 1989;67:449-450.

ADDITIONAL READINGS AND GENERAL REFERENCES

Carayannopoulos L, Capra JD. Immunoglobulins: structure and function. In: Paul WE, ed. *Fundamental Immunology.* 3rd ed. New York, NY: Raven Press; 1993:283-314.

Goodman JW, Parslow TG. Immunoglobulin proteins. In: Stites DP, Terr AI, Parslow TG, eds. *Basic and Clinical Immunology.* 8th ed. Norwalk, Conn: Appleton & Lange; 1994: 66-79.

Max EE. Immunoglobulins: molecular genetics. In: Paul WE, ed. *Fundamental Immunology.* 3rd ed. New York, NY: Raven Press; 1993:315-382.

Parslow TG. Immunoglobulin genes, B cells, and the humoral immune response. In: Stites DP, Terr AI, Parslow TG, eds. *Basic and Clinical Immunology.* 8th ed. Norwalk, Conn: Appleton & Lange; 1994:80-93.

12.8.4 *Lymphocytes.*

The normal adult human body contains on the order of a trillion (10^{12}) lymphocytes. . . . Together, the thymus and marrow produce approximately 10^9 mature lymphocytes each day, which are then released into the circulation.

Tristram G. Parslow[1(p22)]

Plasma cells can produce and release thousands of [antibody] molecules per second. . . .

P. W. Kincade, J. M. Gimble[2(p53)]

Lymphocytes are the cells that carry out antigen-specific immune responses. The 2 main types are the T lymphocyte and the B lymphocyte, also called the T cell and the B cell. A hyphen does not appear in these terms, unless they are used adjectivally (eg, T-cell lymphoma). Historically, the letters T and B reflected the anatomic sites of origin of the 2 groups of cells, the thymus and bursa of Fabricius, respectively. (The bursa of Fabricius is an organ of birds, used investigationally.) Because in human adults B cells originate in the bone marrow, the letter B is sometimes taken as signifying *bone marrow.* The terms *T lymphocyte, T cell, B lymphocyte,* and *B cell* are not customarily expanded.

B Lymphocytes: In the context of B-lymphocyte differentiation, the prefixes pre- and pro- are encountered; note hyphenation:

pro-B cell

pre-B cell

Another group of B cells, formerly known as CD5 B cells or Ly-1 B cells, which comprise a B-cell subset of current interest, are now called:

B1 B cells

T Lymphocytes: The main types of T lymphocyte are:

helper T cells: T_H cells

cytotoxic T cells: T_C cells

Most helper T cells express the cell marker CD4, and most cytotoxic T cells express the cell marker CD8 (see also, CD Cell Markers), giving rise to the following terms:

CD4 cells   CD8 cells

When presence or absence of a marker on a T cell is emphasized, superscript plus and minus signs are used:

$CD4^+$

$CD4^-$

$CD4^+CD8^-$ (a CD4 cell)

$CD4^-CD8^+$ (a CD8 cell)

$CD4^-CD8^-$ ("double-negative lymphocyte")

$CD4^+CD8^+$ ("double-positive lymphocyte")

Subtypes of helper T cells are:

T_H0 T_H1 T_H2

A theoretical precursor to these subtypes is:

$T_{H}p$

The T-cell receptor-CD3 complex (abbreviated TCR-CD3) is a structure that recognizes antigen. Its subunits, or chains, are designated by Greek letters:

α chain γ chain ε chain η chain

β chain δ chain ζ chain

(Although some of these chains are homologous, do not confuse them with the components of major histocompatibility complex [MHC] molecules or the heavy chains of the immunoglobulin [Ig] molecule; see 12.8.2, The Human Leukocyte Antigen [HLA] System, and 12.8.3, Immunoglobulins.)

The α and β chains are also referred to as:

TCRα TCRβ

The linked α and β chains result in these terms:

$\alpha\beta$ dimer

$\alpha\beta$ receptor

$\alpha\beta$ cell

Another type of TCR is the $\gamma\delta$ receptor (and a cell with such a receptor is a $\gamma\delta$ cell).

The γ, δ, ε, ζ, and η chains constitute the CD3 complex.

The CD3 chains are also referred to individually as:

CD3γ CD3δ CD3ε CD3ζ CD3η

The TCR α gene is made up of variable (V), joining (J), and constant (C) segments, as is the β chain, which also has a diversity (D) segment. (These are analogous to segments of the immunoglobulin genes; see 12.8.3, Immunoglobulins.) These segments may also be referred to as

V_α V_β J_α J_β D_β C_α C_β

Various nonallelic forms of the V, D, or J segments are specified numerically, eg:

$V_\alpha2$ $J_\beta7$

Not all cells express all segments. Thus, a T cell expressing a particular segment might be referred to with the name of that segment and a plus sign, eg:

$V_\beta2^+$

As with the immunoglobulins, the terms variable (V) and constant (C) are also used to refer to portions of the TCR protein. By convention, the V, D, and J gene segments together encode the variable (V) region of the protein. Hence, it is unusual to refer to D or J regions of the protein.

Natural Killer Cells: These are a third group of lymphocytes, commonly abbreviated as NK cells.

CD Cell Markers: Clusters of differentiation (CDs) are a system for identifying cellular markers,[3-6] many of which define lymphocyte subsets. The system and its nomenclature were formalized in a 1982 international workshop.[7] Originally CD terms specified the monoclonal antibodies (mAbs) that "clustered" in their reactivities to target cells; more recently, the CD terms apply to the cellular molecules themselves, which are characterized using multiple methods, molecular and functional as well as immunological.[8] CDs, which now number more than 100, are defined at the Human Leukocyte Differentiation Antigen Workshops.

CD markers are designated with CD plus a numeral or a numeral and a letter, eg:

CD1 CD4 CD8 CD11a CD23 CD73

These markers represent many types of molecule and many have other identities (common names), such as:

CD	*Common Name(s)*
CD10	CALLA (common acute lymphoblastic leukemia antigen)
CD16	FcγRIII (an Fc receptor; see also 12.8.3, Immunoglobulins)
CD81	TAPA-1 (target of an antiproliferative antibody)
CD16b	FcRIIIγB
CD42a	GP IX (glycoprotein IX)
CD62L	L-selectin
CD79a	mb-1, Ig-α (see also 12.8.3, Immunoglobulins)
CD79b	B-29, Ig-β
CD120a	type 1 tumor necrosis factor receptor (see also 12.8.5, Cytokines)
CD121b	IL-1R, type 2 (see also 12.8.5, Cytokines)

Because a molecule that is ultimately identified as a CD may have been under study for years under 1 or more recognized designations, it is helpful to mention such terms along with the CD term, especially for new CDs.

As noted previously for CD4 and CD8, presence or absence of a marker may be specifically indicated with a superscript plus or minus sign, and, for a given cell type, several markers may be so specified, eg:

$CD30^+$ lymphoma

$CD2^+CD3^+CD7^+$

The letter R stands for "restricted" tissue distribution, eg:

CD45R

It may be followed by other uppercase or lowercase letters, eg:

CD45RA

CD45RO

A lowercase w ("workshop") signifies a provisional cluster, eg:

CDw84, CDw130

CD nomenclature has displaced previous terms, eg, CD8 for T8, CD4 for T4. (*Note:* These numbers are not always the same, eg, T6 is CD1.) Because, as noted, the CDs now specify the cell markers themselves, rather than the specificities of the monoclonal antibodies first used to identify them, CDs and monoclonal antibody terms are no longer equivalent; eg, the antibodies OKT3 and Leu 4 recognize (but do not stand for) CD3. For therapeutic monoclonal antibody nomenclature, see 12.4, Drugs.

REFERENCES

1. Parslow TG. Lymphocytes and lymphoid tissue. In: Stites DP, Terr AI, Parslow TG, eds. *Basic and Clinical Immunology.* 8th ed. Norwalk, Conn: Appleton & Lange; 1994:22-39.
2. Kincade PW, Gimble JM. B lymphocytes. In: Paul WE, ed. *Fundamental Immunology.* 3rd ed. New York, NY: Raven Press; 1993:43-73.
3. Engel P, Tedder TF. New CD from the B cell section of the Fifth International Workshop on Human Leukocyte Differentiation Antigens. *Leuk Lymphoma.* 1994;13(suppl 1): 61-64.
4. IUIS/WHO Subcommittee on CD Nomenclature. CD antigens 1993: an updated nomenclature for clusters of differentiation on human cells. *Bull World Health Organ.* 1994;72:807-808.
5. IUIS/WHO Subcommittee on CD Nomenclature. Nomenclature for clusters of differentiation (CD) of antigens defined on human leukocyte populations. *Bull World Health Organ.* 1984;62:809-811.
6. Singer NG, Todd RF, Fox DA. Structures on the cell surface: update from the Fifth International Workshop on Human Leukocyte Differentiation Antigens. *Arthritis Rheum.* 1994;37:1245-1248.
7. Bernard A, Boumsell L. The clusters of differentiation (CD) defined by the First International Workshop on Human Leucocyte Differentiation Antigens. *Hum Immunol.* 1984;11:1-10.
8. Springer TA. The next cluster of differentiation (CD) workshop. *Nature.* 1991;354: 415-416.

ADDITIONAL READINGS AND GENERAL REFERENCES

Erber WN. Human leucocyte differentiation antigens: review of the CD nomenclature. *Pathology.* 1990;22:61-69.

Gibco BRL Product Catalogue and Reference Guide 1995-1996. Gaithersburg, Md: Life Technologies Inc; 1995.

Imboden JI. T lymphocytes and natural killer cells. In: Stites DP, Terr AI, Parslow TG, eds. *Basic and Clinical Immunology.* 8th ed. Norwalk, Conn: Appleton & Lange; 1994:94-104.

Parslow TG. Immunoglobulin genes, B cells, and the humoral immune response. In: Stites DP, Terr AI, Parslow TG, eds. *Basic and Clinical Immunology.* 8th ed. Norwalk, Conn: Appleton & Lange; 1994:80-93.

Schlossman SF, Boumsell L, Gilks W, et al. CD antigens 1993. *Immunol Today.* 1994;15:98-99.

Sprent J. T lymphocytes and the thymus. In: Paul WE, ed. *Fundamental Immunology.* 3rd ed. New York, NY: Raven Press; 1993:75-109.

The CD classification of hematopoietic cell surface markers. In: Stites DP, Terr AI, Parslow TG, eds. *Basic and Clinical Immunology.* 8th ed. Norwalk, Conn: Appleton & Lange; 1994:817-818.

12.8.5 ***Cytokines.***—Cytokines are extracellular substances, typically proteins and glycoproteins, usually produced by activated immune and inflammatory cells, which act at short distances in tiny concentrations to produce immune and inflammatory reactions and reparative processes. Each cytokine produces multiple effects and overlaps with other cytokines, even structurally dissimilar ones, in the effects that it produces. Despite this complexity, the nomenclature of cytokines is relatively uncomplicated and, in fact, intentionally so.[1,2]

Lymphokines are cytokines predominantly produced by lymphocytes and *monokines* are cytokines predominantly produced by mononuclear leukocytes (monocytes and macrophages).

Interleukins: The largest group of cytokines are the interleukins. These are designated by number as interleukin 1 through interleukin 16. Specific interleukins are mentioned, most commonly, in their abbreviated form, eg:

IL-1

IL-16

The 2 forms of IL-1 (differing molecularly but producing the same effect) are:

IL-1α

IL-1β

Another entity related to IL-1 is the IL-1 receptor antagonist:

IL-1RA

Receptors for interleukins are designated with the interleukin name plus a capital R, eg:

IL-2R	receptor for IL-2
IL-4R	receptor for IL-4

Receptor names designating subtypes may be even more specific, eg:

IL-1RI

IL-1RII

Greek letters are used for subunits (chains) of the same receptor, eg:

IL-2Rα and IL-2Rβ

IL-6Rα and IL-6Rβ

Discussions may refer to interleukins from different species, but these should be expanded at first mention, eg:

hIL-2	human IL-2
mIL-4	mouse IL-4
vIL-10	viral IL-10

Tumor Necrosis Factor: Tumor necrosis factor (TNF), another cytokine, has retained the name of the property responsible for its discovery. Its major forms are:

TNF-α

TNF-β

Interferons: Another group of cytokines is the interferons, originally discovered because of their interference with viral replication.

The type I interferons (IFNs), also known as *antiviral interferons,* are:

IFN-α

IFN-β

IFN-ω

Type II IFN, also known as *immune interferon,* is:

IFN-γ

For terminology of therapeutic interferons, see 12.4.10, Special Drug Categories.
Other cytokines are shown below:

TGF-β	transforming growth factor β
GM-CSF	granulocyte-monocyte colony-stimulating factor
G-CSF	granulocyte colony-stimulating factor
M-CSF	macrophage (or monocyte) colony-stimulating factor (also known as CSF-1)

Lowercase prefixes such as r (recombinant) and rh (recombinant human) may appear with cytokine terms, which should be expanded at first mention, eg:

rIL-2	recombinant IL-2
rhTNF-α	recombinant human TNF-α

REFERENCES

1. Aarden LA, Brunner TK, Cerottini J-C, et al. Revised nomenclature for antigen-nonspecific T cell proliferation and helper factors [letter]. *J Immunol.* 1979;123:2928-2929.
2. Paul WE, Kishimoto T, Melchers F, et al. Nomenclature for secreted regulatory proteins of the immune system (interleukins). *Clin Exp Immunol.* 1992;88:367.

ADDITIONAL READINGS AND GENERAL REFERENCES

Dexter TM, Moore M. Growth and development in the haemopoietic system: the role of lymphokines and their possible therapeutic potential in disease and malignancy. *Carcinogenesis.* 1986;7:509-516.

Durum SK, Oppenheim JJ. Proinflammatory cytokines and immunity. In: Paul WE, ed. *Fundamental Immunology.* 3rd ed. New York, NY: Raven Press; 1993:801-835.

Haworth C. Multifunctional cytokines in haemopoiesis. *Blood Rev.* 1989;3:263-268.

Howard MC, Miyajima A, Coffman R. T-cell derived cytokines and their receptors. In: Paul WE, ed. *Fundamental Immunology.* 3rd ed. New York, NY: Raven Press; 1993:763-800.

Oppenheim JJ, Ruscetti FW, Faltynek C. Cytokines. In: Stites DP, Terr AI, Parslow TG, eds. *Basic and Clinical Immunology.* 8th ed. Norwalk, Conn: Appleton & Lange; 1994:105-123.

12.9 ■ **ISOTOPES.**—Radiopharmaceuticals administered for therapeutic or diagnostic purposes include isotopes as part of the compound. Because radiopharmaceuticals are drugs, the nomenclature for the isotopes incorporated in radiopharmaceuticals differs from that of isotopes that occur as elements alone.

12.9.1 ***Elements.***—An isotope referred to as an element rather than as part of the name of a chemical compound may be described at first mention by providing the name of the element spelled out followed by the isotope number in the same typeface and type size (no hyphen, subscript, or superscript is used). The element abbreviation may be listed in parentheses at first mention and used thereafter in the article, with the isotope number preceding the element symbol as a superscript.

> Of the 13 known isotopes of iodine, only iodine 128 (^{128}I) is not radioactive. The investigators used ^{128}I to avoid the difficulty and expense of disposing of radioactive waste.

Do not use the symbol representing a single element as an abbreviation for a compound (eg, do not abbreviate the compound sodium arsenate As 74 as ^{74}As).

12.9.2 ***Radiopharmaceuticals.***—The USAN designations for radioactive pharmaceuticals consist of the name of the drug containing the radioactive isotope, the element symbol, the isotope number, and the name of the carrier agent, if any.[1(p10)] Since the nonproprietary name comprises all these components, the complete name should be provided at first mention (the few exceptions to this rule are provided herein). Although the name for the radiopharmaceutical may appear to contain redundant information (eg, potassium bromide Br 82; technetium Tc 99m butilfenin), maintaining consistent terminology is important for clarity. For example, technetium Tc 99m is contained in 21 nonproprietary radiopharmaceuticals manufactured as 35 proprietary preparations.[1(p783)] For drug nomenclature, consult the most recent edition of the *USP Dictionary*.[1] The isotope number appears in the same type (not superscript) as the rest of the drug name, and it is not preceded by a hyphen.

> iodohippurate sodium I 131
>
> sodium iodide I 125
>
> cyanocobalamin Co 60
>
> gallium citrate Ga 67
>
> fibrinogen I 125
>
> indium In 111 altumomab pentetate
>
> In 1993, strontium chloride 89 was approved by the US Food and Drug Administration for the management of pain from skeletal metastases.

Use of nonproprietary and proprietary names for radiopharmaceuticals should follow the guidelines for usage in 12.4, Drugs. Use the nonproprietary name at first mention, particularly when referring to a radiopharmaceutical that is administered to a patient. Subsequently, a shorter term may be used, such as iodinated albumin or gallium scan.

> In an earlier study, 50 patients underwent lung imaging with technetium Tc 99m sulfur colloid.
>
> The patient underwent an exercise stress test with injection of thallous chloride Tl 201 (thallium stress test).

In a discussion that does not refer to administration of a specific drug, the more general term may be used.

> For a patient recuperating from a myocardial infarction who wishes to begin an exercise program, a treadmill test with or without thallium imaging may be useful to determine whether the patient is at high risk for recurrent ischemia.

At the beginning of a sentence, the name rather than the element symbol should be used.

The patient was treated with sodium iodide I 131 after she was found to have hyperthyroidism, to reduce function of her thyroid gland by radiation from ^{131}I. Iodine 131 levels were then monitored by measuring the amount of radioactivity in the patient's urine.

12.9.3 ***Radiopharmaceutical Compounds Without Approved Names.***—A compound without an approved nonproprietary drug name may be referred to in several ways. These guidelines are intended to conform to standard chemical nomenclature; follow 12.9.1, Elements, or consult the *CRC Handbook of Chemistry and Physics*[2] for further information.

After first mention, the name of the substance can be abbreviated. Use the superscript form of the isotope number to the left of the element symbol. Enclose the isotope symbol in brackets and close up with the compound name if the nonradioactive isotope of the element is normally part of the compound.

glucose labeled with radioactive carbon (^{14}C)

(*or* glucose tagged with carbon 14)

[^{14}C]glucose (not glucose C 14)

Use no brackets and separate the element and compound name with a hyphen if the compound does not normally contain the isotope element.

amikacin labeled with iodine 125

^{125}I-amikacin

If uncertain as to whether the isotope element is normally part of a compound, consult the *USP Dictionary*[1] for drugs and *The Merck Index*[3] for other compounds.

12.9.4 ***Radiopharmaceutical Proprietary Names.***—In proprietary names of radiopharmaceuticals, isotope numbers may appear in the same position as in the approved nonproprietary names, but they are usually joined to the rest of the name by a hyphen and are not necessarily preceded by the element symbol. Follow the *USP Dictionary*[1] or the usage of individual manufacturers.

Proprietary	*Nonproprietary*
Iodotope I-131	sodium iodide I 131
Glofil-125	iothalamate sodium I 125

12.9.5 ***Uniform Labeling.***—The abbreviation "ul" (for "uniformly labeled") may be used without expansion in parentheses:

[^{14}C]glucose (ul)

Similarly, terms such *as carrier-free, no carrier added,* or *carrier added* may be used. In general medical publications, these terms should be explained at first mention, since not all readers will be familiar with them.

12.9.6 ***Hydrogen Isotopes.***—Two isotopes of hydrogen have their own specific names, deuterium and tritium, which should be used instead of "hydrogen 2" and "hydrogen 3." In text, the specific names are also preferred to the symbols ^{2}H or D (for deuterium, which is stable) and ^{3}H (for tritium, which is radioactive). The 2 forms of heavy water, D_2O and $^{3}H_2O$, should be referred to by the approved nonproprietary names deuterium oxide and tritiated water, respectively.

12.9.7 ***Metastable Isotopes.***—The abbreviation m, as in krypton Kr 81m (approved nonproprietary name), stands for "metastable." The abbreviation should never be deleted, since the term without the "m" designates a different radionuclide isomer.

REFERENCES

1. Fleeger CA, ed. *USP Dictionary of USAN and International Drug Names.* 34th ed. Rockville, Md: US Pharmacopoeial Convention Inc; 1996.
2. *CRC Handbook of Chemistry and Physics.* 76th ed. Cleveland, Ohio: CRC Press; 1995-1996.
3. Budavari S, ed. *The Merck Index.* 12th ed. Rahway, NJ: Merck & Co Inc; 1996.

12.10 ■ NEUROLOGY.

12.10.1 ***Nerves.***—Most nerves have names (eg, ulnar nerve or nervus ulnaris). English names are preferred to Latin. For terminology, consult a medical dictionary, anatomy text, or *Nomina Anatomica.*[1]

Cranial nerves have names and numbers, and spinal nerves with one exception (the coccygeal nerve) have only numbers.

Cranial Nerves: The cranial nerves are as follows:

Nerve	*English Name*	*Latin Name*
I	olfactory	olfactorius
II	optic	opticus
III	oculomotor	oculomotorius
IV	trochlear	trochlearis
V	trigeminal	trigeminus
VI	abducens	abducens
VII	facial	facialis
VIII	vestibulocochlear (acoustic)	vestibulocochlearis
IX	glossopharyngeal	glossopharyngeus
X	vagus	vagus
XI	accessory	accessorius
XII	hypoglossal	hypoglossus

Use roman numerals or English names when designating cranial nerves:

> Cranial nerves III, IV, and VI are responsible for ocular movement.
>
> The oculomotor, trochlear, and abducens nerves are responsible for ocular movement.

Use ordinals when the numeric adjectival form is used:

> The third, fourth, and sixth cranial nerves are responsible for ocular movement.

Vertebrae, Spinal Nerves, Spinal Levels, and Dermatomes: These entities share a common nomenclature, deriving from spinal anatomic regions: cervical (neck), thoracic (trunk), lumbar (lower back), sacral (pelvis), and coccygeal (coccyx or tailbone). (Spinal nerves C1 through C7 are named for the vertebrae above which they emerge, while T1 through S5 are named for the vertebrae below which they emerge; spinal nerve C8 emerges below vertebra C7, there being no vertebra C8.)

Vertebrae and spinal nerves are as follows:

Region	*Vertebrae*	*Spinal Nerves*
cervical	C1 through C7	C1 through C8
thoracic	T1 through T12	T1 through T12
lumbar	L1 through L5	L1 through L5
sacrum	S1 through S5	S1 through S5
coccyx	4 fused, not individually designated	coccygeal nerve

The alphanumeric terms need not be expanded, and, when clear in context, "vertebra" and "nerve" need not be repeated:

> The first cervical vertebra is also known as the atlas, C2 as the axis, and C7 as the vertebra prominens.

Hyphens are used for intervertebral spaces (including neural foramina) and intervertebral disks, as follows:

Space	*Disk*
C2-3 (space between C2 and C3)	C2-3 disk
T2-3 (space between T2 and T3)	T2-3 disk
L2-3 (space between L2 and L3)	L2-3 disk
C7-T1 (space between C7 and T1)	C7-T1 disk
L5-S1 (space between L5 and S1)	L5-S1 disk

The sacrum, because its vertebrae are fused, does not contain intervertebral spaces. Its 4 paired foramina are commonly referred to as the first sacral foramen, second sacral foramen, etc.

Ranges of vertebrae are expressed as in the following examples; use letters for both the first and last vertebra in the indicated range:

C3 through C7	third through seventh cervical vertebrae (not C3 through 7)
T6 through S1	sixth thoracic through first sacral vertebra

The same abbreviations are used for spinal segments or levels and spinal dermatomes. Text should always indicate unambiguously which is being referred to, eg, vertebra, spinal nerve (or root, radiculopathy, or distribution), spinal level, or dermatome. Within a clear context, the words "vertebra," "nerve," etc, then need not be repeated.

> Serious injury of the cervical cord at the level of the C2 through C5 vertebrae causes respiratory paralysis due to injury of spinal nerves C3 through C5.

> The first patient had herpes zoster in the T9 dermatomal distribution, the second patient in the C5 distribution.

12.10.2 ***Electroencephalographic (EEG) Terms.***—The International 10-20 System specifies placement of electrodes used in electroencephalography. It is so named because electrodes are spaced 10% or 20% apart along the head (see Figure 3).

The terms of the 10-20 System are widely used and recognized. They are systematically named, as follows:

- Letters refer to anatomic areas (primarily of the skull, which do not necessarily coincide with the brain areas from which the electrodes register electrical activity).
- Odd numbers are for electrodes placed on the left side, even numbers for electrodes placed on the right side, and the letter z for midline ("zero") electrodes.

Location	*Designation*
frontal pole or prefrontal electrodes	Fp1, Fp2
superior frontal electrodes	Fz, F3, F4
parietal electrodes	Pz, P3, P4
central electrodes	Cz, C3, C4
lateral frontal (anterior temporal) electrodes	F7, F8
midtemporal electrodes	T3, T4
posterior temporal electrodes	T5, T6
occipital electrodes	O1, O2
earlobe electrodes	A1, A2

Additional electrodes and other placement systems may be used; the following are from the "modified combinatorial nomenclature," which adds electrodes at intermediate 10% positions. This results in additional numeric designations for

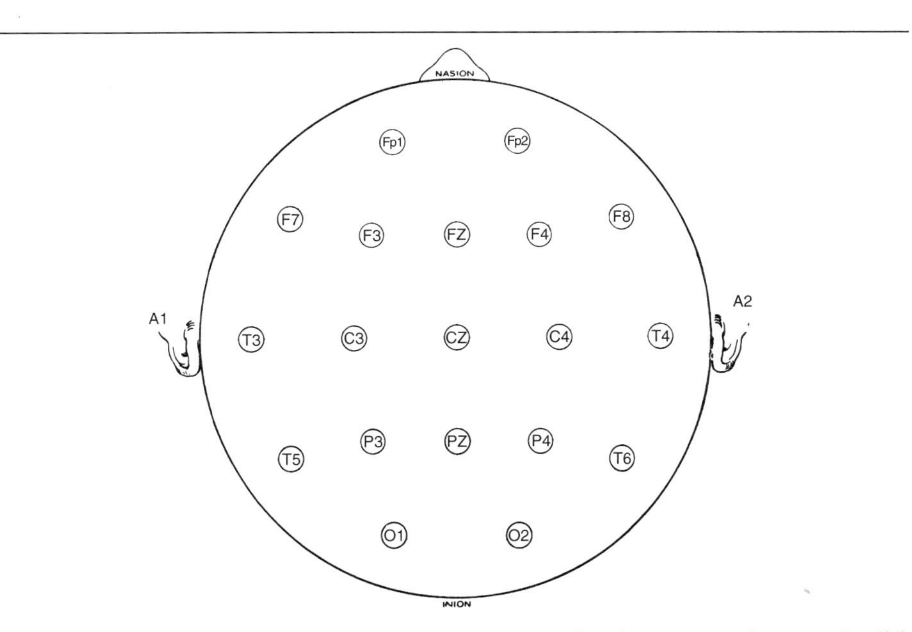

FIGURE 3 Electroencephalographic lead positions. Reprinted with permission from Hughes.[2(p2)]

existing regional electrodes (eg, C5, F10) and in new letters or letter combinations, as in the following examples:

Location	*Designation*
nasion	Nz
midprefrontal	Fpz
anterior frontal	AFz, AF3, AF4, AF7, AF8
frontocentral	FCz, FC1 through FC10
frontotemporal	FT7, FT8, FT9, FT10
centrotemporal	C1, C2, C5, C6, T7 through T10
centroparietal	CPz, CP1 through CP6
temporal-posterior	TP7, TP8, TP9, TP10
parietal-posterior temporal	P1, P2, P5 through P10
parieto-occipital	POz, PO3, PO4, PO7, PO8
midoccipital	Oz
inion	Iz

In figures showing EEGs, electrode symbols will usually be paired. Usually, the symbols will be above or beside and to the left of each channel of the tracing but may be above and below each channel with connecting lines (Figure 4).

Authors should include with tracings a time marker and an indicator of voltage, as in the top tracing above.

Descriptions of EEG potentials include many qualitative terms for waveforms and frequencies. The following are but a few of numerous terms (note that the Greek letters are spelled out in these terms):

> alpha rhythm, beta activity, polymorphic delta activity, sleep spindles, spike-and-slow wave complexes, paroxysms, spikes, sharp waves, delta brush, frontal sharp transient, mu rhythm, lambda waves

A more complete glossary of EEG terms has been provided by the International Societies for Electroencephalography and Clinical Neurophysiology.[3]

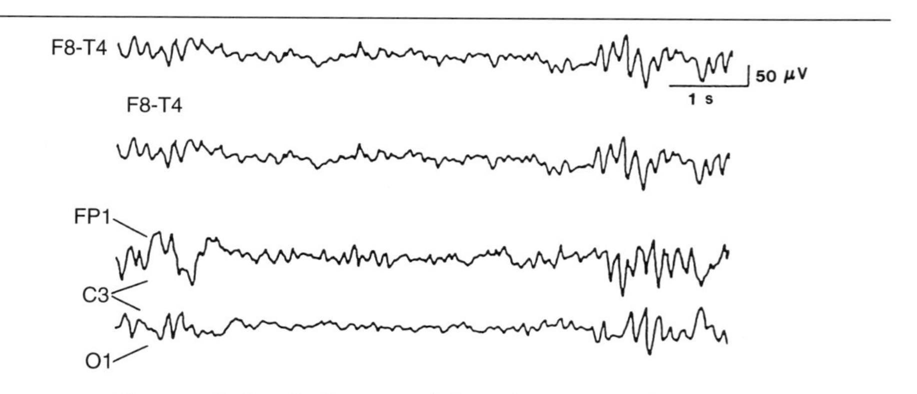

FIGURE 4 Sample electroencephalographic tracings (schematic).

Frequency is given per second (/s); for cycles per second, hertz (Hz) is preferred to c/s (see 15.1, Units of Measure, SI Units), eg:

10-Hz alpha activity

a theta frequency of 5 to 7.5 Hz

14-Hz spindles

60-Hz artifact

background rhythm of 8 to 10 Hz

12.10.3 ***Evoked Potentials.***—Several evoked potentials may be recorded, including visual evoked potentials (VEPs), brainstem auditory evoked potentials (BAEPs), and somatosensory evoked potentials (SSEPs). As in EEG, evoked potential testing uses recording electrodes and produces tracings of various types.

The following examples are included to explain terms from evoked potential testing that are used without expansion.

Electrode terminology resembles that of the 10-20 System for EEGs (see above), with additional or modified electrodes such as the following[4]:

VEP electrodes	
midoccipital	MO
left occipital	LO
right occipital	RO
midfrontal	MF
midparietal	MP
midline of the inion	I
vertex	V
BAEP electrodes	
mastoid processes	M1 M2
external auditory meatus	EAM
ipsilateral electrodes	Ai, Mi, EAMi
contralateral electrodes	Ac, Mc, EAMc
SSEP electrodes	
Erb point	EP
EP ipsilateral	EPi
electrodes midway between C3 or C4 and P3 or P4	CP
contralateral CP electrode	CPc
ipsilateral CP electrode	CPi
anterior cervical	AC
lateral neck	LN
iliac crest	IC
popliteal fossa electrodes (distal, proximal)	Pfd, Pfp
C2 vertebra electrode	C2S

C5 vertebra electrode	C5S
T10 vertebra electrode	T10S
T12 vertebra electrode	T12S
L2 vertebra electrode	L2S
reference electrode	REF

(S, as in C2S, stands for spinous process.)

Waveforms recorded in evoked potential testing are identified with P for positive or N for negative plus a number indicating milliseconds between stimulus and response, eg:

VEP:	N75, P100, N145
SSEP:	N13, P14, N18, N20, N34, P37
LP:	lumbar potential

Other waves, eg, in VEP and BAEP, are designated with roman numerals I through VII.

REFERENCES

1. International Anatomical Nomenclature Committee. *Nomina Anatomica.* 5th ed. Baltimore, Md: Williams & Wilkins; 1983.
2. Hughes JR. *EEG in Clinical Practice.* 2nd ed. Boston, Mass: Butterworth-Heinemann; 1994.
3. Chatrian GE, Begamini L, Dondey M, Klass DW, Lennox-Buchthal M, Petersén I. A glossary of terms most commonly used by clinical electroencephalographers. *Electroencephalogr Clin Neurophysiol.* 1974;37:538-548.
4. Gilmore RL, ed. American Electroencephalographic Society Guidelines in Electroencephalography, Evoked Potentials, and Polysomnography. *J Clin Neurophysiol.* 1994;11:1-148.

ADDITIONAL READINGS AND GENERAL REFERENCES

Adams RD, Victor M. *Principles of Neurology.* 5th ed. New York, NY: McGraw-Hill; 1993:23-32.

Anderson JE. *Grant's Atlas of Anatomy.* 8th ed. Baltimore, Md: Williams & Wilkins; 1983:5-3, 5-13, 5-14.

Ellis H, Feldman S. *Anatomy for Anaesthetists.* 4th ed. Boston, Mass: Blackwell Scientific Publications; 1983:103-119.

Knott JR. Regarding the American Electroencephalographic Society Guidelines for Standard Electrode Position Nomenclature: a commentary on the proposal to change the 10-20 designators [letter]. *J Clin Neurophysiol.* 1993;10:123-124.

Netter FH. *Atlas of Human Anatomy.* Summit, NJ: CIBA-Geigy Corp; 1989. Plates 142, 145, 148-150.

Netter FH. Musculoskeletal system, part I: anatomy, physiology and metabolic disorders. In: *The Ciba Collection of Medical Illustrations.* Vol 8. Summit, NJ: CIBA-Geigy Corp; 1987:9-19.

Nuwer MR. Recording electrode site nomenclature. *J Clin Neurophysiol.* 1987;4:121-133.

Sharbrough FW. Regarding the American Electroencephalographic Society Guidelines for Standard Electrode Position Nomenclature: a commentary on the proposal to change the 10-20 designators [reply]. *J Clin Neurophysiol.* 1993;10:124-128.

12.11 ■ OBSTETRIC TERMS.

12.11 ■ OBSTETRIC TERMS.—Two colloquial types of shorthand expression exist for an individual's obstetric history, "GPA" and "TPAL."

12.11.1 ***GPA.***—The letters G, P, and A (or Ab) accompanied by numbers indicate number of pregnancies, births of viable offspring, and number of spontaneous or induced abortions. In the expansions below, the clinical meaning associated with the GPA shorthand appears, although the Latin terms actually refer to the individual (see any medical dictionary):

Letter	*Expansion of Letter*	*Clinical Meaning*
G	gravida	pregnancies
P	para	births of viable offspring
A or Ab	aborta	abortions

For example, the term G3, P2, A1 would indicate 3 pregnancies, 2 births of viable offspring, and 1 abortion. In published articles, however, it is preferable to write out the expression, eg:

gravida 3, para 2, aborta 1

Although some sources, including medical dictionaries, feature roman numerals with these expressions, use arabic numerals.

12.11.2 ***TPAL.***—The letters of this mode of expression indicate obstetric history as follows:

Letter	*Expansion*
T	term infants
P	premature infants
A	abortions
L	living children

Often, 4 numbers separated by hyphens are recorded, eg:

TPAL: 3-1-1-4

or

3-1-1-4

which would indicate 3 term infants, 1 premature infant, 1 abortion, and 4 living children. However, the text of a manuscript should define the numerical expressions and not give the numbers alone.

Various prefixes combine with the terms gravida and para, eg, nulligravida (gravida 0), primigravida (gravida 1), segundigravida (gravida 2), multigravida, nullipara (para 0), primipara (para 1), multipara. Consult a dictionary or textbook for specific explanations.

The TPAL and GPA expressions are familiar and widely used clinically. However, they are also recognized as imprecise and lacking in standardization, eg, of age of viability.[1-3] Even the Latin-derived terms are etymologically discordant and somewhat imprecise.[4] Therefore, in addition to the use of expansions as recommended previously, further specification (eg, single or multiple births, ectopic pregnancy) is required in scientific articles.

12.11.3 ***Apgar Score.***—This score is an assessment of a newborn's physical well-being based on pulse, breathing, color, tone, and reflex irritability, each of which is rated 0, 1, or 2; the 3 ratings are then summed. The Apgar score is often reported as 2 numbers, from 0 to 10, separated by a virgule, reflecting assessment at 1 minute and 5 minutes after birth. In general medical journals, however, it is best to specify the time intervals, especially as the Apgar score may be assessed at other intervals, such as 10, 15, and 20 minutes.

Ambiguous: Apgar of 9/10

Preferred: Apgar score of 9/10 at 1 and 5 minutes

or

Apgar score of 9 at 1 minute and 10 at 5 minutes.

The score is named after the late anesthesiologist Virginia Apgar, MD, and thus, "Apgar" is *not* printed in all capital letters as though for an acronym (although versions of such an acronym have been created as a mnemonic device).

REFERENCES

1. Ely JW. Summarizing the obstetric history [question]. *JAMA.* 1991;266:3344.
2. Pun TC, Ng JC. "Madame is a 30-year-old housewife, gravida X, para Y. . . ." *Obstet Gynecol.* 1989;73:276-277.
3. Woolley RJ. Parity clarity: proposal for a new obstetric shorthand. *J Fam Pract.* 1993;36:265-266.
4. Dirckx JH. Summarizing the obstetric history [answer]. *JAMA.* 1991;266:3344.

ADDITIONAL READINGS AND GENERAL REFERENCES

Committee on Fetus and Newborn, American Academy of Pediatrics, and Committee on Obstetric Practice, American College of Obstetricians and Gynecologists. Use and abuse of the Apgar score. *Pediatrics.* 1996;98:141-142.

Cunningham FG, MacDonald PC, Gant NF, Leveno KJ, Gilstrap LC III. *Williams Obstetrics.* 19th ed. Norwalk, Conn: Appleton & Lange; 1993:248-249, 444-446.

12.12 ■ ORGANISMS.

> *There is no "official" classification of bacteria. . . . [B]acterial classifications are devised for microbiologists, not for the entities being classified.* Bacteria show little interest in the matter of their classification.
>
> J. T. Staley, N. R. Krieg[1(p3)]

> Serratia *was named to honor Serafino Serrati because it was felt this early inventor of the steamboat concept had not received sufficient recognition. . . .*
>
> S. A. Berger, S. C. Edberg[2(p346)]

Of course, etiquette requires that you not name a taxon for yourself. But the British 19th-century ornithologist John Gould was neither the first nor the last to engage in the transparent device of naming a species—in Gould's case the superb Australian finch Erythrura gouldiae—*"after my wife."*

K. S. Thompson[3(p515)]

. . . [M]icrobiology is a field in flux, and one promise that will not issue from my lips is, "No new taxa."

M. Turck[4(p109)]

I know the scientific names of beings animalculous.

W. S. Gilbert

Biological nomenclature is the scientific naming of organisms. Taxonomy comprises the principles and practices of classifying organisms[5] to reflect their relatedness. Taxonomy and nomenclature are not identical: "Nomenclature is the ***assignment*** of names ***to*** the taxonomic groups according to international rules [emphasis added]."[1(p1)]

Nomenclature of living things derives from the paradigm of the 18th-century taxonomist Linnaeus. Since Linnaeus, international bodies have continued to formalize biological nomenclature, resulting in the current principal codes: the *International Code of Botanical Nomenclature*,[6] the *International Code of Zoological Nomenclature*,[7] and the *International Code of Nomenclature of Bacteria*.[8] (For an explanatory comparison of the codes, see Jeffrey.[5])

Taxonomy is necessarily mutable; new evidence causes organisms to be reclassified. Biological nomenclature is not mutable in the same way, but rather is intended to reflect relatedness and produce stability.[5] Reclassification will cause names of organisms to change, but the names will be derived and applied consistently, according to internationally agreed-upon rules.

Organisms are allotted to taxonomic groups, also called taxa (singular: taxon), within different ranks. For example, in the classification of human beings, *Homo* is the taxon of the rank genus.

Hallmarks of the biological nomenclature descended from Linnaeus include use of Latin for scientific names of all taxa and a binomial (also called binary or binominal) designation for species, eg, *Homo sapiens.* Within a code, the names of ranks above species usually must be unique; the same species name, however, can be used with multiple genera.[3,5,8]

Italics are always used for the genus and species components of the binomial species designation, which is formally called the *specific name* in the botanical and bacteriological codes, and the *binomen* in the zoological code.[5]

According to the international codes, all taxa names are capitalized, except for the second portion of the 2-word species name (called formally the *specific epithet* in the botanical and bacteriological codes and the *specific name* in the zoological code[5]).

In AMA publications taxa above genus are not italicized. The following example of the taxonomic classification of the modern human species illustrates AMA style for capitalization and italicization (see also 8.1.7, Capitalization, Organisms):

Rank	*Taxon*
kingdom	Animalia
phylum	Chordata

Rank	*Taxon*
class	Mammalia
order	Primates
family	Hominidae
genus	*Homo*
species	*Homo sapiens*

Subranks and superranks follow the same style, eg:

subphylum	Vertebrata
suborder	Anthropoidea
superfamily	Hominoidea

In medical publications, uncapitalized anglicized forms are often used for higher orders,[9] eg, primates for Primates, hominids for Hominidae, and vertebrates for Vertebrata.

12.12.1 ***Microorganisms Other Than Viruses.***—Because microorganisms are frequent subjects of medical publications, their nomenclature is presented in more detail.

For the names of microorganisms, consult a reputable medical dictionary or any of the following:

- *Approved Lists of Bacterial Names* and the *International Journal of Systematic Bacteriology:* appropriate sources for names that are valid according to the *International Code of Nomenclature of Bacteria*
- *Bergey's Manual of Determinative Bacteriology*[10]: index includes specific epithets as entries (eg, *Klebsiella pneumoniae* can be found under the specific epithet *pneumoniae* as well as under *Klebsiella*)
- *Bergey's Manual of Systematic Bacteriology*[11]: comprehensive reference source of bacterial nomenclature and taxonomy, but volumes are issued infrequently
- *Clinical Infectious Diseases:* biennial updated lists of microbial names
- *Mandell, Douglas and Bennett's Principles and Practice of Infectious Diseases*[12]: one of several major textbooks that reflect medical usage
- *Manual of Clinical Microbiology*[13]: authoritative source of approved nomenclature; includes fungi and viruses

Protozoal and parasite nomenclature is governed by the *International Code of Zoological Nomenclature* and fungal nomenclature by the *International Code of Botanical Nomenclature.* A special bacterial nomenclature code was proposed with the creation of the International Society for Microbiology in 1930. As a result, formal scientific bacterial nomenclature is defined by the *International Code of Nomenclature of Bacteria.* The code is issued by the International Committee on Systematic Bacteriology, and a judicial commission of the international society is the arbiter of nomenclatural questions and rules.[8]

The bacterial nomenclature code derives from the Linnaean botanical code. Rules of the bacterial code concern the criteria for formal recognition of taxa, including species, and the derivation of names. The nomenclature is stable but not static,[1] and changes in classifications and names of specific organisms occur as necessary. Bacterial species names are backed up by a "gold standard" of nomenclatural type strains maintained in culture.

The code contains principles, rules, and recommendations that govern name derivations, priority, spelling, and so on. For the complete rules, consult the code directly.[8]

To be formally recognized, a taxon must be the subject of a report published in the *International Journal of Systematic Bacteriology* or, if previously reported, the taxon must be announced in that journal. All bacterial nomenclature was revised in 1980. The resulting report, the *Approved Lists of Bacterial Names,* became the baseline for all new approved bacterial names.

As described previously, the genus name is capitalized, and the specific epithet is lowercase. Both are italicized, eg:

Staphylococcus aureus

Giardia lamblia

Cryptococcus neoformans

Pneumocystis carinii

Bacterial taxonomic ranks do not have the phylogenetic meaning of those for plants and animals; ie, rankings do not necessarily reflect evolutionary lines of descent[14] or genomic homology.[15] For bacteria, family, genus, and species are mentioned more frequently than taxa of higher ranks,[14] and bacteria are more often grouped as gram-negative or gram-positive cocci or rods, and so on. Nevertheless, bacterial taxa of all the traditional ranks receive mention in the medical literature, and style for bacterial taxa names follows the tabular example given for animals. Instead of phylum, bacteria are classified by division, as are microorganisms subject to the botanical code (although phylum is also a permitted rank in the botanical code as of 1994). The following table is included as a guide to the endings that typify the various bacterial taxonomic ranks:

Rank	*Bacterial Taxon*
kingdom	Procaryotae
division	Firmicutes
class	Firmibacteria
order	Eubacteriales(?)
family	Micrococcaceae
genus	*Staphylococcus*
species	*Staphylococcus aureus*

(For a comparison of typographic style of viruses and bacteria for various taxonomic ranks, see 12.12.2, Viruses. Fungal ranks higher than order have different endings but follow the above style for capitalization and use of italics.)

Abbreviation of Genus: As described in 11.11, Abbreviations, Clinical and Technical Terms, treat each manuscript portion (title, abstract, text, etc) separately. After first mention of the singular form of a species name, abbreviate genus name (without a period) when used with species *except when the species is other than that given at first mention.* Another genus may be mentioned in the interim. Do not abbreviate species name.

Staphylococcus aureus and *Staphylococcus epidermidis* may be components of normal flora or pathogens in clinically significant infections, although *S aureus* is the more serious pathogen of the two.

Subgenus is designated in parentheses after the genus, eg:

Moraxella (Branhamella) catarrhalis

Moraxella (Moraxella) bovis

Since parentheses are also used to indicate a name change, use quotation marks (for the familiar but unapproved name), the word "formerly," or an equivalent expression, eg:

Helicobacter (formerly *Campylobacter*) *pylori*

Bartonella (formerly *Rochalimaea*) *henselae*

Indicate a change in species name as follows:

Bacteroides ureolyticus (formerly *Bacteroides corrodens*)[4]

The abbreviation sp nov (*species nova*) is used in published proposals of new species designations, eg:

Cellulomonas hominis sp nov[16]

Candida dubliniensis sp nov[17]

Leptotrichia sanguinegens sp nov[18]

Wigglesworthia glossinidia sp nov[19]

The abbreviation gen nov (*genus novum*) is used in published proposals of new genus designations, eg:

Wigglesworthia gen nov[19]

New proposals for higher taxa are handled as in the following example[20,21]:

Cycliophora, new phyllum

Eucycliophora, new class

Symbiida, new order

Symbiidae, new family

Symbion gen nov

Symbion pandora sp nov

The "nov" abbreviations should be mentioned prominently in the article, eg, in the title, but need not be included with every mention of the organism name.

Subspecific Ranks, Ternary Names: Subspecific ranks receive so-called ternary or trinomial names. Subspecific designations are handled differently for bacteria, plants, and animals, as in the following examples. (The term "var" as a synonym for subspecies was removed from the bacterial nomenclature code in 1990.)

Type of Organism	*Subspecific Rank and Designator*	*Example*
bacteria		
bacterium	subspecies ("subsp")	*Campylobacter fetus* subsp *fetus*
plant		
fungus	variety ("var")	*Histoplasma capsulatum* var *duboisii*

Type of Organism	*Subspecific Rank and Designator*	*Example*
animal		
protozoan	subspecies (no designator)	*Plasmodium vinckei petteri*
parasite		*Trypanosoma brucei gambiense*
higher animal		*Mus musculus domesticus*

(In medical contexts, "var" seems the most common subspecific designation. However, plant names may use "var," as above, "subsp," "f" (form), and other infraspecific epithets in ternary names, which are not interchangeable.)

Editors should follow author usage and not attempt to insert or substitute within ternary terms.

Not all terms that appear to be ternary subspecies names are. Terms in which a species name modifies a noun (*Trypanosoma brucei* procyclin), especially a latinate noun (*Schistosoma mansoni* miracidium), may cause confusion in electronic media or electronically generated manuscripts that do not display italics or underlining.

Infrasubspecific Subdivisions, Strains, and Other Practical Groupings: Subdivisions below the subspecies level (infrasubspecific subdivisions) "have no official standing in nomenclature but often have great practical usefulness,"[1(p2)] eg, in epidemiology.[13] These include the serovar (serologically differentiated) and biovar (differentiated according to "special biochemical or physiological properties"). The suffix "type" is most often used, in the clinical literature, eg, serotype, biotype. However, "type" has a specific meaning in the codes of nomenclature (eg, "type strain," discussed earlier), and the suffix "-var" is preferred in microbiologic literature.

Infrasubspecific subdivisions such as biovars and biogroups are designated with various numbers, letters, or terms; follow author usage, eg:

Brucella suis biovar 1

Haemophilus influenzae biovar VIII

Pseudomonas putida biovar A

Serratia odorifera biogroup 1

A hyphenated species name implies 2 species that are indistinguishable in the context in which they are mentioned; neither is a subspecies of the other. For example, the 2 species *Mycobacterium avium* and *Mycobacterium intracellulare* may be referred to as:

Mycobacterium avium-intracellulare complex

or

Mycobacterium avium-intracellulare

or

Mycobacterium avium complex

(includes both species)

Practical groupings according to laboratory analysis for clinical isolates do not necessarily coincide with phylogenetically valid taxonomic relationships[13(p299)] but persist in clinical recognition and importance. Follow author usage. Prominent examples are the clinically important streptococci, differentiated according to laboratory tests, ie, types of hemolytic reaction and Lancefield serologic group.

Descriptor	*Species*
group A β-hemolytic streptococci	These fall within the species *Streptococcus pyogenes*.
group B β-hemolytic streptococci	*S agalactiae*

There is not always a one-to-one correspondence between Lancefield group and streptococcal species (eg, groups C, E), and the one may be a subset of the other.

Strains: These are treated in the bacterial nomenclature code as follows: "A strain is made up of the descendants of a single isolation in pure culture . . . and is often derived from a single colony. . . . A strain may be designated in any manner, eg, by the name of an individual, by a locality, or by a number."[8(pp134-135)] For instance, the chlamydial strain

TWAR

was named "after the laboratory designation of the first 2 isolates—TW-183 and AR-39."[22(p161),23,24] This strain retained the designation TWAR when it was found to represent a new species, resulting in the change from *Chlamydia psittaci* TWAR to *Chlamydia pneumoniae* TWAR.[22-24] Such usage confers consistency in designation of an infectious microorganism, eg, in an epidemiologic context, even when the name of that organism has changed.

In the case of *Escherichia coli,* a serotype profile, the O:K:H serotype, helps designate strains. Such a profile is based on the somatic O antigen, capsular K antigen, and flagellar H antigen,[10(p180)] and is expressed as in the following examples (avoid misprinting the capital letter O as the numeral 0):

Escherichia coli O6:K13:H1

Escherichia coli O157:H7

Escherichia coli strains grouped according to type of diarrheal infection have commonly abbreviated designations, which are expanded here for reference but which, in medical articles, should always be treated in accordance with 11.11, Abbreviations, Clinical and Technical Terms.

EAggEC	enteroaggregative *E coli*
EHEC	enterohemorrhagic *E coli*
EIEC	enteroinvasive *E coli*
EPEC	enteropathogenic *E coli*
ETEC	enterotoxigenic *E coli*

". . . *E. coli* O157:H7 is the prototype EHEC."[25(p450)]

Haemophilus influenzae strains are defined by capsular antigens, designated types a through f,[26] eg:

Haemophilus influenzae type b

The last has conferred a familiar abbreviation (expand at first mention) on its vaccine:

Hib vaccine

Salmonella *Nomenclature:*[12(pp2013-2014),13(pp452-453),27] Nomenclature for bacteria in the genus *Salmonella* is in flux. *Salmonella* bacteria were originally grouped as species and named accordingly, eg, *Salmonella typhi, Salmonella typhimurium.* However, it was subsequently found that what were considered separate species were, in fact, serovars (serotypes). (Bacteria of the former genus *Arizona* also were found to belong in the genus *Salmonella.*) Although terminology appropriate to serovars is preferred in microbiology settings, the binomial specieslike terms predominate in the clinical infectious disease literature.

Terminology using "serotype" or "serovar" is taxonomically correct, but the binomial terminology still predominates in clinical infectious disease literature. Editors, therefore, should follow author preference, using the typographic style in the examples below:

Salmonella typhi
or
Salmonella serovar Typhi
(*Salmonella* serotype Typhi also acceptable)
(*Salmonella* Typhi acceptable on subsequent mentions)

Salmonella typhimurium
or
(*Salmonella* serotype Typhimurium also acceptable)
(*Salmonella* Typhimurium acceptable on subsequent mentions)

When the serotype/serovar form is used, to avoid confusion, it is best to expand *Salmonella,* rather than following style for abbreviating genus.

Serovars are defined by the O (somatic), Vi (capsular), and H (flagellar) antigens. In practice, and in contrast to *E coli* strains, when the serotype is expressed using those antigens, the letters O, H, and Vi are not included in the serotype designation. Colons separate the O, Vi, and H designations, which take a variety of forms (letter, numeric, etc), eg:

Salmonellae subsp *arizonae* serovar $50{:}z_4z_{24}{:}-$

Salmonellae are also allotted to 7 subgroups, represented with roman numerals, as in the following expression:

Salmonella serotype IIIa $41{:}z_4z_{23}{:}-$

O antigen serotypes are A, B, C_1, C_2, D, and E, eg:

Salmonella paratyphi B

Vernacular Plurals and Adjectives: Many bacteria and other organisms possess traditional generic plural designations, which are verifiable in the dictionary. However, if the correct generic plural cannot be determined, add the word "organisms" or "species" to the italicized genus name (see also 7.5, Plurals, Microorganisms). The following are examples:

Genus	*Plural Noun Form*
Chlamydia	chlamydiae
Escherichia	*Escherichia* organisms
Mycobacterium	mycobacteria
Proteus	*Proteus* organisms

Genus	*Plural Noun Form*
Pseudomonas	pseudomonads
Salmonella	salmonellae
Staphylococcus	staphylococci
Streptococcus	streptococci
Treponema	treponemes

Viridans streptococci are another cause of infective endocarditis.

Some of these have special adjectival forms, eg, chlamydial, mycobacterial, staphylococcal, streptococcal, treponemal.

Unspecified Species: The name of a genus used alone implies the genus as a whole, eg:

Toxocara infections are frequently acquired from household pets.

The term *species* is used in cases in which the genus is certain but the species cannot be determined. For instance, if an author knew that a skin test reaction indicated presence of *Toxocara* organisms but was uncertain as to whether the reaction resulted in a particular case from the presence of *Toxocara canis* or *Toxocara cati,* the author might write:

The source of the patient's infection was *Toxocara* species.

In the latter example, *Toxocara* organisms would also be acceptable, but *Toxocara* alone would be incorrect.[28,29] Although use of sp or spp (eg, *Toxocara* sp, *Toxocara* spp) is widespread in such contexts, AMA publications do not use these terms in place of species.

Laboratory Media: Microorganism names applied to laboratory media are given lowercase and roman, eg:

brucella agar

bacteroides bile esculin agar

Capitalization indicates a product name, eg:

Haemophilus ID Quad agar

(Sometimes confused with laboratory media that mention organism names is the the *Limulus* test. This is an assay using the amebocyte lysate of the horseshoe crab, *Limulus polyphemus.* As described previously, capitalize and italicize the genus name *Limulus.*)

Bacterial Gene Nomenclature: See 12.6.5, Animal Genetic Terms.

Usage: In text dealing with infectious conditions, it is important to distinguish between the infectious agent and the condition. Infectious agents, infections, and diseases are not equivalent:

Incorrect: *Haemophilus influenzae* may be a life-threatening disease.
Better: *Haemophilus influenzae* infection may be life-threatening.
Preferred: Infection with *Haemophilus influenzae* may be life-threatening.

Incorrect: *Chlamydia trachomatis* is often an overlooked disease.
Inelegant: *Chlamydia trachomatis* disease is often overlooked.
Preferred: Disease caused by *Chlamydia trachomatis* is often overlooked.

-osis, -iasis.—The Council of the World Federation of Parasitologists recommends that the suffix *-osis* (plural: *-oses*) be used in preference to *-iasis* (plural: *-iases*) in the names of parasitic infections and diseases,[30] eg:

babesiosis

entamoebosis

giardiosis

parasitosis

Traditional parasitic disease terms (malaria, scabies) would be retained. A complete listing of preferred terms has been published.[31] Editors for now, however, may follow author preference, eg, candidiasis, candidosis.

Authors should note that when a fungal name is ambiguous because it does not describe the actual clinical situation, the name should be changed, eg, "fusariosis" should be changed to "hyalohyphomycosis (subcutaneous abscess) caused by *Fusarium* species" or "hyalohyphomycosis (meningitis) caused by *Fusarium* species" (parenthetical description as appropriate). For fungal diseases in which only one presentation by an organism is possible, eg, basidiobolomycosis, retention of the organism name in the disease is permitted (Kevin C. Hazen, PhD, written communication, June 13, 1996).

REFERENCES

1. Staley JT, Krieg NR. Bacterial classification, I: classification of procaryotic organisms: an overview. In: Krieg NR, Holt JF, eds. *Bergey's Manual of Systematic Bacteriology.* Baltimore, Md: Williams & Wilkins; 1984;1:1-4.
2. Berger SA, Edberg SC. Microbial nomenclature: a list of names and origins. *Diagn Microbiol Infect Dis.* 1987;6:343-356.
3. Thompson KS. By any other name. *Am Scientist.* 1995;83:514-517.
4. Turck M. The new taxonomy in infections. *Hosp Pract.* 1989;24:109-118, 120-121.
5. Jeffrey C. *Biological Nomenclature.* 3rd ed. London, England: Edward Arnold; 1989.
6. Greuter W, Barrie FR, Burdet HM, et al. *International Code of Botanical Nomenclature (Tokyo Code).* Königstein, Germany: Koeltz Scientific Books; 1994.
7. Ride WDL, ed. *International Code of Zoological Nomenclature.* 3rd ed. London, England: International Trust for Zoological Nomenclature in association with the British Museum (Natural History)/Berkeley, California, University of California Press; 1995.
8. Lapage SP, Sneath PHA, Lessel EF, Skerman VBD, Seeliger HPR, Clark WA; Sneath PHA, ed. *International Code of Nomenclature of Bacteria and Statutes of the International Committee on Systematic Bacteriology and Statutes of the Bacteriology and Applied Microbiology Section of the International Union of Microbiological Societies, 1990 Revision.* Washington, DC: American Society for Microbiology; 1992.
9. Barnard PC. Zoological nomenclature. In: Enckell PH, ed. *Science Editors' Handbook.* Lund, Sweden: European Association of Science Editors; 1993:D4-1-D4-2.
10. Holt JG, Krieg NR, Sneath PHA, Staley JT, Williams ST. *Bergey's Manual of Determinative Bacteriology.* 9th ed. Baltimore, Md: Williams & Wilkins; 1994.
11. Krieg NR, Holt JF, eds. *Bergey's Manual of Systematic Bacteriology.* Baltimore, Md: Williams & Wilkins; 1984.
12. Mandell GL, Bennett JE, Dolin R. *Mandell, Douglas and Bennett's Principles and Practice of Infectious Diseases.* 4th ed. New York, NY: Churchill Livingstone; 1995.

13. Murray PR, ed. *Manual of Clinical Microbiology.* 6th ed. Washington, DC: ASM [American Society for Microbiology] Press; 1995.

14. Morse SA. Classification of bacteria. In: Brooks GF, Butel JS, Ornston LN, eds. *Jawetz, Melnick and Adelberg's Medical Microbiology.* 20th ed. Norwalk, Conn: Appleton & Lange; 1995:35-43.

15. Kloos WE, Bannerman TL. *Staphylococcus* and *micrococcus.* In: Murray PR, ed. *Manual of Clinical Microbiology.* 6th ed. Washington, DC: ASM [American Society for Microbiology] Press; 1995:282.

16. Funke G, Ramos CP, Collins MD. Identification of some clinical strains of CDC coryneform group A-3 and A-4 bacteria as *Cellulomonas* species and proposal of *Cellulomonas hominis* sp. nov. for some group A-3 strains. *J Clin Microbiol.* 1995;33:2091-2097.

17. Sullivan DJ, Westerneng TJ, Haynes KA, Bennett DE, Coleman DC. *Candida dubliniensis* sp. nov.: phenotypic and molecular characterization of a novel species associated with oral candidosis in HIV-infected individuals. *Microbiology.* 1995;141:1507-1521.

18. Hanff PA, Rosol-Donoghue JA, Spiegel CA, Wilson KH, Moore LH. *Leptotrichia sanguinegens* sp. nov., a new agent of postpartum and neonatal bacteremia. *Clin Infect Dis.* 1995;20(suppl 2):S237-S239.

19. Aksoy S. *Wigglesworthia* gen. nov. and *Wigglesworthia glossinidia* sp. nov., taxa consisting of the mycetocyte-associated, primary endosymbionts of tsetse flies. *Int J Syst Bacteriol.* 1995;45:848-851.

20. Funch P, Kristensen RM. Cycliophora is a new phylum with affinities to Entoprocta and Ectoprocta. *Nature.* 1995;378:711-714.

21. Morris SC. A new phylum from the lobster's lips. *Nature.* 1995;378:661-662.

22. Grayston JT, Kuo C-C, Wang S-P, Altman J. A new *Chlamydia psittaci* strain, TWAR, isolated in acute respiratory tract infections. *N Engl J Med.* 1986;315:161-168.

23. Grayston JT, Kuo C-C, Campbell LA, Wang SP. *Chlamydia pneumoniae* sp. nov. for *Chlamydia* sp: strain TWAR. *Int J Syst Bacteriol.* 1989;39:88-90.

24. Saikku P, Wang SP, Kleemola M, Brander E, Rusanan E, Grayston JT. An epidemic of mild pneumonia due to an unusual strain of *Chlamydia psittaci. J Infect Dis.* 1985;151:832-839.

25. Gray LD. *Escherichia, Salmonella, Shigella,* and *Yersinia.* In: Murray PR, ed. *Manual of Clinical Microbiology.* 6th ed. Washington, DC: ASM [American Society for Microbiology] Press; 1995.

26. Nitta DM, Jackson MA, Burry VG, Olson LC. Invasive *Haemophilus influenzae* type f disease. *Pediatr Infect Dis J.* 1995;14:157-159.

27. Old DC. Nomenclature of *Salmonella. J Med Microbiol.* 1992;37:361-363.

28. *ASM Style Manual for Journals and Books.* Washington, DC: American Society for Microbiology; 1991.

29. Style notes: taxonomic names in microbiology and their adjectival derivatives [editorial]. *Ann Intern Med.* 1989;110:419-420.

30. Kassai T, Burt MDB. A plea for consistency. *Parasitol Today.* 1994;10:127-128.

31. Kassai T, Cordero del Campillo M, Euzeby J, Gaafar S, Hiepe Th, Himonas CA. Standardized Nomenclature of Animal Parasitic Diseases (SNOAPAD). *Vet Parasitol.* 1988;29:299-326. [SNOAPAD was renamed SNOPAD in 1990.[30]]

ADDITIONAL READINGS AND GENERAL REFERENCES

Microbiology Products: Catalog and Price List. Lenexa, Kan: REMEL; April 1995. Catalog No. 104.

Sneath PHA. Bacterial nomenclature. In: Krieg NR, Holt JF, eds. *Bergey's Manual of Systematic Bacteriology.* Baltimore, Md: Williams & Wilkins; 1984;1:19-23.

12.12.2 *Viruses.*

Viruses evolve rapidly. . . . [A]denovirus, for example, may produce 250 000 DNA molecules in an infected cell. . . .
L. Collier, J. Oxford[1(p12)]

A simple cough can generate up to 10,000 small potentially infectious aerosol particles and a sneeze, nearly 2 million!
K. L. Tyler, B. N. Fields[2(p1319)]

Viruses have been classified in varying ways since their discovery, from size and organ tropism to type of nucleic acid.[2-4] The resulting vernacular names reflect the classification approach at the time of discovery, eg, enterovirus (virus causing gastrointestinal tract infection),[2] picornavirus (small [*pico-*] RNA virus).[1]

An attempt to apply traditional biological nomenclature to viruses ended when viral nomenclature left the purview of bacterial nomenclature in 1966. At that time a separate International Committee on Nomenclature of Viruses was established.[5] Viruses were thought to be "of such a special nature that a new and different system of nomenclature should be introduced [and] Linnaean binary names were considered to be inappropriate" for them.[5(pxxvi)]

The committee, which by its second report in 1976 had become the International Committee on Taxonomy of Viruses (ICTV), provides and promotes a mechanism for recognition and approval of viral taxa,[6,7] "a single universal system for the classification and nomenclature of all viruses."[4(preface)] The ICTV approves the taxa of species, genus, subfamily, family, and order (only 1 order, as of this writing, Mononegavirales, has been approved[4,6]). The reports of the ICTV, published in the *Archives of Virology* (Springer-Verlag), provide compendia of known viruses.

(Current viral taxonomy does not reflect phylogeny, but comparative investigations of gene sequence may result in classification reflecting phylogeny; by agreement, this will be at the level of order or above.[4] A universal virus database, *ICTVdB*, is in development.)

Viral family and genus classifications have held up over time.[4] The concept of viral species and its application continue to evolve.[4,8,9] "It seems clear that the species term will eventually be defined somewhat similarly to the term *virus*—although in some cases the term virus matches best with subspecies, strain, or even variant."[4(p3)]

In AMA publications italics are not used for any virus names. As with other organisms, taxa above the rank of genus are capitalized. Genus is capitalized when approved ICTV terms are used but may appear without capitals (in which case, a qualifier is recommended). Viral species names are in the vernacular and are not capitalized (unless containing a proper noun) or italicized. Table 6 features typical endings of viral taxa and typographic style. Bacteria are included in the table for comparision.

Occasionally, 2-part virus names are encountered, eg, herpesvirus aotus, herpesvirus ateles. However, 2-part virus names are not binomial species names as

TABLE 6. TYPICAL ENDINGS AND TYPOGRAPHIC STYLE FOR VIRAL TAXA COMPARED WITH BACTERIA

	Bacteria		Viruses		
Rank*	**Ending***	**Examples***	**Ending**	**Examples**	
Order	-ales	Pseudomonadales	-ales	Mononegavirales	
Suborder	-ineae	Pseudomonadineae	...	...	
Family	-aceae	Pseudomonadaceae	-idae	Paramyxoviridae	Herpesviridae
Subfamily	-oideae	Pseudomonadoideae	-inae	Paramyxovirinae	Betaherpesvirinae
Genus	(Varies)	*Pseudomonas*	-virus	Paramyxovirus (or the genus paramyxovirus)	Cytomegalovirus (or the genus cytomegalovirus)
Species	(Varies)	*Pseudomonas aeruginosa*	(Varies)	human parainfluenza virus 1	human herpesvirus 5

*Adapted from Lapage et al.[5(p14)]

for other microorganisms and therefore are not italicized, capitalized, or abbreviated (eg, not *H aotus*).[10]

(Many virus names are combinations of specific words, eg, *echovirus* [*e*nteric *c*ytopathic *h*uman *o*rphan *virus*], papovavirus [*pa*pilloma *po*lyoma *va*cuolating agent *virus*]. At one time capitalization reflected this, eg, ECHOvirus, PaPoVa virus, but the trend is now for lowercase terms. For derivations of viral terms, consult the reports of the ICTV.)

Formal vs Vernacular Virus Names: The stability of viral family and genus classifications provides a rationale for increased emphasis on use of formal over vernacular viral names. Moreover, while the fifth ICTV report listed vernacular names as well as approved names for viral genus and species, the sixth report lists vernacular names only for species. However, vernacular terms are well entrenched for genus and higher ranks, and viral species names are in the vernacular.

Formal style is unambiguous; consult Table 7 for formal terms.

Vernacular style can be ambiguous, because the ending "-virus" occurs at several taxonomic levels, eg, a group of several families (arboviruses), a family (retroviruses), a genus (hantavirus), and many species. The term "paramyxovirus" could refer to the family, subfamily, genus, or (if worded "a paramyxovirus") one of the species in the genus.[4] Editors should capitalize terms ending in "-idae" and "-inae" and should follow author usage for other terms. English plurals are in the vernacular and are not capitalized (see Table 7).

Authors who use the vernacular should make it unambiguous by including taxonomic rank terms when necessary and by using the exact species name,[4] eg:

the family of retroviruses

the genus hantavirus

Hantaan virus (for the species)

the paramyxovirus family

the paramyxovirus subfamily

the genus paramyxovirus

a paramyxovirus species
(name the species if possible, eg, human parainfluenza virus 1)

Viruses of Humans: Table 7 presents a selection of virus names encountered in medical publications. Names, including abbreviations, and classifications are according to ICTV.

Table 7. Viruses*

Family[†]	Genus[†]	Sample Species	Abbreviation
Adenoviridae adenoviruses	Mastadenovirus mastadenoviruses	human adenoviruses 1 to 47	HAdV-1 to 47
Arenaviridae arenaviruses	Arenavirus	lymphocytic choriomeningitis virus Lassa virus Tacaribe complex viruses, eg, Guanarito virus Sabia virus	LCMV LASV GUAV
Bunyaviridae bunyaviruses	Bunyavirus Hantavirus hantaviruses	Bunyamwera virus California encephalitis virus Hantaan virus Sin Nombre virus	BUNV CEV HTNV
Calciviridae calciviruses	Calcivirus	human calciviruses, eg, Norwalk virus	HuCV NV
Coronaviridae coronaviruses	Coronavirus	human coronavirus 229E human coronavirus OC43	HCV-229E HCV-OC43
Filoviridae filoviruses	Filovirus	Marburg virus Ebola virus Zaire	MBGV EBOV-Z
Flaviviridae flaviviruses	Flavivirus hepatitis C–like viruses[‡]	yellow fever virus tickborne encephalitis virus dengue viruses 1 to 4 St Louis encephalitis virus hepatitis C virus[‡]	YFV TBEV DENV-1 to 4 SLEV HCV
Hepadnaviridae hepadnaviruses	Orthohepadnavirus orthohepadnaviruses	hepatitis B virus[‡]	HBV
Herpesviridae herpesviruses Alphaherpesvirinae[§] alphaherpesviruses	 Simplexvirus herpes simplex viruses Varicellovirus varicella-zoster virus	 human herpesvirus 1 (herpes simplex virus 1) human herpesvirus 2 (herpex simplex virus 2) human herpesvirus 3 (varicella-zoster virus 1)	 HHV-1 HHV-2 HHV-3
Betaherpesvirinae[§] betaherpesviruses	Cytomegalovirus cytomegalovirus Roseolovirus	human herpesvirus 5 (human cytomegalovirus) human herpesvirus 6	HHV-5 HHV-6
Gammaherpesvirinae[§] gammaherpesviruses	Lymphocryptovirus	human herpesvirus 4 (Epstein-Barr virus)	HHV-4
Orthomyxoviridae[‖] orthomyxoviruses	Influenza virus A, B[‖] influenza A viruses, influenza B viruses Influenza virus C[‖] influenza C viruses	influenza A virus strains[‖] influenza B virus strains[‖] influenza C virus strains[‖]	FLUA FLUB FLUC
Papovaviridae papovaviruses	Papillomavirus papillomaviruses	human papillomaviruses JC virus (polyomavirus)	HPV-1a etc JCV
Paramyxoviridae paramyxoviruses Paramyxovirinae[§]	 Paramyxovirus papillomaviruses Morbillivirus morbilliviruses Rubulavirus	 human parainfluenza virus 1 human parainfluenza virus 3 measles virus human parainfluenza virus 2, 41, 4b mumps virus	 HPIV-1 HPIV-3 MeV HPIV-2 etc
Pneumovirinae[§] pneumoviruses	Pneumovirus	human respiratory syncytial virus	HRSV

continued

TABLE 7. VIRUSES* (*cont*)

Family†	Genus†	Sample Species	Abbreviation
Parvoviridae paravoviruses			
Parvovirinae§	Dependovirus dependoviruses	adenoassociated viruses 1 to 5	AAV-1 etc
	Erythrovirus erythroviruses	B19 virus (parvovirus B19)	B19V
Picornaviridae picornaviruses	Enterovirus enteroviruses	human polioviruses 1 to 3	HPV-1 etc
		human coxsackievirus A (various serotypes)	CAV-1 etc
		human coxsackievirus B (various serotypes)	CBV-1 etc
		human echoviruses (various serotypes)	EV-1 etc
		human enteroviruses (various serotypes)	HEV-68 etc
	Hepatovirus‡	hepatitis A virus‡	HAV
	Rhinovirus rhinoviruses	human rhinoviruses (various serotypes)	HRV-1 etc
Poxviridae poxviruses			
Chordopoxvirinae§ vertebrate poxviruses	Orthopoxvirus orthopoxviruses	vaccinia virus	VACV
		variola (smallpox) virus	VARV
	Parapoxvirus parapoxviruses	orf virus	ORFV
		pseudocowpox virus (milker's nodule virus, paravaccinia virus)	PCPV
	Molluscipoxvirus	molluscum contagiosum virus	MOCV
	Yatapoxvirus yatapoxviruses	tanapox virus	TANV
		Yaba monkey tumor virus	YMTV
Reoviridae reoviruses	Orthoreovirus orthoreoviruses	reoviruses 1 to 3	REOV-1
	Orbivirus orbiviruses	bluetongue viruses (various serotypes)	BTV-1
	Coltivirus coltiviruses	Colorado tick fever virus	CTFV
	Rotavirus rotaviruses	group A rotaviruses	ROTAV-A
		group B rotaviruses	ROTAV-B
		group C rotaviruses	ROTAV-C
Retroviridae retroviruses	Spumavirus spumaviruses, foamy viruses	human spumavirus (human foamy virus)	HSRV
	BLV-HTLV retroviruses¶	human T-lymphotropic virus 1	HTLV-1
		human T-lymphotropic virus 2	HTLV-2
	Lentivirus lentiviruses	human immunodeficiency virus 1	HIV-1
		human immunodeficiency virus 2	HIV-2
Rhabdoviridae rhabdoviruses	Lyssavirus lyssaviruses	rabies virus	RABV
	Vesiculovirus vesiculoviruses	vesicular stomatitis Indiana virus	VSIV
		vesicular stomatitis New Jersey virus	VSNJV
Togaviridae togaviruses	Alphavirus alphaviruses	eastern equine encephalitis	EEEV
		western equine encephalitis	WEEV
	Rubivirus	rubella virus	RUBV

**Adapted from Murphy et al[4] and Melnick.[11]*
†Second line, if any, shows vernacular name. Vernacular is shown for highest taxonomic rank to which it could apply. Vernacular is given in plural form, to reflect common usage, except for genuses with only 1 reported species as of this writing.
‡See also Table 8.
§Subfamily.
‖See also influenza entry, this section.
¶BLV indicates bovine leukemia virus.

Special Virus Terminology

HEPATITIS. The major types of viral hepatitis as currently recognized appear in Table 8, along with antigen and antibody terminology (use parenthetic abbreviated terms in accordance with 11.11, Abbreviations, Clinical and Technical Terms).

Terms such as non-A, non-B (often abbreviated NANB) hepatitis and non-A, non-B, non-C (NANBNC) hepatitis are used as diagnoses of exclusion. Such terms are modified as new hepatitis viruses (eg, hepatitis E, hepatitis G) are identified.

The following are examples of additional hepatitis-related terms, which need not be expanded unless indicated:

hepatitis A

VP1, VP2, VP3: viral proteins of the HAV shell (expand at first mention)

(*Note:* The structure of the virion, the coding capacity of the genome, and the designation of proteins of hepatitis A virus are similar to those of other picornaviruses, eg, poliovirus.)

hepatitis B

subdeterminants of hepatitis B surface antigen (use with "subdeterminant" at first mention)

HBsAg/adr

HBsAg/ayr

HbsAg/adw1

HBsAg/ayw1

HBV genes

S (surface)

pre-S1

pre-S2

C (core)

pre-C

P (polymerase)

X

components of HBeAg

HBeAg/1

HBeAg/2

HBeAg/3

HBIG hepatitis B immune globulin (expand at first mention)

HBV2 HBV type 2, a mutant of HBV (expand at first mention)

TABLE 8. HEPATITIS TERMINOLOGY

	Disease					
	Hepatitis A	Hepatitis B	Hepatitis C	Hepatitis D (Formerly Delta Hepatitis)	Hepatitis E	Hepatitis G
Virus	hepatitis A virus (HAV)	hepatitis B virus (HBV)	hepatitis C virus (HCV)	hepatitis D virus (HDV) (formerly delta agent, delta virus)	hepatitis E virus (HEV)	hepatitis G virus (HGV)
Nucleic acid	RNA	DNA	RNA	RNA	RNA	RNA
Virus group	picornavirus	hepadnavirus	flavivirus	...	...	flavivirus
Antigens	HAV antigen (HAV Ag)	hepatitis B surface antigen (HBsAg) hepatitis B core antigen (HBcAg) hepatitis B e antigen (HBeAg) hepatitis B X antigen (HBxAg) HBV DNA HBV bDNA	HCV antigen (HCV Ag) HCV RNA HCV bDNA	HDV antigen (HDV Ag)	HEV antigen (HEV Ag)	HGV RNA
Antibodies	anti-HAV	antibody to HBsAg (anti-HBs) antibody to HBcAg (anti-HBc) antibody to HBeAg (anti-HBe) antibody to HbxAg (anti-HBx)	anti-HCV	anti-HDV	anti-HEV	

additional antigens and antibodies

pre-S1 antigen

pre-S2 antigen

anti-pre-S antibody

hepatitis C

genes/antigens (need not expand)

5′UT	(untranslated)
C	(core)
E1	(envelope)
E2/NSI	
NS2	(nonstructural)
NS3	
NS4	
NS5	
3′UT	

genotype classification[16]:

HCV types 1-5

subtypes: 1a, 1b, 1c, 2a, 2b, 2c, 3a, 3b, 4a, 5a

Older hepatitis terms, such as *infectious hepatitis, short-incubation-period hepatitis, long-incubation-period hepatitis, serum hepatitis, hepatitis-associated antigen (HAA), Australia antigen, MS-1,* and *MS-2* are no longer useful except in historical discussions.

INFLUENZA TYPES AND STRAINS. The 3 types of influenza, as defined by non-cross-reactivity among 2 internal structural proteins[3] are:

influenza A

influenza B

influenza C

Strains of influenza A are often identified by antigenic subtypes, defined by the surface proteins hemagglutinin and neuraminidase, eg:

influenza A(H1N1)	[hemagglutinin subtype 1, neuraminidase subtype 1]

Only influenza A employs the H,N-suffix, but the 3 types of influenza virus may also contain suffixes with terms for the host of origin (if nonhuman), geographic origin (or a proper name in older strains), laboratory strain number, and year of isolation, separated by virgules (and followed by the H and N designations in parentheses in the case of influenza A),[3] eg:

influenza A/swine/Iowa/15/30(H1N1)

influenza A/USSR/90/77

influenza A/Johannesburg/33/94(H3N2)

influenza B/Panama/45/90

influenza C/Taylor/1233/47

influenza C/Ann Arbor/1/50

PHAGES. Phages are viruses that infect bacteria; *phage* is an accepted term, shortened from "bacteriophage." Phage groups or genera are sometimes referred to with terms such as *T-even phages, actinophages,* and *T7 phage group*. Specific bacteriophages tend to be referred to as "phage x," *x* being a letter (usually roman or lowercase Greek), number, or letter-number combination. Examples include the following:

numeric

phage 1307

lowercase letter

phage fd

alphanumeric, lowercase

phage v7

phage 0c1r

alphanumeric, uppercase

phage L17

phage SSV1

phage PR772

L2 phage

T4 phage

roman numeral

phage II

phage ViII

phage PIIBNV6

alphanumeric, uppercase and lowercase

phage Bam35

phage SpV4

with punctuation marks

phage PA-2

phage MAC-1′

phage ZG/2

phage I_2-2

with Greek letters

phage α1

phage Qβ

phage δA

phage ϕI

phage 1ϕ1

phage dϕ3

phage ϕNS11

phage ϕX174

phage ϕCb2

phage λ

phage μ2

Retroviral Genes. See 12.6.5, Animal Genetic Terms, and 12.6.3, Oncogenes and Tumor Suppressor Genes.

References

1. Collier L, Oxford J. *Human Virology: A Text for Students of Medicine, Dentistry and Microbiology*. New York, NY: Oxford University Press; 1993.
2. Tyler KL, Fields BN. Introduction to viruses and viral diseases. In: Mandell GL, Bennett JE, Dolin R, eds. *Mandell, Douglas and Bennett's Principles and Practice of Infectious Diseases.* 4th ed. New York, NY: Churchill Livingstone; 1995:1314-1324.
3. Brooks GF, Butel JS, Ornston LN, Jawetz E, Melnick JL, Adelberg EA. *Jawetz, Melnick & Adelberg's Medical Microbiology*. 20th ed. Norwalk, Conn: Appleton & Lange; 1995:303-325.
4. Murphy FA, Fauquet CM, Bishop DHL, et al. Virus taxonomy: classification and nomenclature of viruses: sixth report of the International Committee on Taxonomy of Viruses. *Arch Virol.* 1995;suppl 10:1-586.
5. Lapage SP, Sneath PHA, Lessel EF, Skerman VBD, Seeliger HPR, Clark WA; Sneath PHA, ed. *International Code of Nomenclature of Bacteria and Statutes of the International Committee on Systematic Bacteriology and Statutes of the Bacteriology and Applied Microbiology Section of the International Union of Microbiological Societies, 1990 Revision.* Washington, DC: American Society for Microbiology; 1992.
6. Francki RIB, Fauquet CM, Knudson DL, Brown F. Classification and nomenclature of viruses: fifth report of the International Committee on Taxonomy of Viruses. *Arch Virol.* 1991;suppl 2:1-450.
7. Jeffrey C. *Biological Nomenclature*. 3rd ed. New York, NY: Edward Arnold; 1989.
8. Van Regenmortel MH. Virus species, a much overlooked but essential concept in virus classification. *Intervirology*. 1990;31:241-254.
9. Van Regenmortel MH, Maniloff J, Calisher C. The concept of virus species [news]. *Arch Virol*. 1991;120:313-314.
10. *ASM Style Manual for Journals and Books*. Washington, DC: American Society for Microbiology; 1991.
11. Melnick JL. Taxonomy of viruses. In: Murray PR, ed. *Manual of Clinical Microbiology.* 6th ed. Washington, DC: ASM [American Society for Microbiology] Press; 1995:859-867.
12. Jeffers LJ, Piatak M, Bernstein DE, et al. Hepatitis G virus infection in patients with

acute and chronic liver disease of unknown etiology [abstract]. *Hepatology*. 1995;22(pt 2):182A.

13. Leevy CM, Sherlock S, Tygstrup N, Zetterman R, for the International Hepatology Informatics Group. *Diseases of the Liver and Biliary Tract: Standardization of Nomenclature, Diagnostic Criteria, and Prognosis*. New York, NY: Raven Press; 1994:20-22, 47-59.

14. Noskin GA. *Prevention, Diagnosis, and Management of Viral Hepatitis: A Guide for Primary Care Physicians*. Chicago, Ill: American Medical Association; 1995.

15. Koff RS. Viral hepatitis. In: Schiff L, Schiff ER, eds. *Diseases of the Liver.* 7th ed. Philadelphia, Pa: JB Lippincott; 1993:492-511.

16. Simmonds P, Alberti A, Alter HJ, et al. A proposed system for the nomenclature of hepatitis C viral genotypes. *Hepatology.* 1994;19:1321-1324.

ADDITIONAL READINGS AND GENERAL REFERENCES

Hsiung GD. Properties and classification of viruses. In: Hsiung GD, Fond CKY, Landry ML, eds. *Hsiung's Diagnostic Virology: As Illustrated by Light and Electron Microscopy.* 4th ed. New Haven, Conn: Yale University Press; 1994:8-11.

Levy JA, Fraenkel-Conrat H, Owens RA. *Virology.* 3rd ed. Englewood Cliffs, NJ: Prentice-Hall; 1994.

Sherlock S, Dooley J. *Diseases of the Liver and Biliary System*. 10th ed. Boston, Mass: Blackwell Scientific Publications; 1997:265-302.

12.13 ■ **PULMONARY AND RESPIRATORY TERMINOLOGY.**—Despite the familiarity of abbreviations in pulmonary and respiratory medicine, authors and editors are encouraged to expand all terms at first mention, except as noted.

Symbols and abbreviations that are usually initialisms are used in pulmonary-respiratory medicine. Symbols consist of separate elements in various combinations whose letters may differ from the initial letters of the expansion, eg, $\dot{Q}$ (perfusion).

12.13.1 ***Symbols.***—The following groupings of pulmonary-respiratory symbols are adapted from West[1] and Fishman.[2] The symbols and the subgroupings into main symbols and modifiers are consistent with the approved nomenclature of the Committee on Respiratory Physiology of the International Union of Physiological Sciences (IUPS) and the Publications Committee of the American Physiological Society.[2,3] The official listing of terms[2] features symbols from respiratory mechanics and gas exchange separately.

Main symbols are usually capital letters set on the line and are the first elements of an expression. The same letter may stand for one entity in respiratory mechanics and another in gas exchange. The following are examples (note dots above some letters used to indicate flow):

C	concentration, compliance
D	diffusing capacity
F	fractional concentration in a dry gas
P	partial pressure, pressure
Q	volume of blood
$\dot{Q}$	perfusion (volume of blood per unit time or blood flow)

R	gas (respiratory) exchange ratio, resistance
S	saturation
sG	specific conductance
V	volume of gas
$\dot{V}$	ventilation (volume per unit time)

Modifiers are set as small capitals (not subscript):

A	alveolar
B	barometric
DS	dead space
E	expired, expiratory
ET	end-tidal
I	inspired, inspiratory
L	lung
T	tidal

Lowercase-letter modifiers (not subscript) follow small-capital modifiers, if both appear; note bar in last term:

a	arterial
aw	airway
b	blood, in general
c	capillary
c′	pulmonary end-capillary
i	ideal
max	maximum
v	venous
$\bar{v}$	mixed venous

Gas abbreviations are usually the last element of the symbol, given as small capitals. (*Note:* In IUPS terminology, they are given as subscripts.)

CO	carbon monoxide
CO_2	carbon dioxide
N_2	nitrogen
O_2	oxygen

The main symbols and modifiers are combined in various ways to derive terms; common examples are the following:

PCO_2	partial pressure of carbon dioxide
$PaCO_2$	partial pressure of carbon dioxide, arterial
PO_2	partial pressure of oxygen
PaO_2	partial pressure of oxygen, arterial

(*Note:* The above 4 terms may be given without expansion at first mention; see also 11.11, Abbreviations, Clinical and Technical Terms.)

P_{AO_2}	partial pressure of oxygen in the alveoli
$P_{\bar{V}O_2}$	partial pressure of oxygen, mixed venous
P_B	barometric pressure
$P_{AO_2} - P_{aO_2}$	alveolar-arterial difference in partial pressure of oxygen (preferred to AaD_{O_2})
C_{aO_2}	oxygen concentration, arterial
$C_{c'O_2}$	oxygen concentration, pulmonary end-capillary
C_L	lung compliance
D_{LCO}	diffusing capacity of lung for carbon monoxide
F_{EN_2}	fractional concentration of nitrogen in expired gas
F_{IO_2}	fraction of inspired oxygen
$P_{E}max$	maximum expiratory pressure
$P_{I}max$	maximum inspiratory pressure
Raw	airway resistance
S_{aO_2}	oxygen saturation, arterial
sGaw	specific airway conductance
S_{pO_2}	oxygen saturation as measured by pulse oximetry (a more recent term)
V_{DS}	volume of dead space
$\dot{V}_E$	expired volume per unit time
$\dot{V}_{O_2}$	oxygen consumption per unit time
$\dot{V}_{O_2}max$	maximum oxygen consumption
$\dot{V}/\dot{Q}$	ventilation-perfusion ratio (also $\dot{V}_A/\dot{Q}$)
V_T	tidal volume

12.13.2 ***Abbreviations.***—The following are some common abbreviations from pulmonary function testing; they should always be expanded at first mention:

CC	closing capacity
CV	closing volume
ERV	expiratory reserve volume
$FEF_{25\%-75\%}$	forced expiratory flow, midexpiratory phase (formerly midmaximal expiratory flow rate [MMEFR]; midflow; midmaximal flow [MMF] or midexpiratory flow rate [MEFR])
$FEF_{200-1200}$	forced expiratory flow between 200 and 1200 mL of FVC
FEV	forced expiratory volume
FEV_1	forced expiratory volume in 1 second; forced expiratory volume in the first second
FIVC	forced inspiratory vital capacity
FRC	functional residual capacity
FVC	forced vital capacity

IRV	inspiratory reserve volume
IVC	inspiratory vital capacity
MVV	maximum voluntary ventilation
PEF, PEFR	peak expiratory flow rate
RV	residual volume
TLC	total lung capacity
VC	vital capacity

12.13.3 ***Mechanical Ventilation.***—The following should be expanded at first mention:

ACMV	assist/control mode ventilation
CPAP	continuous positive airway pressure
PCV	pressure-control ventilation
PEEP	positive end-expiratory pressure
PSV	pressure-support ventilation
SIMV	synchronized intermittent mandatory ventilation

In pulmonary-respiratory nomenclature, certain letters often stand for more than one entity. For instance, capital C stands for *concentration* in the context of gas exchange and for *closing*, *capacity*, or *compliance* in pulmonary mechanics. Moreover, the lists are condensed from the IUPS nomenclature and are not exhaustive. Therefore, authors and editors should be cautious in expanding terms and should not assume that the letters in the above lists always stand for the terms indicated.

REFERENCES

1. West JB. *Respiratory Physiology: The Essentials.* 5th ed. Baltimore, Md: Williams & Wilkins; 1994.
2. Fishman AP, ed. *Handbook of Physiology: A Critical, Comprehensive Presentation of Physiological Knowledge and Concepts.* Vol 2, section 3, pt 1. Bethesda, Md: American Physiological Society; 1986:endpapers.
3. Macklem PT. Symbols and abbreviations. In: Fishman AP, ed. *Handbook of Physiology: A Critical, Comprehensive Presentation of Physiological Knowledge and Concepts.* Vol 2, section 3, pt 1. Bethesda, Md: American Physiological Society; 1986:ix.

ADDITIONAL READING AND GENERAL REFERENCE

Pappenheimer JR, Comroe JH, Cournand A, et al. Standardization of definitions and symbols in respiratory physiology. *Fed Proc.* 1950;9:602-605.

CHAPTER 13

13.0 EPONYMS

Eponyms are phrases or names derived from or including the name of a person or place. These terms are used in an adjectival sense[1] in medical and scientific writing to describe entities such as conditions or diseases, tests, methods, and procedures. These terms should be distinguished from literal possessives (eg, Rachel Carson's *Silent Spring*).

In relation to diseases or conditions, eponyms historically have indicated the name of the describer or discoverer of the disease (eg, Alzheimer disease), the name of a person or kindred found to have the disease described (eg, Duncan disease[2]), or, when based on the name of a place (technically, toponyms), the geographic location in which the disease was found to occur (eg, Lyme disease). Traditionally, eponyms named after the discoverer took the possessive form (-'*s*) and those in the latter 2 categories took the nonpossessive form. These distinctions are beginning to fade.

Correct usage of eponyms should be considered with a view toward clarity and consistency, the awareness that meaning changes over time and across cultures, and a desire to minimize misunderstanding in an increasingly global medical community.

13.1 ■ **EPONYMOUS VS NONEPONYMOUS TERMS.**—Use of eponyms in the biomedical literature should be considered with regard to their usefulness in transmitting medical information. Although many eponyms are evanescent, some will be permanently integrated into the body of medical knowledge. Eponyms have a certain historical and cultural value[3] and may serve an educational purpose as a mnemonic device.

The international nature of much biomedical communication provides an added incentive to use a term that has meaning common to all. The use of the noneponymous term, consisting of a descriptive word or phrase related to a disease or condition, which may provide information about location and function,[3] may represent progress toward this goal and whenever possible is preferred. This will also avoid confusing distinctly different disease entities with similar eponymous names (eg, Paget disease of bone, Paget disease of the nipple).

However, in some cases the author may believe that readers would be more familiar with the eponymous term. To insist on the use of either the noneponymous or the eponymous term would be contrary to a major purpose of scientific writing, which is to disseminate information that can be understood quickly by all. Placing the less familiar descriptive term(s) in parentheses after first mention of the eponymous/noneponymous term may be helpful, for example:

Turner syndrome (gonadal dysgenesis)

The eponym, but not the noun or adjective that accompanies it, should be capitalized (see 8.1.5, Capitalization, Eponyms):

Osler nodes

Adjectival and derivative forms of proper names used in terms are not capitalized, eg:

parkinsonian gait (from Parkinson disease)

13.2 ■ **POSSESSIVE FORM.**—There is continuing debate over the use of the possessive form; however, a transition toward the nonpossessive form may be gradually taking place, as illustrated by the change from *Down's* to *Down* syndrome.

The National Down Syndrome Society advocates the use of *Down syndrome,* arguing that the syndrome does not actually *belong* to anyone.[4] Some dictionaries may list *Down's syndrome* as a primary or variant entry, but *Dorland's Illustrated Medical Dictionary* (28th edition) and a new edition of a reference book for medical editors, *Scientific Style and Format* (the sixth edition of the Council of Biology Editors [CBE] style manual), have dropped the possessive for *Down syndrome.* The CBE manual recommends that the possessive form of eponymous terms be eliminated altogether so they can be distinguished from true possessives.[5] *Dorland's* continues to show the possessive form for many eponymous terms, reflecting perceived current usage and the stated policy to consider eponyms as an example of a stylistic matter left up to the individual.[6]

A possessive form of a term may have multiple meanings, including a literal possessive sense and an adjectival sense.[1] In eponyms, the adjectival sense is predominant.[1] For example, the name *Addison,* as used in describing "Addison's disease," is used as a noun modifier, with the sense of the modifier being clearly nonpossessive.[1] Although eponyms are possessive nouns, they are structurally adjectival, in addition to being so in a semantic sense.[1] Further evidence of this is the evolution of some possessive eponyms into the form of derived adjectives, as exemplified in the term *addisonian crisis.*[1] Thus, avoidance of the possessive form may contribute to clarity in usage from a linguistic perspective.

The English language readily accommodates unmarked attribution as in "shopkeeper" (proper nouns may also be unmarked when attributive, eg, "Nobel Prize," "Heimlich maneuver") and has often lost case endings over time, eg, "Petri's dish" is now "Petri dish."[1] Thus, the transition of eponyms to the nonpossessive form is consistent with trends in English usage.[1]

Use of the nonpossessive form of eponyms is often the case in medical genetics, and such usage, recommended by McKusick in *Mendelian Inheritance in Man: A Catalog of Human Genes and Genetic Disorders,*[7] may be applied to other areas of medicine. McKusick's reasons for avoiding the possessive form of eponyms include the suggestion that "the eponym is merely a 'handle'; often the person whose name is used was not the first to describe the condition . . . or did not describe the full syndrome as it has subsequently become known."[7] Hence, even the initial description may not belong to the named individual.

The following recommendations provide a rationale for a preference for the nonpossessive form in particular categories of eponymous terms. These recommendations promote mellifluous usage and minimize misspellings.

- When the word following begins with a sibilant *c, s,* or *z* (eg, *syndrome, sign, zone*)[7]:

Schwann cell	Korsakoff psychosis
Bitot spots	Cullen sign
Looser zones	Reye syndrome

- When an eponym ends in *ce, s,* or *z*[7]:

Meigs syndrome	Graves disease
Colles fracture	Wilms tumor
Homans sign	legionnaires disease
Fordyce disease	Grawitz tumor
Betz cell	

- When 2 or more names are involved:

  Charcot-Marie-Tooth disease

  Dejerine-Sottas dystrophy

  Pierre Robin syndrome

- When an article (*a, an, the*) precedes the term:

  a Schatzki ring

  an Opie paradox

There may be instances in which current English idiomatic usage or author preference would suggest that a possessive form is preferable:

Ringer's lactate solution

Occasionally, in certain usages, the nonpossessive eponymous term may appear awkward. This can be addressed by using *the* before the term:

the Avogadro number	the Starling law
the Pascal principle	the Tukey test

Alternative stylings for terms may include the use of *of*:

circle of Willis

In view of the rationale given for preferring the nonpossessive form in particular instances, recommendations of authorities, and in keeping with the desire to promote clarity and consistency in scientific writing, we recommend that the possessive form be omitted in eponymous terms.

ACKNOWLEDGMENT

Principal author: Jeanette M. Smith, MD

REFERENCES

1. Anderson JB. The language of eponyms. *J R Coll Physicians Lond.* 1996;30:174-177.
2. Firkin BG, Whitworth JA, eds. *Dictionary of Medical Eponyms.* Park Ridge, NJ: Parthenon Publishing Group Inc; 1990:134.

3. Leaf-Brock S. Encore on eponyms. *Mayo Alumnus.* Winter 1992;28:2-6.

4. Thumbs-up on Down syndrome? *Copy Editor.* April/May 1994:1, 7.

5. Council of Biology Editors Style Manual Committee. *Scientific Style and Format: The CBE Manual for Authors, Editors, and Publishers.* 6th ed. New York, NY: Cambridge University Press; 1994:97.

6. *Dorland's Illustrated Medical Dictionary.* 28th ed. Philadelphia, Pa: WB Saunders Co; 1994:v.

7. McKusick VA. *Mendelian Inheritance in Man: A Catalog of Human Genes and Genetic Disorders.* 11th ed. Baltimore, Md: The Johns Hopkins University Press; 1994:xl, xlii.

CHAPTER 14

14.0 GREEK LETTERS

Greek letters are frequently used in statistical formulas and notations, in mathematical composition, in certain chemical names for drugs, and in clinical and technical terms (see 11.11, Abbreviations, Clinical and Technical Terms, 11.12, Abbreviations, Units of Measure, 12.0, Nomenclature, 17.0, Statistics, and 18.0, Mathematical Composition).

β-adrenergic κ light chain γ-globulin

14.1 ■ **GREEK LETTER VS WORD.**—Editors of AMA publications prefer the use of Greek letters rather than words, unless usage dictates otherwise. Consult *Stedman's* and *Dorland's* medical dictionaries for general terms. These sources may differ in the representation of terms, ie, α-fetoprotein (*Stedman's*) and alpha-fetoprotein (*Dorland's*). If the Greek letter, rather than the word, is found in either of these sources for the item in question, use the letter in preference to the word. For chemical terms, the use of Greek letters is almost always preferred. For electroencephalographic terms, use the word (see 12.10.2, Nomenclature, Electroencephalographic [EEG] Terms). For drug names that contain Greek letters, consult the sources listed in 12.4, Nomenclature, Drugs, for preferred usage. In some cases, when the Greek letter is part of the word, as in *betamethasone,* the Greek letter is spelled out and set closed up. In addition, for some names, the approved nonproprietary name takes the word, not the Greek letter, eg, beta carotene, with an intervening space. (*Note:* The chemical name would be β-carotene, however.)

A Greek letter used in the name of a molecule does not always correspond to the Roman letter in an equivalent term, as in the following names for the same compound:

δ-sialoglycoprotein = glycophorin B

14.2 ■ **CAPITALIZATION AFTER A GREEK LETTER.**—In titles, subtitles (except in references), centered heads, sideheads, table column heads, line art, and at the beginning of sentences, the first non-Greek letter after a lowercase Greek letter should be capitalized. Do not capitalize the Greek letter itself, unless the capital is specifically intended, in which case the first non-Greek letter after the capital Greek letter should be set lowercase. For hyphenation in words that contain Greek letters, consult 6.3.1, Punctuation, Hyphen, Special Combinations.

Title:	Liver Disease in α_1-Antitrypsin Deficiency
Table title:	Table 1. Effectiveness of Various β-Blockers in Migraine

Beginning of a sentence: β-Hemolytic streptococci were identified.

Δ^1-3,4-*trans*-tetrahydrocannabinol is 1 of 2 psychoactive isomeric principles in cannabis.

14.3 ■ **GREEK ALPHABET.**—Capital and lowercase Greek letters are listed below, in a table adapted from *The Chicago Manual of Style*[1] (copyright 1993, University of Chicago). Alternative fonts exist for some Greek letters. Many computerized systems are available for generating and typesetting these characters.

Name of Letter	*Greek Alphabet*		*Transliteration*
Alpha	Α	α	a
Beta	Β	β	b
Gamma	Γ	γ	g
Delta	Δ	δ ∂*	d
Epsilon	Ε	ε	e
Zeta	Ζ	ζ	z
Eta	Η	η	ē
Theta	Θ	θ ϑ*	th
Iota	Ι	ι	i
Kappa	Κ	κ	k
Lambda	Λ	λ	l
Mu	Μ	μ	m
Nu	Ν	ν	n
Xi	Ξ	ξ	x
Omicron	Ο	ο	o
Pi	Π	π	p
Rho	Ρ	ρ	r; *initially,* rh
Sigma	Σ	σ ς†	s
Tau	Τ	τ	t
Upsilon	Υ	υ	u; *except after* a, e, ē, i, it is *often* y
Phi	Φ	ϕ φ*	ph
Chi	Χ	χ	kh
Psi	Ψ	ψ	ps
Omega	Ω	ω	ō

*Old-style character. Usually used in mathematical formulas; should not be combined with other fonts.

†Final letter.

14.4 ■ **TYPESETTING GREEK LETTERS.**—Greek letters in copy should be marked for the typesetter's attention by writing the letters "GK" in the margin, followed by a description of the character, eg, lowercase mu; similar notation should appear with text provided on disk. (Consult 20.1, Copyediting and Proofreading Marks, Copyediting Marks, regarding the marking of Greek letters in copy.)

ACKNOWLEDGMENT

Principal author: Jeanette M. Smith, MD

REFERENCE

1. *The Chicago Manual of Style.* 14th ed. Chicago, Ill: University of Chicago Press; 1993:350.

Measurement and Quantitation

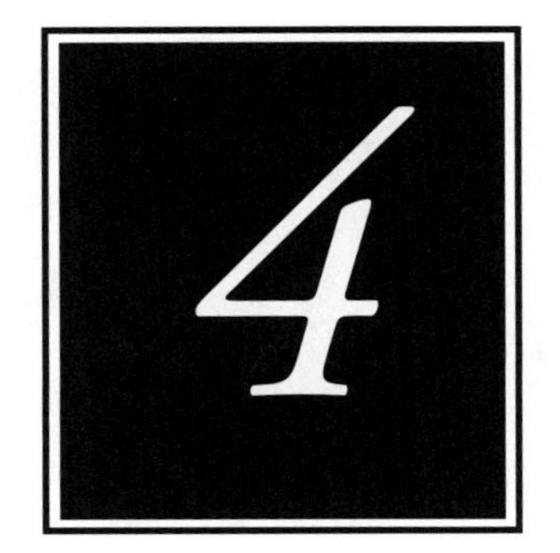

CHAPTER 15

15.0 UNITS OF MEASURE

The presentation of quantitative information is an integral component of biomedical publications. Accurate communication of scientific knowledge and data requires an informative and universal system of units of measure.

15.1 ■ SI UNITS.

—The International System of Units (*Le Système International d'Unites* or SI) represents a modernized version of the metric system. The SI is considered the universal measurement standard and has been adopted as the official measurement system of most nations. The SI units simplify international communication, promote uniformity of quantities and units, minimize the number of units and multiples used in other measurement systems, and unambiguously express virtually any measurement in science, medicine, industry, and commerce.

In 1977, the World Health Organization recommended adoption of the SI by the international scientific community.[1] Since then, many biomedical publications throughout the world have adopted SI units as their preferred units of measure. Although many clinical laboratories in the United States continue to report measurements in conventional units, many leading US biomedical publications have recognized the importance of SI units and now either publish SI values alone or dual-report values, providing both SI units and conventional units.[2,3] Since 1988, AMA scientific publications have used SI units as the primary method for reporting scientific measurements.[4] Currently, *JAMA* and the AMA *Archives* Journals report SI values as their standard units for scientific information and require SI measurements for submitted manuscripts. However, dual-reported values are provided for selected analytes (eg, blood glucose, cholesterol; see 15.5.2, Dual Reporting) and SI unit conversion factors are supplied for selected other values. Authors, scientists, clinicians, editors, and others involved in preparing, reviewing, and processing manuscripts for biomedical publication should become familiar with SI nomenclature and should take responsibility for the conversion from conventional units to SI units.

15.1.1 ***SI Base Units.***—The SI is based on 7 fundamental units (*base units*) that refer to 7 basic quantities of measurement (Table 1). These units are dimensionally independent and are the elements from which other measurement quantities are composed. Although not included among the 7 base units, the liter (the equivalent of 1000 cm^3) is used in the SI as a fundamental measure of capacity or volume. The liter is the recommended unit for measurement of volume for liquids and gases, whereas the cubic meter is the SI unit of volume for solids. Although the kelvin is the SI unit for thermodynamic temperature, the degree Celsius is used with the SI for temperature measurement in biomedical settings.[5]

TABLE 1. SI BASE UNITS

Quantity	Base Unit Name	SI Unit Symbol
Length	meter	m
Mass	kilogram	kg
Time	second	s
Electric current	ampere	A
Thermodynamic temperature	kelvin	K
Luminous intensity	candela	cd
Amount of substance	mole	mol

15.1.2 ***SI Derived Units.***—Other SI measurement quantities are referred to as *derived units* and are expressed as products or quotients of the 7 base units. Certain SI derived units have special names and symbols and may be used in algebraic relationships to express other derived units (Table 2).

15.1.3 ***SI Prefixes.***—Prefixes are combined with base units and derived units to form multiples of SI units. The factors designated by prefixes are powers of 10, and most prefixes involve exponents that are simple multiples of 3, thereby facilitating conversion procedures by means of successive multiplications by 10^3 or 10^{-3} (Table 3). Compound prefixes formed by the combination of 2 or more SI prefixes are not used. It is preferable to use an expression with a single prefix.

nm (nanometer), not mμm (millimicrometer)

The kilogram (kg) is the only SI base unit with a prefix as part of its name. Because compound prefixes are not recommended, prefixes relating to mass are combined with gram (g) rather than kilogram (kg).

10^{-6} kg is 1 mg (milligram), not 1 μkg (microkilogram)

TABLE 2. SI DERIVED UNITS*

Quantity	Name	SI Symbol	Derivation From SI Base Unit
Derived units			
Area	square meter	m^2	m^2
Volume	cubic meter	m^3	m^3
Velocity, speed	meter per second	m/s	m/s
Acceleration	meter per second squared	m/s^2	m/s^2
Density, mass density	kilogram per cubic meter	kg/m^3	kg/m^3
Specific volume	cubic meter per kilogram	m^3/kg	m^3/kg
Concentration	mole per cubic meter	mol/m^3	mol/m^3
Luminance	candela per square meter	cd/m^2	cd/m^2
Derived units with special names			
Frequency	hertz	Hz	s^{-1}
Force	newton	N	$m \cdot kg \cdot s^{-2}$
Pressure, stress	pascal	Pa	$kg \cdot m^{-1} \cdot s^{-2}$ (N/m^2)
Work, energy, quantity of heat	joule	J	$kg \cdot m^2 \cdot s^{-2}$ ($N \cdot m$)
Power, radiant flux	watt	W	$m^2 \cdot kg \cdot s^{-3}$ (J/s)
Electric potential	volt	V	$m^2 \cdot kg \cdot s^{-3} \cdot A^{-1}$ (W/A)
Electric charge	coulomb	C	$A \cdot s$
Electric resistance	ohm	Ω	$m^2 \cdot kg \cdot s^{-3} \cdot A^{-2}$ (V/A)
Capacitance	farad	F	$m^{-2} \cdot kg^{-1} \cdot s^4 \cdot A^2$ (C/V)
Magnetic flux	weber	Wb	$m^2 \cdot kg \cdot s^{-2} \cdot A^{-1}$ ($V \cdot s$)
Magnetic flux density	tesla	T	$kg \cdot s^{-2} \cdot A^{-1}$ (Wb/m^2)
Inductance	henry	H	$m^2 \cdot kg \cdot s^{-2} \cdot A^{-2}$ (Wb/A, $V \cdot A^{-1} \cdot s^{-1}$)

**Data from* The International System of Units (SI).[5]

TABLE 3. SI PREFIXES*

Factor	Prefix	Symbol
10^{24}	yotta	Y
10^{21}	zetta	Z
10^{18}	exa	E
10^{15}	peta	P
10^{12}	tera	T
10^{9}	giga	G
10^{6}	mega	M
10^{3}	kilo	k
10^{2}	hecto	h†
10^{1}	deka (deca)	da†
10^{-1}	deci	d†
10^{-2}	centi	c†
10^{-3}	milli	m
10^{-6}	micro	μ
10^{-9}	nano	n
10^{-12}	pico	p
10^{-15}	femto	f
10^{-18}	atto	a
10^{-21}	zepto	z
10^{-24}	yocto	y

**Data from* The International System of Units (SI).[5]
† Does not follow the preferred incremental intervals of 10^3 and 10^{-3}, but may be used with SI units.

15.2 ■ **EXPRESSING SI UNIT NAMES AND SYMBOLS.**—The SI includes rules for expressing unit names and abbreviations (often referred to as symbols), along with conventions for displaying them in text.

15.2.1 ***Capitalization.***—The SI unit names are written lowercase (eg, kilogram), except for Celsius (as in "degrees Celsius"), which is capitalized. Abbreviations or symbols for SI units also are written lowercase, with the following exceptions:

- Abbreviations derived from a proper name should be capitalized (eg, N for newton, K for kelvin, A for ampere), although the nonabbreviated SI unit names are not capitalized (eg, newton, ampere).
- An uppercase letter L is used as the abbreviation for liter to avoid confusion with the lowercase letter l and the number 1.
- Two SI prefixes, M and P, are capitalized to distinguish them from similar lowercase abbreviations. The letter M denotes the prefix *mega* (10^6), whereas m signifies *milli* (10^{-3}). Accordingly, the abbreviation mg denotes milligram (10^{-3} g), whereas MHz denotes megahertz (10^6 Hz). The letter P denotes the prefix *peta* (10^{15}), whereas p signifies *pico* (10^{-12}).

15.2.2 ***Products and Quotients of SI Unit Symbols.***—The *product* of 2 or more SI units should be indicated by a thin space or a centered multiplication dot between them.[6] The multiplication dot must be positioned properly to distinguish it from a decimal point, which is set on the baseline (see 18.6, Mathematical Composition, Expressing Multiplication and Division). When the unit of measure is the product of 2 or more units and appears without a numeral expressing quantity, either abbreviations (symbols) or nonabbreviated units should be used. Abbreviated and nonabbreviated forms should not be combined in products.

> newton meter may be expressed as newton meter, newton-meter, N m, or N · m (not as newton · m or N · meter).

When numerals are used to denote a quantity of measurement, the abbreviated form of the SI unit should be used.

> 50 N · m (not 50 newton meter).

The *quotient* of SI unit symbols may be expressed by the virgule (/) or by the use of negative exponents. If the derived unit is formed by 2 abbreviated units of measure, the quotient may be expressed by means of the virgule or negative exponent.

> μg/L or μg · L^{-1} or μg L^{-1}
> (not μg per L)

When the unit names are spelled out in a quotient, the word *per* should be used.

> The power output was measured in joules per second.
> (not joules/second)

To ensure clarity in SI unit quotients with more than 2 units of measure, no more than 1 virgule should be used. The mathematical relationships among the units should be specified by means of dot products, negative exponents, or parentheses (see 18.6, Mathematical Composition, Expressing Multiplication and Division).

> mL · kg^{-1} · min^{-1} or mL/(kg · min) (not mL/kg/min)

> m^2 · kg · s^{-2} · A^{-2} or (mg^2 · kg)/(s^2 · A^2)

15.3 ■ SI FORMAT, STYLE, AND PUNCTUATION.

15.3.1 ***Exponents.***—The SI reporting style uses exponents rather than the abbreviations cu and sq.

m^2, not sq m

m^3, not cu m

15.3.2 ***Plurals.***—The same SI symbol is used for single and multiple quantities. SI unit symbols are not expressed in the plural form.

1 L, 70 L (not 70 Ls)

1 g, 1500 g (not 1500 gs)

15.3.3 ***Subject-Verb Agreement.***—Units of measure are treated as collective singular (not plural) nouns and require a singular verb.

15.3.4 ***Beginning of Sentence, Title, Subtitle.***—A unit of measure that follows a number (as a quantity) at the beginning of a sentence, title, or subtitle should not be abbreviated, even though the same unit of measure is abbreviated if it appears elsewhere in the same sentence (see 16.2.1, Numbers and Percentages, Beginning a Sentence, Title, Subtitle, or Heading).

Seventy-five milligrams of lidocaine was administered on admission and 100 mg was given 20 minutes later.

15.3.5 ***Abbreviations.***—Most units of measure are abbreviated when used with numerals or in a virgule construction. Certain units of measure should be spelled out at first mention, with the abbreviated form in parentheses. Thereafter, the abbreviated form should be used in the text (see 11.12, Abbreviations, Units of Measure).

15.3.6 ***Punctuation.***—Symbols or abbreviations of units of measure are not followed by a period unless the symbol occurs at the end of a sentence.

80 kg (not 80 kg.)

15.3.7 ***Hyphens.***—A hyphen may be used to join 2 spelled-out units of measure.

pascal-second

A hyphen is used to join a unit of measure and the number associated with it when the combination is used as an adjective (see 6.3.1, Punctuation, Hyphens and Dashes, Temporary Compounds).

an 8-L container

a 10-cm visual analog scale

15.3.8 ***Spacing.***—With the exception of the percent sign, the degree sign (for angles), and the °C symbol, a full space should appear between the arabic numeral indicating the quantity and the unit of measure.

140 nmol/L (not 140nmol/L)

40% compliance rate

45° angle

temperature of 37.5°C (not 37.5° C or 37.5 °C)

15.4 ■ USE OF NUMERALS WITH SI UNITS.

15.4.1 ***Expressing Quantities.***—Arabic numerals are used for all quantities with units of measure (see 16.1, Numbers and Percentages, Use of Numerals). By SI convention, it is preferable to use numbers between 0.1 and 1000 for expressing quantities and to use the appropriate prefix.

0.003 mL is expressed 3 μL

15 000 g is expressed 15 kg

For large numbers, the use of scientific notation is acceptable with SI units.

20 000 000 A may be expressed as 20 MA or 2×10^7 A

Reported SI values must follow recommendations for preserving the proper number of significant digits (see 17.3.2, Statistics, Rounding Off). Laboratory values should be rounded based on the number of digits recommended to reflect the precision of the reported results. The use of significant digits is intended to prevent reporting results beyond the sensitivity of the procedure performed.

15.4.2 ***Decimal Format.***—The decimal format is recommended for numbers used with units of measure. Numerical values less than 1 require placement of a zero before the decimal marker (see also 16.7.1, Numbers and Percentages, Decimals).

0.123 (not .123)

Fractions should not be used with SI units.

2.5 kg (not 2½ kg)

Mixed fractions are not used in scientific format, but occasionally are used in less formal text to indicate less precise measurements, most commonly with units of measure representing time.

After more than 7½ years of investigation, the effort to develop a new vaccine was abandoned.

15.4.3 ***Number Spacing.***—By SI convention, the decimal marker is the only punctuation mark used in numerals and it is used to separate the integer and decimal parts of the number. Although the comma is used internationally as the decimal sign, the SI does not use commas in numbers. Integers (whole numbers) with more than 4 digits are separated into groups of 3 (by means of a half-space) with respect to the decimal marker. Four-digit integers are typeset closed up (without a space). Decimal numbers also are grouped in sets of 3 digits beginning at the decimal sign, with the same closed-up spacing for 4-digit groups.

1,234	becomes	1234
12,345	becomes	12 345
123,456	becomes	123 456
12,345.678901	becomes	12 345.678 901
1,234.56789	becomes	1234.567 89
1,234,567.8901	becomes	1 234 567.8901

However, there are exceptions for certain types of numerals that have more than 4 digits. For instance, spacing is not used for street addresses, postal codes (eg,

5-digit ZIP codes), patent numbers, page numbers, or numerals combined with letters (eg, grant numbers).

> Chicago, IL 60610
>
> US patent 4942516
>
> This study was supported by grant MCH-110624.

15.4.4 ***Multiplication of Numbers.***—Multiplication of numbers should be indicated by the multiplication sign (×) and may be used to express area (eg, a 15×35-cm^2 burn), volume (eg, a 5.2×3.7×6.9-mm^3 mass), matrices (eg, 2×2 table), magnification (eg, ×30 000), or scientific notation (eg, 3.6×10^9/L).

15.4.5 ***Percentage Replaced by Values Expressed as a Decimal.***—In the SI, values for mass fraction, volume fraction, and other relative quantities, such as white blood cell differential counts, are expressed as a decimal rather than as a percentage.

hematocrit	0.40 (not 40%)
differential cell count	0.30 band cells (not 30% band cells)

15.5 ■ SI UNITS AND CONVENTIONAL UNITS.

15.5.1 ***SI Conversion Tables.***—Despite the use of SI units by the scientific community in most countries, many laboratories in the United States currently report clinical laboratory values in conventional units. Consequently, many US physicians, clinicians, researchers, authors, and readers may not be familiar with SI units. Depending on the reporting requirements of the publication, authors, editors, or readers may have to convert conventional values to SI units or vice versa.

Table 4 provides reference ranges and SI unit conversion factors for clinical laboratory measurements. Several articles[7,8] and textbooks[9-13] also contain useful information for converting values between conventional units and SI units. Computer programs[14] and online resources[15] for SI unit conversion also are available. Values provided in Table 4 are intended to facilitate conversion from SI units to conventional units and vice versa. Values are derived from several authoritative sources[9-12] and represent accepted normal ranges for adults. However, these values are provided only as a guide, since reference values and ranges may vary substantially among individual laboratories and are highly dependent on the analytic method used. Table 5 includes factors for converting from English to metric measurements.

15.5.2 ***Dual Reporting.***—Some biomedical publications have adopted a system of dual reporting, in which both SI and traditional units are presented. In AMA journals, SI units are the standard method of reporting. However, because of the continued widespread clinical use of conventional units in the United States and to facilitate readers' understanding and encourage education about SI units, some of the more common analytes (including α_1-antitrypsin, ammonia, bilirubin, calcium, cholesterol, creatinine, creatinine clearance, digoxin, estradiol, glucose, iron, iron binding capacity, lead, lipids [total], lipoproteins, magnesium, phosphate, testosterone,

TABLE 4. CONVERSIONS FROM CONVENTIONAL UNITS TO SYSTÈME INTERNATIONAL (SI) UNITS*

Component	System	Reference Range, Conventional Units	Conventional Units	Conversion Factor (Multiply by)	Reference Range, SI Units	SI Units
Acetaminophen (therapeutic)	Serum, plasma	10-30	μg/mL	6.62	70-200	μmol/L
Acetoacetic acid	Serum, plasma	<1	mg/dL	0.098	<0.1	mmol/L
Acetone	Serum, plasma	<2.0	mg/dL	0.172	<0.34	mmol/L
Acetylcholinesterase	Red blood cells	30-40	U/g of hemoglobin	0.0645	2.13-2.63	MU/mol of hemoglobin
Acid phosphatase (prostatic)	Serum	0.0-0.6	U/L	1.0	0.0-0.6	U/L
Activated partial thromboplastin time (APTT)	Whole blood	25-40	s	1.0	25-40	s
Adenosine deaminase	Serum	11.5-25.0	U/L	1.0	11.5-25.0	U/L
Adrenocorticotropic hormone (ACTH) (see Corticotropin)						
Alanine	Plasma	1.87-5.89	mg/dL	112.2	210-661	μmol/L
Alanine aminotransferase (ALT, previously SGPT)	Serum	10-40	U/L	1.0	10-40	U/L
Albumin	Serum	3.5-5.0	g/dL	10	35-50	g/L
Alcohol (see Ethanol, Isopropanol, Methanol)						
Alcohol dehydrogenase	Serum	<2.8	U/L	1.0	<2.8	U/L
Aldolase	Serum	1.0-7.5	U/L	1.0	1.0-7.5	U/L
Aldosterone	Serum, plasma	7-30	ng/dL	0.0277	0.19-0.83	nmol/L
	Urine	3-20	μg/24 h	2.77	8-55	nmol/d
Alkaline phosphatase	Serum	50-120	U/L	1.0	50-120	U/L
Alprazolam (therapeutic)	Serum, plasma	10-50	ng/mL	3.24	32-162	nmol/L
Aluminum	Serum	0-6	ng/mL	0.0371	0.00-0.22	nmol/L
Amikacin (therapeutic) (peak)	Serum, plasma	20-30	μg/mL	1.71	34-52	μmol/L

Aminobutyric acid (α-aminobutyric acid)	Plasma	0.08-0.36	mg/dL	97	8-35	μmol/L
Amiodarone (therapeutic)	Serum, plasma	0.5-2.5	μg/mL	1.55	0.8-3.9	μmol/L
Aminolevulinic acid (δ-aminolevulinic acid)	Urine	1.0-7.0	mg/24 h	7.626	8-53	μmol/d
Amitriptyline (therapeutic)	Serum, plasma	80-250	ng/mL	3.61	289-903	nmol/L
Ammonia (as NH_3)	Plasma	15-45	μg/dL	0.714	11-32	μmol/L
Amobarbital (therapeutic)	Serum	1-5	μg/mL	4.42	4-22	μmol/L
Amoxapine (therapeutic)	Plasma	200-600	ng/mL	1.0	200-600	μg/L
Amylase	Serum	25-85	U/L	1.0	25-85	U/L
Androstenedione						
Adult male	Serum	75-205	ng/dL	0.0349	2.6-7.2	nmol/L
Adult female	Serum	85-275	ng/dL	0.0349	3.0-9.6	nmol/L
Angiotensin I	Plasma	<25	pg/mL	1.0	<25	ng/L
Angiotensin II	Plasma	10-60	pg/mL	1.0	10-60	ng/L
Angiotensin-converting enzyme (ACE)	Serum	8-52	U/L	1.0	8-52	U/L
Anion gap $Na^+ - (Cl^- + HCO_3^-)$	Serum, plasma	8-16	mEq/L	1.0	8-16	mmol/L
Antidiuretic hormone (ADH, vasopressin) (varies with osmolality)						
285-290 mOsm/kg	Plasma	1-5	pg/mL	0.926	0.9-4.6	pmol/L
Antithrombin III	Plasma	21-30	mg/dL	10	210-300	mg/L
α_1-Antitrypsin	Serum	126-226	mg/dL	0.01	1.26-2.26	g/L
Apolipoprotein A						
Male	Serum	80-151	mg/dL	0.01	0.8-1.5	g/L
Female	Serum	80-170	mg/dL	0.01	0.8-1.7	g/L
Apolipoprotein B						
Adult male	Serum, plasma	50-123	mg/dL	0.01	0.5-1.2	g/L
Adult female	Serum, plasma	25-120	mg/dL	0.01	0.25-1.20	g/L
Arginine	Plasma	0.37-2.40	mg/dL	57.4	21-138	μmol/L

TABLE 4. CONVERSIONS FROM CONVENTIONAL UNITS TO SYSTÈME INTERNATIONAL (SI) UNITS* (*cont*)

Component	System	Reference Range, Conventional Units	Conventional Units	Conversion Factor (Multiply by)	Reference Range, SI Units	SI Units
Arsenic (As)	Whole blood	<23	μg/L	0.0133	<0.31	μmol/L
Acute poisoning	Whole blood	600-9300	μg/L	0.0133	7.98-123.7	μmol/L
Ascorbate, ascorbic acid (see Vitamin C)						
Asparagine	Plasma	0.40-0.91	mg/dL	75.7	30-69	μmol/L
Aspartate aminotransferase (AST, previously SGOT)	Serum	20-48	U/L	1.0	20-48	U/L
Aspartic acid	Plasma	<0.3	mg/dL	75.1	<25	μmol/L
Atrial natriuretic hormone	Plasma	20-77	pg/mL	1.0	20-77	ng/L
Bands (see White blood cell count)						
Barbiturates (see Pentobarbital, Phenobarbital, Thiopental)						
Basophils (see White blood cell count)						
Benzodiazepines (see Alprazolam, Chlordiazepoxide, Diazepam, Lorazepam)						
Bicarbonate	Plasma	21-28	mEq/L	1.0	21-28	mmol/L
Bile acids (total)	Serum	0.3-2.3	μg/mL	2.448	0.73-5.63	μmol/L
Bilirubin						
Total	Serum	0.3-1.2	mg/dL	17.1	5-21	μmol/L
Direct (conjugated)	Serum	<0.2	mg/dL	17.1	<3.4	μmol/L
Biotin	Whole blood, serum	200-500	pg/mL	0.0041	0.82-2.05	nmol/L
Bismuth	Whole blood	1-12	μg/L	4.785	4.8-57.4	nmol/L
Blood gases						
P_{CO_2}	Arterial blood	35-45	mm Hg	1.0	35-45	mm Hg
pH	Arterial blood	7.35-7.45	. . .	1.0	7.35-7.45	. . .
P_{O_2}	Arterial blood	80-100	mm Hg	1.0	80-100	mm Hg

Bromide	Serum	<5	mg/dL	0.125	<0.63	mmol/L
C1 esterase inhibitor	Serum	12-30	mg/dL	0.01	0.12-0.30	g/L
C3 complement	Serum	1200-1500	μg/mL	0.001	1.2-1.5	g/L
C4 complement	Serum	350-600	μg/mL	0.001	0.35-0.60	g/L
Cadmium (nonsmoker)	Whole blood	0.3-1.2	μg/L	8.897	2.7-10.7	nmol/L
Calcitonin	Serum, plasma	<19	pg/mL	1.0	<19	ng/L
Calcium						
Ionized	Serum	4.60-5.08	mg/dL	0.25	1.15-1.27	mmol/L
	Serum	2.30-2.54	mEq/L	0.50	1.15-1.27	mmol/L
Total	Serum	8.2-10.2	mg/dL	0.25	2.05-2.55	mmol/L
Normal diet	Urine	<250	mg/24 h	0.025	<6.2	mmol/d
Carbamazepine (therapeutic)	Serum, plasma	8-12	μg/mL	4.23	34-51	μmol/L
Carbon dioxide	Serum, plasma, venous blood	22-28	mEq/L	1.0	22-28	mmol/L
Carboxyhemoglobin (carbon monoxide) (as proportion of hemoglobin saturation)						
Nonsmoker	Whole blood	<2.0	%	0.01	<0.02	Proportion of 1.0
Toxic	Whole blood	>20	%	0.01	>0.2	Proportion of 1.0
Carcinoembryonic antigen (CEA)	Serum	<3.0	ng/mL	1.0	<3.0	μg/L
β-Carotene	Serum	10-85	μg/dL	0.0186	0.2-1.6	μmol/L
Ceruloplasmin	Serum	20-40	mg/dL	10	200-400	mg/L
Chloramphenicol (therapeutic)	Serum	10-25	μg/mL	3.1	31-77	μmol/L
Chlordiazepoxide (therapeutic)	Serum, plasma	0.7-1.0	μg/mL	3.34	2.3-3.3	μmol/L
Chloride	Serum, plasma	96-106	mEq/L	1.0	96-106	mmol/L
	CSF	118-132	mEq/L	1.0	118-132	mmol/L
Chlorpromazine (therapeutic)	Plasma	50-300	ng/mL	3.14	157-942	nmol/L
Chlorpropamide (therapeutic)	Plasma	75-250	mg/L	3.61	270-900	μmol/L
Cholecalciferol (see Vitamin D)						

TABLE 4. CONVERSIONS FROM CONVENTIONAL UNITS TO SYSTÈME INTERNATIONAL (SI) UNITS* (*cont*)

Component	System	Reference Range, Conventional Units	Conventional Units	Conversion Factor (Multiply by)	Reference Range, SI Units	SI Units
Cholesterol (total)						
Desirable	Serum	<200	mg/dL	0.02586	<5.17	mmol/L
Borderline high	Serum	200-239	mg/dL	0.02586	5.17-6.18	mmol/L
High	Serum	≥240	mg/dL	0.02586	≥6.21	mmol/L
Cholesterol, high-density lipoproteins (HDL) (see High-density lipoprotein cholesterol)						
Cholesterol, low-density lipoproteins (LDL) (see Low-density lipoprotein cholesterol)						
Cholesterol esters (as plasma fraction of total cholesterol)	Plasma	60-75	%	0.01	0.60-0.75	Proportion of 1.0
Chromium	Whole blood	0.7-28.0	μg/L	19.2	13.4-538.6	nmol/L
Citrate	Serum	1.2-3.0	mg/dL	52.05	60-160	μmol/L
Citrulline	Plasma	0.2-1.0	mg/dL	57.1	12-55	μmol/L
Clonazepam (therapeutic)	Serum	10-50	ng/mL	3.17	32-158	nmol/L
Coagulation factor I	Plasma	0.15-0.35	g/dL	29.41	4.4-10.3	μmol/L
(fibrinogen)	Plasma	150-350	mg/dL	0.01	1.5-3.5	g/L
Coagulation factor II (prothrombin)	Plasma	70-130	%	0.01	0.70-1.30	Proportion of 1.0
Coagulation factor V	Plasma	70-130	%	0.01	0.70-1.30	Proportion of 1.0
Coagulation factor VII	Plasma	60-140	%	0.01	0.60-1.40	Proportion of 1.0
Coagulation factor VIII	Plasma	50-200	%	0.01	0.50-2.00	Proportion of 1.0
Coagulation factor IX	Plasma	70-130	%	0.01	0.70-1.30	Proportion of 1.0
Coagulation factor X	Plasma	70-130	%	0.01	0.70-1.30	Proportion of 1.0

Coagulation factor XI	Plasma	70-130	%	0.01	0.70-1.30	Proportion of 1.0
Coagulation factor XII	Plasma	70-130	%	0.01	0.70-1.30	Proportion of 1.0
Cobalt	Serum	4.0-10.0	μg/L	16.97	67.9-169.7	nmol/L
Cocaine (toxic)	Serum	>1000	ng/mL	3.3	>3300	nmol/L
Codeine (therapeutic)	Serum	10-100	ng/mL	3.34	33-334	nmol/L
Copper	Serum	70-140	μg/dL	0.1574	11.0-22.0	μmol/L
Coproporphyrin	Urine	<200	μg/24 h	1.527	<300	nmol/d
Corticotropin	Plasma	<120	pg/mL	0.22	<26	pmol/L
Cortisol	Plasma	5-25	μg/dL	27.59	140-690	nmol/L
	Urine	30-100	μg/24 h	2.759	80-280	nmol/d
Cotinine (smoker)	Plasma	16-145	ng/mL	5.68	91-823	nmol/L
C peptide	Serum	0.5-2.5	ng/mL	0.333	0.17-0.83	nmol/L
Creatine	Serum	0.1-0.4	mg/dL	76.25	8-31	μmol/L
Creatine kinase (CK)	Serum	50-200	U/L	1.0	50-200	U/L
Creatine kinase-MB fraction (isoenzymes; proportion of total CK)	Serum	<6	%	0.01	<0.06	Proportion of 1.0
	Serum	<10	U/L	1.0	<10	U/L
Creatinine	Serum, plasma	0.6-1.2	mg/dL	88.4	53-106	μmol/L
	Urine	1-2	g/24 h	8.8	8.8-17.7	mmol/d
Creatinine clearance	Serum, urine	75-125	mL/min	0.01667	1.24-2.08	mL/s
Cyanide (toxic)	Whole blood	>1.0	μg/mL	38.4	>38.4	μmol/L
Cyanocobalamin (see Vitamin B_{12})						
Cyclic adenosine monophosphate (cAMP)	Plasma	4.6-8.6	ng/mL	3.04	14-26	nmol/L
Cystine	Plasma	0.40-1.40	mg/dL	83.3	33-117	μmol/L
Dehydroepiandrosterone (DHEA) (unconjugated, adult male)	Plasma, serum	180-1250	ng/dL	3.47	6.2-43.3	nmol/L
Dehydroepiandrosterone sulfate (DHEA-S) (adult male)	Plasma, serum	50-450	μg/dL	0.027	1.6-12.2	μmol/L
Desipramine (therapeutic)	Plasma, serum	50-200	ng/mL	3.75	170-700	nmol/L

TABLE 4. CONVERSIONS FROM CONVENTIONAL UNITS TO SYSTÈME INTERNATIONAL (SI) UNITS* (*cont*)

Component	System	Reference Range, Conventional Units	Conventional Units	Conversion Factor (Multiply by)	Reference Range, SI Units	SI Units
Diazepam (therapeutic)	Plasma, serum	100-1000	ng/mL	0.00351	0.35-3.51	μmol/L
Digoxin (therapeutic)	Plasma	0.5-2.0	ng/mL	1.281	0.6-2.6	nmol/L
Disopyramide (therapeutic)	Plasma, serum	2.8-7.0	mg/L	2.95	8-21	μmol/L
Doxepin (therapeutic)	Plasma, serum	150-250	ng/mL	3.58	540-890	nmol/L
Electrophoresis (protein)						
Proportion of total protein						
Albumin	Serum	52-65	%	0.01	0.52-0.65	Proportion of 1.0
α_1-Globulin	Serum	2.5-5.0	%	0.01	0.025-0.05	Proportion of 1.0
α_2-Globulin	Serum	7.0-13.0	%	0.01	0.07-0.13	Proportion of 1.0
β-Globulin	Serum	8.0-14.0	%	0.01	0.08-0.14	Porportion of 1.0
γ-Globulin	Serum	12.0-22.0	%	0.01	0.12-0.22	Proportion of 1.0
Concentration						
Albumin	Serum	3.2-5.6	g/dL	10.0	32-56	g/L
α_1-Globulin	Serum	0.1-0.4	g/dL	10.0	1-10	g/L
α_2-Globulin	Serum	0.4-1.2	g/dL	10.0	4-12	g/L
β-Globulin	Serum	0.5-1.1	g/dL	10.0	5-11	g/L
γ-Globulin	Serum	0.5-1.6	g/dL	10.0	5-16	g/L
Eosinophils (see White blood cell count)						
Epinephrine	Plasma	<60	pg/mL	5.46	<330	pmol/L
	Urine	<20	μg/24 h	5.46	<109	nmol/d
Erythrocyte count (see Red blood cell count)						
Erythrocyte sedimentation rate	Whole blood	0-20	mm/h	1.0	0-20	mm/h
Erythropoietin	Serum	5-36	mU/mL	1.0	5-36	IU/L
Estradiol (E_2, unconjugated) (varies with age and menstrual cycle)	Serum	30-400	pg/mL	3.67	110-1470	pmol/L

Estriol (E_3, unconjugated) (varies with length of gestation)	Serum	5-40	ng/mL	3.47	17.4-138.8	nmol/L
Estrogens (total)	Serum	60-400	pg/mL	1.0	60-400	ng/L
Estrone (E_1) (varies with day of menstrual cycle)	Plasma, serum	1.5-25.0	ng/dL	37	55-925	pmol/L
Ethanol (ethyl alcohol)	Serum, whole blood	<100	mg/dL	0.2171	<21.7	mmol/L
Ethchlorvynol (toxic)	Plasma, serum	>20	μg/mL	6.92	>138	μmol/L
Ethylene glycol (toxic)	Plasma, serum	>30	mg/dL	0.1611	>5	mmol/L
Fatty acids (nonesterified)	Plasma	300-480	μEq/L	1.00	300-480	μmol/L
Fecal fat (as stearic acid)	Stool	2.0-6.0	g/d	1.0	2-6	g/d
Ferritin	Plasma	15-200	ng/mL	1.0	15-200	μg/L
α_1-Fetoprotein	Serum	<10	ng/mL	1.0	<10	μg/L
Fibrinogen (see Coagulation factor I)	Plasma	0.15-0.35	g/dL	29.41	4.4-10.3	μmol/L
Fibrin breakdown products (fibrin split products)	Serum	<10	μg/mL	1.0	<10	mg/L
Fluoride	Whole blood	<0.05	mg/dL	0.5263	<0.027	mmol/L
Folate (folic acid)	Red blood cells	166-640	ng/mL	2.266	376-1450	nmol/L
	Serum	5-25	ng/mL	2.266	11-57	nmol/L
Follicle-stimulating hormone (FSH)	Serum	1-100	mIU/mL	1.0	1-100	IU/L
(follitropin)	Urine	5-30	IU/24 h	1.0	5-30	IU/d
Fructosamine	Serum	1.5-2.7	mmol/L	1.0	1.5-2.7	mmol/L
Fructose	Serum	1-6	mg/dL	55.5	55.5-333	μmol/L
Galactose	Plasma, serum	<20	mg/dL	0.0555	<1.10	mmol/L
Gastrin (fasting)	Serum	<100	pg/mL	0.477	47.7	pmol/L
Gentamicin (therapeutic)	Serum	6-10	μg/mL	2.1	12-21	μmol/L
Glucagon	Plasma	20-100	pg/mL	1.0	20-100	ng/L
Glucose	Serum, plasma	70-110	mg/dL	0.05551	3.9-6.1	mmol/L
	CSF	50-80	mg/dL	0.05551	2.8-4.4	mmol/L

Table 4. Conversions From Conventional Units to Système International (SI) Units* (*cont*)

Component	System	Reference Range, Conventional Units	Conventional Units	Conversion Factor (Multiply by)	Reference Range, SI Units	SI Units
Glucose-6-phosphate dehydrogenase	Red blood cells	10-14	U/g of hemoglobin	0.0645	0.65-0.90	MU/mol of hemoglobin
Glutamic acid	Plasma	0.2-2.8	mg/dL	67.97	15-190	μmol/L
Glutamine	Plasma	6.1-10.2	mg/dL	68.42	420-700	μmol/L
γ-Glutamyltransferase (GGT; γ-glutamyl transpeptidase)	Serum	0-30	U/L	1.0	0-30	U/L
Glutethimide (therapeutic)	Plasma, serum	<6	μg/mL	4.60	<28	μmol/L
Glycerol (free)	Serum	<1.5	mg/dL	0.1086	<0.16	mmol/L
Glycine	Plasma	0.9-4.2	mg/dL	133.3	120-560	μmol/L
Glycosylated hemoglobin (glycated hemoglobin; hemoglobin A_1, A_{1c})	Whole blood	4-7	% of total hemoglobin	0.01	0.04-0.07	Proportion of total hemoglobin
Gold (therapeutic)	Serum	100-200	μg/dL	0.050 77	5.1-10.2	μmol/L
Growth hormone (GH, somatotropin)	Plasma, serum	<20	ng/mL	44	<880	pmol/L
Haloperidol (therapeutic)	Serum, plasma	5-20	ng/mL	2.6	13-52	nmol/L
Haptoglobin	Serum	40-180	mg/dL	0.01	0.4-1.8	g/L
Hematocrit						
Adult male	Whole blood	41-50	%	0.01	0.41-0.50	Proportion of 1.0
Adult female	Whole blood	35-45	%	0.01	0.35-0.45	Proportion of 1.0
Hemoglobin						
Mass concentration						
Adult male	Whole blood	14.0-17.5	g/dL	10.0	140-175	g/L
Adult female	Whole blood	12.0-15.0	g/dL	10.0	120-150	g/L
Substance concentration (Hb (Fe])						
Adult male	Whole blood	13.6-17.2	g/dL	0.6206	8.44-10.65	mmol/L
Adult female	Whole blood	12.0-15.0	g/dL	0.6206	7.45-9.30	mmol/L
Mean corpuscular hemoglobin (MCH)						
Mass concentration	Red blood cells	27-33	pg	1.0	27-33	pg
Substance concentration (Hb (Fe])	Red blood cells	27-33	pg	0.062 06	1.70-2.05	fmol

Mean corpuscular hemoglobin concentration (MCHC)						
Mass concentration	Red blood cells	33-37	g/dL	10	330-370	g/L
Substance concentration (Hb [Fe])	Red blood cells	33-37	g/dL	0.6206	20-23	mmol/L
Hemoglobin A_{1c} (see Glycosylated hemoglobin)						
Hemoglobin A_2	Whole blood	2.0-3.0	%	0.01	0.02-0.03	Proportion of 1.0
High-density lipoprotein cholesterol (HDL-C)						
Male	Plasma	35-65	mg/dL	0.02586	0.91-1.68	mmol/L
Female	Plasma	35-80	mg/dL	0.02586	0.91-2.07	mmol/L
Histidine	Plasma	0.5-1.7	mg/dL	64.5	32-110	μmol/L
Homocysteine (total)	Plasma, serum	0.68-2.02	mg/L	7.397	5.0-15	μmol/L
Homovanillic acid	Urine	<8	mg/24 h	5.489	<45	μmol/d
Human chorionic gonadotropin (HCG) (adult female, not pregnant)	Serum	<3	mIU/mL	1.0	<3	IU/L
Hydroxybutyric acid (as β-hydroxybutyric acid)	Serum	0.21-2.81	mg/dL	96.05	20-270	μmol/L
5-Hydroxyindoleacetic acid (5-HIAA)	Urine	<25	mg/24 h	5.23	<131	μmol/d
17α-Hydroxyprogesterone (adult female)	Serum	20-300	ng/dL	0.03	0.6-9.0	nmol/L
Hydroxyproline	Plasma	<0.55	mg/dL	76.3	<42	μmol/L
Imipramine (therapeutic)	Plasma	150-250	ng/mL	3.57	536-893	nmol/L
Immunoglobulin A (IgA)	Serum	113-563	mg/dL	0.01	1.1-5.6	g/L
Immunoglobulin D (IgD)	Serum	0.5-3.0	mg/dL	10	5-30	mg/L
Immunoglobulin E (IgE)	Serum	0.01-0.04	mg/dL	10	0.1-0.4	mg/L
Immunoglobulin G (IgG)	Serum	800-1800	mg/dL	0.01	8.0-18.0	g/L
Immunoglobulin M (IgM)	Serum	54-222	mg/dL	0.01	0.5-2.2	g/L
Insulin	Plasma	11-240	μU/mL	7.175	79-1722	pmol/L
Insulin C peptide (see C peptide)						
Insulinlike growth factor	Plasma	130-450	ng/mL	1.0	130-450	ng/mL

TABLE 4. CONVERSIONS FROM CONVENTIONAL UNITS TO SYSTÈME INTERNATIONAL (SI) UNITS* (*cont*)

Component	System	Reference Range, Conventional Units	Conventional Units	Conversion Factor (Multiply by)	Reference Range, SI Units	SI Units
Ionized calcium (see Calcium)						
Iron (total)	Serum	60-150	μg/dL	0.179	10.7-26.9	μmol/L
Iron binding capacity	Serum	250-400	μg/dL	0.179	44.8-71.6	μmol/L
Isoleucine	Plasma	0.5-1.3	mg/dL	76.24	40-100	μmol/L
Isoniazid (therapeutic)	Plasma	1-7	μg/mL	7.29	7-51	μmol/L
Isopropanol (toxic)	Plasma, serum	>400	mg/L	0.0166	>6.64	mmol/L
Lactate (lactic acid)	Arterial blood	3-7	mg/dL	0.1110	0.3-0.8	mmol/L
	Venous blood	4.5-19.8	mg/dL	0.1110	0.5-2.2	mmol/L
Lactate dehydrogenase (LDH)	Serum	50-200	U/L	1.0	50-200	U/L
Lactate dehydrogenase isoenzymes						
LD_1	Serum	17-27	%	0.01	0.17-0.27	Proportion of 1.0
LD_2	Serum	27-37	%	0.01	0.27-0.37	Proportion of 1.0
LD_3	Serum	18-25	%	0.01	0.18-0.25	Proportion of 1.0
LD_4	Serum	3-8	%	0.01	0.03-0.08	Proportion of 1.0
LD_5	Serum	0-5	%	0.01	0.00-0.05	Proportion of 1.0
Lead	Whole blood	<25	μg/dL	0.0483	<1.21	μmol/L
Leucine	Plasma	1.0-2.3	mg/dL	76.3	75-175	μmol/L
Leukocyte count (see White blood cell count)						
Lidocaine (therapeutic)	Serum, plasma	1.5-6.0	μg/mL	4.27	6.4-25.6	μmol/L
Lipase	Serum	14-280	mIU/mL	1.0	14-280	U/L
Lipoprotein(a) [Lp(a)]	Serum, plasma	10-30	mg/dL	0.01	0.1-0.3	g/L
Lithium (therapeutic)	Serum	0.6-1.2	mEq/L	1.0	0.6-1.2	mmol/L
Lorazepam (therapeutic)	Serum, plasma	50-240	ng/mL	3.11	156-746	nmol/L
Low-density lipoprotein cholesterol (LDL-C)	Plasma	60-130	mg/dL	0.025 86	1.55-3.37	mmol/L

Luteinizing hormone (LH)	Serum	6-30	mIU/mL	1.0	6-30	IU/L
Lymphocytes (see White blood cell count)						
Lysine	Plasma	1.2-3.5	mg/dL	68.5	80-240	μmol/L
Lysozyme (muramidase)	Serum	4-13	mg/L	1.0	4-13	mg/L
Magnesium	Serum	1.5-2.3	mg/dL	0.4114	0.60-0.95	mmol/L
	Serum	1.3-2.1	mEq/L	0.50	0.65-1.05	mmol/L
Manganese	Whole blood	10-12	μg/L	18.2	182-218	nmol/L
Maprotiline (therapeutic)	Plasma	200-600	ng/mL	1.0	200-600	μg/L
Mean corpuscular hemoglobin (see Hemoglobin)						
Mean corpuscular hemoglobin concentration (see Hemoglobin)						
Meperidine (therapeutic)	Serum, plasma	0.4-0.7	μg/mL	4.04	1.6-2.8	μmol/L
Meprobamate (therapeutic)	Serum	6-12	μg/mL	4.58	28-55	μmol/L
Mercury	Whole blood	0.6-59.0	μg/L	4.99	3.0-294.4	nmol/L
Metanephrines (total)	Urine	<1.0	mg/24 h	5.07	<5	μmol/d
Methadone (therapeutic)	Serum, plasma	100-400	ng/mL	0.003 23	0.32-1.29	μmol/L
Methanol	Whole blood, serum	<1.5	mg/L	0.0312	<0.05	mmol/L
Methaqualone (therapeutic)	Serum, plasma	2-3	μg/mL	4.00	8-12	μmol/L
Methemoglobin	Whole blood	<0.24	g/dL	155	<37.2	μmol/L
	Whole blood	<1.0	% of total hemoglobin	0.01	<0.01	Proportion of total hemoglobin
Methionine	Plasma	0.1-0.6	mg/dL	67.1	6-40	μmol/L
Methsuximide (therapeutic)	Serum	10-40	μg/mL	5.29	53-212	μmol/L
Methyldopa (therapeutic)	Serum, plasma	1-5	μg/mL	4.73	5-24	μmol/L
Metoprolol (therapeutic)	Serum, plasma	75-200	ng/mL	3.74	281-748	nmol/L
β_2-Microglobulin	Serum	<2	μg/mL	85	<170	nmol/L
Morphine (therapeutic)	Serum, plasma	10-80	ng/mL	3.50	35-280	nmol/L
Muramidase (see Lysozyme)						

TABLE 4. CONVERSIONS FROM CONVENTIONAL UNITS TO SYSTÈME INTERNATIONAL (SI) UNITS* (*cont*)

Component	System	Reference Range, Conventional Units	Conventional Units	Conversion Factor (Multiply by)	Reference Range, SI Units	SI Units
Myoglobin	Serum	5-70	μg/L	1.0	5-70	μg/L
Niacin (nicotinic acid)	Urine	2.4-6.4	mg/24 h	7.30	17.5-46.7	μmol/d
Nickel	Whole blood	1.0-28.0	μg/L	17	17-476	nmol/L
Nicotine (smoker)	Plasma	0.01-0.05	mg/L	6.16	0.062-0.308	μmol/L
Nitrogen (nonprotein)	Serum	20-35	mg/dL	0.714	14.3-25.0	mmol/L
Norepinephrine	Plasma	110-410	pg/mL	5.91	650-2423	nmol/L
	Urine	15-80	μg/24 h	5.91	89-473	nmol/d
Nortriptyline (therapeutic)	Serum, plasma	50-150	ng/mL	3.80	190-570	nmol/L
Ornithine	Plasma	0.4-1.4	mg/dL	75.8	30-106	μmol/L
Osmolality	Serum	275-295	mOsm/kg H_2O	1.0	275-295	mmol/kg H_2O
	Urine	250-900	mOsm/kg H_2O	1.0	250-900	mmol/kg H_2O
Osteocalcin	Serum	3.0-13.0	ng/mL	1.0	3.0-13.0	μg/L
Oxalate	Serum	1.0-2.4	mg/L	11.4	11-27	μmol/L
Oxazepam (therapeutic)	Serum, plasma	0.2-1.4	μg/mL	3.49	0.7-4.9	μmol/L
Oxygen, partial pressure (Po_2)	Arterial blood	80-100	mm Hg	1.0	80-100	mm Hg
Pantothenic acid (see Vitamin B_3)						
Parathyroid hormone						
Intact	Serum	10-50	pg/mL	0.1053	1.1-5.3	pmol/L
N-terminal specific	Serum	8-24	pg/mL	0.1053	0.8-2.5	pmol/L
C-terminal (mid-molecule)	Serum	0-340	pg/mL	0.1053	0-35.8	pmol/L
Pentobarbital (therapeutic)	Serum, plasma	1-5	μg/mL	4.42	4.0-22	μmol/L
Pepsinogen I	Serum	28-100	ng/mL	1.0	28-100	μg/L
pH (see Blood gases)						
Phenobarbital (therapeutic)	Serum, plasma	15-40	μg/mL	4.31	65-172	μmol/L
Phenylalanine	Plasma	0.6-1.5	mg/dL	60.5	35-90	μmol/L

Phenytoin (therapeutic)	Serum, plasma	10-20	μg/mL	3.96	40-79	μmol/L
Phosphorus (inorganic)	Serum	2.3-4.7	mg/dL	0.3229	0.74-1.52	mmol/L
	Urine	0.9-1.3	g/24 h	32.29	29-42	mmol/d
Phospholipid phosphorus (total)	Serum	8.0-11.0	mg/dL	0.3229	2.58-3.55	mmol/L
Placental lactogen (5- to 38-wk gestation)	Serum	0.5-11	μg/mL	46.30	23-509	nmol/L
Plasminogen	Plasma	20	mg/dL	10	200	mg/L
	Plasma	80-120	%	0.01	0.80-1.20	Proportion of 1.0
Plasminogen activator inhibitor	Plasma	<15	IU/mL	1.0	15	IU/L
Platelet count (thrombocytes)	Whole blood	150-450	$\times 10^3/\mu L$	1.0	150-450	$\times 10^9/L$
Porphobilinogen deaminase	Red blood cells	>7.0	nmol/s/L	1.0	>7.0	$nmol \cdot s^{-1} \cdot L^{-1}$
Porphyrins (total)	Urine	<320	nmol/L	1.0	<320	nmol/L
Potassium	Plasma	3.5-5.0	mEq/L	1.0	3.5-5.0	mmol/L
Pregnanediol	Urine	<2.6	mg/24 h	3.12	<8	μmol/d
Pregnanetriol	Urine	<2.5	mg/24 h	2.97	<7.5	μmol/d
Primidone (therapeutic)	Plasma	5-12	μg/mL	4.58	23-55	μmol/L
Procainamide (therapeutic)	Serum, plasma	4-10	μg/mL	4.23	17-42	μmol/L
Progesterone (first trimester)	Serum	>1000	ng/dL	0.0318	>32	nmol/L
Prolactin (nonlactating subject)	Serum	1-25	ng/mL	1.0	1-25	μg/L
Proline	Plasma	1.2-3.9	mg/dL	86.9	104-340	μmol/L
Propoxyphene (therapeutic)	Serum	0.1-0.4	μg/mL	2.946	0.3-1.2	μmol/L
Propranolol (therapeutic)	Serum	50-100	ng/mL	3.86	190-390	nmol/L
Prostate-specific antigen	Serum	<4.0	ng/mL	1.0	<4.0	ng/mL
Prostatic acid phosphatase (see Acid phosphatase)						
Protein (total)	Serum	6.0-8.0	g/dL	10.0	60-80	g/L
Prothrombin time (PT)	Plasma	10-13	s	1.0	10-13	s
Protoporphyrin	Red blood cells	15-50	mg/dL	0.0177	0.27-0.89	μmol/L
Pyridoxine (see Vitamin B_6)						
Pyruvate (as pyruvic acid)	Whole blood	0.3-0.9	mg/dL	113.6	34-102	μmol/L

TABLE 4. CONVERSIONS FROM CONVENTIONAL UNITS TO SYSTÈME INTERNATIONAL (SI) UNITS* (*cont*)

Component	System	Reference Range, Conventional Units	Conventional Units	Conversion Factor (Multiply by)	Reference Range, SI Units	SI Units
Quinidine (therapeutic)	Serum	2.0-5.0	μg/mL	3.08	6.2-15.4	μmol/L
Red blood cell count						
Female	Whole blood	3.9-5.5	$\times 10^6/\mu L$	1.0	3.9-5.5	$\times 10^{12}/L$
Male	Whole blood	4.6-6.0	$\times 10^6/\mu L$	1.0	4.6-6.0	$\times 10^{12}/L$
Red cell folate (see Folate)						
Renin	Plasma	1.0-6.0	ng/mL/h	0.77	0.77-4.6	$nmol \cdot L^{-1} \cdot h^{-1}$
Reticulocyte count	Whole blood	25-75	$\times 10^3/\mu L$	1.0	25-75	$\times 10^9/L$
	Whole blood	0.5-1.5	% of red blood cells	0.01	0.005-0.015	Proportion of red blood cells
Retinol (see Vitamin A)						
Riboflavin (see Vitamin B_2)						
Salicylates (therapeutic)	Serum, plasma	15-30	mg/dL	0.07240	1.08-2.17	mmol/L
Sedimentation rate (see Erythrocyte sedimentation rate)						
Selenium	Whole blood	58-234	μg/L	0.0127	0.74-2.97	μmol/L
Serine	Plasma	0.7-2.0	mg/dL	95.2	65-193	μmol/L
Serotonin (5-hydroxytryptamine)	Whole blood	50-200	ng/mL	0.00568	0.28-1.14	μmol/L
Sex hormone binding globulin	Serum	0.5-1.5	μg/dL	34.7	17.4-52.1	nmol/L
Sodium	Plasma	136-142	mEq/L	1.0	136-142	mmol/L
Somatostatin	Plasma	<25	pg/mL	1.0	<25	ng/L
Somatomedin C (see Insulinlike growth factor)						
Strychnine (toxic)	Whole blood	>0.5	mg/L	2.99	>1.5	μmol/L
Substance P	Plasma	<240	pg/mL	1.0	<240	ng/L
Sulfmethemoglobin	Whole blood	<1.0	% of total hemoglobin	0.01	<0.010	Proportion of total hemoglobin

Taurine	Plasma	0.3-2.1	mg/dL	80	24-168	μmol/L
Testosterone	Plasma, serum	300-1200	ng/dL	0.0347	10.4-41.6	nmol/L
Theophylline (therapeutic)	Plasma, serum	10-20	μg/mL	5.55	56-111	μmol/L
Thiamin(e) (see Vitamin B_1)						
Thiocyanate (nonsmoker)	Plasma, serum	1-4	mg/L	17.2	17-69	μmol/L
Thiopental (therapeutic)	Plasma, serum	1-5	μg/mL	4.13	4-21	μmol/L
Thioridazine (therapeutic)	Plasma, serum	1.0-1.5	μg/mL	2.70	2.7-4.1	μmol/L
Threonine	Plasma	0.9-2.5	mg/dL	84	75-210	μmol/L
Thrombocytes (see Platelet count)						
Thyroglobulin	Serum	3-42	ng/mL	1.0	3-42	μg/L
Thyrotropin (thyroid-stimulating hormone, TSH)	Serum	0.5-5.0	μIU/mL	1.0	0.5-5.0	μIU/L
Thyroxine						
Free (FT_4)	Serum	0.9-2.3	ng/dL	12.87	12-30	pmol/L
Total (T_4)	Serum	5.5-12.5	μg/dL	12.87	71-160	nmol/L
Thyroxine-binding globulin (TBG)	Serum	10-26	μg/dL	10	100-260	μg/L
Tissue plasminogen activator	Plasma	<0.04	IU/mL	1000	<40	IU/L
Tobramycin (therapeutic)	Plasma, serum	5-10	μg/mL	2.14	10-21	μmol/L
Tocainide (therapeutic)	Plasma, serum	4-10	μg/mL	5.20	21-52	μmol/L
α-Tocopherol (see Vitamin E)						
Tolbutamide (therapeutic)	Plasma	80-240	μg/mL	3.70	296-888	μmol/L
Transferrin (siderophilin)	Serum	200-380	mg/dL	0.01	2.0-3.8	g/L
Triglycerides (as triolein)	Plasma, serum	10-190	mg/dL	0.01129	0.11-2.15	mmol/L
Triiodothyronine						
Free (FT_3)	Serum	260-480	pg/dL	0.0154	4.0-7.4	pmol/L
Resin uptake	Serum	25-35	%	0.01	0.25-0.35	Proportion of 1.0
Total (T_3)	Serum	70-200	ng/dL	0.0154	1.08-3.14	nmol/L
Troponin I (cardiac)	Serum	<0.6	mg/mL	1.0	<0.6	μg/L
Troponin T (cardiac)	Serum	<0.2	μg/L	1.0	<0.2	μg/L
Tryptophan	Plasma	0.5-1.5	mg/dL	48.97	25-73	μmol/L

TABLE 4. CONVERSIONS FROM CONVENTIONAL UNITS TO SYSTÈME INTERNATIONAL (SI) UNITS* (*cont*)

Component	System	Reference Range, Conventional Units	Conventional Units	Conversion Factor (Multiply by)	Reference Range, SI Units	SI Units
Tyrosine	Plasma	0.4-1.6	mg/dL	55.19	20-90	μmol/L
Urea nitrogen	Serum	8-23	mg/dL	0.357	2.9-8.2	mmol/L
Uric acid	Serum	4.0-8.5	mg/dL	0.0595	0.24-0.51	mmol/L
Urobilinogen	Urine	0.05-2.5	mg/24 h	1.693	0.1-4.2	μmol/d
Valine	Plasma	1.7-3.7	mg/dL	85.5	145-315	μmol/L
Valproic acid (therapeutic)	Plasma, serum	50-100	μg/mL	6.93	346-693	μmol/L
Vancomycin (therapeutic)	Plasma, serum	20-40	μg/mL	0.690	14-28	μmol/L
Vanillylmandelic acid (VMA)	Urine	2.1-7.6	mg/24 h	5.046	11-38	μmol/d
Vasoactive intestinal polypeptide	Plasma	<50	pg/mL	1.0	<50	ng/L
Verapamil (therapeutic)	Plasma, serum	100-500	ng/mL	2.2	220-1100	nmol/L
Vitamin A	Serum	30-80	μg/dL	0.0349	1.05-2.80	μmol/L
Vitamin B_1	Whole blood	2.5-7.5	μg/dL	29.6	74-222	nmol/L
Vitamin B_2	Plasma, serum	4-24	μg/dL	26.6	106-638	nmol/L
Vitamin B_3	Whole blood	0.2-1.8	μg/mL	4.56	0.9-8.2	μmol/L
Vitamin B_6	Plasma	5-30	ng/mL	4.046	20-121	nmol/L
Vitamin B_{12}	Serum	160-950	pg/mL	0.7378	118-701	pmol/L
Vitamin C	Plasma, serum	0.4-1.5	mg/dL	56.78	23-85	μmol/L
Vitamin D						
1,25-Dihydroxyvitamin D	Plasma, serum	16-65	pg/mL	2.6	42-169	pmol/L
25-Hydroxyvitamin D	Plasma, serum	14-60	ng/mL	2.496	35-150	nmol/L
Vitamin E	Plasma, serum	0.5-1.8	mg/dL	23.22	12-42	μmol/L
Vitamin K	Plasma, serum	0.13-1.19	ng/mL	2.22	0.29-2.64	nmol/L

Warfarin (therapeutic)	Plasma, serum	1.0-10	μg/mL	3.24	3.2-32.4	μmol/L
White blood cell count	Whole blood	4500-11 000	10^3/μL	0.001	4.5-11.0	×10^9/L
Differential count						
Neutrophils	Whole blood	1800-7800	/μL	0.001	1.8-7.8	×10^9/L
Bands	Whole blood	0-700	/μL	0.001	0.00-0.70	×10^9/L
Lymphocytes	Whole blood	1000-4800	/μL	0.001	1.0-4.8	×10^9/L
Monocytes	Whole blood	0-800	/μL	0.001	0.00-0.80	×10^9/L
Eosinophils	Whole blood	0-450	/μL	0.001	0.00-0.45	×10^9/L
Basophils	Whole blood	0-200	/μL	0.001	0.00-0.20	×10^9/L
Differential count (number fraction)						
Neutrophils	Whole blood	56	%	0.01	0.56	Proportion of 1.00
Bands	Whole blood	3	%	0.01	0.03	Proportion of 1.00
Lymphocytes	Whole blood	34	%	0.01	0.34	Proportion of 1.00
Monocytes	Whole blood	4	%	0.01	0.04	Proportion of 1.00
Eosinophils	Whole blood	2.7	%	0.01	0.027	Proportion of 1.000
Basophils	Whole blood	0.3	%	0.01	0.003	Proportion of 1.000
Xylose absorption test (25-g dose)	Whole blood	25-40	mg/dL	0.066 61	1.67-2.66	mmol/L
Zidovudine (therapeutic)	Plasma, serum	0.15-0.27	μg/mL	3.7	0.56-1.01	μmol/L
Zinc	Serum	50-150	μg/dL	0.153	7.7-23.0	μmol/L

* *The information in this table is from the following sources: (1) Tietz NW, ed.* Clinical Guide to Laboratory Tests. *3rd ed. Philadelphia, Pa: WB Saunders Co; 1995; (2) Jacobs DS, Demott WR, Grady HJ, Horvat RT, Huestis DW, Kasten BL, eds.* Laboratory Test Handbook. *4th ed. Hudson, Ohio: Lexi-Comp Inc; 1996; (3) Henry JB, ed.* Clinical Diagnosis and Management by Laboratory Methods. *19th ed. Philadelphia, Pa: WB Saunders Co; 1996; (4) Laposata M.* SI Unit Conversion Guide. *Boston, Mass: NEJM Books; 1992. The reference values are provided for illustration only and are not intended to be comprehensive or definitive. Each laboratory determines its own values, and reference ranges are highly method dependent. Reference values given are for adults, unless otherwise specified. For some entries for which specific molecular masses are not known (eg, proteins), reference values in SI are given as mass amounts per liter.*

TABLE 5. CONVERSIONS FROM ENGLISH TO METRIC MEASUREMENTS

Symbol	Known Quantity	Conversion Factor (Multiply by)	To Find	Metric Symbol
Length				
in	inches	2.54	centimeters	cm
ft	feet	30	centimeters	cm
ft	feet	0.3	meters	m
yd	yards	0.9	meters	m
mi	miles	1.6	kilometers	km
Area				
sq in	square inches	6.5	square centimeters	cm^2
sq ft	square feet	0.09	square meters	m^2
sq yd	square yards	0.8	square meters	m^2
sq mi	square miles	2.6	square kilometers	km^2
Mass				
oz	ounces	28	grams	g
lb	pounds	0.45	kilograms	kg
Volume				
tsp	teaspoons	5	milliliters	mL
tbsp	tablespoons	15	milliliters	mL
fl oz	fluid ounces	30	milliliters	mL
c	cups	0.24	liters	L
pt	US pints	0.47	liters	L
qt	US quarts	0.95	liters	L
gal	US gallons	3.8	liters	L
cu ft	cubic feet	0.03	cubic meters	m^3
cu yd	cubic yards	0.76	cubic meters	m^3
Temperature				
°F	Fahrenheit	*	Celsius	°C

* *To convert from degrees Fahrenheit to degrees Celsius, use the following formula:*

$$(°F - 32)(0.556) = °C.$$

thyroxine [T_4], triglycerides, and urea nitrogen) currently are dual-reported, with the SI value and unit listed first, followed by the conventional value and unit in parentheses.

blood glucose level of 7.8 mmol/L (140 mg/dL)

lead level of 0.97 μmol/L (20 mg/dL)

total cholesterol level of 6.85 mmol/L (265 mg/dL)

Analytes with a one-to-one conversion between SI and conventional values or a conversion factor that is a multiple of 10 are not dual-reported. Also, because dual-reporting in figures and tables can clutter the presentation, the values within the figures and tables may be presented in SI units only (although the analytes listed above commonly are dual-reported). Information on how to convert to conventional units may be given in the table footnote or the figure legend.

To convert ethanol from millimoles per liter to milligrams per deciliter, divide millimoles per liter by 0.217.

15.6 ■ **NON-SI REPORTING OF COMMON MEASUREMENTS.**—Exceptions for several non-SI units are permitted and are used with the SI. These include measurements for temperature, pressure, pH, enzyme activity, and time.

15.6.1 ***Temperature.***—The Celsius scale (°C) is used for temperature measurement rather than the base SI unit for temperature, the kelvin (K), which has little application in medicine. Although both kelvin and Celsius scales have the same interval value for temperature differences, they differ in their absolute values.

15.6.2 ***Pressure.***—The pascal (newton per square meter [N/m^2]) is the recommended SI unit for pressure measurement. However, the pascal is not used for reporting common physiologic pressure measurements. Blood pressure, intraocular pressure, and partial pressures (eg, oxygen, carbon dioxide) are reported in millimeters of mercury (mm Hg); cerebrospinal fluid pressure is reported as centimeters of water (cm H_2O).

15.6.3 ***pH.***—Although SI nomenclature could be used to express values of hydrogen ion concentration (nmol/L), the pH scale has been retained in scientific reporting.

15.6.4 ***Enzyme Activity.***—The katal (the amount of enzyme generating 1 mol of product per second) has been provisionally recommended as the SI unit for catalytic or enzymatic activity but has not been adopted widely. The international unit (the amount of enzyme generating 1 μmol of product per minute) continues to be commonly used for reporting enzymatic activity.[5,9]

15.6.5 ***Time.***—The SI unit for time is the second, although minute, hour, and day also are used. Other units of time, such as week, month, and year, are not part of the SI but are used occasionally. The abbreviations for second, minute, hour, and day are s, min, h, and d, respectively, and the abbreviations for week, month, and year are wk, mo, and y. These abbreviations should be used only in tables, line art, and virgule constructions.

15.6.6 ***Visual Acuity.***—Visual acuity should be reported based on how the measurement was determined. For example, the commonly used English units for visual acuity notations of 20/20 or 20/100 indicate that the person being evaluated can see at 20 ft what a person with "normal visual acuity" can see at 20 ft or at 100 ft, respectively. The equivalent metric measurement for visual acuity is 6/6 or 6/30, respectively, which should be specified as using meters for the acuity measurement.

15.6.7 ***Informal Text.***—In less formal, nontechnical text, such as essays, references to non-SI units, such as miles or inches, and the use of idioms or proverbs, such as "An ounce of prevention is worth a pound of cure," are acceptable.

15.7 ■ **SI UNITS FOR IONIZING RADIATION.**—SI units for measurement of ionizing radiation and radioactivity have been established (Table 6). In radiation exposure, dose refers to the energy deposited by an amount of radiation per mass unit. One rad (radiation absorbed dose) is equivalent to 100 erg of energy deposited in 1 g of material. The SI unit for absorbed dose of radiation is the gray (Gy) (1 Gy = 100 rad). The rem (roentgen equivalent man) is the quantity of radiation that has the same biological activity as 1 rad of x-rays. The rem is a calculated radiation unit of this equivalent dose in which the absorbed dose (in grays) is multiplied by a factor to account for the different types of radiation. For dose equivalent, the SI unit used to indicate the detrimental effects of an absorbed radiation dose on biological tissue is the sievert (Sv) (1 Sv = 100 rem). The SI unit of radiation

TABLE 6. SI UNITS FOR IONIZING RADIATION

Quantity	SI Name (Symbol)	SI Unit	Traditional Unit	Application	Conversion Factor
Activity (radionuclide)	becquerel (Bq)	s^{-1}	curie (Ci)	Radionuclide activity	1 Bq = 2.7×10^{-11} Ci (approx) 1 Ci = 3.7×10^{10} Bq 1 mCi = 37 MBq 1 μCi = 0.037 MBq
Absorbed dose	gray (Gy)	J/kg ($m^2 \cdot s^{-2}$)	rad	Imparted dose of ionizing radiation	1 Gy = 100 rad 1 rad = 0.01 Gy*
Exposure (in air)	No SI name	C/kg	roentgen	Radiation exposure	1 C/kg = 3876 R (approx) 1 R = 2.58×10^{-4} C/kg
Dose equivalent	sievert (Sv)	J/kg ($m^2 \cdot s^{-2}$)	rem	Protection against detrimental effects of radiation	1 Sv = 100 rem 1 rem = 0.01 Sv

* *Although 1 rad = 1 cGy, the "centi-" prefix generally is not preferred in SI. Therefore, despite the appeal of one-to-one conversion, rad should be converted to gray, not centigray.*

exposure is the coulomb per kilogram (C/kg), and the SI unit for activity of a radionuclide is the becquerel (Bq).

15.8 ■ **SI UNITS AND ENERGY.**—In SI units, the joule, rather than the calorie, is used as the unit of energy.

1 calorie = 4.184 J

1 kilocalorie = 4.184 kJ

In articles dealing with nutrition and diet, food energy content provided as calories and kilocalories should be converted to joules (J) and kilojoules (kJ).

A former distinction was made between the "small" calorie (=4.184 J) and the large calorie, denoted as Calorie (ie, with a capital C) and abbreviated Cal, which was equivalent to 1000 small calories or 1 kilocalorie. This large calorie is used in nutrition to indicate the energy content of food. In this instance, calorie (now written with a small c) indicates kilocalorie when specifying the energy content of foods.[16]

15.9 ■ **SI UNITS AND LEUKOCYTE COUNTS.**—With the use of the liter as the SI reference volume, the numerical values for white blood cell (WBC) counts are increased by 10^6 compared with values expressed by means of conventional reference units (ie, microliters or cubic millimeters). For instance, for the leukocyte count, the SI reference interval is 4.5 to 11.0×10^9/L; the conventional reference interval is 4500 to 11 000/μL.

In SI, the WBC differential count is reported as a proportion of 1.0, rather than as a percentage of the number of total WBC count. The absolute values for various leukocyte cell types, such as neutrophils, band forms, and lymphocytes (including $CD4^+$ cells), also may be reported. With the use of conventional units, these cell counts are reported as number of cells per microliter (or number of cells per cubic millimeter). In SI, cell counts are reported as number of cells $\times$ 10^9/L, although some laboratories and publications report these values as number of cells $\times$ 10^6/L.

The $CD4^+$ cell count was less than 0.20×10^9/L (200/μL).

The $CD4^+$ cell count was less than 200×10^6/L (200/μL).

15.10 ■ **DRUG DOSAGES.**—Drug dosages most likely will continue to be expressed in conventional metric mass units (eg, milligrams or milligrams per kilogram), although expressing drug doses in molar units is possible. However, drug dispensing and administration is standardized worldwide with the use of mass units (eg, 5 mg). There is little justification for converting to molar terms because drug dosages are not subject to the lack of standardization that exists for reporting conventional units vs SI units for laboratory values. However, even if the SI system were used for drug dosages, dual units would be necessary to avoid errors in prescribing and dispensing. Moreover, certain forms of some drugs (such as heparin and insulin) are mixtures, thereby precluding their expression in molar units. Besides standard metric mass units for drug doses (eg, milligrams or milligrams per kilogram), other drug dosage units such as drops (for ophthalmic preparations), grains (for aspirin), and various apothecary system measurements (eg, teaspoonfuls, ounces, and drams) may be encountered clinically. However, these units generally should be avoided in scientific writing.

15.11 ■ **SOLUTIONS.**—A *molar* solution contains 1 mol (1 gram molecular weight) of solute in 1 L of solution. The SI style for reporting molar concentration is mol/L; for solutions with millimolar concentrations, mmol/L; and for solutions with micromolar concentrations, μmol/L. This is the style followed by AMA publications.

> The gel was incubated at 40°C by applying 10 mL of a solution of 4-mmol/L potassium chloride and 5 mL of a solution of 1-mol/L sodium chloride.

Some scientific publications express molar concentration of solutions and reagents by means of another scientifically valid approach. Molar is designated by M and SI prefixes are used to denote concentration (eg, mM, for millimolar; μM, for micromolar concentrations).

> After harvesting, the cells were lysed by sonication in homogenizing buffer (50mM NaH_2PO_4 and 0.1mM EDTA).

A *normal* solution contains a concentration of 1 gram-equivalent of solute per liter. To show the concentration of a solution in relation to normality, the abbreviation N is used, with no space between the numerical value and the N. The term *normal saline* has been superseded. The preferred term is isotonic sodium chloride solution.

15.12 ■ **INDEXES.**—An index usually refers to a quantity derived from a ratio of 2 measurable quantities and is used to compare individuals with each other or with normal ranges. Except for products or quotients that represent derived SI units of measure, the ratio of SI units used to create indexes does not represent an SI convention.

At first mention in the text, the formula used to calculate an index should be given; thereafter, the numerical value for the index may be given without units. Some commonly used indexes are as follows:

> body mass index (BMI or the Quetelet index); calculated as weight in kilograms divided by the square of height in meters: weight (kg)/[height (m)]^2

> cardiac index (CI); calculated as cardiac output in liters per minute divided by body surface area in square meters

15.13 ■ **CURRENCY.**—Amounts of currency generally are expressed as a decimal number or whole number preceded by the symbol for the unit of measure for the currency.

> The cost-effectiveness analysis suggested a $700 difference between the 2 treatment strategies.
>
> The estimated cost of the new research laboratory was £25 million.

Because the dollar is the unit of currency in many nations, the country abbreviation should be designated for cases in which ambiguity is possible.

> The surgeon's fee of Can $3000 (US $2800) was disputed by the patient.

For some types of currency, abbreviations rather than symbols may be used to denote the unit of measure (eg, DM for *deutsche marks*; Fr for *francs*). Examples of commonly used types of currency and their abbreviations are listed below:

Currency	*Country*	*Abbreviation or Symbol*
Canadian dollar	Canada	Can $
yuan	China	¥
franc	France	Fr
deutsche mark	Germany	DM
lira	Italy	Lit
yen	Japan	¥
peso	Mexico	Mex$
krone	Norway	NKr
pound sterling	United Kingdom	£
dollar	United States	$, US $

ACKNOWLEDGMENTS

Principal author: Phil B. Fontanarosa, MD

Paul Frank, Electronic Editing Specialist, AMA Scientific Publications, provided an electronic file of the previous version of the SI conversion table; Gwenn Gregg, *JAMA* Department of Editorial Affairs, provided assistance with manuscript preparation.

REFERENCES

1. Lehmann HP. Recommended SI units for the clinical laboratory. *Lab Med.* 1980;11:473-480.
2. Huth EJ. The American shift to medical SI units. *Ann Intern Med.* 1987;106:149-150.
3. Campion EW. A retreat from SI units. *N Engl J Med.* 1992;327:49.
4. Lundberg GD. SI unit implementation—the next step. *JAMA.* 1986;260:73-76.
5. *The International System of Units (SI)*. Washington, DC: US Dept of Commerce, National Institute of Standards and Technology (NIST); 1991. Special Publication 330.
6. Baron DN. *Units, Symbols, and Abbreviations*. 5th ed. London, England: Royal Society of Medicine Press; 1994.

7. Young DS. Implementation of SI units for clinical laboratory data. *Ann Intern Med.* 1987;106:114-129.

8. Jordan CD, Flood JG, Laposata M, Lewandrowski KB. Normal reference laboratory values. *N Engl J Med.* 1992;327:718-724.

9. Laposata M. *SI Unit Conversion Guide*. Boston, Mass: NEJM Books; 1992.

10. Henry JB. *Clinical Diagnosis and Management by Laboratory Methods.* 19th ed. Philadelphia, Pa: WB Saunders Co; 1996.

11. Jacobs DS, Demott WR, Grady HJ, Horvat RT, Huestis DW, Kasten BL. *Laboratory Test Handbook*. 4th ed. Hudson, Ohio: Lexi-Comp Inc; 1996.

12. Tietz NW. *Clinical Guide to Laboratory Tests*. 3rd ed. Philadelphia, Pa: WB Saunders Co; 1995.

13. Metric Commission Canada, Sector 9.10 Health and Welfare. *The SI Manual in Health Care.* 2nd ed. Toronto, Ontario: Metric Commission Canada; 1982.

14. Boyko EJ, Hoke DG. Beat the Système [computer program]. Bainbridge Island, Wash: Edward J Boyko; 1993.

15. SI Unit Conversion Table. Available at: http://www.techexpo.com/techdata/techcntr.html. Accessed August 21, 1997.

16. *Dorland's Illustrated Medical Dictionary.* 28th ed. Philadelphia, Pa: WB Saunders Co; 1994.

CHAPTER 16

16.0 NUMBERS AND PERCENTAGES

Any policy on the use of numbers in text must take into account the reader's impression that numbers written as numerals (symbols) appear to emphasize quantity more strongly than those spelled out as words. Hence, literary style is to spell out most numbers, whereas the style of technical works is to use numerals when a degree of accuracy is intended or, as recommended in *Scientific Style and Format: The CBE Manual for Authors, Editors, and Publishers,*[1] to use numerals for nearly all numbers. Inevitably, when a publication chooses to use words in some instances and numerals in others, usage may appear inconsistent. The guidelines outlined in this section attempt to reduce these inconsistencies while avoiding use of numerals that may be jarring to the reader's eye. In the application of these guidelines, however, common sense and editorial judgment should prevail over dogma.

16.1 ■ **USE OF NUMERALS.**—Numerals should be used to express numbers in most circumstances. Exceptions are numbers that begin a sentence, title, subtitle, or heading; common fractions; accepted usage such as idiomatic expressions, numbers used as pronouns, and other uses of the number "one" in running text; ordinals *first* through *ninth;* and numbers spelled out in quotations or published titles (see 16.2, Spelling Out Numbers).

> The relative risk of exposed individuals was nearly 3 times that of the controls.
>
> In the second phase of the study, 3 of the investigators administered the 5 tests to the 7 remaining subjects. The test scores revealed a 2-fold to 2.4-fold improvement over the first phase.
>
> In 2 of the 17 patients in whom both ears were tested, we were unable to obtain responses from either ear. While testing patient 3, we experienced technical problems consisting of unmanageable electrical artifacts.
>
> Groups 1 and 2 were similar in terms of demographic and clinical characteristics (Table 1). Table 2 lists the 4 tests that were performed: auditory deprivation, wave V latency, EABR threshold, and speech recognition scores.

A 3-member committee from the Food and Drug Administration visited the researchers.

16.1.1 ***Numbers of 4 or More Digits to Either Side of the Decimal Point.***—According to SI convention, commas are not used in numbers. In numbers of 4 digits, the digits are typeset closed up. For numbers of 10 000 or greater, a half-space is used to separate every 3 digits starting from the left of the decimal point. For numbers with 5 or more digits to the right of the decimal point, a half-space is used between every 3 digits starting from the right of the decimal point (see also 15.4, Units of Measure, Use of Numerals With SI Units).

The weight of the salt was 8.453 98 g, but the value was rounded off to 8.4540 g when recorded in the laboratory book.

16.1.2 ***Mixed Fractions.***—For less precise measurements, mixed fractions may be used instead of decimals. These expressions usually involve time (see also 16.2.2, Common Fractions).

The surgery lasted 3¼ hours.

The patient was hospitalized for 5½ days.

16.1.3 ***Measures of Time.***—Measures of time usually are expressed as numerals (see also 11.3, Abbreviations, Days of the Week, Months, Eras). When dates are provided, numerals should be used for day and year; the month should be spelled out unless listed in a table. Conventional form for time and dates (11:30 PM on February 25, 1961) is preferred to European or military form (2330 on 25 February 1961). However, use of military time may clarify the time course in figures that depict a 24-hour experiment, times of drug dosing, and the like. For time, if the hour of the day is given, AM or PM is used and set in small capitals (see also 19.0, Typography). With 12 o'clock, simply use noon or midnight, whichever is intended. When referring to a position as it would appear on a clock face, express the position by means of numerals, eg, "The needle was inserted at the 9-o'clock position."

The 6 case subjects ranged in age from 2 to 5 years.

At 5:45 AM, October 15, 1994, the researchers completed the final experiment.

16.1.4 ***Measures of Temperature.***—Use the degree sign with Celsius or Fahrenheit measures of temperature.

The plates were cultured at 20°C, 3°C lower than usual.

16.1.5 ***Measures of Currency.***—For sums of money, use the appropriate symbol to indicate the type of the currency (eg, $, £; see also 15.13, Units of Measure, Currency).

His charge for the medication was $55.60 plus $0.95 for shipping.

The equivalent sum in British currency was £30.

16.2 ■ **SPELLING OUT NUMBERS.**—Use words to express numbers that occur at the beginning of a sentence, title, subtitle, or heading; for common fractions; for accepted usage and numbers used as pronouns; for ordinals *first* through *ninth;* and when part of a published quotation or title in which the number is spelled out. When spelling out numerals, hyphenate *twenty-one* through *ninety-nine* when these numbers occur alone or as part of a larger number. When numbers greater than 100 are spelled out, do not use commas or *and* (eg, one hundred thirty-two).

16.2.1 ***Beginning a Sentence, Title, Subtitle, or Heading.***—Use words for any number that begins a sentence, title, subtitle, or heading. However, it may be better to reword the sentence so that it does not begin with a number.

> Three hundred twenty-eight men and 126 women were included in the study.
> *Better:* The study population comprised 328 men and 126 women.
>
> Five patients were identified; 2 had hypertension and 1 had diabetes.

However, numerals may be used in sentences that begin with a specific year.

> 1995 marked the 50th anniversary of the bombing of Hiroshima.
>
> 2005 will be the medical school's centennial year.

When a unit of measure follows a number that begins a sentence, it too must be written out, even if the same unit is abbreviated elsewhere in the same sentence. Because this construction can be cumbersome, rewording the sentence may be preferable (see 15.3, Units of Measure, SI Format, Style, and Punctuation).

> Two milligrams of haloperidol was administered at 9 PM, followed by 1 mg at 3:30 AM.
> *Better:* At 9 PM, 2 mg of haloperidol was administered, followed by 1 mg at 3:30 AM.

16.2.2 ***Common Fractions.***—Common fractions are expressed with words. Hyphens are used only if the fraction modifies a noun.

> There was a half-second delay before the concert hall was illuminated.
>
> We require a two-thirds majority for consensus.
>
> Of those attending, nearly three fourths were members of the association.

A *quarter* may be used in place of *one fourth.*

> A quarter of the consensus panel dissented.

16.2.3 ***Numbers Used as Pronouns.***—Spell out numbers when used as pronouns.

> The investigators compared a new laboratory method with the standard one.
>
> These differences may be concealed if one looks only at the total group.
>
> William James uses the idea of the one and the many as the great challenge of the philosophical mind.

16.2.4 ***Accepted Usage.***—Spell out numbers for generally accepted usage, such as idiomatic expressions. *One* frequently appears in running text without referring to a quantity per se and may appear awkward to the author and reader if expressed as a numeral. When *one* may be replaced by *a* or *a single* without changing the meaning, the word *one* rather than the numeral is usually appropriate. Other numbers, most often *zero, two,* and large rounded numbers, also may be written as words in circumstances in which use of the numeral would place an unintended emphasis on a precise quantity or would be confusing.

> Twelve individuals were selected, any one of whom could have been the chair. [In this example, *one* is superfluous. The following is an equivalent sentence: Twelve individuals were selected, any of whom could have been the chair.]

When one numerical expression immediately follows another, spell out the one that can be more easily expressed in words or reword the sentence. [In this example, "one numerical expression" is equivalent to "a numerical expression." "One" is also used as a pronoun.]

The study was plagued by one problem after another.

One researcher estimates that firearms are used for protective purposes in the United States several hundred thousand times annually.

Models were developed to allow for the inclusion of one-time variables.

We appear to be moving from one extreme to another.

On the one hand, the blood glucose concentrations were substantially improved; on the other hand, the patient felt worse.

During one of the laboratory runs, it was observed that samples from cases 1, 3, and 9 had faint electrophoretic bands due to suboptimal DNA quality.

Medical futility has become one of the dominant topics in medical ethics in recent years.

In one recent case, the bonus amounted to $1 billion.

We ought to bring together in one place all that we have learned on a given subject.

The outcome was a zero-sum gain.

A zero should not be placed to the left of the decimal point of a *P* value. [Here, use of the numeral 0 could be confused with the letter O.]

Conventional wisdom has it that there are at least two sides to every issue.

Please include an example or two of the following scales.

I would like to ask the patient a question or two about her perception of her illness.

Given a choice among antihypertensive drugs, I would choose the other two.

He quoted the Ten Commandments.

Many of the mass-vaccination campaigns have been large, with tens of thousands of persons immunized, and expensive, costing as much as a half million dollars.

16.2.5 ***Ordinals.***—Ordinals generally are used to express order or rank rather than to emphasize quantity, and so ordinals *first* through *ninth* are spelled out. Exceptions are ordinals that are part of a series that includes an ordinal greater than *ninth.* Ordinals greater than *ninth* are expressed as numerals (10th, 11th, and so on) except at the beginning of a sentence, title, subtitle, or heading. Use the following suffixes: *-st, -nd, -rd, -th.*

The third patient was not available for reevaluation.

The 5th and 12th editions each had new editors.

Eleventh-hour negotiations settled the strike.

The pandemic will continue well into the 21st century.

(*But:* Some forms are spelled out by convention, eg, Twenty-fifth Amendment.)

16.3 ■ COMBINING NUMERALS AND WORDS.

—Use a combination of numerals and words to express rounded large numbers and consecutive numerical expressions.

16.3.1 ***Rounded Large Numbers.***—Rounded large numbers, such as those starting with *million,* should be expressed with numerals and words.

The disease afflicts 5 million to 6 million people.

The word *billion* signifies 2 different quantities, depending on one's location. In Britain, billion traditionally has signified 10^{12} (1 million million), whereas billion means 10^9 (1 thousand million) in North America. However, British usage is changing,[2] and the distinction may become moot. The CBE manual, *Scientific Style and Format,* avoids use of *billion* altogether, preferring all numerals or scientific notation.[1(p198)] Since most articles may be read by international readers, wherever possible avoid the use of *billion* and instead use numerals with million or scientific notation, depending on context. *Trillion* may also be confused, and the same rule should apply.

The projected budget is $2500 million.

The budget deficit is expected to expand to $1 trillion ($10^{12}$) by 2020.

16.3.2 ***Consecutive Numerical Expressions.***—When one numerical expression immediately follows another and the consecutive numerical expressions may create confusion or hinder ease of reading, reword the sentence or spell out the one that can more easily be expressed in words.

Study participants were provided with twenty 5-mL syringes.

In the cohort of fifteen hundred, 690 were men.
Better: In the cohort, 690 of the 1500 subjects were men.

The envelope contained 3 copies of the manuscript and one 3.5-inch diskette.

A similar situation arises when abbreviations or symbols follow numbers. In this case, if there is potential for misunderstanding, it is preferable to reword the sentence.

All subjects had 2 D_2 dopamine receptor genes.
Better: All subjects had 2 genes for the D_2 dopamine receptor.

The investigators were able to identify 3 γ-aminobutyric acid–mediated sites.
Better: The investigators were able to identify 3 sites mediated by γ-aminobutyric acid.

16.4 ■ **USE OF DIGIT SPANS AND HYPHENS.**—Digits should not be omitted when indicating a span of years or page numbers in the text. Hyphens may be used in text when a year span is used as the identifying characteristic of a study (eg, the 1982-1984 NHANES survey), but only when the actual dates of the study have been defined previously in the text; if the dates are not defined in the text, the hyphen is ambiguous and may or may not mean that the dates indicated are inclusive. If a title includes a span indicated by a hyphen, the meaning of the hyphen should be defined in the abstract (where applicable).

Trends in Drug-Resistant Tuberculosis in the United States, 1993-1996

In certain circumstances, such as fiscal year or academic year, the actual span may be understood and no definition is required; in these cases, the hyphen is acceptable at first mention and throughout the text.

The students participated in the study during the 1994-1995 academic year.

Substantial profits were anticipated for fiscal years 1996-1998.

Use of *to* also may introduce ambiguity. *To* should be used rather than *through* only when the final digit is not included in the span and *through* instead of *to* when the final digit is included in the span. However, in some circumstances, such as life span, historical periods, fiscal or academic year, page numbers in text, or age ranges, the meaning is clear without making a distinction between *to* and *through,* and *to* may be used.

> The subjects ranged in age from 23 to 56 years.
>
> The second enrollment period spanned January 30, 1991, to September 1, 1993. [In this example, the enrollment period ended on August 31.]
>
> We looked at the following 3 time periods: 1964 through 1967, 1968 through 1978, and 1979 through 1992.

In the last example, for brevity the time spans may be referred to by means of hyphens between years once the meaning has been made clear at the first mention.

> The mortality rate ratio of 2.01 (95% confidence interval, 1.80-2.24) indicates that the mortality rate during 1968-1978 was about twice that during 1979-1992.

A hyphen may be used within parentheses or in tables to indicate spans without further definition, provided the meaning is clear. However, if one of the values in the span includes a minus sign (most commonly found in confidence intervals), the word *to* should be used to avoid ambiguity. The word *to* should then be used in place of the hyphen throughout the table for consistency (see also 6.3, Punctuation, Hyphens and Dashes, and 17.3, Statistics, Significant Digits and Rounding Numbers).

> The mean number of years of life gained was 1.7 (95% confidence interval, 1.3-2.1).
>
> The mean number of years of disease-free life gained was 0.4 (95% confidence interval, −0.1 to 0.9).
>
> After the drug was injected, the seizures continued for a brief period (20-30 seconds), then ceased.
>
> The fourth edition contains a discussion of recommended preventive measures (pp 1243-1296).
>
> The median age of the individuals surveyed was 56 years (range, 31-92 years).

If the unit of measure for the quantity is set closed up with the number, the unit should be repeated for each number.

> The temperature remained normal throughout the day (96.5°C-97.3°C).
>
> The differences between groups were relatively small (5%-8%).
>
> *But:* The pressure gradient varied widely (10-60 mm Hg) throughout the day.

If the unit of measure changes within the parentheses, *to* is used.

> The subject's blood pressure was measured every 30 seconds while the drug was being injected (from 30 seconds to 5 minutes during injection).

16.5 ■ **ENUMERATIONS.**—Indicate a short series of enumerated items by numerals or lowercase italic letters run in and enclosed within parentheses in the text (see also 6.5, Punctuation, Parentheses and Brackets).

> The testing format focused on 6 aspects: (1) alertness and concentration, (2) language, (3) naming, (4) calculations, (5) construction, and (6) memory.

For long or complex enumerations, indented numbers without parentheses followed by a period may be used. Bullets without enumeration may be used for emphasis and clarity when the specific order of the items is not important.

The current labeling of allergenic extracts provides the following instructions:

- use should be limited to physicians experienced in their use and in emergency treatment of anaphylaxis;
- initial dosage should be based on skin testing;
- the patient should be observed for at least 20 minutes after injection;
- immunotherapy should be withheld when a β-blocker is used.

16.6 ■ ABBREVIATING *NUMBER*.

—The word *number* may be abbreviated *No.* in the body of tables and line art (not in the title, footnotes, or legend) or in the text when used as a specific designator. Do not use the number sign (#) in place of the abbreviation.

	Drug	**Placebo**
No. of subjects	49	48

Polyethylene No. 10 catheters were placed in both femoral arteries.

16.7 ■ FORMS OF NUMBERS

16.7.1 *Decimals.*

—The decimal form should be used when a fraction is given with an abbreviated unit of measure (eg, 0.5 g, 2.7 mm) or whenever a precise measurement is intended (see also 15.4.2, Units of Measure, Decimal Format).

The patient was receiving gentamicin sulfate, 3.5 mg/kg, every 8 hours. Her serum gentamicin level reached a peak of 12.2 μmol/L and a trough of 1.5 μmol/L after the third dose.

Place a zero before the decimal point in numbers less than 1, except when expressing *P* values, α , and β. These values cannot equal 1, except when values are rounded (see 17.4, Statistics, Glossary of Statistical Terms), and appear frequently; thus eliminating the zero can save substantial space in tables and text. (Although other statistical values also may never equal 1, their use is less frequent, and to simplify usage, the zero before the decimal point is included.)

$P = .16$ $\kappa = 0.87$ $1 - \beta = .80$

Our predetermined α level was .05.

By convention, a zero is not used in front of the decimal point of the measure of the bore of a firearm.

.22-caliber rifle

16.7.2 *Percentages.*

—The term *percent* derives from the Latin *per centum,* meaning by the hundred, or in, to, or for every hundred. The term *percent* and symbol % should be used with a specific number, whereas *percentage* is an extension of the term and refers in general to a number or amount stated in percent. *Percentile* is defined as the value on a scale of 100 that indicates the percent of the distribution within which the value falls.

Ten percent of the work remained to be done.

Heart disease was present in a small percentage of the subjects.

Her body mass index placed her in the upper fifth percentile of the study group.

Use arabic numerals and the symbol % for specific percentages. The symbol is set close to the numeral and is repeated with each number in a series or range of percentages. Include the symbol % with a percentage of zero.

A 5% incidence (95% confidence interval, 1%-9%) was reported.

The prevalence in the populations studied varied from 0% to 20%.

At the beginning of a sentence, spell out both the number and the word *percent*, even if the percentage is part of a series or range. Often it is preferable to reword the sentence so that a comparison between percentages is more readily apparent.

Twenty percent to 30% of patients reported gastrointestinal symptoms.
Better: Gastrointestinal symptoms were reported in 20% to 30% of patients.

When referring to a percentage derived from a study sample, include with the percentage the numbers from which the percentage is derived. This is particularly important when the sample size is less than 100 (see also 17.3, Statistics, Significant Digits and Rounding Numbers). To give primacy to the original data, it is preferable to place the percentage in parentheses.

Of the 26 cases, 19 (73%) occurred in infants.

Any discrepancy in the sum of percentages in a tabulation (eg, errors in rounding off numbers, missing values, or multiple procedures) should be explained in the text, table footnote, or figure legend.

The term *percent change* is often used in place of *percentage of change.* While the less formal term is acceptable, its usage must be precise. *Percent change* must be differentiated from *percentage point change.* For example, a change in rate from 20% to 30% can be referred to either as an increase of 10 percentage points, as in "the intervention group improved 10 percentage points," or as a 50% increase (percent change), as in "the intervention group showed a 50% improvement" ([30% − 20%]/20%). The 2 terms are *not* interchangeable. Since the percent change does not indicate the magnitude of change for the population, providing the actual values in addition to the percent change is preferred.

16.7.3 ***Proportions and Rates.***—Use the virgule construction for proportions or rates when placed in parentheses (eg, 1/2). A colon is used for ratios (eg, 1 : 2). When a proportion, rate, ratio, or percentage is stated in addition to the numerator (*n*) and denominator (*d*) from which it is derived, it is preferable to place the proportion, rate, ratio, or percentage in parentheses after the numerator.

Death occurred in 3 (1%) of the 300 patients.

This format is also acceptable in text in which the denominator is clear from the context and does not have to be repeated within the sentence.

Death occurred in 3 patients (1%).

Placing the proportion inside parentheses in *n/d* form also is acceptable, but the *n/d* form should never be used in running text.

Death occurred in 3% (6/200) of the patients.
Avoid: Death occurred in 6/200 (3%) of the patients.
Better: Death occurred in 6 (3%) of the 200 patients.

Rates should use the decimal format when the denominator is understood to be 100; otherwise, the denominator should be specified.

Of all individuals exposed, children were affected at a rate of 0.05.

The infant mortality rate was 3 per 10 000 live births.

16.7.4 ***Roman Numerals.***—Roman numerals should be marked "roman" for the typesetter. Use roman numerals with proper names (eg, Henry Ford III). No comma is used before the numeral. Avoid the use of roman numerals except when part of established nomenclature (see 12.0, Nomenclature).

Schedule II drug	level I trauma center
Step I diet	Axis I diagnosis

But:

type 2 diabetes	phase 3 study

Use roman numerals for cancer stages and arabic numerals for cancer grades (see also 12.2, Nomenclature, Cancer). In pedigree charts, use roman numerals to indicate generations and arabic numerals to indicate families or individual family members. Roman numerals also may be used in outline format (see 2.13, Manuscript Preparation, Tables).

In bibliographic material (eg, references or book reviews), do not use roman numerals to indicate volume number, even though roman numerals may have been used in the original. However, if roman numerals were used in the original title or in an outline, refer to the title or outline as it was published, with roman numerals. Retain lowercase roman numerals that refer to pages in a foreword, preface, or introduction. Roman numerals may also be used to number supplements to journals, so that roman numerals appear adjacent to page numbers in references to the work. In this case, the roman numerals should be retained.

For the use of roman numerals in biblical and classical references, follow the most recent edition of *The Chicago Manual of Style*[3] (see also 2.12, Manuscript Preparation, References).

The following table indicates the roman equivalent for arabic numerals 1 through 5000. In general, roman numerals to the right of the greatest numeral are added to that numeral, and numerals to the left are subtracted. A horizontal bar over a roman numeral multiplies its value by 1000.

1	I	11	XI	30	XXX	300	CCC
2	II	12	XII	40	XL	400	CD
3	III	13	XIII	50	L	500	D
4	IV	14	XIV	60	LX	600	DC
5	V	15	XV	70	LXX	700	DCC
6	VI	16	XVI	80	LXXX	800	DCCC
7	VII	17	XVII	90	XC	900	CM
8	VIII	18	XVIII	100	C	1000	M
9	IX	19	XIX	200	CC	5000	$\bar{V}$
10	X	20	XX				

ACKNOWLEDGMENT

Principal author: Margaret A. Winker, MD

REFERENCES

1. Council of Biology Editors Style Manual Committee. *Scientific Style and Format: The CBE Manual for Authors, Editors, and Publishers.* 6th ed. New York, NY: Cambridge University Press; 1994.

2. Billion bites the dust [Opinion]. *Nature.* 1992;358:2.

3. *The Chicago Manual of Style.* 14th ed. Chicago, Ill: University of Chicago Press; 1993.

ADDITIONAL READING AND GENERAL REFERENCE

American Psychological Association. *Publication Manual of the American Psychological Association.* 4th ed. Washington, DC: American Psychological Association; 1994.

CHAPTER 17

The essence of life is statistical improbability on a grand scale.
Richard Dawkins[1]

There are three kinds of lies: lies, damn lies, and statistics.
Attributed to Disraeli by Mark Twain[1]

17.0 STATISTICS

We encounter statistical concepts every day, such as the margin of error in a presidential poll or the probability that a catastrophic event will occur, but, just as one may understand how the heart functions and how blood circulates but not be able to perform a cardiac catheterization, an understanding of statistical concepts does not enable one to perform the work of a statistician. Although the concepts may be familiar, the tools of statistics may be misapplied and the results misinterpreted without a statistician's help.

In medical research, the quality of the statistical analysis and clarity of presentation of statistical results are critical to the validity and impact of the study. The cardiologist's knowledge can help the patient more before a myocardial infarction than after the damage is done; the statistician's knowledge is more effective at the beginning of the study than resuscitating the results at the end. Regardless of the statistician's role, authors (who may include statisticians) are responsible for the appropriate design, analysis, and presentation of the study's results.

Many excellent statistical texts are available, and a comprehensive approach is far beyond the scope of this chapter. However, authors, editors, and copy editors should have a general understanding of statistical terms, concepts, and the use of statistical tests and presentation. Although few rules exist to guide how statistics should be presented, presenting statistics briefly but completely and consistently should improve the reader's understanding of the analysis.

17.1 ■ THE MANUSCRIPT: PRESENTING STUDY DESIGN, RATIONALE, AND STATISTICAL ANALYSIS.—Each portion of the manuscript should contribute to the reader's understanding of why and how the study was done and should persuade the reader that (1) the hypothesis or study question is clearly stated, carefully considered, and important, (2) the methods are designed to answer the question and the analysis is appropriate, (3) the results are credible and convincing, and (4) the implications are placed in context and the limitations do not preclude interpretation of the results. Words used herein that are defined in the glossary are given in a different `font`.

17.1.1 ***Abstract and Introduction.***—The structured abstract enables the reader to assess the study hypothesis and methods quickly and easily. The context for the study question and the hypothesis (objective) should be clearly stated (eg, To determine whether enalapril reduces left ventricular mass. . . .), the study design and population and setting from which the sample was drawn described, and the main outcome measures explained. The results should include some explanation of effect size, if appropriate, with point estimates and confidence intervals used to describe the results. The conclusions should follow from the results without overinterpreting the data. Abstract format is too brief to permit detailed explanation of statistical analyses, but a basic description may be appropriate (eg, The screening test was validated using a bootstrap procedure and performance tested using an ROC curve.).

The introduction should include a concise review of the relevant literature to provide a context for the study question and a rationale for the choice of a particular method. The study `hypothesis` or purpose should be clearly stated in the last sentence(s) before the methods section. Results or conclusions do not belong in the introduction.

17.1.2 ***Methods.***—The methods section should include enough information to enable a knowledgeable reader to reproduce the study and, given the original data, verify the reported results. Components should include as many of the following as are applicable to the study design:

- Study design (see 17.2, Types of Study Design).
- Year(s) (and month if appropriate) in which the study was conducted.
- Disease or condition to be studied—how was it defined?
- Setting in which subjects were studied (community based, referral population, primary care clinic, volunteers).
- Subjects studied—who was eligible; `inclusion` and `exclusion criteria`; if all subjects were not included in each analysis, reason for exclusions; informed consent and institutional review board approval when appropriate (see 3.8.1, Ethical and Legal Considerations, Informed Consent and Ethics Review Committees). If results for any of the subjects have been previously described, provide citations for all reports or ensure that different reports of the same study can be easily identified (eg, by using a unique study name).
- Intervention, including length of intervention and enough information to allow a knowledgeable reader to reproduce the intervention, or define the exposure adequately to allow comparison of different studies.
- Outcomes and how they were measured, including reliability of measures and whether investigators determining outcomes were blinded to which group received the intervention or underwent the exposure.
- Independent variables and how they were measured—for example, demographic variables and risk factors for the disease.
- Preliminary analyses: if the study is a preliminary analysis of an ongoing study, the reason for publishing data before the end of the study should be clearly stated, along with information regarding when the study is to be completed.
- Source to obtain original or additional data if somewhere other than from the authors. For example, data tapes are often obtained from the US government;

the source should be stated. The National Auxiliary Publications Service (NAPS; see 2.10.6, Manuscript Preparation, National Auxiliary Publications Service [NAPS] or Availability in Other Forms or Databases) and the World Wide Web can be used to store or display data or information that could not be included in the manuscript. The source also may be listed in the acknowledgment.

- Statistical methods, including which procedures were used for which analyses, what α level was considered acceptable, power of the study (if calculated before the study was conducted), assumptions made, any data transformations or multiple comparisons procedures performed, steps used for developing a model in multivariate analysis, and pertinent references for statistical tests and type of software used. Results should be presented in terms of confidence intervals wherever possible.
- If the study has been registered in a central trial registry, the name of the registry and the trial number should be provided.

17.1.3 ***Results.***—The results section should include the number of subjects in the study at its inception, statistics describing the study population, and the number of subjects who were excluded, dropped out, or were lost to follow-up at any point in the study. Primary outcome measures should be discussed after the study population is described, followed by secondary outcome measures. Post hoc analyses may be discussed, but they should be identified as such. Post hoc analyses should be used for generating rather than testing hypotheses (see type I error). If one statistical test has been used throughout the manuscript, the test should be clearly stated in the methods section. If more than one statistical test has been used, the statistical tests performed should be discussed in the methods and the specific test used reported along with the results.

17.1.4 ***Discussion (Comment).***—Whether the hypothesis was supported or refuted by the results should be addressed. The study results should be placed in context with published literature. The limitations of the study should be discussed, including possible sources of bias and how these problems might affect conclusions and generalizability. Evidence to support or refute the problems introduced by the limitations should be provided. The implications for clinical practice, if any, and specific directions for future research may be offered. The conclusions should not go beyond the data and should be based on the study results and population.

17.2 ■ TYPES OF STUDY DESIGN.

—There are many types of study design; the most commonly used types are provided here (see 17.4, Glossary of Statistical Terms, for additional study designs).

17.2.1 ***Randomized Controlled Trial.***—The parallel-design, double-blind, randomized controlled trial (RCT) is often the optimal study design to compare 2 or more types of drug or other therapy, since known and unknown potentially confounding factors are randomly distributed between intervention and control groups. RCTs are not appropriate to answer some questions, such as efficacy of a treatment in which a comparison group would be unethical, or when testing effects of exposure of the population to potentially harmful substances. In addition, RCTs often are criticized because they assess efficacy of the treatment intervention in the controlled and highly monitored setting of a clinical trial and may not reflect effectiveness of the treatment in real-world settings, and they are often performed in highly selected patient populations, making the results difficult to extrapolate to subpopulations not enrolled in the trial. One consideration when interpreting RCTs is that the distribution of subject characteristics may not be equal in the treatment arms; some inequality of distribution is expected by chance alone and is more frequent with a small sample size. If unequal distribution of certain critical characteristics is likely (such as tumor stage when evaluating efficacy of cancer treatment), the potential for such confounding can be reduced by stratifying the groups according to 1 or 2 important characteristics before randomization is performed.

The methods of RCTs must be described in detail to allow the reader to judge the quality of the study, reproduce the study intervention, and abstract pertinent information for comparison with other studies. The CONSORT statement[2] provides a checklist (Table 1) to help ensure complete reporting of RCTs. *JAMA* and many other journals require that authors complete the checklist showing the subjects enrolled at each phase of the study and where subjects were excluded, were lost to follow-up, or dropped out. While completing the checklist does not guarantee that a study has been performed well, it can help ensure that the information critical to interpretation of the study is provided and accessible to editors, reviewers, and, if published, readers. A flow diagram is also helpful to outline the flow of subjects in the study, including when and why subjects dropped out or were lost to follow-up and how many subjects were evaluated for the study end points. When authors submit manuscripts reporting RCTs to journals that use the CONSORT guidelines, such a flow diagram (Figure 1) should be included and, if the manuscript is accepted for publication, the flow diagram is published with the study. The number of arms after randomization shown in the diagram should correspond to the number of intervention and control arms in the study.

The report of an RCT should include a comparison of characteristics of the subjects in the different arms of the trial, usually as a table. However, performing significance testing on the characteristics to determine whether significant differences exist is controversial. First, the problem of multiple comparisons arises, so that for every comparison of 20 characteristics, 1 would be expected to be different at $P < .05$ by chance alone. Further, if randomization were competently done, any differences between groups would be based on chance alone and a test of the null hypothesis (the product of which is the *P* value) is not appropriate (John C. Bailar III, MD, PhD, written communication, June 26, 1996).

The decision to perform interim analyses with stopping rules (specific criteria used to define prospectively what interim results would be necessary to stop the study) is made before the study begins.[3(pp130,258)] If the criteria for the stopping rules have not been met, the results of interim analyses should not be reported unless the treatment has important adverse effects and reporting is necessary for patient safety. If a report is an interim analysis, it should be clearly stated in the manuscript with the reason for reporting the interim results. The plans for interim analyses and reports contained in the original study protocol should be provided, and, if the interim analysis deviates from those, the reasons for the change should be justified. If a manuscript reports the final results of a study for which an interim analysis was previously published, the reason for publishing both reports should be stated and the interim analysis referenced.

17.2.2 ***Crossover Trial.***—The crossover trial is a prospective trial, usually with both the subject and investigator unaware of the treatment assignment (double blinded), used for evaluating drug treatments. The individual serves as his or her own control, thereby eliminating intersubject variability when comparing treatment effects and reducing the sample size needed to detect a significant effect. Most considerations of parallel-design randomized trials apply (including

TABLE 1. CONSORT CHECKLIST

Checklist for Authors Submitting Reports of Randomized Controlled Trials to *JAMA*

This checklist of 21 items is intended to assist authors, editors, and reviewers by ensuring that information pertinent to the trial is included in the study report. Adapted from Begg C, Cho M, Eastwood S, et al. Improving the quality of reporting of randomized controlled trials: the CONSORT statement. *JAMA*. 1996;276:637-639.

First Author's Name and Manuscript Title ______________________________

Heading	**Subheading**	**Descriptor**	**Was It Reported? Yes or No**	**If Yes, What Page No.?**
TITLE		1. Identify the study as a randomized trial.	______	______
ABSTRACT		2. Use a structured format.	______	______
INTRODUCTION		3. State prospectively defined hypothesis, clinical objectives, and planned subgroup or covariate analyses.	______	______
METHODS	**Protocol**	Describe		
		4. Planned study population, together with inclusion/exclusion criteria.	______	______
		5. Planned interventions and their timing.	______	______
		6. Primary and secondary outcome measure(s) and the minimum important difference(s), and how the target sample size was projected.	______	______
		7. Rationale and methods for statistical analyses, detailing main comparative analyses and whether they were completed on an intention-to-treat basis.	______	______
		8. Prospectively defined stopping rules (if warranted).	______	______
	Assignment	Describe		
		9. Unit of randomization (eg, individual, cluster, geographic).	______	______
		10. Method used to generate the allocation schedule.	______	______
		11. Method of allocation concealment and timing of assignment.	______	______
		12. Method to separate the generator from the executor of assignment.	______	______
	Masking (Blinding)	13. Describe mechanism (eg, capsules, tablets); similarity of treatment characteristics (eg, appearance, taste); allocation schedule control (location of code during trial and when broken); and evidence for successful masking (blinding) among participants, person doing intervention, outcome assessors, and data analysts.	______	______
RESULTS	**Participant Flow and Follow-up**	14. Provide a trial profile (see Figure of flow diagram on page 77) summarizing participant flow, numbers and timing of randomization assignment, interventions, and measurements for each randomized group.	______	______
	Analysis	15. State estimated effect of intervention on primary and secondary outcome measures, including a point estimate and measure of precision (confidence interval).	______	______
		16. State results in absolute numbers when feasible (eg, 10/20, not 50%).	______	______
		17. Present summary data and appropriate descriptive and inferential statistics in sufficient detail to permit alternative analyses and replication.	______	______
		18. Describe prognostic variables by treatment group and any attempt to adjust for them.	______	______
		19. Describe protocol deviations from the study as planned, together with the reasons.	______	______
COMMENT		20. State specific interpretation of study findings, including sources of bias and imprecision (internal validity) and discussion of external validity, including appropriate quantitative measures when possible.	______	______
		21. State general interpretation of the data in light of the totality of the available evidence.	______	______

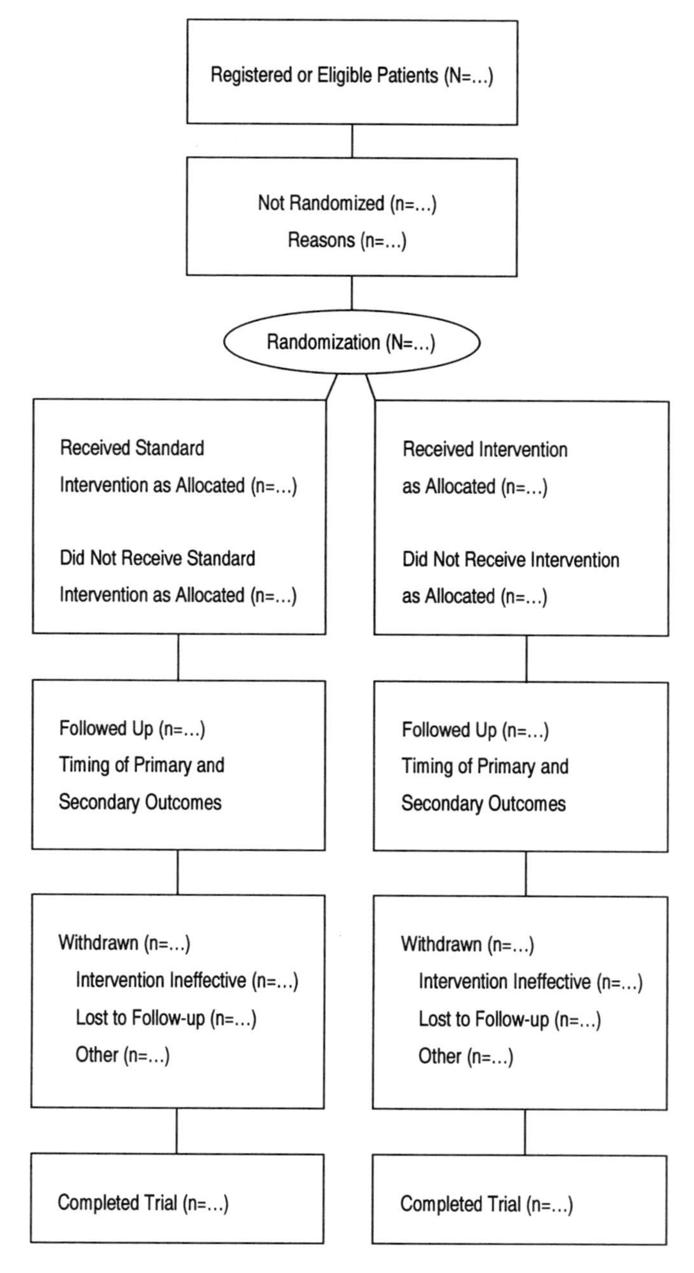

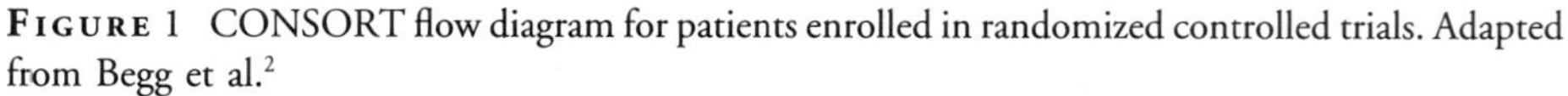
FIGURE 1 CONSORT flow diagram for patients enrolled in randomized controlled trials. Adapted from Begg et al.[2]

the items listed in the CONSORT checklist, except item 14, the trial profile, and item 18), and new considerations arise. Information important to this study design includes possible carryover effects (ie, effect of intervention persists after completion of intervention) and length of washout period (intervention effects should have ended completely before crossover to the other treatment). If the actual period of crossover differs from the original study protocol, how and why decisions were made to cross over to the alternate treatment and when the crossover occurred should be stated. The initial treatment should be randomized to ensure that investigators remain blinded and that no systematic differences arise because of treatment order. Otherwise, unblinding is likely, treatment order may confound the analysis, and carryover effects will be more difficult to assess. If carryover effects are significant, or if a washout period with no treatment is undesirable or unethical, a parallel group design (with a larger sample size) may be necessary.

17.2.3 ***Cohort Study.***—A prospective cohort study is a study that follows a group or cohort of individuals initially free of the outcome of interest. The study is usually conducted for a predetermined period, long enough for some members of the cohort to develop the outcome of interest. Individuals who developed the outcome are compared with those who did not. The report of the study should include a description of the cohort and the length of follow-up, what independent variables were measured and how, and what outcomes were measured and how. The number of subjects unavailable for follow-up and whether they differed from those with complete follow-up should also be included. All adverse events should be reported. Any previous publications reporting results from the same cohort should be cited in the text or should be clear from the study name; all previous reports on the same or similar outcomes should be cited. Retrospective cohort studies may be appropriate if investigators are blinded to study outcomes when formulating the hypothesis and determining the dependent and independent variables, but many of the strengths of prospective cohort studies are lost with retrospective studies, such as identifying the population to study and defining the variables and outcomes before the events occur.

17.2.4 ***Case-Control Study.***—A case-control study is retrospective and matches those who have had an event (cases) with those who have not (controls). Cases and controls generally are matched according to specific characteristics (eg, age, sex, or duration of disease) to reduce confounding by these variables. However, if the matched variables are inextricably linked with the exposure of interest (not necessarily with the disease or outcome of interest), matching may confound the analysis (see also overmatching). The independent variable is exposure to an item of interest (eg, a drug or disease). Information about the source of both cases and controls must be included, and inclusion and exclusion criteria must be listed for each. Cases and controls should be drawn from the same or similar populations to avoid selection bias. Each pair (1:1 match) or group (eg, 1:2 or 1:3 match) of cases and controls may be matched on 1 or more variable. The analysis generally is unpaired, because of the inability to match on every important characteristic. However, paired analysis reduces the necessary sample size to detect a difference may be justified if subjects are well matched. Recall bias is common in this and other types of retrospective studies and is especially a concern when participants believe that a factor related to the independent variable may be associated with the outcome. If recall bias may have occurred, how the investigators dealt with this possibility should be discussed.

17.2.5 ***Cross-sectional Study.***—Cross-sectional studies assess the characteristics of a sample of subjects at a given point or period in time and generally do not attempt to determine which characteristics or events occurred first. A cross-sectional study can be used to determine whether variables are associated with each other but, unlike a prospective study, cannot be used to test a hypothesis of causation.

17.2.6 ***Case Series.***—A case series describes characteristics of a group of patients with a particular disease or patients who have undergone a particular procedure. Case series may be used to formulate a case definition of a disease or describe the experience of an individual or institution in treating a disease or performing a type of procedure. Case series should comprise consecutive patients seen by the individual or institution to minimize selection bias. A case series is not used to test a hypothesis because no group is compared with it. (Occasionally comparisons are made with historical controls or published studies, but these comparisons are informal and should not include formal statistical analysis.) A report of a case series should include the rationale for publishing the population description and inclusion and exclusion criteria.

17.2.7 ***Meta-analysis.***—Meta-analysis is a systematic overview of studies that pools results of 2 or more studies to obtain an overall answer to a question of interest or hypothesis. According to Moher and Olkin,[4]

> [Meta-analyses] provide a systematic and explicit method for synthesizing evidence, a quantitative overall estimate (and confidence intervals) derived from the individual studies, and early evidence as to the effectiveness of treatments, thus reducing the need for continued study. They also can address questions in specific subgroups that individual studies may not have examined.

Meta-analysis summarizes quantitatively the evidence regarding a treatment, procedure, or association. It is a more statistically powerful test of the null hypothesis than is provided by the separate studies themselves since the sample size is substantially larger than those in the individual studies. However, a number of issues make meta-analysis a much-debated form of statistics.[4-7] Sacks et al[8] defined 6 basic content areas that should be addressed in meta-analyses—study design, combinability, control of bias, statistical analysis, sensitivity analysis, and problems of applicability—and found that only 24 of 86 meta-analyses they reviewed addressed all 6 content areas. Jadad and McQuay[9] found that lower-quality meta-analyses were more likely to have a positive result than higher-quality meta-analyses.

To ensure that the meta-analysis accurately reflects the available evidence, the methods of identifying possible studies for inclusion should be explicitly stated (eg, literature search, reference search, and contacting authors regarding other or unpublished work). A search strategy that includes several approaches to identify articles is preferable to a single database search.[10] Publication bias, or the tendency of authors to publish articles with positive results, is a potential limitation of any systematic review of the literature.[11] *JAMA* permits inclusion of unpublished studies in meta-analyses, provided the studies meet the same inclusion criteria as the published studies. One approach to addressing whether publication bias might affect the result is to define the number of negative studies that would be needed to change the results of a meta-analysis from positive to negative.

Other issues debated by meta-analysts and others include which study designs are acceptable for inclusion, whether and how studies should be rated for quality,[12] and whether and how to combine results from studies with disparate study characteristics. While few would disagree that meta-analysis of randomized controlled trials is most appropriate when possible, many areas include too few randomized trials to permit meta-analysis or cannot be studied in a trial. Gerbarg and Horiwitz[13] have suggested that criteria for combining studies should be similar to criteria for multicenter trials and should include similar prognostic factors, such as severity of illness, equal potency and administration of the intervention, equal detection of outcome events, and sufficient similarity of study subjects to justify combining them. Few of the meta-analyses they reviewed met these criteria. Whether studies can be appropriately combined can be determined statistically by analyzing the degree of heterogeneity, taking into account the effect size (the population effect = z), the sample size in each group, and whether the effect sizes from different studies are homogeneous. If statistically significant heterogeneity is found (measured by means of the Q statistic), then combining the studies into a single analysis may not be valid.[14] A final concern is the influence 1 or 2 large trials may have on the results—large trials in a small pool of studies can dominate the analysis, and the meta-analysis may reflect little more than the individual large trial.

Meta-analyses are often analyzed using both `fixed-effects` and `random-effects` models to determine how different assumptions affect the results. An example of how results of a meta-analysis may be depicted graphically is shown in 2.14.1, Manuscript Preparation, Types of Figures, Example F14.

Ultimately, a meta-analysis is useful only as long as it reflects current literature. Thus, a concern of meta-analysts and clinicians is that the meta-analyses be updated as new studies are published. One international effort, the Cochrane Collaboration, has been developed to provide constantly updated systematic reviews and meta-analyses in a variety of fields.[15]

17.2.8 ***Cost-effectiveness Analysis, Cost-benefit Analysis.***—As pressures to contain health care costs have mounted, emphasis in research has shifted from simply establishing that a treatment is effective to assessing the costs vs benefits of that treatment. Cost-effectiveness analysis "compares the net monetary costs of a health care intervention with some measure of clinical outcome or effectiveness such as mortality rates or life-years saved."[16] Cost-benefit analysis is similar but the clinical measures of outcomes are converted into monetary units, so that costs and benefits are both expressed in terms of monetary units.[16] The results of a cost-effectiveness analysis are usually expressed in terms of a cost-effectiveness ratio, for example, the cost per year of life gained.[17] The use of `quality-adjusted life-years`, or QALYs, permits one to directly compare different types of interventions using the same measure for outcomes.[17] Unfortunately, no standard method for performing or reporting cost-effectiveness analyses has been established. The complexity of the analyses and the many decisions required when selecting data and choosing assumptions are particularly concerning when the analysis is performed by an investigator or company with financial interest in the treatment being evaluated.[18]

One approach frequently used by cost-effectiveness analysts is to define a base case that represents the choices to be considered, perform an analysis for the base case, and then perform `sensitivity analyses` to determine how varying the data used and assumptions made for the base case affects the results.[17] A number of journals have published guidelines and approaches to cost-effectiveness analysis, but consensus has yet to emerge.[16-20]

17.3 ■ SIGNIFICANT DIGITS AND ROUNDING NUMBERS.

—When numbers are expressed in scientific and biomedical articles, they should reflect the degree of accuracy of the original measurement. Numbers obtained from mathematical calculations should be rounded off to reflect the original degree of precision.

17.3.1 ***Significant Digits.***—The use of a numeral in a numbers column (eg, the ones column) implies that the method of measurement is accurate to that level of precision. For example, when a reporter attempts to estimate the size of a crowd, the estimate might be scores of people, but would not be expressed as 86 unless each individual was counted. Similarly, when an author provides a number with numerals to the right of the decimal point, the numerals imply that the measurement used to obtain the number is accurate to the last place a numeral is shown. Therefore, numbers should be rounded to reflect the precision of the instrument or measurement; for example, for a scale accurate to 0.1 kg, a weight should be expressed as 75.2 kg, not 75.23 kg. Similarly, for SI units, the instrument used to measure a concentration is accurate only to a given fraction of the concentration, for example, 15.6 mg/L, not 15.638 mg/L (see 15.5.1, Units of Measure, SI Conversion Tables, for the appropriate number of significant digits). Numbers that result from calculations, such as means and SDs, should be expressed to no more than 1 significant digit beyond the accuracy of the instrument. Thus, the mean (SD) of weights of individuals weighed on a scale accurate to 0.1 kg should be expressed as 62.45 (4.13) kg. Adult age is reported rounded off to 1-year increments, so the mean would be expressed as, for example, 47.7 years.

17.3.2 ***Rounding Off.***—The digits to the right of the last significant digit are rounded off. If the digit to the right of the last significant digit is less than 5, the last significant digit is not changed. If the digit is greater than 5, the last significant digit is rounded up to the next higher digit. (For example, 47.746 years is rounded to 47.7 years and 47.763 years is rounded to 47.8 years.) If the digit immediately to the right of the last significant digit is 5, with either no digits or all zeros after the 5, the last significant digit is rounded up if it is odd and down if it is even. (For example, 47.7500 would become 47.8; 47.65 would become 47.6.) If the digit to the right of the last significant digit is 5 followed by numbers other than 0, the last significant digit is rounded up (47.6501 would become 47.7).

`P values` and other statistical expressions raise particular issues about rounding. For more information about how and why to round *P* values and other statistical terms, see the individual section pertaining to the statistical term in 17.4, Glossary of Statistical Terms. Briefly, *P* values should be expressed to 2 digits to the right of the decimal point (regardless of whether the *P* value is significant), unless $P < .01$, in which case the *P* value should be expressed to 3 digits to the right of the decimal point. (One exception to this rule is when rounding *P* from 3 digits to 2 digits would result in *P* appearing nonsignificant, such as $P = .046$. In this case, expressing the *P* value to 3 places may be preferred by the author. The same holds true for rounding confidence intervals that are significant before rounding but nonsignificant after rounding.) The smallest *P* value that should be expressed is $P < .001$, since additional zeros do not convey useful information.[21]

17.4 ■ **GLOSSARY OF STATISTICAL TERMS.**—In the glossary, terms defined elsewhere in the glossary are printed in `this font`. An arrow (⇒) indicates points to consider in addition to the definition. For detailed discussion of these terms, the referenced texts or the resource list at the end of the chapter are useful sources.

Eponymous names for statistical procedures often differ from one text to another (for example, the Newman-Keuls and Student-Newman-Keuls test). The names provided in this glossary follow the *Dictionary of Statistical Terms*[22] published for the International Statistical Institute. Although statistical texts use the possessive form for most eponyms, the possessive form for eponyms is not used in AMA journals (see 13.0, Eponyms).

abscissa: horizontal or x-axis of a graph.

absolute risk: probability of an event occurring during a specified period. The absolute risk equals the relative risk times the average probability of the event during the same time, if the risk factor is absent.[23(p327)] See absolute risk reduction.

absolute risk reduction: proportion in the control group experiencing an event minus the proportion in the intervention group experiencing an event. The inverse of the absolute risk reduction is the number needed to treat. See absolute risk.

accuracy: ability of a test to produce results that are close to the true measure of the phenomenon.[23(p327)] Generally, assessing accuracy of a test requires that there be a criterion standard with which to compare the test results. Accuracy encompasses a number of measures including reliability, validity, and lack of bias.

actuarial life-table method: see life table, Cutler-Ederer method.

adjustment: techniques used after the collection of data to control for the effect of known or potential confounding variables.[23(p327)] A typical example is adjusting a result for the independent effect of age of the subjects (age is the independent variable).

aggregate data: data accumulated from disparate sources.

agreement: statistical test performed to determine the equivalence of the results obtained by 2 tests when 1 test is compared with another (of which 1 is usually but not always a criterion standard).

⇒Agreement should not be confused with correlation. Correlation is used to test whether 2 variables are interdependent, whereas agreement tests whether 2 variables are equivalent. For example, an investigator compares results obtained by 2 methods of measuring hematocrit. Method A gives a result that is exactly twice that of method B. The correlation between A and B is perfect since A is always twice B, but the agreement is very poor; method A is not equivalent to method B (written communication, George W. Brown, MD, September 1993). One appropriate way to assess agreement has been described by Bland and Altman.[24]

algorithm: systematic process that consists of an ordered sequence of steps; each step depends on the previous step.[25(p6)] An algorithm may be used clinically to guide treatment decisions for an individual patient on the basis of the patient's clinical outcome or result.

α (alpha), α level: size of the likelihood acceptable to the investigators that a relationship observed between 2 variables is due to chance (the probability of a type I error); usually $\alpha = .05$. If $\alpha = .05$, $P \leq .05$ will be considered significant.

analysis: process of mathematically summarizing and comparing data to confirm or refute a hypothesis. Analysis serves 3 functions: (1) to test hypotheses regarding differences in large populations based on samples of the populations, (2) to control for confounding variables, and (3) to measure the size of differences between groups or the strength of the relationship between variables in the study.[23(p25)]

analysis of covariance (ANCOVA): statistical test used to examine data that include both continuous and nominal independent variables and a continuous dependent variable. It is basically a hybrid of multiple regression (used for continuous independent variables) and analysis of variance (used for nominal independent variables).[23(p299)]

analysis of residuals: see linear regression.

analysis of variance (ANOVA): statistical method used to compare a continuous dependent variable and more than one nominal independent variable. The null hypothesis in ANOVA is tested by means of the F test.

The most commonly used type of ANOVA is the 1-way ANOVA, in which there are more than 2 mutually exclusive categories for a nominal independent variable (eg, systolic blood pressure for the continuous variable and race/ethnicity as the nominal variable, categorized as non-Hispanic black, non-Hispanic white, or Hispanic). If there are 2 mutually exclusive categories for the nominal independent variable (eg, Hispanic or non-Hispanic), the 1-way ANOVA is equivalent to the *t* test.

A 2-way ANOVA is used if there are 2 categorical variables with a continuous variable (eg, systolic blood pressure for the continuous variable, with race/ethnicity categorized as non-Hispanic white, non-Hispanic black, or Hispanic, and age categorized as 20-40 years, 40-60 years, and 60 years and older as the 2 categorical variables). Three- and 4-way ANOVAs may also be performed.

If more than 1 nonexclusive independent variable is analyzed (eg, race and sex in addition to systolic blood pressure), the process is called factorial ANOVA. (An analysis of main effects in this analysis would assess the independent effects of either race or sex; an association between female sex and systolic blood pressure that exists in one race but not another would mean that an interaction between race and sex exists.)

If repeated measures are made on an individual (such as measuring blood pressure over time) so that a matched form of analysis is appropriate, but potentially confounding factors (such as age) are to be controlled for simultaneously, repeated-measures ANOVA is used. Randomized-block ANOVA is used if treatments are assigned by means of block randomization.[23(pp291-295)]

⇒ANOVA can establish only whether a significant difference exists among groups, not which groups are significantly different from each other. To determine which groups differ significantly, a pairwise analysis of a continuous dependent variable and more than 1 nominal variable is performed by the Newman-Keuls test or Tukey test. These multiple comparisons procedures avoid the potential of a type I error that might occur if the *t* test were applied at this stage.

⇒The F ratio is the statistical result of ANOVA and is a number between 1 and infinity. The F ratio is compared with tables of the F distribution, taking into account the α level and degrees of freedom (df) for the numerator and denominator, to determine the P value.

> *Example:* The difference was found to be significant by 1-way ANOVA ($F_{2,63} = 61.07$; $P < .001$).[26]

The *df* are provided along with the F statistic. The first subscript (2) is the *df* for the numerator; the second subscript (63) is the *df* for the denominator. The *P* value is obtained from an F statistic table that provides the *P* value that corresponds to a given F and *df*. Because ANOVA does not determine which groups are significantly different from each other, this example would normally be accompanied by the results of the multiple comparisons procedure.[26] Other models such as Latin square may also be used.

ANCOVA: see abbreviation for analysis of covariance.

ANOVA: see abbreviation for analysis of variance.

Ansari-Bradley dispersion test: rank test to determine whether 2 distributions known to be of identical shape (but not necessarily of normal distribution) have equal parameters of scale.[22(p6)]

area under the curve (AUC): technique used to measure the performance of a test plotted on a receiver operating characteristic (ROC) curve or to measure drug clearance in pharmacokinetic studies.[27(p12)] When measuring test performance, the larger the AUC, the better the test performance. When measuring drug clearance, the AUC assesses the total exposure of the individual, as measured by levels of the drug in blood or urine, to a drug over time. The curve of drug clearance used to calculate the AUC is also used to calculate the drug half-life.

⇒ The method used to determine the AUC should be specified (eg, the trapezoidal rule).

artifact: difference or change in measure of occurrence of a condition that results from the way the disease or condition is measured, sought, or defined.[23(p327)]

> *Example:* An artifactual increase in the incidence of acquired immunodeficiency syndrome (AIDS) was expected because the definition of AIDS was changed to include a larger number of AIDS-defining illnesses.

assessment: in the statistical sense, evaluating the outcome(s) of the study and control groups.

assignment: process of distributing individuals to study and control groups. See also randomization.

association: statistically significant relationship between 2 variables in which one does not necessarily cause the other. When 2 variables are measured simultaneously, association rather than causation generally is all that can be assessed.

> *Example:* After controlling for confounding factors by means of multivariate regression, a significant association remained between age and disease prevalence.

attributable risk: disease that can be attributed to a given risk factor; conversely, if the risk factor were eliminated entirely, the amount of the disease that could be eliminated.[23(pp327-328)] Attributable risk assumes a causal relationship (ie, the factor to be eliminated is a cause of the disease and not merely associated with the disease). An attributable risk of 1 indicates that the factor does not contribute, an attributable risk of less than 1 indicates that the factor reduces risk, and an attributable risk of greater than 1 indicates that the factor increases risk. See `attributable risk percentage` and `attributable risk reduction`.

attributable risk percentage: the percentage of risk associated with a given factor among those with the risk factor.[23(pp327-328)] For example, risk of stroke in an older person who smokes and has hypertension and no other risk factors can be divided among the risks attributable to smoking, hypertension, and age. Attributable risk percentage is often determined for a population and is the percentage of the disease related to the risk factor. See `population attributable risk percentage`.

attributable risk reduction: the number of events that can be prevented by eliminating a particular risk factor from the population. Attributable risk reduction is a function of 2 factors: the strength of the association between the risk factor and the disease (ie, how often the risk factor causes the disease) and the frequency of the risk factor in the population (ie, a common risk factor may have a lower attributable risk in an individual than a less common risk factor, but could have a higher attributable risk reduction because of the risk factor's high prevalence in the population). Attributable risk reduction is a useful concept for public health decisions. The inverse of attributable risk reduction is the `number needed to treat`, a number more useful for clinical practice. See also `attributable risk`.

average: sum of all measurements divided by the total number of measurements. Mathematically synonymous with `mean`, but mean is preferred since the term *average* is often used loosely.

Bayesian analysis: theory of statistics involving the concept of `prior probability`, conditional probability or `likelihood`, and `posterior probability`.[22(p16)] For interpreting studies, the prior probability is based on previous studies and may be informative, or, if none exists or those that exist are not useful, one may assume a `uniform prior`. The study results are then incorporated with the prior probability to obtain a posterior probability. Bayesian analysis can be used to interpret how likely it is that a positive result indicates presence of a disease, by incorporating the prevalence of the disease in the population under study and the sensitivity and specificity of the test in the calculation.

⇒Bayesian analysis has been criticized because the weight a particular study is given when prior probability is calculated can be a subjective decision, but the process most closely approximates how studies are considered when they are incorporated into clinical practice. When Bayesian analysis is used to assess posterior probability for an individual patient in a clinic population, the process may be less subjective than usual practice because the prior probability, equal to the prevalence of the disease in the clinic population, is more accurate than if the prevalence for the population at large were used.[20]

β (beta), β level: probability of showing no significant difference when a true difference exists; a false acceptance of the `null hypothesis`.[25(p57)] $1 - \beta$ is the statistical power of the test to detect a true difference, so the smaller the β, the greater the power. A value of .2 for β is equal to .8 or 80% power. A β of .1 or .2 is most frequently used in power calculations. The β error is synonymous with `type II error`.[26]

bias: situation or condition that causes a result to depart from the true value in a consistent direction. Bias refers to defects in study design (often selection bias) or measurement.[23(p328)] One method to reduce measurement bias is to ensure that the investigator measuring outcomes for a subject is unaware of the group to which the subject belongs (ie, blinded assessment).

bimodal distribution: nonnormal distribution with 2 peaks, or modes. The mean and median may be equivalent, but neither will describe the data accurately.

binary variable: variable that has 2 mutually exclusive subgroups, such as male/female or pregnant/not pregnant; synonym for dichotomous variable.[27(p75)]

binomial distribution: probability with 2 possible mutually exclusive outcomes; used for modeling cumulative incidence and prevalence rates[25(p17)] (for example, the probability of a person having a stroke in a given population over a given period; the outcome must be stroke or no stroke).

biological plausibility: evidence that an independent variable can be expected to exert a biological effect on a dependent variable with which it is associated. For example, studies in animals were used to establish the biological plausibility of adverse effects of passive smoking.

bivariable analysis: see bivariate analysis.

bivariate analysis: used when 1 dependent and 1 independent variable are to be assessed.[23(p263)] Common examples include the t test for 1 continuous variable and 1 binary variable and χ^2 test for 2 binary variables. Bivariate analyses can be used for hypothesis testing in which only 1 independent variable is taken into account, to compare baseline characteristics of 2 groups, or to develop a model for multivariate regression. See also univariate and multivariate analysis.

⇒Bivariate analysis is the simplest form of hypothesis testing but is often used incorrectly, either because it is used too frequently, resulting in an increased likelihood of a type I error, or because tests that assume a normal distribution (eg, the t test) are applied to nonnormally distributed data.

Bland-Altman plot: a method to assess agreement (eg, between 2 tests) developed by Bland and Altman.[24]

blinded (masked) assessment: evaluation or categorization of an outcome in which the person assessing the outcome is unaware of the treatment assignment. Masked assessment is the term preferred by some investigators and journals, particularly those in ophthalmology.

⇒ Blinded assessment is important to prevent bias on the part of the investigator performing the assessment, who may be influenced by the study question and consciously or unconsciously expect a certain test result.

blinded (masked) assignment: assignment of individuals participating in a prospective study (usually random) to a study group and a control group without the investigator or the subjects being aware of the group to which they are assigned. Studies may be single-blind, in which either the subject or the investigator does not know the treatment assignment, or double-blind, in which neither knows the treatment assignment. The term masked assignment is preferred by some investigators and journals, particularly those in ophthalmology.

block randomization: type of randomization in which the unit of randomization is not the individual but a larger group, sometimes stratified on particular variables such as age or severity of illness to ensure even distribution of the variable between randomized groups.

Bonferroni adjustment: statistical adjustment applied when multiple comparisons are made. The α level (usually .05) is divided by the number of comparisons to determine the α level that will be considered statistically significant. Thus if 10 comparisons are made, and α of .05 would become $\alpha = .005$ for the study. Alternatively, the *P* value may be multiplied by the number of comparisons, while retaining the α of .05.[27(pp31-32)] Alternatively, the *P* value may be multiplied by the number of comparisons, while retaining the α of .05. For example, a *P* value of .02 obtained for 1 of 10 comparisons would be multiplied by 10 to get the final result of $P = .20$, a nonsignificant result.

⇒The Bonferroni test is a conservative adjustment for large numbers of comparisons (ie, less likely than other methods to give a significant result) but is simple and used frequently.

bootstrap method: statistical method for validating a new diagnostic parameter in the same group from which the parameter was derived. Thus, the validation of the method is based on a simulated sample, rather than a new sample. The parameter is first derived from the entire group, then applied sequentially to subsegments of the group to see if the parameter performs as well for the subgroups as it does for the entire group (derived from "pulling oneself up by one's own bootstraps").[27(p32)]

For example, a number of prognostic indicators are measured in a cohort of hospitalized patients to predict mortality. To determine if the model using the indicators is equally predictive of mortality for subsegments of the group, the bootstrap method is applied to the subsegments and confidence intervals are calculated to determine the predictive ability of the model. The jackknife dispersion test also uses the same sample for both derivation and validation.

⇒ Although the preferable means for validating a model is to apply the model to a new sample (eg, a new cohort of hospitalized patients in the example listed), the bootstrap method can be used to reduce the time, effort, and expense necessary to complete the study. However, the bootstrap method provides less assurance than validation in a new sample that the model is generalizable to another population.

Brown-Mood procedure: test used with a regression model that does not assume normally distributed data or common variance of the errors.[22(p26)] It is an extension of the median test.

case: individual with the outcome or disease of interest.

case-control study: retrospective study in which subjects with the disease (cases) are compared with those who do not have the disease (controls). Cases and controls are identified without knowledge of exposure to the risk factors under study. Cases and controls are matched on certain important variables, such as age, sex, and year in which the individual was treated or identified. A case-control study conducted within a cohort study is referred to as a nested case-control study.[25(p111)] This type of case-control study may be an especially strong study design if characteristics of the cohort have been carefully ascertained. See also 17.2.4, Case-Control Study.

⇒ Cases and controls should be selected from the same population to minimize confounding by factors other than those under study. Matching cases and controls on too many characteristics may obscure the association of interest, since if cases and controls are too similar, their exposures may be too similar to detect a difference (see overmatching).

case-fatality rate: probability of death among people diagnosed as having a disease. The rate is calculated as the number of deaths during a specific period divided by the number of persons with the disease at the beginning of the period.[27(p38)]

case series: retrospective descriptive study in which clinical experience with a number of patients is described. See 17.2.6, Case Series.

categorical data: counts of members of a category or class; for the analysis each member or item should fit into only 1 category or class[22(p29)] (eg, sex or race/ethnicity). The categories have no numerical significance. Categorical data are summarized by means of proportions, percentages, fractions, or simple counts. Categorical data is synonymous with nominal data.

cause, causation: something that brings about an effect or result. To be distinguished from association, especially in cohort studies. To establish something as a cause it must be known to precede the effect. The concept of causation includes the contributing cause, the direct cause, and the indirect cause.

censored data: for continuous data, defining a cutoff for measuring or reporting data. Censoring data reduces the problem of extreme outliers skewing distribution of the data and is also used for individuals for whom the final outcome is not known, such as in survival analyses for individuals who have not experienced the outcome (usually death) at the time the analysis is conducted. The term left-censored data means that data were censored from the low end or left of the distribution; right-censored data come from the high end or right of the distribution[25(p26)] (eg, in survival analyses). For example, if data for falls are categorized as individuals who have 0, 1, or 2 or more falls, falls exceeding 2 have been right-censored.

central limit theorem: theorem that states that the mean of a number of samples with variances that are not large relative to the entire sample will increasingly approximate a normal distribution as the sample size increases. This is the basis for the importance of the normal distribution in statistical testing.[22(p30)]

central tendency: property of the distribution of data, usually measured by mean, median, or mode.[25(p41)]

χ^2 test (chi-square test): a test of significance based on the χ^2 statistic, usually used for categorical data. The observed values are compared with the expected values under the assumption of no association. The χ^2 goodness-of-fit test compares the observed with expected frequencies. The χ^2 test can also compare an observed variance with hypothetical variance in normally distributed samples.[22(p33)] In the case of a continuous independent variable and a nominal dependent variable, the χ^2 test for trend can be used to determine whether a linear relationship exists (for example, the relationship between systolic blood pressure and stroke).[23(p284-285)]

⇒ The *P* value is determined from χ^2 tables with the use of the specified α level and the *df* calculated from the number of cells in the χ^2 table. The χ^2 statistic should be reported to no more than 1 decimal place; if Yates correction was used, that should be specified. See also contingency table.

> *Example:* The exercise intervention group was least likely to have suffered a fall in the previous month ($\chi^2_3 = 17.7$, $P = .02$).

Note that the *df* for χ^2 (subscript 3) is specified; it is derived from the number of cells in the χ^2 table (for this example, 4 cells in a 2×2 table). The value 17.7 is the χ^2 value. The *P* value is determined from the χ^2 value and *df*.

choropleth map: map of a region or country that uses shading to display quantitative data.[25(p28)] See also 2.14, Manuscript Preparation, Figures.

chunk sample: subset of a population selected for convenience without regard to whether the sample is random or representative of the population.[22(p32)] A synonym is convenience sample.

Cochran *Q* test: method used to compare percentage results in matched samples, often used to test whether the observations made by 2 observers vary in a systematic manner. The analysis results in a *Q* statistic, which, with the *df*, determines the *P* value; if significant, the variation between the 2 observers cannot be explained by chance alone.[22(p25)] See also interobserver bias.

coefficient of determination: square of the correlation coefficient, used in linear or multiple regression analysis. This statistic indicates the proportion of the variation of the dependent variable that is explained by the independent variable.[23(p328)] If the analysis is bivariate, the correlation coefficient is r and the coefficient of determination is r^2. If the correlation coefficient is derived from multivariate analysis, the correlation coefficient is R and the coefficient of determination is R^2. See also correlation coefficient.

> *Example:* The sum of the R^2 values for age and body mass index was 0.23. [Twenty-three percent of the variance could be explained by those 2 variables.]

⇒ When R^2 values of the same dependent variable total more than 1.0 or 100%, then the independent variables have an interactive effect on the dependent variable.

coefficient of variation: ratio of the standard deviation [SD] to the mean. The coefficient of variation is expressed as a percentage and is used to compare dispersions of different samples. The smaller the coefficient of variation, the greater the precision.[26] The coefficient of variation is also used when the SD is dependent on the mean; eg, the increase in height with age is accompanied by an increasing SD of height in the population.

cohort: term to describe a group of individuals who share a common exposure, experience, or characteristic, or a group of individuals followed up or traced over time in a cohort study.[25(p31)]

cohort effect: change in rates that can be explained by the common experience or characteristic of a group or cohort of individuals. A cohort effect implies that a current pattern of variables may not be generalizable to a different cohort.[23(p328)]

Example: The decline in socioeconomic status with age was a cohort effect explained by fewer years of education among the older individuals.

cohort study: study of a group of individuals, some of whom are exposed to a variable of interest (eg, a drug treatment or environmental exposure), in which subjects are followed up over time to determine who develops the outcome of interest and whether the outcome is associated with the exposure. Cohort studies may be concurrent (prospective) or nonconcurrent (retrospective).[23(pp328-329)] See also 17.2.3, Cohort Study.

⇒ Whenever possible, a subject's outcome should be assessed by an individual(s) without knowledge of whether the subject was exposed (see `blinded assessment`).

concordant pair: pair in which both individuals have the same trait or outcome (as opposed to `discordant pair`). Used frequently in twin studies.[25(p35)]

conditional probability: `probability` that an event *E* will occur given the occurrence of *F*, called the conditional probability of *E* given *F*. The reciprocal is not necessarily true: the probability of *E* given *F* may not be equal to *F* given *E*.[27(p55)]

confidence interval (CI): range of numerical expressions within which one can be confident (usually 95% confident, to correspond to an α `level` of .05) the population value the study is intended to estimate lies.[23(p329)] The CI is an indication of the precision of an estimated population value.

⇒ Confidence intervals used to estimate a population value usually are symmetric or nearly symmetric around a value, but CIs used for relative risks and odds ratios may not be. Confidence intervals are preferable to `P values` since they convey information about precision as well as statistical significance. If the CI does not overlap 1, the result is significant ($P<.05$); if the CI overlaps 1, the results are consistent with the null hypothesis (equivalent to $P>.05$). If a CI value equals 1, then generally $P=.05$. In all cases, the point estimate should be contained within the CI (although if the CIs are very close to the point estimate, the rounded-off CI may be identical to the point estimate).

⇒ Confidence intervals are expressed with *to* or a hyphen separating the 2 values. To avoid confusion, hyphens are not used if 1 of the values is a negative number. Units that are closed up with the numeral are repeated for each CI; those not closed up are repeated only with the last numeral. See also 17.3, Significant Digits and Rounding Numbers, and 16.4, Numbers and Percentages, Use of Digit Spans and Hyphens.

Example: The odds ratio was 3.1 (95% CI, 2.2-4.8). The prevalence of disease in the population was 1.2% (95% CI, 0.8%-1.6%).

confidence limits (CLs): upper and lower boundaries of the `confidence interval`, expressed with a comma separating the 2 values.[25(p35)]

Example: The mean (95% confidence limits) was 30% (28%, 32%).

confounding: confounding has 3 possible meanings when used in a statistical sense: (1) the apparent effect of an exposure on risk is caused by an association with other factors that can influence the outcome; (2) the effects of 2 or more causal factors as observed by a set of data cannot be separated to identify the cause of any single causal factor; (3) the measure of the effect of an exposure on risk is distorted because of the association of exposure with another factor(s) that influences the outcome under study.[25(p35)] See also confounding variable.

confounding variable: variable that can cause or prevent the outcome of interest, is not an intermediate variable and is associated with the factor under investigation. Unless it is possible to adjust for confounding variables, their effects cannot be distinguished from those of the factors being studied. Bias can occur when adjustment is made for any factor that is caused in part by the exposure and also is correlated with the outcome.[25(p35)] Multivariate analysis is used to control the effects of confounding variables that have been measured.

contingency coefficient: the coefficient, *C*, is used to measure the strength of association between 2 characteristics in a contingency table.[27(pp56-57)]

contingency table: table created when categorical variables are used to calculate expected frequencies in an analysis and to present data, especially for a χ^2 test (2-dimensional data) or log-linear models (data with at least 3 dimensions). A 2×3 contingency table has 2 rows and 3 columns. The *df* are calculated as (number of rows − 1)(number of columns − 1). Thus, a 2×3 contingency table has 6 cells and 2 *df*.

continuous data: data with an unlimited number of equally spaced values[23(p329)] (eg, weight, systolic blood pressure, cholesterol), as opposed to categorical, nominal, ordinal, or dichotomous data. Parametric statistics require that continuous data have a normal distribution.

contributory cause: independent variable (cause) that is thought to contribute to the occurrence of the dependent variable (effect). That a cause is contributory should not be assumed unless all of the following have been established: (1) an association exists between the putative cause and effect, (2) the cause precedes the effect in time, and (3) altering the cause alters the probability of occurrence of the effect.[23(p329)] Other factors that may contribute to establishing a contributory cause include the concept of biological plausibility, the existence of a dose-response relationship, and consistency of the relationship when evaluated in different settings.

control: in a case-control study, the designation for an individual without the disease or outcome of interest; in a cohort study, the individuals not exposed to the independent variable of interest; in a randomized controlled trial, the group receiving a placebo or standard treatment rather than the intervention under study.

controlled clinical trial: study in which a group receiving an experimental treatment is compared with a control group receiving a placebo or an active treatment. See also 17.2.1, Randomized Controlled Trial.

convenience sample: sample of subjects selected because they were available for the researchers to study, not because they are necessarily representative of a particular population.

⇒Use of a convenience sample limits generalizability and can confound the analysis depending on the source of the sample. For instance, cardiac auscultation are compared with the results obtained from echocardiography and cardiac catheterization in a group of patients who have undergone all 3 procedures. The patients studied, simply by virtue of their having undergone cardiac catheterization and echocardiography, likely are not comparable to an unselected population.

correlation: description of the strength of an association among 2 or more variables, each of which has been sampled by means of a representative or naturalistic method from a population of interest.[23(p329)] The association is described by the `correlation coefficient`. See also `agreement`.

⇒ The `Kendall τ rank correlation` test is used when testing 2 ordinal variables: the `Pearson product moment correlation` is used when testing 2 normally distributed continuous variables, and the `Spearman rank correlation` is used when testing 2 nonnormally distributed continuous variables.[26]

⇒ Correlation is often depicted graphically by means of a scatterplot of the data (see 2.14, Manuscript Preparation, Figures). The more circular a scatter plot, the smaller the correlation; the more linear a scatterplot, the greater the correlation.

correlation coefficient: measure of the association between 2 variables. The coefficient falls between -1 and 1; the sign indicates the direction of the relationship and the number the magnitude of the relationship. A positive sign indicates that the 2 variables increase or decrease together; a negative sign indicates that one increases while the other decreases. A value of 1 or -1 indicates that the sample values fall in a straight line, while a value of 0 indicates no relationship.[19(p38)] The correlation coefficient should be followed by a measure of the significance of the correlation, and the statistical test used to measure correlation should be specified.

> *Example:* Body mass index increased with age (Pearson $r = 0.61$; $P < .001$); years of education decreased with age (Pearson $r = -0.48$; $P = .01$).

⇒ When 2 variables are compared, the correlation coefficient is expressed by r; when more than 2 variables are compared by multivariate analysis, the correlation coefficient is expressed by R. The symbol r^2 or R^2 is termed the `coefficient of determination` and indicates the amount of variation in the `dependent variable` that can be explained by knowledge of the `independent variable`.

cost-benefit analysis: economic analysis that compares the costs accruing to an individual for some treatment, process, or procedure and the ensuing medical consequences, with the benefits of reduced loss of earnings resulting from prevention of death or premature disability. The cost-benefit ratio is the ratio of marginal benefit (financial benefit of preventing 1 case) to marginal cost (cost of preventing 1 case).[25(p38)] See also 17.2.8, Cost-effectiveness Analysis, Cost-benefit Analysis.

cost-effectiveness analysis: comparison of interventions to determine which provides the most clinical value for the cost.[26] The preferred intervention is the one that will cost the least for a given result or be the most effective for a given cost.[25(pp38-39)] Outcomes are expressed by the cost-effectiveness ratio, such as cost per year of life saved. See also 17.2.8, Cost-effectiveness Analysis, Cost-benefit Analysis.

cost-utility analysis: form of economic evaluation in which the outcomes of alternative procedures are expressed in terms of a single utility-based measurement, most often the quality-adjusted life-year (QALY).[25(p39)]

Cox-Mantel test: method for comparing 2 survival curves that does not assume a particular distribution of data,[27(p63)] similar to the log-rank test.[28(p113)]

Cox proportional hazards regression model (Cox proportional hazards model): in survival analysis, a procedure used to determine relationships between survival time and treatment and prognostic independent variables such as age.[21(p290)] The hazard function is modeled on the set of independent variables without making assumptions that the hazard function is dependent on time. Estimates depend only on the order in which events occur, not on the times they occur.[27(p64)]

criterion standard: test considered to be the diagnostic standard for a particular disease or condition, used as a basis of comparison for other (usually noninvasive) tests. Ideally, the sensitivity and specificity of the criterion standard for the disease should be 100%. (A commonly used synonym, gold standard, is considered jargon,[25(p70)] and thus criterion standard is preferred.) See also diagnostic discrimination.

Cronbach α: index of the internal consistency of a test,[27(p65)] which assesses the correlation between the total score across a series of items and the comparable score that would have been obtained had a different series of items been used.[25(p39)] The Cronbach α is often used for psychological tests.

cross-design synthesis: method for evaluating outcomes of medical interventions, developed by the US General Accounting Office, that pools results from databases of randomized controlled trials and other study designs. It is a form of meta-analysis (see 17.2.7, Meta-analysis).[25(p39)]

crossover design: method of comparing 2 or more treatments or interventions. Individuals initially are randomized to 1 treatment or the other; after completing 1 treatment they are crossed over to the other randomization arm and undergo the other course of treatment. Advantages are that a smaller sample size is needed to detect a difference between treatments, since a paired analysis is used to compare the treatments in each individual, but the disadvantage is that an adequate washout period is needed after the initial course of treatment to avoid carryover effect from the first to the second treatment. Order of treatments should be randomized to avoid potential bias.[27(pp65-66)] See 17.2.2, Crossover Trial.

cross-sectional study: study that identifies subjects with and without the condition or disease under study and the characteristic or exposure of interest at the same point in time.[23(p329)] See 17.2.5, Cross-sectional Study.

⇒ Causality is difficult to establish in a cross-sectional study because the outcome of interest and associated factors are assessed simultaneously.

crude death rate: total deaths during a year divided by the midyear population. Deaths are usually expressed per 100 000 persons.[27(p66)]

cumulative incidence: number of people who experience onset of a disease or outcome of interest during a specified period; may also be expressed as a rate or ratio.[25(p40)]

Cutler-Ederer method: form of `life-table` analysis that uses actuarial techniques. The method assumes that the times at which follow-up ended (because of death or the outcome of interest) are uniformly distributed during the time period, as opposed to the `Kaplan-Meier method`, which assumes that termination of follow-up occurs at the end of the time block. Therefore, Cutler-Ederer estimates of risk tend to be slightly higher than Kaplan-Meier estimates.[23(p308)] Often an intervention and control group are depicted on 1 graph and the curves are compared by means of a `log-rank` test. This is also known as the actuarial method.

cut point: in testing, the arbitrary level at which "normal" values are separated from "abnormal" values, often selected at the point 2 SDs from the mean. See also `receiver operating characteristic curve`.[25(p40)]

data: collection of items of information.[25(p42)] (Datum, the singular form of this word, is rarely used.)

data dredging (aka "fishing expedition"): jargon meaning `post hoc analysis`, with no a priori `hypothesis`, of several variables collected in a study to identify which have a statistically significant association for purposes of publication.

⇒ Although post hoc analyses occasionally can be useful to generate hypotheses, data dredging increases the likelihood of a `type I error` and should be avoided. If post hoc analyses are performed, they should be declared as such and the number of post hoc comparisons performed specified.

decision analysis: process of identifying all possible choices and outcomes for a particular set of decisions to be made regarding patient care. Decision analysis uses epidemiologic data to estimate the likelihood of occurrence of each outcome. The process is displayed as a decision tree, with each node depicting a branch point representing a decision in treatment or intervention to be made (usually represented by a square at the branch point) or possible outcomes (usually represented by a circle at the branch point). The relative worth of each outcome may be expressed as a utility, such as the `quality-adjusted life-year`[25(p44)] (Figure 2).

degrees of freedom (*df*): see *df*.

dependent variable: outcome variable of interest in any study; the outcome that one intends to explain or estimate[23(p329)] (for example, death, myocardial infarction, or reduction in blood pressure). When investigating the dependent variable, `independent variables` that might modify the occurrence of the dependent variable (eg, age, sex, and other medical diseases or risk factors) are controlled for using `multivariate analysis.`

descriptive statistics: method used to summarize or describe data with the use of the `mean, median, SD, SE, or range`, or to convey in tabular form (eg, by using a histogram, shown in 2.14, Manuscript Preparation, Figures) for purposes of data presentation and analysis.[27(p73)]

***df* (degrees of freedom)** (*df* is not expanded at first mention): the number of independent comparisons that can be made among members of a sample. In a

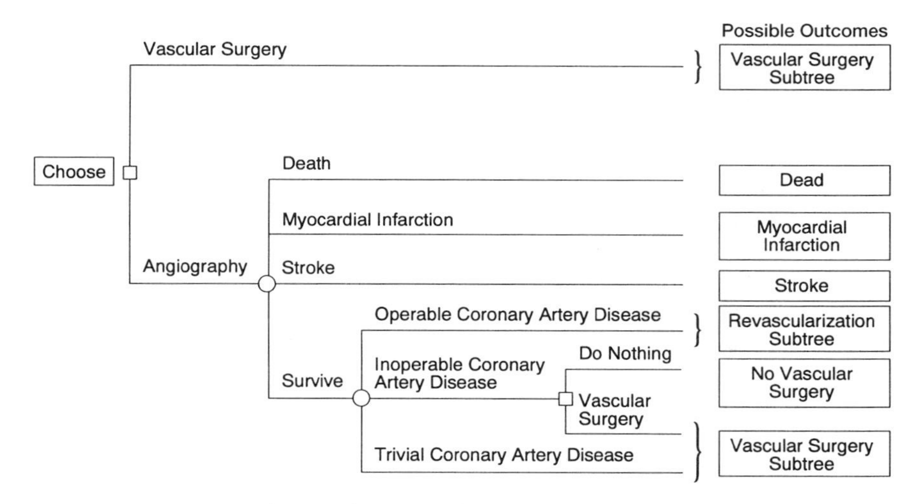

FIGURE 2 Decision tree showing decision nodes (squares) and chance outcomes (circles). End branches are labeled with outcome states. The subtrees to which the decision tree refers are depicted in a separate figure for simplicity. Adapted from Mason JJ, Owens DK, Harris RA, Cooke JP, Hlatky MA. The role of coronary angiography and coronary revascularization before noncardiac vascular surgery. *JAMA*. 1995;273:1919-1925.

contingency table, *df* is calculated as (number of rows − 1)(number of columns − 1).

⇒ The *df* should be reported as a subscript after the related statistic, such as the *t* test, analysis of variance, and χ^2 test (eg, $\chi^2_3 = 17.7$, $P = .02$; in this example, the subscript 3 is the number of *df*).

diagnostic discrimination: statistical assessment of how the performance of a clinical diagnostic test compares with the criterion standard. To assess a test's ability to distinguish an individual with a particular condition from one without the condition, the researcher must (1) determine the variability of the test, (2) define a population free of the disease or condition and determine the normal range of values for that population for the test (usually the central 95% of values, but in tests that are quantitative rather than qualitative, a receiver operating characteristic curve may be created to determine the optimal cut point for defining normal and abnormal), and (3) determine the criterion standard for a disease (by definition, the criterion standard should have 100% sensitivity and specificity for the disease) with which to compare the test. Diagnostic discrimination is reported with the performance measures sensitivity, specificity, positive predictive value, and negative predictive value, false-positive rate, and the likelihood ratio.[23(pp151-163)] See Table 2.

⇒ Because the values used to report diagnostic discrimination are ratios, they can be expressed either as the ratio, using the decimal form, or as the percentage, by multiplying the ratio by 100.

> *Example:* The test had a sensitivity of 0.80 and a specificity of 0.95; the false-positive rate was 0.05.

> *Or:* The test had a sensitivity of 80% and a specificity of 95%; the false-positive rate was 5%.

TABLE 2. DIAGNOSTIC DISCRIMINATION

Test Result	Disease by Criterion Standard	Disease-Free by Criterion Standard
Positive	a (true positives)	b (false positives)
Negative	c (false negatives)	d (true negatives)
	a + c = total number of persons with disease	b + d = total number of persons without disease
	Sensitivity $= \frac{a}{a+c}$	Specificity $= \frac{d}{b+d}$
	Positive predictive value $= \frac{a}{a+b}$	Negative predictive value $= \frac{d}{c+d}$

⇒When the diagnostic discrimination of a test is defined, the individuals tested should represent the full spectrum of the disease and reflect the population on whom the test will be used. For example, if a test is proposed as a screening tool, it should be assessed in the general population.

dichotomous variable: a variable with 2 possible answers (eg, male/female); synonym for binary variable.[27(p75)]

⇒ The variable may have a continuous distribution during data collection but is made dichotomous for purposes of analysis (eg, age < 65 years/age ≥ 65 years). This is done most often for nonnormally distributed data.

direct cause: contributory cause that is believed to be the most direct cause of a disease. The direct cause is dependent on the current state of knowledge and may change as more immediate mechanisms are discovered.[23(p330)]

Example: Although several other causes were suggested when the disease was first described, the human immunodeficiency virus is the direct cause of acquired immunodeficiency syndrome.

discordant pair: pair in which the individuals have different outcomes. In twin studies, only the discordant pairs are informative about the association between exposure and disease.[25(pp47-48)] Antonym is concordant pair.

discrete variable: variable that is counted as an integer; no fractions are possible.[27(p77)] Examples are numbers of pregnancies or surgical procedures.

discriminant analysis: analytic technique used to classify subjects according to their characteristics (eg, the independent variables, signs, symptoms, and diagnostic test results) to the appropriate outcome or dependent variable[27(pp77-78)] This is also referred to as discriminatory analysis[22(pp59-60)] and tests the ability of the independent variable model to correctly classify an individual in terms of outcome.

dispersion: degree of scatter shown by observations; may be measured by SD, quantile, or range.[22(p60)]

distribution: group of ordered values; the frequencies or relative frequencies of all possible values of a characteristic.[23(p330)] Distributions may have a normal distribution (bell-shaped curve) or a nonnormal distribution (eg, binomial or Poisson distribution).

dose-response relationship: relationship in which changes in levels of exposure are associated with changes in the frequency of an outcome in a consistent direction. This supports the idea that the agent of exposure (most often a drug) is responsible for the effect seen.[23(p330)] May be tested statistically by using a χ^2 test for trend.

Duncan multiple range test: modified form of the Newman-Keuls test for multiple comparisons.[27(p82)]

Dunnett test: multiple comparisons procedure intended for comparing each of a number of treatments with a single control.[27(p82)]

Dunn test: multiple comparisons procedure based on the Bonferroni adjustment.[27(p84)]

Durbin-Watson test: test to determine whether the residuals from linear regression or multiple regression are independent or, alternatively, are serially correlated.[27(p84)]

ecological fallacy: error that occurs when the existence of a group association is used to imply, incorrectly, the existence of a relationship at the individual level.[23(p330)]

effectiveness: extent to which a treatment is beneficial when implemented under the usual conditions of clinical care for a group of patients,[23(p330)] as distinguished from efficacy (the degree of beneficial effect seen in a clinical trial) and efficiency (the treatment effect achieved relative to the effort expended in time, money, and resources).

effect of observation: bias that results when the process of observation alters the outcome of the study.[23(p330)] See also Hawthorne effect.

effect size: observed or expected change in outcome as a result of an intervention. Expected effect size is used when the sample size necessary to achieve a given power is estimated, since, given a similar amount of variability, a large effect size will require a smaller sample size to detect a difference than will a smaller effect size.

efficacy: degree to which a treatment produces a beneficial result under the ideal conditions of an investigation,[23(p330)] usually in a randomized controlled trial; to be distinguished from effectiveness.

efficiency: effects achieved in relation to the effort expended in money, time, and resources. Statistically, the precision with which a study design will estimate a parameter of interest.[25(pp52-53)]

effort-to-yield measures: amount of resources needed to produce a unit change in outcome, such as number needed to treat[26]; used in cost-effectiveness and cost-benefit analyses. See 17.2.8, Cost-effectiveness Analysis, Cost-benefit Analysis.

error: difference between a measured or calculated value and the true value. Three types are seen in scientific research: a false or mistaken result obtained in a study; measurement error, a random form of error; and systematic error that skews results in a particular direction.[25(pp56-57)]

estimate: value or values calculated from sample observations that are used to approximate the corresponding value for the population.[23(p330)]

event: end point or outcome of a study; usually the dependent variable. The event should be defined before the study is conducted and assessed by an individual blinded to the intervention or exposure category of the study subject.

exclusion criteria: characteristics of potential study subjects that will exclude them from the study sample (such as being younger than 65 years, history of cardiovascular disease, expected to move within 6 months of the beginning of the study). Exclusion criteria are defined before subjects are enrolled.

explanatory variable: synonymous with independent variable, but preferred by some since *independent* in this context does not refer to statistical independence.[22(p98)]

extrapolation: conclusions drawn about the meaning of a study for a target population that includes types of individuals or data not represented in the study sample.[23(p330)]

factor analysis: procedure used to group related variables to reduce the number of variables needed to represent the data. This analysis is used to explain correlations among groups of variables or factors,[26] especially for developing scoring systems for rating scales and questionnaires.

false negative: negative test result in an individual who has the disease or condition as determined by the criterion standard.[23(p330)] See also diagnostic discrimination.

false-negative rate: proportion of test results found or expected to yield a false-negative result; equal to 1 − sensitivity.[26] See also diagnostic discrimination.

false positive: positive test result in an individual who does not have the disease or condition as determined by the criterion standard.[23(p330)] See also diagnostic discrimination.

false-positive rate: proportion of tests found to or expected to yield a false-positive result; equal to 1 − specificity.[26] See also diagnostic discrimination.

F distribution: ratio of the distribution of 2 normally distributed independent variables; synonymous with variance ratio distribution.[25(p61)]

Fisher exact test: assesses the independence of 2 variables by means of a 2×2 contingency table, used when the frequency in at least 1 cell is small[27(p96)] (usually <6). This test is also known as the Fisher-Yates test and the Fisher-Irwin test.[22(p77)]

fixed-effects model: model used in meta-analysis that assumes that differences in treatment effect in each study all estimate the same true difference. This is not often the case, but the model assumes that it is close enough to the truth that the results will not be misleading.[29(p349)] Antonym is random-effects model.

Friedman test: a nonparametric test for a design with 2 factors that uses the ranks rather than the values of the observations.[22(p80)] Nonparametric analog to analysis of variance.

Friedman urn model: an alternative to random allocation of patients in a clinical trial to avoid imbalance in the number of patients in each group when the number of subjects is small. The model considers an urn filled with balls; each color of ball represents a treatment arm of the study, and the number of balls of each color is proportional to the number of patients to be enrolled in that treatment arm. If the number of balls greatly exceeds the number of patients to be enrolled, selecting a ball to determine which treatment arm the patient will be enrolled in will approach random assignment. However, if the number of balls is similar to the total number of patients, after most of the balls have been selected the remaining balls will tend to even out the total number of patients in each treatment arm and treatment will not be based on random assignment.[27(p101)]

F test (score): alternative name for the variance ratio test,[25(p74)] which results in the F score. Often encountered in analysis of variance.[27(p101)]

> *Example:* There were differences by academic status in perceptions of the quality of both primary care training ($F_{1,682} = 6.71$, $P = .01$) and specialty training ($F_{1,682} = 6.71$, $P = .01$). [The numbers set as subscripts are the *df* for the analysis.]

Gaussian distribution: see normal distribution.

gold standard: see criterion standard.

goodness of fit: agreement between an observed set of values and a second set that is derived wholly or partly on a hypothetical basis.[22(p86)] The Kolmogorov-Smirnov test is one example.

group association: situation in which a characteristic and a disease both occur more frequently in 1 group of individuals than another. The association does not mean that individuals with the characteristic also have the disease.[23(p331)]

group matching: process of matching during assignment in a study to ensure that the groups have a nearly equal distribution of particular variables; also known as frequency matching.[23(p331)]

Hartley test: test for the equality of variances of a number of populations that are normally distributed, based on the ratio between the largest and smallest sample variations.[22(p90)]

Hawthorne effect: effect produced in an experiment because of the awareness of the study subjects that they are participating in a study. The term usually refers to an effect on the control group that changes the group in the direction of the outcome, resulting in a smaller effect size.[27(p115)] A related concept is effect of observation.

hazard rate, hazard function: theoretical measure of the likelihood that an individual will experience an event within a given period.[25(p73)] A number of hazard rates for specific intervals of time can be combined to create a hazard function.

heterogeneity: inequality of a quantity of interest (such as variance) in a number of groups or populations. Antonym is homogeneity.

histogram: graphical representation of data in which the frequency (quantity) within each class or category is represented by the area of a rectangle centered on the class interval. The heights of the rectangles are proportional to the observed frequencies. See also 2.14, Manuscript Preparation, Figures.

Hoeffding independence test: bivariate test of nonnormally distributed continuous data to determine whether the elements of the 2 groups are independent of each other.[25(p93)]

Hollander parallelism test: determines whether 2 regression lines for 2 independent variables plotted against a dependent variable are parallel. The test does not require a normal distribution, but there must be an equal and even number of observations corresponding to each line. If the lines are parallel, then both independent variables predict the dependent variable equally well. The Hollander parallelism test is a special case of the signed rank test.[22(p94)]

homogeneity: equality of a quantity of interest (such as variance) specifically in a number of groups or populations.[22(p94)] Antonym is heterogeneity.

homoscedasticity: statistical determination that the variance of the different variables under study is equal.[25(p78)] See also heterogeneity.

Hosmer-Lemeshow goodness-of-fit test: a series of statistical steps used to assess goodness of fit; approximates the χ^2 statistic.[30]

Hotelling *T* statistic: generalization of the *t* test for use with multivariate data; results in a *T* statistic. Significance can be tested with the variance ratio distribution.[22(p94)]

hypothesis: supposition that leads to a prediction that can be tested to be either supported or refuted.[25(p80)] The null hypothesis is that no such relationship exists, and any association is based strictly on chance. Hypothesis testing includes (1) generating the study hypothesis and defining the null hypothesis, (2) determining the level below which results are considered statistically significant, or α level (usually $\alpha = .05$), and (3) identifying and applying the appropriate statistical test to accept or reject the null hypothesis.

incidence: number of new cases of disease that occur over time,[25(p82)] as contrasted with prevalence, which is the total number of persons with the disease at any given time. Incidence is usually expressed as a percentage of individuals who will be affected during a year, or as a rate calculated as the number of individuals who develop the disease during a period divided by the number of person-years at risk.

Example: The incidence rate for the disease was 1.2 cases per 100 000 people per year.

inclusion criteria: characteristics a study subject must possess to be included in the study population (such as age 65 years or older at the time of study enrollment and willing and able to provide informed consent). Inclusion criteria are defined before subjects are enrolled.

independence, assumption of: assumption that the occurrence of 1 event is in no way linked to another event. Many statistical tests depend on the assumption that each outcome is independent.[25(p83)] This may not be a valid assumption if repeated tests are performed on 1 individual (eg, blood pressure is measured sequentially over time), if more than 1 outcome is measured for a given individual (eg, myocardial infarction and death or all hospital admissions), or if more than 1 intervention is made on the same individual (eg, blood pressure is measured during 3 different drug treatments). Tests for `repeated measures` may be used in those circumstances.

independent variable: variable postulated to influence the `dependent variable` within the defined area of relationships under study.[25(p83)] The term does not refer to statistical independence, so some use the term `explanatory variable` instead.[22(p98)]

Example: Age, sex, systolic blood pressure, and cholesterol were the independent variables entered into the multiple logistic regression.

indirect cause: contributory cause that acts through the biological mechanism that is the direct cause.[23(p331)]

Example: Overcrowding in the cities facilitated transmission of the tubercle bacillus and precipitated the tuberculosis epidemic. [Overcrowding is an indirect cause; the tubercle bacillus is the direct cause.]

inference: process of passing from observations to generalizations, usually with calculated degrees of uncertainty.[25(p85)]

Example: Intake of a high-fat diet was significantly associated with cardiovascular mortality; therefore, we infer that eating a high-fat diet increases the risk of cardiovascular death.

instrument error: error introduced in a study when the testing instrument is not appropriate for the conditions of the study or is not accurate enough to measure the study outcome[23(p331)] (may be due to deficiencies in such factors as calibration, `accuracy`, and `precision`).

intention-to-treat analysis, intent-to-treat analysis: analysis of outcomes for individuals based on the treatment arm to which they were randomized, rather than which treatment they actually received and whether they completed the study. The intention-to-treat analysis preserves the process of randomization and should be the main analysis of a randomized trial.[27(p125)] See 17.2.1, Randomized Controlled Trials.

⇒Although other analyses, such as evaluable patient analysis, are often performed to evaluate outcomes based on treatment actually received, the intention-to-treat analysis should be presented regardless of other analyses because the intervention may influence whether treatment was changed and whether subjects dropped out.

interaction: see `interactive effect.`

interaction term: variable used in `analysis of covariance` in which 2 independent variables interact with each other (for example, when assessing the effect of energy expenditure on cardiac output, the increase in cardiac output per unit increase in energy expenditure might differ between men and women; the interaction term would enable the analysis to take this difference into account).[23(p301)]

interactive effect: effect of 2 or more `independent variables` on a `dependent variable` in which the effect of an independent variable is influenced by the presence of another.[22(p101)] The interactive effect may be additive (ie, equal to the sum of the 2 effects present separately), synergistic (ie, the 2 effects together have a greater effect than the sum of the effects present separately), or antagonistic (ie, the 2 effects together have a smaller effect than the sum of the effects present separately).

interim analysis: data analysis carried out during a clinical trial to monitor treatment effects. Interim analysis should be determined as part of the study protocol prior to patient enrollment and specify the `stopping rules` if a particular treatment effect is reached.[3(p130)]

interobserver bias: likelihood that one observer is more likely to give a particular response than another observer because of factors unique to the observer or instrument. For example, one physician may be more likely than another to identify a particular set of signs and symptoms as indicative of religious preoccupation on the basis of his or her beliefs, or a physician may be less likely than another physician to diagnose alcoholism in a patient because of the physician's expectations.[28(p25)] The `Cochran Q test` is used to assess interobserver bias.[28(p25)]

interobserver reliability: test used to measure agreement among observers about a particular measure or outcome.

⇒Although the proportion of times that 2 observers agree can be reported, this does not take into account the number of times they would have agreed by chance alone. For example, if 2 observers must decide whether a factor is present or absent, they should agree 50% of the time according to chance. The κ statistic assesses agreement while taking chance into account and is described by the equation [(observed agreement) − (agreement expected by chance)]/(1 − agreement expected by chance). The value of κ may range from 0 (poor agreement) to 1 (perfect agreement) and may be classified by various descriptive terms, such as slight (0-0.20), fair (0.21-0.40), moderate (0.41-0.60), substantial (0.61-0.80), and near perfect (0.81-0.99).[28(pp27-29)]

⇒ In cases in which disagreement may render especially grave consequences, such as one pathologist rating a slide "negative" and another rating a slide "invasive carcinoma," a weighted κ may be used to grade disagreement according to the severity of the consequences.[28(p29)] See also Pearson product moment correlation.

interobserver variation: see interobserver reliability.

interquartile range: range used to describe the dispersion of values; describes the variate distance between the upper and lower quartiles. This and other quantiles are used to describe nonnormally distributed data, since SD does not accurately describe such data. The interquartile range describes the inner 50% of values; the interquintile range describes the inner 60% of values; the interdecile range describes the inner 80% of values.[22(pp102-103)]

interrater reliability: reproducibility among raters or observers; synonymous with interobserver reliability.

interval estimate: see confidence interval.[23(p331)]

intraobserver reliability (or variation): reliability (or, conversely, variation) in measurements by the same person at different times.[23(p331)] Similar to interobserver reliability, intraobserver reliability is the agreement between measurements by 1 individual beyond that expected by chance and can be measured by means of the κ statistic or the Pearson product moment correlation.

intrarater reliability: synonym for intraobserver reliability.

jackknife dispersion test: technique for estimating the variance and bias of an estimator, applied to a predictive model derived from a study sample to determine whether the model fits subsamples from the model equally well. The estimator or model is applied to subsamples of the whole, and the differences in the results obtained from the subsample compared with the whole are analyzed as a jackknife estimate of variance. This method uses a single data set to derive and validate the model.[27(p131)]

⇒ Although validating a model in a new sample is preferable, investigators often use techniques such as jackknife dispersion or the bootstrap method to validate a model to save the time and expense of obtaining an entirely new sample for purposes of validation.

Kaplan-Meier method: nonparametric method of compiling life tables. Unlike the Cutler-Ederer method, the Kaplan-Meier method assumes that termination of follow-up occurs at the end of the time block. Therefore, Kaplan-Meier estimates of risk tend to be slightly lower than Cutler-Ederer estimates.[23(p308)] Often an intervention and control group are depicted on one graph and the curves are compared by a log-rank test. This method is also known as the product-limit method.

κ (kappa) statistic: statistic used to measure nonrandom agreement between observers or measurements.[25(p94)] See interobserver and intraobserver reliability.

Kendall τ (tau) rank correlation: rank correlation coefficient for ordinal data. The coefficient is τ.[27(p134)]

Kolmogorov-Smirnov test: comparison of 2 independent samples of continuous data without requiring that the data be normally distributed[27(p136)]; may be used to test goodness of fit.[26]

Kruskal-Wallis test: comparison of 3 or more groups of nonnormally distributed data to determine whether they differ significantly.[27(p137)] The Kruskal-Wallis test is a nonparametric analog of analysis of variance and generalizes the 2-sample Wilcoxon rank sum test to the multiple-sample case.[22(p111)]

kurtosis: the way in which a unimodal curve deviates from a normal distribution; may be more peaked (leptokurtic) or more flat (platykurtic) than a normal distribution.[27(p137)]

Latin square: form of complete treatment crossover design used for crossover drug trials that eliminates the effect of treatment order. Each patient receives each drug, but each drug is followed by another drug only once in the array. For example, in the following 4 × 4 array, letters A through D correspond to each of 4 drugs, each row corresponds to a patient, and each column corresponds to the order in which the drugs are given[3(p142)]:

	First Drug	*Second Drug*	*Third Drug*	*Fourth Drug*
Patient 1	C	D	A	B
Patient 2	A	C	B	D
Patient 3	D	B	C	A
Patient 4	B	A	D	C

See also 17.2.2, Crossover Trial.

lead-time bias: artifactual increase in survival time that results from earlier detection of a disease, usually cancer, during a time when the disease is asymptomatic. Lead-time bias produces longer survival from the time of diagnosis but not longer survival from the time of onset of the disease.[23(p331)] See also length-time bias.

⇒Lead-time bias may give the appearance of a survival benefit from screening, when in fact the increased survival is only artifactual. Lead-time bias is used more generally to indicate a systematic error arising when follow-up of groups does not begin at comparable stages in the natural course of the condition.

least significant difference test: test for comparing mean values arising in analysis of variance. An extension of the *t* test.[22(p115)]

least squares method: method of estimation, particularly in regression analysis, that minimizes the differences between the observed response and the values predicted by the model.[27(p140)] The regression line is created so that the sum of the squares of the residuals is as small as possible.

left-censored data: see censored data.

length-time bias: bias that arises when a sampling scheme is based on patient visits, because patients with more frequent clinic visits are more likely to be selected than those with less frequent visits. In a screening study of cancer, for example, screening patients with frequent visits is more likely to detect slow-growing tumors than would sampling patients who visit a physician only when symptoms arise.[27(p140)] See also lead-time bias.

life table: method of organizing data that allows examination of the experience of 1 or more groups of individuals over time with varying periods of follow-up. For each increment of the follow-up period, the number entering, the number leaving, and the number dying of disease or developing disease can be calculated. An assumption of the life-table method is that an individual not completing follow-up is exposed for half the incremental follow-up period.[27(p143)] (The Kaplan-Meier method and the Cutler-Ederer method are also forms of life-table analysis but make different assumptions about the length of exposure.) See Figure 3.

⇒ The *clinical life table* describes the outcomes of a cohort of individuals classified according to their exposure or treatment history. The *cohort life table* is used for a cohort of individuals born at approximately the same time and followed up until death. The *current life table* is a summary of mortality of the population over a brief (1- to 3-year) period, classified by age, often used to estimate life expectancy for the population at a given age.[25(p97)]

likelihood ratio: probability of getting a certain test result if the patient has the condition compared with the probability of getting the result if the patient does not have the condition. Calculated as sensitivity/(1 − specificity). The greater the likelihood ratio, the more likely that a positive test result will occur in a patient who has the disease. A ratio of 2 means a person with the disease is twice as likely to have a positive test result as a person without the disease.[26] The

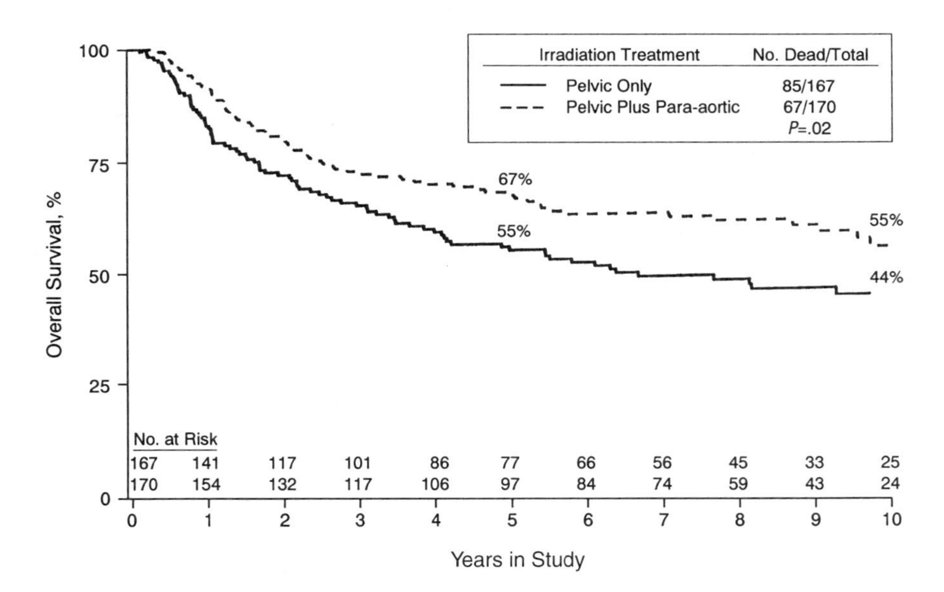

FIGURE 3 Survival curve showing outcomes for 2 treatments groups with number at risk at each time point. While numbers at risk are not essential to include in a survival analysis figure, this presentation conveys more information than the curve alone would. Adapted from Rotman M, Pajak TF, Choi K, et al. Prophylactic extended-field irradiation of para-aortic lymph nodes in stages IIB and bulky IB and IIA cervical carcinomas. *JAMA*. 1995;274:387-393.

likelihood ratio test is based on the ratio of 2 likelihood functions.[22(p118)] See also diagnostic discrimination.

Likert scale: scale often used to assess opinion or attitude, ranked by attaching a number to each response such as 1, strongly approve; 2, approve; 3, undecided or neutral; 4, disapprove; 5, strongly disapprove. The score is a sum of the numerical responses to each question.[27(p144)]

Lilliefors test: test of normality (using the Kolmogorov-Smirnov test statistic) in which mean and variance are estimated from the data.[22(p118)]

linear regression: statistical method used to compare continuous dependent and independent variables. When the data are depicted on a graph as a regression line, the independent variable is plotted on the x-axis and the dependent variable on the y-axis. The residual is the vertical distance from the data point to the regression line[26(p110)]; analysis of residuals is a commonly used procedure for linear regression. (See 2.14, Manuscript Preparation, Figures, Example F13.) This method is frequently performed using least squares regression.[21(pp202-203)]

⇒ The description of a linear regression model should include the equation of the fitted line with the slope and 95% confidence interval if possible, the fraction of variation in y explained by the x variables (correlation), and the variances of the fitted coefficients a and b (and their SDs).[21(p227)]

> *Example:* The regression model identified a significant positive relationship between the dependent variable weight and height (slope = 0.25; 95% CI, 0.19-0.31; $y = 12.6 + 0.25x$; $t_{451} = 8.3$, $P < .001$; $r^2 = 0.67$).[26]

[In this example, the slope is positive, indicating that as one variable increases the other increases; the t test with 451 *df* is significant; the regression line is described by the equation and includes the slope 0.25 and the constant 12.6, and the coefficient of determination r^2 demonstrates that 67% of the variance in weight is explained by the height.][26]

⇒ Four important assumptions are made when linear regression is conducted: the dependent variable is sampled randomly from the population, the spread or dispersion of the dependent variable is the same regardless of the value of the independent variable (this equality is referred to as homogeneity of variances or homoscedasticity), the relationship between the 2 variables is linear, and the independent variable is measured with complete precision.[23(pp273-274)]

location: central tendency of a normal distribution, as distinguished from dispersion. The location of 2 curves may be identical (means are the same) but the kurtosis may vary (one may be peaked and the other flat, producing small and large SDs, respectively).[31(p28)]

logistic regression: type of regression model used to analyze the relationship between a binary dependent variable (expressed as a natural log after a *logit transformation*) and 1 or more independent variables. Often used to determine the independent effect of each of several explanatory variables by controlling for several factors simultaneously in a multiple logistic regression analysis. Results are usually expressed by odds ratios or relative risks and 95% confidence intervals.[23(pp311-312)] (The multiple logistic regression equation may also be provided but is substantially more complicated than the linear regression equation.

Therefore, in AMA publications, the equation is generally not published but can be made available on request from authors. Alternatively, it may be placed in NAPS [see 2.10.6, Manuscript Preparation, National Auxiliary Publications Service (NAPS)] or on the World Wide Web.)

⇒To be valid, a multiple regression model must have an adequate sample size for the number of variables examined. A rough rule of thumb is to have at least 25 individuals in the study for each explanatory variable examined.

log-linear model: linear models used in the analysis of categorical data.[22(p122)]

log-rank test: method of using the relative death rates in subgroups to compare overall differences between survival curves for different treatments; same as the Mantel-Haenszel test.[22(pp122,124)]

main effect: estimate of the independent effect of an explanatory (independent) variable on a dependent variable in analysis of variance.[27(p153)]

Mann-Whitney test: nonparametric equivalent of the *t* test, used to compare ordinal dependent variables with either nominal independent variables or continuous independent variables converted to an ordinal scale.[25(p100)] Alternative name for Wilcoxon rank sum test.

MANOVA: multivariate analysis of variance.

Mantel-Haenszel test: another name for the log-rank test.

Markov process: process of modeling possible events or conditions over time that assumes that the probability that a given state or condition will be present depends only on the state or condition immediately preceding it and that no additional information about previous states or conditions would create a more accurate estimate.[27(p155)] If the assumptions are appropriate, it can be used instead of decision analysis.

masked assessment: synonymous with blinded assessment, preferred by some investigators and journals to the term *blinded*, especially in ophthalmology.

masked assignment: synonymous with blinded assignment, preferred by some investigators and journals to the term *blinded*, especially in ophthalmology.

matching: process of making study and control groups comparable with respect to factors other than the factors under study, generally as part of a case-control study. Matching can be done in several ways, including frequency matching (matching on frequency distributions of the matched variable[s]), category (matching in broad groups such as young and old), individual (matching on individual rather than group characteristics), and pair matching (matching each study individual with a control individual).[25(p101)]

McNemar test: form of the χ^2 test for binary responses in comparisons of matched pairs.[25(p103)] The ratio of discordant to concordant pairs is determined; the greater the number of discordant pairs with the better outcome being associated with the treatment intervention, the greater the effect of the intervention.[27(p158)]

mean: sum of values measured for a given variable divided by the number of values; a measure of central tendency appropriate for normally distributed data.[31(p29)]

⇒ If the data are not normally distributed, the median is preferred. See also average.

measurement error: estimate of the variability of a measurement. Variability of a given parameter (eg, weight) is the sum of the true variability of what is measured (eg, day-to-day weight fluctuations) plus the variability of the instrument or observer measurement, or variability caused by measurement error (error variability, eg, the scale used for weighing). The intraclass correlation coefficient R measures the relationship of these 2 types of variability: as the error variability declines with respect to true variability, R increases, up to 1 when error variance is 0. If all variability is a result of error variability, then $R = 0$.[28(p30)]

median: midpoint of a distribution chosen so that half the values for a given variable appear above and half occur below.[23(p332)] For nonnormally distributed data, the median provides a better measure of central tendency than does the mean, since it is less influenced by outlying values.[30(p29)]

median test: nonparametric rank-order test for 2 groups.[22(p128)]

meta-analysis: See 17.2.7, Meta-analysis.

mode: in a series of values of a given variable, the number that occurs most frequently; used most often when a distribution has 2 peaks (bimodal distribution).[31(p29)]

mortality rate: death rate described by the following equation: [(number of deaths during period) × (period of observation)]/(number of individuals observed). For values such as the crude mortality rate, the denominator is the number of individuals observed at the midpoint of observation. See also crude death rate.[27(p66)]

⇒ Mortality rate is often expressed in terms of a standard ratio, such as deaths per 100 000 persons per year.

Moses ranklike dispersion test: rank test of the equality of scale of 2 identically shaped populations, applicable when the population medians are not known.[22(p134)]

multiple analyses problem: problem that occurs when several statistical tests are performed on one group of data because of the potential to introduce a type I error. The problem is particularly an issue when the analyses were not specified as primary outcome measures. Multiple analyses can be appropriately adjusted for by means of a Bonferroni adjustment or any of several multiple comparisons procedures.

multiple comparisons procedures: any of several tests used to determine which groups differ significantly after another more general test has identified that a significant difference exists but not between which groups. These tests are intended to avoid the problem of a type I error caused by sequentially applying tests such as the *t* test not intended for repeated use.

⇒Some tests result in more conservative estimates (less likely to be significant) than others. More conservative tests include the Tukey test and the Bonferroni adjustment; the Duncan multiple range test is less conservative. Other tests include the Scheffé test, the Newman-Keuls test, and the Gabriel test.[22(p137)]

multiple regression: general term for multivariate analysis procedures used to estimate values of the dependent variable for all measured independent variables that are found to be associated. The procedure used depends on whether the variables are continuous or nominal. When all variables are continuous variables, multiple linear regression is used and the mean of the dependent variable is expressed using the equation $Y = \alpha + \beta_1\chi_1 + \beta_2\chi_2 + \ldots + \beta_k\chi_k$. When independent variables may be either nominal or continuous and the dependent variable is continuous, analysis of covariance is used. (Analysis of covariance often requires an interaction term to account for differences in the relationship between the independent and dependent variables.) When all variables are nominal and the dependent variable is time-dependent, life-table methods are used. When the independent variables may be either continuous or nominal and the dependent variable is nominal and time-dependent (such as incidence of death), the Cox proportional hazards model may be used. Nominal dependent variables that are not time-dependent are analyzed using logistic regression or discriminant analysis.[23(pp296-312)]

multivariable analysis: another name for multivariate analysis.

multivariate analysis: any statistical test that deals with 1 dependent variable and at least 2 independent variables. It may include nominal or continuous variables, but ordinal data must be converted to a nominal scale for analysis. The multivariate approach has 3 advantages over bivariate analysis: (1) it allows for investigation of the relationship between the dependent and independent variables while controlling for the effects of other independent variables, (2) it allows several comparisons to be made statistically without increasing the likelihood of a type I error, and (3) it can be used to compare how well several independent variables individually can estimate values of the dependent variable.[23(pp289-291)] Examples include analysis of variance, multiple (logistic or linear) regression, analysis of covariance, Kruskal-Wallis test, Friedman test, life table, and Cox proportional hazards model.

N: entire population under study.

> *Example:* We assessed the diagnoses of admission all patients admitted from the emergency department during a 1-month period (N = 127).

n: sample of the population under study.

> *Example:* Of the patients admitted from the emergency department (N = 127), the most frequent admission diagnosis was unstable angina (n = 38).

natural experiment: investigation in which a change in a risk factor or exposure occurs in one group of individuals but not in another. The distribution of individuals into a particular group is nonrandom and, as opposed to controlled clinical trials, the change is not brought about by the investigator.[23(p332)] The natural experiment is often used to study effects that cannot be studied in a controlled trial, such as the incidence of medical illness immediately after an earthquake. This is also referred to as a "found" experiment.

naturalistic sample: set of observations obtained from a sample of the population in such a way that the distribution of independent variables in the sample is representative of the distribution in the population.[23(p332)]

necessary cause: characteristic whose presence is required to bring about or cause the disease or outcome under study.[32(p332)]

negative predictive value: the probability that an individual does not have the disease (as determined by the criterion standard) if the test result is negative.[23(p334)] This measure takes into account the prevalence of the condition or the disease. A more general term is posttest probability. See diagnostic discrimination.

nested case-control study: case-control study in which cases and controls are drawn from a cohort study. The advantages of a nested case-control study over a case-control study are that the controls are selected from subjects at risk at the time of occurrence of each case that arises in a cohort, thus avoiding the confounding effect of time in the analysis, and that cases and controls are by definition drawn from the same population.[25(p111)] See also 17.2.4, Case-Control Study, and 17.2.3, Cohort Study.

Newman-Keuls test: type of multiple comparisons procedure, used to compare more than 2 groups, that first compares the 2 groups that have the highest and lowest means, then sequentially compares the next most extreme groups, and stops when a comparison is not significant.[33(p92)]

n-of-1 trial: randomized controlled trial that uses a single patient and an outcome measure agreed on by the patient and physician. The n-of-1 trial may be used by clinicians to assess which of 2 possible treatment options is superior for the individual patient.[32]

nominal variable: variable with named categories. If nominal data have more than 2 categories, the categories are not ordered (for example, gene alleles, race, or eye color). The nominal or discrete variable usually is assessed to determine its frequency within a population.[23(p332)] The variable can have either a binomial (equal chance for each category) or Poisson (the nominal event is extremely rare, eg, a genetic mutation) distribution.

nonconcurrent cohort study: cohort study in which an individual's group assignment is determined by information that exists at the time a study begins. The extreme of a nonconcurrent cohort study is one in which the outcome is determined retrospectively from existing records.[23(p332)]

nonnormal distribution: data that do not have a normal (bell-shaped curve) distribution; includes binomial or Poisson distribution.

⇒ Nonnormally distributed continuous data must be either transformed to a normal distribution to use parametric methods or, more commonly, analyzed by nonparametric methods.

nonparametric statistics: statistical procedures used for data that do not have a normal distribution. Nonparametric tests are most often used for ordinal or nominal data, or for nonnormally distributed continuous data converted to an ordinal scale[23(p332)] (for example, weight classified by tertile).

normal distribution: continuous data distributed in a symmetrical, bell-shaped curve with the mean value corresponding to the highest point of the curve. This distribution of data is assumed in many statistical procedures.[23(p330)] This is also called a Gaussian distribution.

⇒Descriptive statistics such as mean and SD can be used to accurately describe data only if the values are normally distributed or can be transformed into a normal distribution. Parametric statistics assume that data are normally distributed.

normal range: measure of the range of values on a particular test among those without the disease. Cut points for abnormal tests are arbitrary and are often defined as the central 95% of values, or the mean of values ±2 SDs.

null hypothesis: the assertion that no true association or difference in the study outcome or comparison of interest between comparison groups exists in the larger population from which the study samples are obtained.[23(p332)] The hypothesis is expressed as the null hypothesis to be proved (no significant difference) or disproved (a statistically significant difference) by statistical analysis.

number needed to treat (NNT): number of patients who must be treated with an intervention for a specific period of time to prevent 1 bad outcome or result in 1 good outcome.[23(pp332-333)] The NNT is the reciprocal of the absolute risk reduction, the difference between event rates in the intervention and placebo groups in a clinical trial.

⇒ The study patients from whom the NNT is calculated should be representative of the population to whom the numbers will be applied. The NNT does not take into account adverse effects of the intervention.

odds ratio (OR): ratio of 2 odds. Odds ratio may have different definitions depending on the study and therefore should be defined. For example, it may be the odds of having the disease if a particular risk factor is present to the odds of not having the disease if the risk factor is not present, or the odds of having a risk factor present if the person has the disease to the odds of the risk factor being absent if the person does not have the disease.

The odds ratio typically is used for a case-control or cohort study. For a study of incident cases with an infrequent disease (for example, <2% incidence), the odds ratio approximates the relative risk.[25(p118)]

⇒ The odds ratio is usually expressed by a point estimate and 95% confidence interval (CI). An odds ratio for which the CI includes 1 indicates no statistically significant effect on risk; if the point estimate and CI are both less than 1, there is a statistically significant reduction in risk; if the point estimate and CI are both greater than 1, there is a statistically significant increase in risk.

1-tailed test: test of statistical significance in which deviations from the null hypothesis in only 1 direction are considered.[23(p333)] Most commonly used for the *t* test.

⇒One-tailed tests are more likely to produce a statistically significant result than are 2-tailed tests. Since the use of a 1-tailed test implies that the intervention could have only 1 direction of effect, ie, beneficial or harmful, the justification for the use of a 1-tailed test must be provided.

ordinal data: type of data with a limited number of categories with an inherent ordering of the category from lowest to highest, but without fixed or equal spacing between increments.[23(p333)] Examples are Apgar scores, heart murmur rating, and cancer stage and grade. Discrete variables, such as family size, parity, or number of teeth, are special forms of ordinal data. Ordinal data can be summarized by means of the median and quantiles or range.

⇒ Since increments between the numbers for ordinal data generally are not fixed (eg, the difference between a grade 1 and a grade 2 heart murmur is not quantitatively the same as the difference between a grade 3 and a grade 4 heart murmur), ordinal data should be analyzed by nonparametric statistics.

ordinate: vertical or y-axis of a graph.

outcome: dependent variable or end point of an investigation. In retrospective studies such as case-control studies, the outcome occurs before the study; in prospective studies such as cohort studies and controlled trials, the outcome occurs during the study.[23(p333)]

outliers (outlying values): values at the extremes of a distribution. The median is preferred to describe data with outliers that influence the mean.

⇒If outliers are excluded from an analysis, the exclusion should be explained in the text.

overmatching: obscuring by the matching process of a case-control study a true causal relationship between the independent and dependent variables because the variable used for matching is strongly related to the mechanism by which the independent variable exerts its effect.[25(pp119-120)] For example, matching cases and controls on residence within a certain area could obscure an environmental cause of a disease. Overmatching may also be used to refer to matching on variables that have no effect on the dependent variable, and therefore are unnecessary, or the use of so many variables for matching that no suitable controls can be found.[25(p120)]

paired samples: form of matching that can include self-pairing, when each subject serves as his or her own control, or artificial pairing, when 2 subjects are matched on prognostic variables.[27(p186)] Paired analyses provide greater power to detect a difference for a given sample size than do nonpaired analyses, since interindividual differences are minimized or eliminated. Pairing may also be used to match subjects in case-control or cohort studies. See Table 3.

paired *t* test: *t* test for paired data.

parameter: measurable characteristic of a population. One purpose of statistical analysis is to estimate population parameters from sample observations.[23(p333)] The statistic is the numerical characteristic of the sample; the parameter is the numerical characteristic of the population. *Parameter* is also used to refer to aspects of a model (eg, a regression model).

parametric statistics: tests used for continuous data and that require the assumption that the data being tested are `normally distributed`, either as collected initially or after transformation to the ln or log of the value or other mathematical conversion.[25(p121)] The `t test` is a parametric statistic. See Table 3.

Pearson product moment correlation: test of `correlation` between 2 groups of normally distributed data. See `diagnostic discrimination`.

point estimate: single value calculated from sample observations that is used as the estimate of the population value, or parameter[23(p333)]; in most circumstances accompanied by an interval estimate (eg, 95% confidence interval).

Poisson distribution: distribution that occurs when a `nominal` event (often disease or death) occurs rarely.[25(p125)] The Poisson distribution is used instead of a binomial distribution when sample size is calculated for a study of events that occur rarely.

population: any finite or infinite collection of subjects from which a sample is drawn for a study to obtain estimates to approximate the values that would be obtained if the entire population were sampled.[27(p197)]

population attributable risk percentage: percentage of risk within a population that is associated with exposure to the risk factor. Population `attributable risk` takes into account the frequency with which a particular event occurs and the frequency with which a given risk factor occurs in the population. Population attributable risk does not necessarily imply a cause-and-effect relationship. It is also called *attributable fraction, attributable proportion*, and *etiologic fraction*.[23(p333)]

positive predictive value: proportion of those with a positive test result who have the condition or disease as measured by the `criterion standard`. This measure takes into account the prevalence of the condition or the disease. Clinically, it is the probability that an individual has the disease if the test is positive[23(p334)] (synonym: `posttest probability`). See Table 2 and `diagnostic discrimination`.

posterior probability: in `Bayesian analysis`, the probability obtained after the `prior probability` is combined with the probability from the study of interest.[25(p128)] If one assumes a `uniform prior` (no useful information for estimating probability exists before the study), the posterior probability is the same as the probability from the study of interest alone.

post hoc analysis: analysis performed after completion of a study and not based on a hypothesis considered before the study. Such analyses should be performed without prior knowledge of the relationship between the `dependent` and `independent variables`. A potential hazard of post hoc analysis is the `type I error`.

⇒While post hoc analyses may be used to explore intriguing results and generate new hypotheses for future testing, they should not be used to test hypotheses, since the comparison is not hypothesis-driven. See also `data dredging`.

posttest probability: the probability that an individual has the disease if the test result is positive (positive predictive value) or that the individual does not have the disease if the test result is negative (negative predictive value).[23(p158)]

power: ability to detect a significant difference with the use of a given sample size and variance; determined by frequency of the condition under study, magnitude of the effect, study design, and sample size.[25(p128)] Power should be calculated before a study is begun. If the sample is too small to have a reasonable chance (usually 80% or 90%) of rejecting the null hypothesis if a true difference exists, then a negative result may indicate a type II error rather than a true acceptance of the null hypothesis.

⇒ Power calculations are important to perform when designing a study; a statement providing the power of the study should be included in the methods section of all randomized controlled trials (see Table 1) and is appropriate for many other types of studies. A power statement is especially important if the study results are negative, to demonstrate that a type II error was not the reason for the negative result. Performing a post hoc power analysis is controversial, especially if it is based on the study results, but, if included, it should be placed in the discussion section and the fact that it was performed post hoc clearly stated.

> *Example:* We determined that a sample size of 800 patients would have 80% power to detect the clinically important difference of 10% at $\alpha = .05$.

precision: inverse of the variance in measurement (see measurement error)[25(p129)]; the degree of accuracy with which an instrument can make measurements.

pretest probability: see prevalence.

prevalence: proportion of persons with a particular disease at a given point in time. Prevalence can also be interpreted to mean the likelihood that a person selected at random from the population will have the disease (synonym: pretest probability).[23(p334)] See also incidence.

principal components analysis: procedure used to group related variables to help describe data. The variables are grouped so that the original set of correlated variables is transformed into a smaller set of uncorrelated variables called the *principal components*.[25(p131)] Variables are not grouped according to dependent and independent variables, unlike many forms of statistical analysis. Principal components analysis is similar to factor analysis.

prior probability: in Bayesian analysis, the probability of an event based on previous information before the study of interest is considered. The prior probability may be informative, based on previous studies or clinical information, or not, in which case the analysis uses a uniform prior (no information is known before the study of interest). A *reference prior* is one with minimal information, a *clinical prior* is based on expert opinion, and a *skeptical prior* is used when large treatment differences are not expected.[27(p201)] When Bayesian analysis is used to determine the posterior probability of a disease after a patient has undergone a diagnostic test, the prior probability is the prevalence of the disease in the population from which the patient is drawn (usually the clinic or hospital population).

probability: in clinical studies, the number of times an event occurs in a study group divided by the number of individuals being studied.[23(p334)]

product-limit method: see Kaplan-Meier method.

proportionate mortality ratio: number of individuals who die of a particular disease during a span of time divided by the number of individuals who die of all diseases during the same period.[23(p334)] This ratio may also be expressed as a rate if corrected to a standard unit of time (eg, cardiovascular deaths per total deaths per year).

prospective study: study in which subjects with and without an exposure are identified and then followed up over time; the outcomes of interest have not occurred at the time the study commences.[27(p205)] *Prospective* is most commonly used in the context of a cohort study.

pseudorandomization: assigning of individuals to 1 of 2 groups in a nonrandom manner, eg, selecting every other individual for an intervention or assigning subjects by Social Security number or birth date.

publication bias: tendency of articles reporting positive and/or "new" results to be published, and studies with negative or confirmatory results to not be submitted or published; especially important in meta-analysis, but also in other systematic reviews. Substantial publication bias has been demonstrated from the "file-drawer" problem.[34]

purposive sample: set of observations obtained from a population in such a way that the sample distribution of independent variable values is determined by the researcher and is not necessarily representative of distribution of the values in the population.[23(p334)]

***P* value:** probability of obtaining the observed data (or data that are more extreme) if the null hypothesis were exactly true.[27(p206)]

⇒While hypothesis testing often results in the *P* value, *P* values themselves can only provide information about whether the null hypothesis is accepted or rejected. Confidence intervals (CIs) are much more informative since they provide a plausible range of values for an unknown parameter, as well as some indication of the power of the study as indicated by the width of the CI.[21(pp186-187)] (For example, an odds ratio of 0.5 with a 95% CI of 0.05-4.5 indicates to the reader the [im]precision of the estimate, whereas $P = .63$ does not provide such information.) Confidence intervals are preferred whenever possible. Including both the CI and the *P* value provides more information than either alone.[21(p187)] This is especially true if the CI is used to provide an interval estimate and the *P* value to provide the results of hypothesis testing.

⇒ When any *P* value is expressed, it should be clear to the reader what parameters and groups were compared, what statistical test was performed, and the degrees of freedom (*df*) and whether the test was 1-tailed or 2-tailed (if these distinctions are relevant for the statistical test).

⇒ For expressing *P* values in manuscripts and articles, the actual value for *P* should be expressed to 2 digits for $P \geq .01$, whether or not *P* is significant. (When rounding a *P* value expressed to 3 digits would make the *P* value nonsignificant, such as $P = .049$ rounded to .05, the *P* value can be left as 3 digits.) If $P < .01$,

P should be expressed to 3 digits. The actual P value should be expressed ($P = .04$), rather than expressing a statement of inequality ($P < .05$), unless $P < .001$. Expressing P to more than 3 significant digits does not add useful information to $P < .001$, since precise P values with extreme results are sensitive to biases or departures from the statistical model.[21(p198)]

P values should not be listed simply as not significant (NS), since for meta-analysis the actual values are important and not providing exact P values is a form of incomplete reporting.[21(p195)] Because the P value represents the result of a statistical test and not the strength of the association or the clinical importance of the result, P values should be referred to simply as statistically significant or not significant; terms such as highly significant or very highly significant should be avoided.

⇒The AMA style does not use a zero to the left of the decimal point, since statistically it is not possible to prove or disprove the null hypothesis completely when only a sample of the population is tested (P cannot equal 0 or 1, except by rounding). If $P < .00001$, P should be expressed as $P < .001$ as discussed. If $P > .999$, P should be expressed as $P > .99$.

qualitative data: data that fit into discrete categories according to their attributes, such as nominal or ordinal data, as opposed to quantitative data.[25(p136)]

qualitative study: form of study based on observation and interview with individuals that uses inductive reasoning and a theoretical sampling model, with emphasis on validity rather than reliability of results. Qualitative research is used traditionally in sociology, psychology, and group theory, but also occasionally in clinical medicine to explore beliefs and motivations of patients and physicians.[35]

quality-adjusted life-year (QALY): method used in economic analyses to reflect the existence of chronic conditions that cause impairment, disability, and loss of independence. Numerical weights representing severity of residual disability are based on assessments of disability by study subjects, parents, physicians, or other researchers made as part of utility analysis.[25(p136)]

quantile: method used for grouping and describing dispersion of data. Commonly used quantiles are the tertile (3 equal divisions of data into lower, middle, and upper ranges), quartile (4 equal divisions of data), quintile (5 divisions), and decile (10 divisions). Quantiles are also referred to as *percentiles*.[22(p165)]

⇒ Data may be expressed as median (quantile range), eg, length of stay was 7.5 days (interquartile range, 4.3-9.7 days). See also interquartile range.

quantitative data: data in numerical quantities such as continuous data or counts[25(p137)] (as opposed to qualitative data).

quasi-experiment: experimental design in which variables are specified and subjects assigned to groups, but interventions cannot be controlled by the experimenter. One type of quasi-experiment is the natural experiment.[25(p137)]

***r*:** correlation coefficient for bivariate analysis.

***R*:** correlation coefficient for multivariate analysis.

r^2: coefficient of determination for bivariate analysis. See also correlation coefficient.

R^2: coefficient of determination for multivariate analysis. See also correlation coefficient.

random-effects model: model used in meta-analysis that assumes that there is a universe of conditions and that the effects seen in the studies are only a sample, ideally a random sample, of the possible effects.[29(p349)] Antonym is fixed-effects model.

randomization: method of assignment in which individuals have a random chance of being assigned to a particular study or control. Individuals may be randomly assigned at a 2:1 or 3:1 frequency, in addition to the usual 1:1 frequency. Subjects may or may not be representative of a larger population.[23(p334)] Simple methods of randomization include coin flip or use of a random numbers table. See also block randomization.

randomized controlled trial: see 17.2.1, Randomized Controlled Trial.

random sample: method of obtaining a sample that ensures that every individual in the population has a known (but not necessarily equal, eg, in weighted sampling techniques) chance of being selected for the sample.[23(p335)]

range: the highest and lowest values of a variable measured in a sample.

> *Example:* The mean age of the participants was 45.6 years (range, 20-64 years).

rank sum test: see Mann-Whitney test or Wilcoxon rank sum test.

rate: measure of the occurrence of a disease or outcome per unit of time, usually expressed as a decimal if the denominator is 100 (eg, the surgical mortality rate was 0.02). See also 16.7.3, Numbers and Percentages, Proportions and Rates.

ratio: fraction in which the numerator is not necessarily a subset of the denominator, unlike a proportion[23(p335)] (eg, the assignment ratio was 1:2:1 for each drug dose [twice as many individuals were assigned to the second group as to the first and third groups]).

recall bias: systematic error resulting from individuals in one group being more likely than individuals in the other group to remember past events.[25(p141)]

⇒Recall bias is especially common in case-control studies that assess risk factors for serious illness in which individuals are asked about past exposures or behaviors, such as environmental exposure in an individual who has cancer.[23(p335)]

receiver operating characteristic curve (ROC curve): graphic means of assessing the extent to which a screening test can be used to discriminate between persons with and without disease,[25(p142)] and to select an appropriate cut point for defining normal vs abnormal results. The ROC curve is created by plotting sensitivity vs (1 - specificity). The area under the curve provides some

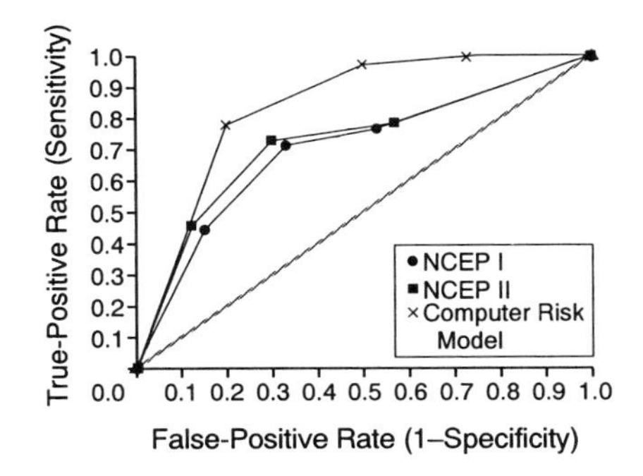

FIGURE 4 Receiver operating characteristic curve. The 45° line represents the point at which the test is no better than chance. The area under the curve measures the performance of the test; the larger the area under the curve, the better the test performance. Adapted from Grover SA, Coupal L, Hu X-P. Identifying adults at increased risk of coronary disease: how well do the current cholesterol guidelines work? *JAMA.* 1995;274:801-806.

measure of how well the test performs; the larger the area, the better the test. See Figure 4.

⇒ The appropriate cut point is a function of the test. A screening test would require high `sensitivity`, whereas a diagnostic test would require high `specificity`. See Table 2 and `diagnostic discrimination`.

reference group: group of presumably disease-free individuals from which a sample of individuals is drawn and tested to establish a range of normal values for a test.[23(p335)]

regression analysis: statistical techniques used to describe a `dependent variable` as a function of 1 or more `independent variables`; often used to control for `confounding variables`.[23(p335)] See also `linear regression`, `logistic regression`.

regression line: diagrammatic presentation of a `linear regression` equation, with the `independent variable` plotted on the x-axis and the `dependent variable` plotted on the y-axis. As many as 3 variables may be depicted on one graph.[25(p145)]

regression to the mean: principle that unusual events are unlikely to recur. A common example is blood pressure measurement; on repeated measurements individuals who are initially hypertensive often will have a blood pressure closer to the population mean than the initial measurement was.[23(p335)]

relative risk (RR): probability of developing an outcome within a specified period if a risk factor is present, divided by the probability of developing the outcome in that same period if the risk factor is absent. The relative risk is applicable to randomized clinical trials and `cohort studies`[23(p335)]; for `case-control studies` the `odds ratio` can be used to approximate the relative risk if the outcome is infrequent.

⇒ The relative risk should be accompanied by confidence intervals.

Example: The individuals with untreated mild hypertension had a relative risk of 2.4 (95% confidence interval, 1.9-3.0) for stroke or transient ischemic attack.

[In this example, individuals with untreated mild hypertension were 2.4 times more likely than the rest of the cohort to have a stroke or transient ischemic attack.]

relative risk reduction: proportion of the control group experiencing a given outcome minus the proportion of the treatment group experiencing the outcome, divided by the proportion of the control group experiencing the outcome.

reliability: ability of a test to replicate a result given the same measurement conditions, as distinguished from validity, which is the ability of a test to measure what it is intended to measure.[25(p145)]

repeated measures: analysis designed to take into account the lack of independence of events when measures are repeated in each subject over time (eg, blood pressure, weight, or test scores). This type of analysis emphasizes the change measured for a subject over time, rather than the differences between subjects over time.

repeated-measures ANOVA: see analysis of variance.

reporting bias: a bias in assessment that can occur when individuals in one group are more likely than individuals in another group to report past events. Reporting bias is especially likely to occur when different groups have different reasons to report or not report information.[23(pp335-336)] For example, when examining behaviors, adolescent girls may be less likely than adolescent boys to report being sexually active. See also recall bias.

reproducibility: ability of a test to produce consistent results when repeated under the same conditions and interpreted without knowledge of the first test results[23(p336)]; same as reliability.

residual: measure of the discrepancy between observed and predicted values. The residual SD is a measure of the goodness of fit of the regression line to the data and gives the uncertainty of estimating a point y from a point x.[22(p176)]

response rate: number of individuals who respond to a survey divided by the number of individuals who are contacted for the survey, usually expressed as a percentage.

⇒In general, response rates of less than 60% may not reflect the population surveyed and results may be unreliable.

retrospective study: study performed after the outcomes of interest have already occurred[25(p147)]; most commonly a case-control study, but also may be a retrospective cohort study or case series.

right-censored data: see censored data.

risk: probability that an event will occur during a specified period. Risk is equal to the number of individuals who develop the disease during the period divided by the number of disease-free persons at the beginning of the period.[23(p336)]

risk factor: characteristic or factor that is associated with an increased probability of developing a condition or disease. Also called a risk marker, a risk factor does not necessarily imply a causal relationship. A modifiable risk factor is one that can be modified through an intervention[25(p148)] (eg, stopping smoking or treating elevated cholesterol level, as opposed to a genetically linked characteristic for which there is no effective treatment).

robust: term used to indicate that a statistical procedure's assumptions (most commonly, normal distribution of data) can be violated without a substantial effect on its conclusions.[25(p149)]

root-mean-square: see `standard deviation`.

rule of three: method used to estimate the number of observations required to have a 95% chance of observing at least 1 episode of a serious adverse effect. For example, to observe at least 1 case of penicillin anaphylaxis that occurs in about 1 in 10 000 cases treated, 30 000 treated cases must be observed. If an adverse event occurs 1 in 15 000 times, 45 000 cases need to be treated and observed.[23(p114)]

sample: subset of a larger population, selected for investigation to draw conclusions or make estimates about the larger population.[34(p336)]

sampling error: error introduced by chance differences between the estimate obtained from the sample and the true value in the population from which the sample was drawn. Sampling error is inherent in the use of sampling methods and is measured by the `standard error`.[23(p336)]

Scheffé test: see `multiple comparisons procedures`.

SD: see `standard deviation`.

SE: see `standard error`.

SEE: see `standard error of the estimate`.

selection bias: bias in assignment that occurs when the way the study and control groups are chosen causes them to differ from each other by at least 1 factor that affects the outcome of the study.[23(p336)]

⇒A common type of selection bias occurs when individuals from the study group are drawn from one population (eg, patients seen in an emergency department or admitted to a hospital) and the control subjects are drawn from another (eg, clinic patients). Regardless of the disease under study, the clinic patients will be healthier overall than the patients seen in the emergency department or hospital and will not be comparable controls.

SEM: see `standard error of the mean`.

sensitivity: proportion of those with the disease or condition as measured by the `criterion standard` who have a positive test result (true positives divided by all positives).[23(p336)] See Table 2 and `diagnostic discrimination`.

sensitivity analysis: method to determine the robustness of an assessment by examining the extent to which results are changed by differences in methods, values of variables, or assumptions[25(p154)]; applied in decision analysis to test the robustness of the conclusion to changes in the assumptions.

signed rank test: see Wilcoxon signed rank test.

significance: statistically, the testing of an hypothesis that an effect is not present. A significant result rejects the null hypothesis. Statistical significance is highly dependent on sample size and provides no information about the clinical significance of the result. Clinical significance, on the other hand, involves a judgment as to whether the risk factor or intervention studied would affect a patient's outcome enough to make the intervention worthwhile. The level of clinical significance considered important is sometimes defined prospectively (often by consensus of a group of physicians) as the minimal clinically important difference, but the cutoff is arbitrary.

sign test: a nonparametric test of significance that depends on the signs (positive or negative) of variables and not on their magnitude; used when combining the results of several studies, as in meta-analysis.[25(p156)] See also Cox-Stuart trend test.

skewed distribution: asymmetric frequency distribution. Data for a given variable with a longer tail on the right of the distribution curve are referred to as positively skewed; data with a longer left tail are negatively skewed.[27(pp238-239)]

Spearman rank correlation (*ρ*): statistical test used to determine the covariance between 2 nominal or ordinal variables.[27(p243)] The nonparametric equivalent to the Pearson product moment correlation, it can also be used to calculate the coefficient of determination.

specificity: proportion of those without the disease or condition as measured by the criterion standard who have negative results by the test being studied[23(p326)] (true negatives divided by all negatives). See Table 2 and diagnostic discrimination.

standard deviation (SD; does not need to be expanded at first mention): commonly used descriptive measure of the spread or dispersion of data; the positive square root of the variance.[23(p336)] The mean ±2 SDs represents the middle 95% of values obtained.

⇒Describing data by means of SD implies that the data are normally distributed; if not, then the interquartile range or a similar measure is more appropriate to describe the data. If the interquantile range cannot be provided, and particularly if the mean ±2 SDs would be impossible (eg, length of stay 9 ± 15 days or age at evaluation 4 ± 5.3 days), it is preferable to use the format mean (SD) rather than the ± construction.[36]

standard error (SE; does not need to be expanded at first mention): positive square root of the variance of the sampling distribution of the statistic.[22(p195)] There are several types of SE; the type intended should be clear.

⇒The SE is not interchangeable with SD. The SD is a descriptive statistic; SE is an inferential statistic. In text and tables that provide descriptive statistics, SD is usually appropriate; in figures where the SE is frequently depicted for error bars, the 95% confidence interval is preferred (see 2.14, Manuscript Preparation, Figures).[37]

standard error of the difference: measure of the dispersion of the differences between samples of 2 populations, usually the differences between the means of 2 samples; used in the `t test`.

standard error of the estimate (SEE): SD of the observed values about the regression line.[22(p195)]

standard error of the mean (SEM): quantification of the certainty with which the mean computed from a random sample estimates the true mean of the population from which the sample was drawn.[33(p21)] If multiple samples of a population were taken, then 95% of the sample means (equal to the 95% `confidence interval`) would fall within the sample mean ±2 SEMs.

standard error of the proportion: SD of the population of all possible values of the proportion computed from samples of a given size.[33(p109)]

standardization (of a rate): adjustment of a rate to account for factors such as age or sex[23(pp336-337)]; also referred to as *age-adjusted rate*.

standardized mortality ratio: ratio in which the numerator contains the observed number of deaths and the denominator contains the number of deaths that would be expected in a comparison population. This ratio implies that confounding factors have been controlled for by means of indirect `standardization`. It is distinguished from `proportionate mortality ratio`, which is the mortality rate for a specific disease.[23(p337)]

standard normal distribution: `normal distribution` in which the mean has a `z score` of 0 and the SD has a z score of 1.[27(p245)] By definition, 68% of the curve is contained within 1 SD and 95% within 2 SDs. The `mean`, `median`, and `mode` are equal.

standard score: `z score`.[22(p196)]

statistic: value calculated from sample data that is used to estimate a value or parameter in the larger population from which the sample was obtained,[23(p337)] as distinguished from `data`, which refers to the actual values obtained via measurement, chart review, patient interview, and the like.

stochastic: type of measure that implies the presence of a random variable.[22(p197)]

stopping rule: rule, based on a test statistic or other function, specified as part of the design of the trial and established before patient enrollment, that specifies a limit for the observed treatment difference for the primary outcome measure, which, if exceeded, will lead to the termination of the trial or one of the study arms.[3(p258)] The stopping rules are designed to ensure that a study does not continue to enroll patients after a significant treatment difference has been demonstrated that would still exist regardless of the treatment results of subsequently enrolled patients.

stratification: division into groups. Stratification may be used to compare groups separated according to similar confounding characteristics. Stratified sampling may be used to increase the number of individuals sampled in rare categories of independent variables, or to obtain an adequate sample size to examine differences among individuals with certain characteristics of interest.[17(p337)] One example is stratified sampling of blacks and Hispanics in epidemiologic studies to ensure that adequate numbers of individuals are included for comparisons of study characteristics by race.

Student-Newman-Keuls test: see Newman-Keuls test.

Student *t* test: see *t* test. Student is not the name of the originator of the test; W. S. Gossett wrote under the name Student since his employment precluded individual publication.[25(p166)]

study group: in a controlled clinical trial, the group of individuals who undergo an intervention; in a cohort study, the group of individuals with the exposure or characteristic of interest; and in a case-control study, the group of cases.[23(p337)]

sufficient cause: characteristic that will bring about or cause the disease.[23(p337)]

supportive criteria: substantiation of the existence of a contributory cause. Potential supportive criteria include the strength and consistency of the relationship, the presence of a dose-response relationship, and biological plausibility.[23(p337)]

survey: method of study that depends on self-report, conducted with the use of a form mailed or otherwise distributed to individuals, or completed by an interviewer in person or on the telephone. A survey is used to collect information regarding an individual's demographic characteristics, medical history, attitudes, knowledge, and behaviors.[25(p163)] Methods that describe a survey should include how the survey was developed and performed, how the sample was selected, and the response rate.

⇒The most important factors to consider when a survey is assessed include the validity of the survey instrument, how the study sample was obtained, and the response rate. Measures of the validity of the survey instrument should be included in the methods section. The method of sampling (patients attending a clinic, individuals with a telephone, people responding to a mailing) affects the generalizability of the results. A low response rate (eg, $<60\%$) may also affect the generalizability of results, since those surveyed may not be representative of the population regardless of the representativeness of the initial sample.

⇒If more than one attempt to reach individuals was made, each response rate should be reported individually. If the overall response rate is low, a comparison can be made between the different waves of respondents. If significant differences exist between groups of respondents, the individuals who responded may not be representative of the overall group that was surveyed.

survival analysis: statistical procedures for estimating the survival function and for making inferences about how it is affected by treatment and prognostic factors.[25(p163)] See life table.

target population: group of individuals to whom one wishes to apply or extrapolate the results of an investigation, not necessarily the population studied.[23(p337)] If the target population is different from the population studied, whether the study results can be extrapolated to the target population should be discussed.

τ (tau): see Kendall τ rank correlation.

trend, test for: see χ^2 test.

trial: controlled experiment with an uncertain outcome[22(p208)]; used most commonly to refer to a randomized study.

true negative: negative test result in an individual who does not have the disease or condition as determined by the criterion standard.[23(p338)] See also Table 2.

true-negative rate: number of individuals who have a negative test result and do not have the disease by the criterion standard, divided by the total number of individuals who do not have the disease as determined by the criterion standard; usually expressed as a decimal (eg, the true-negative rate was 0.85). See also Table 2.

true positive: positive test result in an individual who has the disease or condition as determined by the criterion standard.[23(p338)] See also Table 2.

true-positive rate: number of individuals who have a positive test result and have the disease as determined by the criterion standard, divided by the total number of individuals who have the disease as measured by the criterion standard; usually expressed as a decimal (eg, the true-positive rate was 0.92). See also Table 2.

***t* test:** statistical test used when the dependent variable is continuous and the parameter of interest is the location of the variable. Use of the *t* test assumes that the variable has a normal distribution; if not, nonparametric statistics must be used.[23(p266)]

⇒ Usually the *t* test is unpaired, unless the data have been measured in the same individual over time. A paired *t* test is appropriate to assess the change of the parameter in the individual from baseline to final measurement; in this case the dependent variable is the change from one measurement to the next.

⇒ Presentation of the *t* statistic should include the degrees of freedom (*df*), whether the *t* test was paired or unpaired, and whether a 1- or 2-tailed test was used. Since a 1-tailed test assumes that the study effect has only 1 possible direction (ie, either beneficial or harmful), justification for use of the 1-tailed test must be provided. (The 1-tailed test is similar to testing at $\alpha = .10$ for a 2-tailed test and therefore is more likely to give a significant result.)

> *Example:* The difference was significant by a 2-tailed test for paired samples ($t_{15} = 2.78$, $P = .05$).

⇒ The *t* test can also be used to compare different coefficients of variation.

Tukey test: a type of multiple comparisons procedure.

2-tailed test: test of statistical significance in which deviations from the null hypothesis in either direction are considered.[23(p338)] For most outcomes, the 2-

tailed test is appropriate unless there is a plausible reason why only 1 direction of effect is considered and a 1-tailed test is appropriate. Commonly used for the *t* test.

2-way analysis of variance: see analysis of variance.

type I error: data demonstrating a statistically significant result, although no true association or difference exists in the population.[23(p338)] The α level is the size of a type I error that will be permitted, usually .05.

⇒A frequent cause of a type I error is performing multiple comparisons, which increase the likelihood that a significant result will be found by chance. To avoid a type I error, one of several multiple comparisons procedures can be used.

type II error: failure of the data to demonstrate a statistically significant result although a true association or difference exists in the population.[23(p338)]

⇒A frequent cause of a type II error is insufficient sample size. Therefore, a power calculation should be performed when a study is planned to determine the sample size needed to avoid a type II error.

uncensored data: continuous data reported as collected, without adjustment, as opposed to censored data.

uniform prior: assumption that no useful information regarding the outcome of interest is available prior to the study. See Bayesian analysis.

unity: number 1; a relative risk of 1 is a relative risk of unity, and a regression line with a slope of 1 is said to have a slope of unity.

univariable analysis: another name for univariate analysis.

univariate analysis: statistics involving 1 dependent variable and no independent variables; uses measures of central tendency (mean or median) and location or dispersion. The purpose of the analysis is to describe the sample, determine how the sample compares with the population, and determine whether chance has skewed 1 or more of the variables in the study. If the characteristics of the sample do not reflect those of the population from which the sample was drawn, the results may not be generalizable to the population.[23(pp245-246)]

unpaired analysis: method that compares 2 treatment groups when the 2 treatments are not given to the same individual. Most case-control studies also use unpaired analysis..

unpaired *t* test: see *t* test.

***U* test:** see Wilcoxon rank sum test.

utility: in decision theory and clinical decision analysis, a scale used to judge the importance of achieving a particular outcome (used in studies to quantify the importance of an outcome vs the discomfort of the intervention to a patient) or the discomfort experienced by the patient with a disease.[25(p170)] Commonly used methods are the *time trade-off* and the *standard gamble*. The result is expressed as a single number along a continuum from death (0) to full health or absence of disease (1.0). This quality number can then be multiplied by the number of years a patient is in the health state produced by a particular treatment to obtain the quality-adjusted life-year. See also 17.2.8, Cost-effectiveness Analysis, Cost-benefit Analysis.

validity (of a measurement): degree to which a measurement is appropriate for the question being addressed or measures what it is intended to measure. For example, a test may be highly consistent and reproducible over time, but unless it is compared with a criterion standard or other validation method, the test cannot be considered valid (see also diagnostic discrimination). *Construct validity* refers to the extent to which the measurement corresponds to theoretical concepts (eg, a measure thought to change over time does change). *Content validity* is the extent to which the measurement incorporates the domain under study (eg, a measurement to assess delirium evaluates cognition). *Criterion validity* is the extent to which the measurement is correlated with an external criterion of the phenomenon under study. Validity can be *concurrent* (assessed simultaneously) or *predictive* (eg, ability of a standardized test to predict school performance).[25(p171)]

⇒Validity of a test is sometimes mistakenly used as a synonym of reliability; the two are distinct statistical concepts and should not be used interchangeably.

validity (of a study): *internal validity* means that the observed differences between the control and comparison groups may, apart from sampling error, be attributed to the effect under study; *external validity* or generalizability means that a study can produce unbiased inferences regarding the target population, beyond the subjects in the study.[25(p171)]

Van der Waerden test: nonparametric test that is sensitive to differences in location for 2 samples from otherwise identical populations.[22(p216)]

variable: characteristic measured as part of a study. Variables may be dependent (usually the outcome of interest) or independent (characteristics of individuals that may affect the dependent variable).

variance: variation measured in a set of data for 1 variable, defined as the sum of squares of the deviation of each data point from the mean for the data, divided by the *df* (sample observation − 1).[27(p266)]

variance components analysis: process of isolating the sources of variability in the outcome variable for the purpose of analysis.

variance ratio distribution: synonym for F distribution.[25(p61)]

visual analog scale: scale used to quantify subjective factors such as pain or satisfaction. Subjects are asked to indicate where their current feelings fall by marking a straight line with 1 extreme, such as "worst pain ever experienced," at 1 end of the scale and the other extreme, such as "pain-free," at the other end. The feeling (eg, degree of pain) is quantified by measuring the distance from the mark on the scale to the end of the scale.[25(p268)]

TABLE 3. STATISTICAL METHODS FREQUENTLY USED TO TEST HYPOTHESES*

Scale of Measurement	2 Treatment Groups	3 or More Treatment Groups	Before and After 1 Treatment in the Same Individual	Multiple Treatments in the Same Individual	Association Between 2 Variables
Interval (assumes normally distributed data)†	Unpaired *t* test	Analysis of variance	Paired *t* test	Repeated-measures analysis of variance	Linear regression and Pearson product moment correlation
Nominal‡	χ^2 analysis-of-contingency table	χ^2 analysis-of-contingency table	McNemar test	Cochran *Q*	Contingency coefficients
	Fisher exact test if ≤ 6 in any cell	Fisher exact if ≤ 6 in any cell	Wilcoxon signed rank test	Friedman statistic	Spearman rank correlation
Ordinal	Mann-Whitney rank sum test	Kruskal-Wallis statistic			

* *Adapted with permission from Glantz SA.* Primer of Biostatistics. *2nd ed. New York, NY: McGraw-Hill Book Co Inc; 1981.*[33]

† *If data are not normally distributed, then rank the observations and use the methods for data measured on an ordinal scale.*

‡ *For a nominal dependent variable that is time dependent (such as mortality over time), use life-table analysis for nominal independent variables and Cox regression for continuous and/or nominal independent variables.*

Wilcoxon rank sum test: a nonparametric test that ranks and sums observations from combined samples and compares the result with the sum of ranks from 1 sample.[22(p20)] *U* is the statistic that results from the test. Alternative name for the Mann-Whitney test.

Wilcoxon signed rank test: nonparametric test in which 2 treatments that have been evaluated by means of matched samples are compared. Each observation is ranked according to size and given the sign of the treatment difference (ie, positive if the treatment effect was positive and vice versa) and the ranks are summed.[22(p220)]

Wilks λ (lambda): a test used in multivariate analysis of variance (MANOVA).

x-axis: horizontal axis of a graph. By convention, the dependent variable is plotted on the x-axis.

Yates correction: continuity correction used to bring a distribution based on discontinuous frequencies closer to the continuous χ^2 distribution from which χ^2 tables are derived.[25(p176)]

y-axis: vertical axis of a graph. By convention, the independent variable is plotted on the y-axis.

z-axis: third axis of a 3-dimensional graph, generally placed so that it appears to project out toward the reader. The z- and y-axes are both used to plot independent variables and are often used to demonstrate that the 2 independent variables each contribute independently to the dependent variable. See x-axis and y-axis.

***z* score:** score used to analyze continuous variables that represents the deviation of a value from the mean value, expressed as the number of SDs from the mean. This score is frequently used to compare children's height and weight measurements and for behavioral scores.[25(p176)]

17.5 ■ STATISTICAL SYMBOLS AND ABBREVIATIONS

■ STATISTICAL SYMBOLS AND ABBREVIATIONS.—The following may be used without expansion except where noted by an asterisk. For a term expanded at first mention, the abbreviation may be placed in parentheses after the expanded term and the abbreviation used thereafter (see also 11.11, Abbreviations, Clinical and Technical Terms). Most terms other than mathematical symbols can also be found in 17.4, Glossary of Statistical Terms.

Symbol or Abbreviation	*Description*
$\lvert x \rvert$	absolute value
Σ	sum
$>$	greater than
$\geq$	greater than or equal to
$<$	less than
$\leq$	less than or equal to

Symbol or Abbreviation	*Description*
^	hat, used to denote an estimate
ANOVA	analysis of variance*
ANCOVA	analysis of covariance*
α	alpha, probability of type I error
$1 - \alpha$	confidence coefficient
β	beta, probability of type II error; or population regression coefficient
$1 - \beta$	power of a statistical test
b	sample regression coefficient
CI	confidence interval*
CV	coefficient of variation $(s/\bar{x}) \times 100$*
D	difference
df	degrees of freedom (v is the international symbol[38] and also may be used if familiar to readers)
D^2	Mahalanobis distance, distance between the means of 2 groups
Δ	delta, change
δ	delta, true sampling error
ε	epsilon, true experimental error
e	exponential
$E(x)$	expected value of the variable x
f	frequency; or a function of, usually followed by an expression in parentheses, eg, $f(x)$
$F_{v_1,v_2}(1 - \alpha)$	F test, ratio of 2 variances, with $df = v_1, v_2$ for numerator and denominator, respectively, and $(1 - \alpha)$ = confidence coefficient
$G^2(df)$	likelihood ratio χ^2
H_0	null hypothesis
H_1	alternate hypothesis; specify whether 1- or 2-sided
κ	kappa statistic
λ_i	lambda, hazard function for interval i; eigenvalue; or estimate of parameter for log-linear models
Λ	Wilks lambda
ln	natural logarithm
log	logarithm to base 10
MANOVA	multivariate analysis of variance*
μ	population mean
n	size of a subsample

Symbol or Abbreviation	*Description*
N	total sample size
$n!$	(n) factorial
OR	odds ratio*
P	statistical probability
χ^2	Yates corrected χ^2 (1 *df*)
χ^2	χ^2 test
r	bivariate correlation coefficient
R	multivariate correlation coefficient
r^2	bivariate coefficient of determination
R^2	multivariate coefficient of determination
RR	relative risk*
ρ	rho, population correlation coefficient
S_D	standard deviation of a difference D
s^2	sample variance
σ^2	sigma squared, population variance
σ	sigma, population SD
SD	standard deviation of a sample
SE	standard error
SEM	standard error of the mean
t	Student t; specify α level, *df*, 1-tailed vs 2-tailed
τ	Kendall tau
T^2	Hotelling T^2 statistic
U	Mann-Whitney U (Wilcoxon) statistic
$\|x\|$	arithmetic mean
z	z score

ACKNOWLEDGMENTS

Principal author: Margaret A. Winker, MD

Dedicated to George W. Brown, MD, whose patient, but persistent, teaching led to this chapter.

Many thanks to John C. Bailar III, MD, PhD, Thomas B. Cole, MD, MPH, Theodore Colton, ScD, and Naomi Vaisrub, PhD, for reviewing this chapter.

REFERENCES

1. Partington A, ed. *The Oxford Dictionary of Quotations.* 4th ed. Oxford, England: Oxford University Press; 1992.

2. Begg C, Cho M, Eastwood S, et al. Improving the quality of reporting randomized controlled trials: the CONSORT statement. *JAMA.* 1996,276:637-639.

3. Meinert CL. *Clinical Trials Dictionary: Terminology and Usage Recommendations.* Baltimore, Md: Harbor Duvall Graphics; 1996.

4. Moher D, Olkin I. Meta-analysis of randomized controlled clinical trials: a concern for standards. *JAMA.* 1995;274:1962-1964.

5. Bailar JC III. The practice of meta-analysis. *J Clin Epidemiol.* 1995;48:149-157.

6. Shapiro S, Petitti DB, Greenland S. Meta-analysis of observational studies. *Am J Epidemiol.* 1994;140:771-791. Point/Counterpoint.

7. Chalmers TC, Lau J. Meta-analytic stimulus for changes in clinical trials. *Stat Methods Med Res.* 1993;2:161-172.

8. Sacks HS, Berrier J, Reitman D, Ancona-Berk VA, Chalmers TC. Meta-analyses of randomized controlled trials. *N Engl J Med.* 1987;316:450-455.

9. Jadad AR, McQuay HJ. Meta-analyses to evaluate analgesic interventions: a systematic qualitative review of their methodology. *J Clin Epidemiol.* 1996;49:245-243.

10. Dickersin K, Hewitt P, Mutch L, Chalmers I, Chalmers TC. Revising the literature: comparison of MEDLINE searching with a perinatal clinical trials database. *Control Clin Trials.* 1985;6:306-317.

11. Easterbrook PJ, Berlin J, Gopalan R, Matthews DR. Publication bias in clinical research. *Lancet.* 1991;337:867-872.

12. Dickersin K, Scerer R, Lefebvre C. Identifying relevant studies for systematic reviews. *BMJ.* 1994;309:1286-1291.

13. Gerbarg ZB, Horiwitz RI. Resolving conflicting clinical trials: guidelines for meta-analysis. *J Clin Epidemiol.* 1988;41:502-509.

14. Thompson SG. Why sources of heterogeneity in meta-analysis should be investigated. *BMJ.* 1994;309:1351-1355.

15. Bero L, Rennie D. The Cochrane Collaboration: preparing, maintaining, and disseminating systematic reviews of the effects of health care. *JAMA.* 1995;274:1935-1938.

16. Udvarhelyi IS, Colditz GA, Rai A, Epstein AM. Cost-effectiveness and cost-benefit analyses in the medical literature: are the methods being used correctly? *Ann Intern Med.* 1992;116:238-244.

17. Russell LB, Gold MR, Siegel JE, Daniels N, Weinstein MC. The role of cost-effectiveness analysis in health and medicine. *JAMA.* 1996;276:1172-1177.

18. Kassirer JP, Angell M. The *Journal*'s policy on cost-effectiveness analyses. *N Engl J Med.* 1994;331:669-670.

19. Drummond MF, Jefferson TO. Guidelines for authors and peer reviewers of economic submissions to the *BMJ*. *BMJ.* 1996;313:275-283.

20. Drummond MF, Richardson WS, O'Brien BJ, Levine M, Heyland D, for the Evidence-Based Medicine Working Group. Users' guides to the medical literature: how to use an article on economic analyses of clinical practice, A: are the results of the study valid? *JAMA.* 1996;277:1552-1557.

21. Bailar JC, Mosteller F. *Medical Uses of Statistics.* 2nd ed. Boston, Mass: NEJM Books; 1992.

22. Marriott FHC. *A Dictionary of Statistical Terms.* 5th ed. Essex, England: Longman Scientific & Technical; 1990.

23. Reigelman RK, Hirsch RP. *Studying a Study and Testing a Test.* 2nd ed. Boston, Mass: Little Brown & Co Inc; 1989.

24. Bland JM, Altman DG. Statistical methods for assessing agreement between two methods of clinical measurement. *Lancet.* 1986;1:307-310.

25. Last JM. *A Dictionary of Epidemiology*. 3rd ed. New York, NY: Oxford University Press; 1995.

26. Lang TA, Secic M. *Reporting Statistical Information in Medicine: Annotated Guide for Authors, Editors, and Reviewers*. Philadelphia, Pa: American College of Physicians; 1997.

27. Everitt BS. *The Cambridge Dictionary of Statistics in the Medical Sciences*. Cambridge, England: Cambridge University Press; 1995.

28. Everitt BS. *Statistical Methods for Medical Investigations*. 2nd ed. New York, NY: John Wiley & Sons Inc; 1994.

29. Ingelfinger JA, Mosteller F, Thibodeau LA, Ware JH. *Biostatistics in Clinical Medicine.* 3rd ed. New York, NY: McGraw-Hill Book Co Inc; 1994.

30. Hosmer DW, Lemeshow S. *Applied Logistic Regression.* New York, NY: John Wiley & Sons Inc; 1989.

31. Colton T. *Statistics in Medicine*. Boston, Mass: Little Brown & Co Inc; 1974.

32. Guyatt G, Sackett D, Taylow DW, et al. Determining optimal therapy: randomized trial in individual patients. *N Engl J Med.* 1986;314:889-892.

33. Glantz SA. *Primer of Biostatistics*. 2nd ed. New York, NY: McGraw-Hill Book Co Inc; 1981.

34. Scherer RW, Dickersin K, Langenberg P. Full publication of results initially presented as abstracts: a meta-analysis. *JAMA.* 1994;272:158-162.

35. Pope C, Mays N. Reaching the parts other methods cannot reach: an introduction to qualitative methods in health and health services research. *BMJ*. 1995;331:42-45.

36. Brown GW. a±b: keeping the meaning clear. *Diagn Med*. July/August 1983:1-3.

37. Brown GW. Standard deviation, standard error: which "standard" should we use? *AJDC.* 1982;136:937-941.

38. Geng D. Conventions in statistical symbols and abbreviations. *CBE Views*. 1992;15:95-96.

Additional Readings and General References

Friedman LM, Furberg CD, DeMets DL. *Fundamentals of Clinical Trials.* 3rd ed. St Louis, Mo: Mosby-Year Book Inc; 1996.

Norman GR, Streiner DL. *PDQ Statistics*. Philadelphia, Pa: BC Decker Inc; 1986.

Sackett DL, Haynes RB, Guyatt GH, Tugwell P. *Clinical Epidemiology: A Basic Science for Clinical Medicine*. 2nd ed. Boston, Mass: Little Brown & Co Inc; 1991.

Streiner DL, Norman GR. *PDQ Epidemiology*. 2nd ed. St Louis, Mo: Mosby-Year Book Inc; 1996.

CHAPTER 18

18.0 MATHEMATICAL COMPOSITION

Mathematical formulas and other expressions involving special symbols, character positions, and relationships may present difficulties in typesetting and in clarity. Careful markup (clarifying the symbols used and superior and inferior characters), avoidance of ambiguity through proper use of parentheses and brackets, and adherence to typographic conventions and capitalization rules in equations require special note (see also 6.5, Punctuation, Parentheses and Brackets, and 19.0, Typography).

18.1 ■ **COPY MARKING.**—It is essential to mark carefully each character, letter, and symbol that may be mistaken for another form (eg, x, X, χ^2, $\times 2$, $2x$, x_2).

The following examples show correct markup for complex relations between elements of equations:

Superior	x 2	x^2
Inferior	x 2	x_2
Inferior to superior	x x i	x^{x_i}
Superior to superior	x x 2	x^{x^2}
Inferior to inferior	x r i	x_{r_i}
Superior to inferior	x r 2 (set subscript directly under superscript)	x_{r^2}
Inferior with superior and subinferior	x 2 x i	$x_2^{x_i}$

Usually, in expressions that involve both superscripts and subscripts, the subscript is aligned directly under the superscript.

18.2 ■ **DISPLAYED VS RUN-IN.**—Simple formulas may remain in the text of the manuscript if they can be set on the line:

> The pulmonary vascular resistance index (PVRI) was calculated as follows: PVRI = (MPAP − PCWP)/CI, where MPAP indicates mean pulmonary artery pressure; PCWP, pulmonary capillary wedge pressure; and CI, cardiac index.

Long or complicated formulas should be centered on a separate line. In both cases, symbols and signs should be marked in detail. Such formulas may be handled either as copy or as prepared art, depending on the availability of special characters and use of software for equation preparation.

If there are numerous equations in a manuscript, or if equations are related to each other or are referred to after initial presentation, they should be numbered consecutively. Numbered equations should each be set on a separate line, centered, with the parenthetical numbers set flush left.

(1) $$x = r \cos \theta$$

(2) $$y = r \sin \theta$$

(3) $$z = (x + y)$$

Standard abbreviations should be used in expressing units of measure (see 11.12, Abbreviations, Units of Measure). For short, simple equations, it may be preferable to express an equation as words in the running text, rather than to set it off as an actual formula:

> Attributable risk is calculated by subtracting the incidence among the nonexposed from the incidence among the exposed.

18.3 ■ **STACKED VS UNSTACKED.**—A virgule should be used to avoid stacking of fractions unless "unstacking" sacrifices clarity (see 6.4.4, Punctuation, Virgule [Solidus], In Equations).

$$y = (x_1 + x_2)/(x_1 - x_2) \text{ instead of } y = \frac{x_1 + x_2}{x_1 - x_2}$$

Whenever a fraction is unstacked, parentheses or brackets, or both, should be used appropriately to avoid ambiguity. The expression

$$a + \frac{b + c}{d} + e,$$

if written as $a + b + c/d + e$, is ambiguous and could have several interpretations, such as

$$\frac{a + b + c}{d + e}$$

or

$$a + b + \frac{c}{d} + e.$$

The expression's meaning is unambiguous if set off as follows:

$$a + [(b + c)/d] + e.$$

18.4 ■ **EXPONENTS.**

18.4.1 ***Fractional Exponents vs Radicals.***—Use of radicals may sometimes be avoided by substituting a fractional exponent:

$$(a^2 - b^2)^{1/2} \text{ instead of } \sqrt{a^2 - b^2}.$$

As with unstacking fractions, if clarity is sacrificed by making the equation fit within the text, it is preferable to set it off.

For example, $E = 1.96\{[P(1 - P)]/m\}^{1/2}$ fits within the text, but the centered

$$E = 1.96\sqrt{\frac{P(1-P)}{m}}$$

might be more easily understood. Note the use of parentheses, brackets, and braces to remove ambiguity in unstacking fractions. In mathematical formulas, parentheses are the *innermost* symbol: {[( )]} (see 6.5.2, Punctuation, Brackets, In Formulas).

18.4.2 ***Negative Exponents.***—A negative exponent denotes the reciprocal of the expression, as illustrated in these examples:

$$x^{-n} = 1/x^n \qquad A^{-1} = 1/A \qquad B^{-2} = 1/B^2$$

A negative exponent may simplify some expressions within running text:

$$\frac{A}{(x+y)^2} \text{ may also be written as } A(x+y)^{-2}.$$

18.5 ■ LONG FORMULAS.

18.5 ■ **LONG FORMULAS.**—Long formulas may be given in 2 or more lines by breaking them at operation signs outside brackets or parentheses and keeping the indention the same whenever possible (since some formulas may be too long to permit indention).

$$\begin{aligned} Y = {} & [(a_1 + b_1)/(a_2 - b_2)] \\ & + [(\sigma_1 + \sigma_2)/(\sigma_2 - \sigma_1)] \\ & + [(s_1 + s_2)/(t_1 + t_2)] \end{aligned}$$

However, if a formula loses comprehensibility by being unstacked and broken up, and/or if it fits the width of the column, it is preferable to leave it stacked.

$$\text{Percent Excess Weight Loss} = \frac{\text{(Baseline Weight} - \text{Ideal Weight)} - \text{(Follow-up Weight} - \text{Ideal Weight)}}{\text{Baseline Weight} - \text{Ideal Weight}} \times 100$$

18.6 ■ **EXPRESSING MULTIPLICATION AND DIVISION.**—The product of 2 or more units of measure is conventionally indicated by a raised multiplication dot (·) (eg, 7 kg · m²). However, in scientific notation the times sign (×) is used (eg, 3×10^{-10} cm) (see 15.4.4, Units of Measure, Multiplication of Numbers). An asterisk should not be used to represent multiplication, despite its use in this role in computer programming languages. *Note:* However, there may be occasions on which the asterisk may be used to provide the reader with the exact equation used in the analysis (eg, regression models).

A virgule or solidus (/), a horizontal line, or a negative exponent may be used to express division of one unit by another, eg:

$$\mathrm{m/s} \quad \text{or} \quad \frac{\mathrm{m}}{\mathrm{s}} \quad \text{or} \quad \mathrm{m \cdot s^{-1}}$$

The virgule should not be used twice in the same expression. For example, the expression 2 mL/kg/min is unclear. Instead, use 2 mL/kg per minute. Negative exponents may also be used to clarify such an expression: 2 mL · $\mathrm{kg^{-1}}$ · $\mathrm{min^{-1}}$ (see 15.2.2, Units of Measure, Products and Quotients of SI Unit Symbols).

18.7 **■ COMMONLY USED SYMBOLS.**—Some commonly used symbols are as follows:

Symbol	*Description*
$>$	greater than
$\geq$	greater than or equal to
$>>$	much greater than
$<$	less than
$\leq$	less than or equal to
$<<$	much less than
$\pm$	plus or minus
$\int_a^b$	integral from value of a to value of b
$\sum_{a=1}^{\infty}$	summation from $a = 1$ to $a = \infty$
Δ	delta (change, difference between values)
f	function
$\neq$	not equal to
$\approx$	approximately equal to
$\sim$	similar to (reserve for use in geometry and calculus; use words in other cases where "approximately" is meant)
$\cong$	congruent to
$\equiv$	defined as
∞	infinity
!	factorial, eg, $n! = n(n - 1)\ (n - 2). . .1$

The following are examples of these commonly used mathematical expressions:

$>10^5$ CFUs/mL	24.5 ± 0.5	$L \approx 2 \times 10^{10}$ m
$f(x) = x + \Delta x$	$y = dx/dt$	$P < .01$
$\sum_{i=0}^{n} a_i x_i$	$\int_{10}^{13} 2x\, dx$	$F \sim \frac{m_1 m_2}{r^2}$
$r!(n - r)!$	$(e^x + e^{-x})/2$	
$\mathrm{kg \cdot m \cdot s^{-2}}$	$x + \frac{x^2}{2} + \frac{x^3}{3} + \frac{x^4}{4} + \ldots + \frac{x^n}{n}$	

18.8 ■ **TYPOGRAPHY AND CAPITALIZATION.**—In general, lines, variables, unknown quantities, and constants (eg, x, y, z, A, B, C) are set in italics, while units of measure (eg, kg, mL, s, m), symbols (including Greek characters [see 14.0, Greek Letters]), and numbers are set roman. Also, subscripts or superscripts used as modifiers are set roman: $\mathrm{C_{in}}$ = clearance of inulin. Arrays (**A**) and vectors (**V**) should be set boldface. Mathematical functions, such as sin, cos, ln, and log, are set roman.

$$\mathbf{V} = ai + bj + ck$$

$$\mathbf{A} = \begin{bmatrix} a_{11} & a_{12} & a_{13} \\ a_{21} & a_{22} & a_{23} \\ a_{31} & a_{32} & a_{33} \end{bmatrix}$$

For equations that are set off from the text, the words and letters should be set roman and the equation should be capitalized by the same rules that apply to titles (see 8.4, Capitalization, Titles and Headings):

$$U = \frac{\text{Efficacy}}{\text{Toxicity} - \text{Risk}} \times \frac{\text{Money Saved by Its Use}}{\text{Cost of Contrast Medium}}$$

$$\text{Age-Specific Attributable Risk} = (\text{RR}_i - 1)/\text{RR}_i$$

18.9 ■ **PUNCTUATION.**—Punctuation after a set-off equation is helpful and often clarifies the meaning. Display equations are often preceded by punctuation.

> In the linear quadratic equation model, the survival probability for cells receiving an increment of radiation, D_i, is as follows:
>
> $$S = e^{(-\alpha D_i - \beta D_i{}^2)},$$
>
> where α and β are the parameters of the linear quadratic equation model.

Do not use periods after a set-off equation if the equation is preceded by a period.

18.10 ■ **SPACING WITH MATHEMATICAL SYMBOLS.**—The AMA uses a thin space before and after the following mathematical symbols: $\pm$, $=$, $+$, $-$, $\div$, $\times$, $\cdot$, $\approx$, and $\sim$.

$$a \pm b \qquad a = b \qquad a + b \qquad a - b \qquad a \div b \qquad a \times b \qquad a \cdot b$$

Symbols are set close to numbers, superscripts and subscripts, greater than or less than signs, and parentheses, brackets, and braces.

$$2a \qquad a^2 \qquad x_2 \qquad a{<}b \qquad a{>}b$$

$$(a + b) \qquad [a - b] \qquad \{a + b\}$$

ACKNOWLEDGMENT

Principal author: Cheryl Iverson, MA

ADDITIONAL READINGS AND GENERAL REFERENCES

Council of Biology Editors Style Manual Committee. *Scientific Style and Format: The CBE Manual for Authors, Editors, and Publishers.* 6th ed. New York, NY: Cambridge University Press; 1994.

Swanson E. *Mathematics Into Type: Copy Editing and Proofreading of Mathematics for Editorial Assistants and Authors.* Rev ed. Providence, RI: American Mathematical Society; 1979.

Technical Information

CHAPTER 19

19.0 TYPOGRAPHY

Typography is broadly defined as the arrangement and appearance of printed matter and involves elements of design as well as the appearance of letters on the printed page. The editor and graphic designer often cooperate in the process of creating the typography and design for a book, monograph, or journal, with the goal of achieving a balance of form and readability.

19.1 ■ **BASIC ELEMENTS OF DESIGN.**—Good design will lead the reader through the printed material. There are 5 basic elements of design.

- The first is contrast—the contrast between dark and light type and large and small units of information (such as title and byline, sideheads and subheads, and text).
- The second element is the rhythm of the design as in repetition of similar units, in both opposition and juxtaposition, eg, spacing and proportion of type, and repetition of graphic contrasts or similarities.
- The third element is the size relationships within the design. These relationships refer to the optical image, the way the type and graphic material appear on the page.
- The fourth element is color, which attracts attention and creates associations. In scholarly publishing, however, the use of color for these purposes is limited.
- The fifth element is movement and focal points. Several elements may be present on a page, and the reader's eye follows the lines of composition unconsciously, from large to small, from top to bottom, from left to right, from dark to light, or vice versa for any of these elements.

In scholarly publishing, a number of typography and design elements, such as prescribed text format, titles and headings, bylines, tables and figures, equations and block quotations, and reference citations and lists, must be considered and incorporated.

The examples of journal pages (Figures 1 and 2) include some of these elements of design used in AMA journals.

19.2 ■ **TYPEFACES AND FONTS.**—A font of type is the complete assortment of type sizes and styles of a particular typeface (Figure 3). Serif type is generally used for body copy on account of its readability; sans serif type is used for contrasting and complementary elements. The size of type is conventionally referred to as its

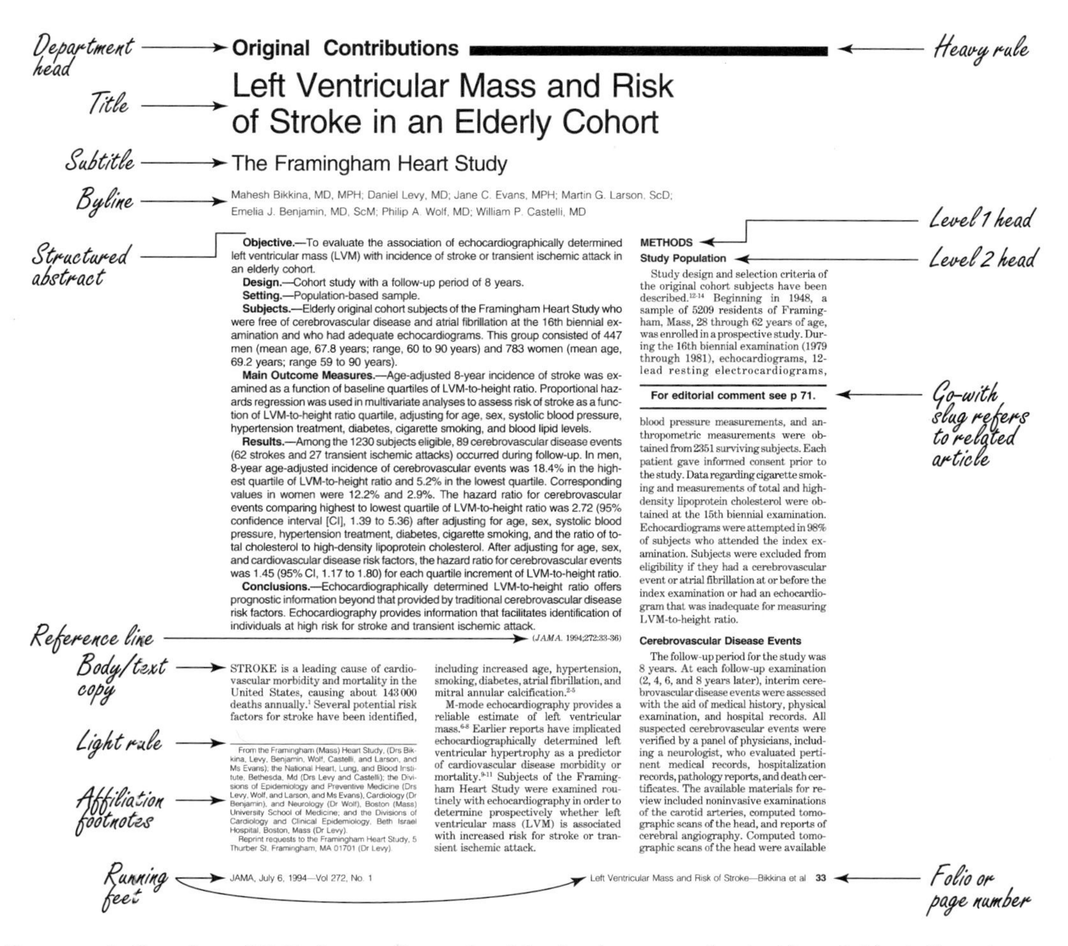

Original Contributions

Left Ventricular Mass and Risk of Stroke in an Elderly Cohort

The Framingham Heart Study

Mahesh Bikkina, MD, MPH; Daniel Levy, MD; Jane C. Evans, MPH; Martin G. Larson, ScD; Emelia J. Benjamin, MD, ScM; Philip A. Wolf, MD; William P. Castelli, MD

Objective.—To evaluate the association of echocardiographically determined left ventricular mass (LVM) with incidence of stroke or transient ischemic attack in an elderly cohort.

Design.—Cohort study with a follow-up period of 8 years.

Setting.—Population-based sample.

Subjects.—Elderly original cohort subjects of the Framingham Heart Study who were free of cerebrovascular disease and atrial fibrillation at the 16th biennial examination and who had adequate echocardiograms. This group consisted of 447 men (mean age, 67.8 years; range, 60 to 90 years) and 783 women (mean age, 69.2 years; range 59 to 90 years).

Main Outcome Measures.—Age-adjusted 8-year incidence of stroke was examined as a function of baseline quartiles of LVM-to-height ratio. Proportional hazards regression was used in multivariate analyses to assess risk of stroke as a function of LVM-to-height ratio quartile, adjusting for age, sex, systolic blood pressure, hypertension treatment, diabetes, cigarette smoking, and blood lipid levels.

Results.—Among the 1230 subjects eligible, 89 cerebrovascular disease events (62 strokes and 27 transient ischemic attacks) occurred during follow-up. In men, 8-year age-adjusted incidence of cerebrovascular events was 18.4% in the highest quartile of LVM-to-height ratio and 5.2% in the lowest quartile. Corresponding values in women were 12.2% and 2.9%. The hazard ratio for cerebrovascular events comparing highest to lowest quartile of LVM-to-height ratio was 2.72 (95% confidence interval [CI], 1.39 to 5.36) after adjusting for age, sex, systolic blood pressure, hypertension treatment, diabetes, cigarette smoking, and the ratio of total cholesterol to high-density lipoprotein cholesterol. After adjusting for age, sex, and cardiovascular disease risk factors, the hazard ratio for cerebrovascular events was 1.45 (95% CI, 1.17 to 1.80) for each quartile increment of LVM-to-height ratio.

Conclusions.—Echocardiographically determined LVM-to-height ratio offers prognostic information beyond that provided by traditional cerebrovascular disease risk factors. Echocardiography provides information that facilitates identification of individuals at high risk for stroke and transient ischemic attack.

(*JAMA*. 1994;272:33-36)

STROKE is a leading cause of cardiovascular morbidity and mortality in the United States, causing about 143 000 deaths annually.[1] Several potential risk factors for stroke have been identified, including increased age, hypertension, smoking, diabetes, atrial fibrillation, and mitral annular calcification.[2-5]

M-mode echocardiography provides a reliable estimate of left ventricular mass.[6-8] Earlier reports have implicated echocardiographically determined left ventricular hypertrophy as a predictor of cardiovascular disease morbidity or mortality.[9-11] Subjects of the Framingham Heart Study were examined routinely with echocardiography in order to determine prospectively whether left ventricular mass (LVM) is associated with increased risk for stroke or transient ischemic attack.

From the Framingham (Mass) Heart Study, (Drs Bikkina, Levy, Benjamin, Wolf, Castelli, and Larson, and Ms Evans); the National Heart, Lung, and Blood Institute, Bethesda, Md (Drs Levy and Castelli); the Divisions of Epidemiology and Preventive Medicine (Drs Levy, Wolf, and Larson, and Ms Evans), Cardiology (Dr Benjamin), and Neurology (Dr Wolf), Boston (Mass) University School of Medicine; and the Divisions of Cardiology and Clinical Epidemiology, Beth Israel Hospital, Boston, Mass (Dr Levy).

Reprint requests to the Framingham Heart Study, 5 Thurber St, Framingham, MA 01701 (Dr Levy).

METHODS

Study Population

Study design and selection criteria of the original cohort subjects have been described.[12-14] Beginning in 1948, a sample of 5209 residents of Framingham, Mass, 28 through 62 years of age, was enrolled in a prospective study. During the 16th biennial examination (1979 through 1981), echocardiograms, 12-lead resting electrocardiograms,

For editorial comment see p 71.

blood pressure measurements, and anthropometric measurements were obtained from 2351 surviving subjects. Each patient gave informed consent prior to the study. Data regarding cigarette smoking and measurements of total and high-density lipoprotein cholesterol were obtained at the 15th biennial examination. Echocardiograms were attempted in 98% of subjects who attended the index examination. Subjects were excluded from eligibility if they had a cerebrovascular event or atrial fibrillation at or before the index examination or had an echocardiogram that was inadequate for measuring LVM-to-height ratio.

Cerebrovascular Disease Events

The follow-up period for the study was 8 years. At each follow-up examination (2, 4, 6, and 8 years later), interim cerebrovascular disease events were assessed with the aid of medical history, physical examination, and hospital records. All suspected cerebrovascular events were verified by a panel of physicians, including a neurologist, who evaluated pertinent medical records, hospitalization records, pathology reports, and death certificates. The available materials for review included noninvasive examinations of the carotid arteries, computed tomographic scans of the head, and reports of cerebral angiography. Computed tomographic scans of the head were available

JAMA, July 6, 1994—Vol 272, No. 1

Left Ventricular Mass and Risk of Stroke—Bikkina et al 33

FIGURE 1 Page from *JAMA*. Sans serif type (used in the department head, title, subtitle, byline, abstract, footnotes, sideheads and subheads, go-with slug, and running feet) is used to contrast with serif type in the body copy.

point size. A point is approximately 1/72 of an inch; 12 points equals 1 pica; 6 picas equals 1 inch. Points are also used to measure the space between lines of type. The pica is used to measure the length of a line and the depth of the type area. Typefaces are commonly available and used in 6-point to 72-point sizes. The font for a publication usually includes 7 alphabets: roman capitals, roman lowercase letters, italic capitals, italic lowercase letters, boldface capitals, boldface lowercase letters, and small capitals. Each font may also include numerals, punctuation marks, commonly used symbols and diacritical marks, and ligatures and diphthongs (2 or more letters joined together, such as ff, fi, and æ; ligatures may be vowels and consonants, diphthongs are vowels only). Not all typefaces include all fonts, and the requirements of the text often will determine which font will be chosen depending on the alphabets needed.

19.3 ■ SPACING.

19.3.1 ***Letterspacing.***—Ideally, the spacing between letters should be optically balanced. There are no absolute values for optimal letterspacing, but column width and type size are interdependent in design. One convention suggests that the type

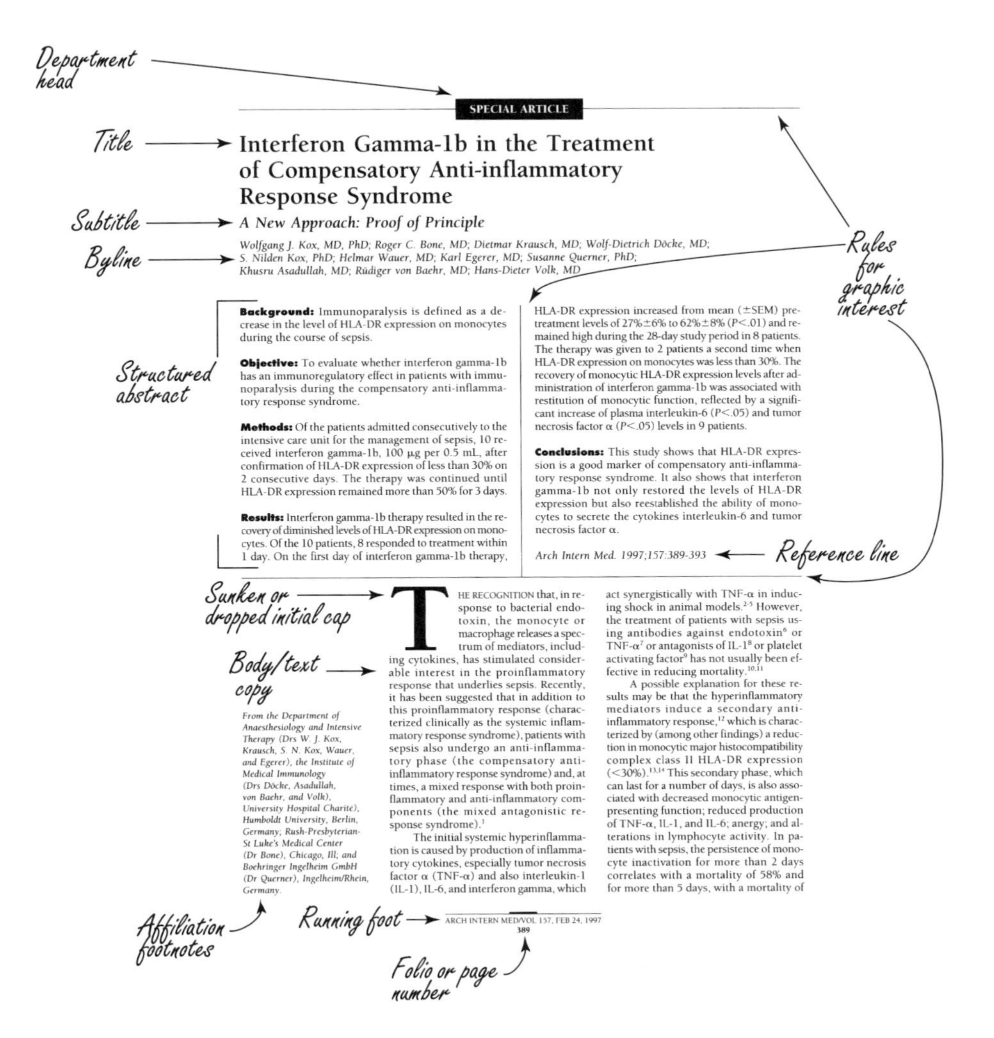

SPECIAL ARTICLE

Interferon Gamma-1b in the Treatment of Compensatory Anti-inflammatory Response Syndrome

A New Approach: Proof of Principle

Wolfgang J. Kox, MD, PhD; Roger C. Bone, MD; Dietmar Krausch, MD; Wolf-Dietrich Döcke, MD; S. Nilden Kox, PhD; Helmar Wauer, MD; Karl Egerer, MD; Susanne Querner, PhD; Khusru Asadullah, MD; Rüdiger von Baehr, MD; Hans-Dieter Volk, MD

Background: Immunoparalysis is defined as a decrease in the level of HLA-DR expression on monocytes during the course of sepsis.

Objective: To evaluate whether interferon gamma-1b has an immunoregulatory effect in patients with immunoparalysis during the compensatory anti-inflammatory response syndrome.

Methods: Of the patients admitted consecutively to the intensive care unit for the management of sepsis, 10 received interferon gamma-1b, 100 μg per 0.5 mL, after confirmation of HLA-DR expression of less than 30% on 2 consecutive days. The therapy was continued until HLA-DR expression remained more than 50% for 3 days.

Results: Interferon gamma-1b therapy resulted in the recovery of diminished levels of HLA-DR expression on monocytes. Of the 10 patients, 8 responded to treatment within 1 day. On the first day of interferon gamma-1b therapy, HLA-DR expression increased from mean (±SEM) pretreatment levels of 27%±6% to 62%±8% (*P*<.01) and remained high during the 28-day study period in 8 patients. The therapy was given to 2 patients a second time when HLA-DR expression on monocytes was less than 30%. The recovery of monocytic HLA-DR expression levels after administration of interferon gamma-1b was associated with restitution of monocytic function, reflected by a significant increase of plasma interleukin-6 (*P*<.05) and tumor necrosis factor α (*P*<.05) levels in 9 patients.

Conclusions: This study shows that HLA-DR expression is a good marker of compensatory anti-inflammatory response syndrome. It also shows that interferon gamma-1b not only restored the levels of HLA-DR expression but also reestablished the ability of monocytes to secrete the cytokines interleukin-6 and tumor necrosis factor α.

Arch Intern Med. 1997;157:389-393

THE RECOGNITION that, in response to bacterial endotoxin, the monocyte or macrophage releases a spectrum of mediators, including cytokines, has stimulated considerable interest in the proinflammatory response that underlies sepsis. Recently, it has been suggested that in addition to this proinflammatory response (characterized clinically as the systemic inflammatory response syndrome), patients with sepsis also undergo an anti-inflammatory phase (the compensatory anti-inflammatory response syndrome) and, at times, a mixed response with both proinflammatory and anti-inflammatory components (the mixed antagonistic response syndrome).[1]

The initial systemic hyperinflammation is caused by production of inflammatory cytokines, especially tumor necrosis factor α (TNF-α) and also interleukin-1 (IL-1), IL-6, and interferon gamma, which act synergistically with TNF-α in inducing shock in animal models.[2-5] However, the treatment of patients with sepsis using antibodies against endotoxin[6] or TNF-α[7] or antagonists of IL-1[8] or platelet activating factor[9] has not usually been effective in reducing mortality.[10,11]

A possible explanation for these results may be that the hyperinflammatory mediators induce a secondary anti-inflammatory response,[12] which is characterized by (among other findings) a reduction in monocytic major histocompatibility complex class II HLA-DR expression (<30%).[13,14] This secondary phase, which can last for a number of days, is also associated with decreased monocytic antigen-presenting function; reduced production of TNF-α, IL-1, and IL-6; anergy; and alterations in lymphocyte activity. In patients with sepsis, the persistence of monocyte inactivation for more than 2 days correlates with a mortality of 58% and for more than 5 days, with a mortality of

From the Department of Anaesthesiology and Intensive Therapy (Drs W. J. Kox, Krausch, S. N. Kox, Wauer, and Egerer), the Institute of Medical Immunology (Drs Döcke, Asadullah, von Baehr, and Volk), University Hospital Charité, Humboldt University, Berlin, Germany; Rush-Presbyterian-St Luke's Medical Center (Dr Bone), Chicago, Ill; and Boehringer Ingelheim GmbH (Dr Querner), Ingelheim/Rhein, Germany.

ARCH INTERN MED/VOL 157, FEB 24, 1997
389

FIGURE 2 Page from *Archives of Internal Medicine.* Type varies among design elements to create graphic interest.

size should be chosen so that 40 to 50 characters fit on 1 line of the column. Another convention specifies that the column width chosen should accommodate 1½ alphabets (approximately 39 characters) of the typeface per line. A column width too narrow to accommodate about 40 characters creates a problem of excessive hyphenation at line endings. A column width that holds more than 50 or so characters creates a problem of readability—the reader's eye does not easily follow a line of type across too great a column width. See Figure 4 for examples of changes in the appearance of a line of type that occur by changing the letterspacing.

19.3.2 ***Word Spacing.***—Word spacing is similar to letterspacing. Conventionally, a line of type includes 8 to 10 words.

19.3.3 ***Line Spacing.***—Optimal line spacing requires consideration of the type size, layout density, and line length. Generally, longer lines call for increased line spacing (traditionally called *leading,* for the strips of lead between lines of type) for optimal

Palatino Light
Palatino Light Italic
Palatino Regular
Palatino Regular Italic
Palatino Medium
Palatino Medium Italic
Palatino Bold
Palatino Bold Italic
Palatino Black
Palatino Black Italic
Palatino Regular Condensed
Palatino Regular Condensed Italic
PALATINO REGULAR SMALL CAPS

FIGURE 3 A family of type.

readability. See Figure 5 for examples of changes in line spacing that change the appearance of the text. More open line spacing also calls for wider margins; tighter line spacing can be done within narrower margins.

The conventions for letterspacing and word and line spacing vary depending on the amount of spacing between lines and whether the text is justified (set as a squared-off block) or unjustified (set with a ragged right margin). For example, a smaller type size may be used on a wider column if the line spacing (also called white space) is adequate for readability. The nature of the printed material will suggest whether variations in typography may be adapted to the piece.

19.4 ■ **LAYOUT.**—Layout is the arrangement of all the elements of design and typography on the page for optimal readability, taking into account the context and aesthetic requirements of the text. To create emphasis, complementary typefaces and various fonts within a typeface may be used. The type size and weight create emphasis or continuity, as needed. Headings and subheadings create the outline within the text to frame the article. In page layout, all the elements of design and typography come together. See Figures 1 and 2 for examples.

Many of the technical terms and concepts of typography, typesetting, and computer-assisted composition are listed in 21.0, Glossary of Publishing Terms. Examples of some specific uses of italic and boldface fonts, as well as small capital

No letterspacing

Letterspacing. Note that the typesize

2-Point letterspacing

Letterspacing. Note that the typesize

4-Point letterspacing

Letterspacing. Note that the typesize

FIGURE 4 Letterspacing. Note that the type size and style are identical in each line; only the letterspacing changes.

No line spacing
Line spacing (or leading). Note that the type size and style are identical in each line; only the space between the lines changes.

1-Point line spacing
Line spacing (or leading). Note that the type size and style are identical in each line; only the space between the lines changes.

2-Point line spacing
Line spacing (or leading). Note that the type size and style are identical in each line; only the space between the lines changes.

FIGURE 5 Line spacing (or leading). Note that the type size and style are identical in each line; only the space between the lines changes.

letters, are provided in 19.5, Specific Uses of Fonts, with cross-references to other chapters and sections.

19.5 ■ SPECIFIC USES OF FONTS.

19.5.1 ***Boldface.***—A general scheme of heads and sideheads may call for the use of boldface type for first- and second-level heads and for first-level sideheads in the text, although heading styles and formats vary among journals (see also 2.8, Manuscript Preparation, Parts of a Manuscript, Headings, Subheadings, and Side Headings). For example:

METHODS (level 1 head, flush left, bold caps)

Statistical Analysis (level 2 head, bold caps and lowercase)

Clustering Data.—(level 3 head or first-level sidehead, paragraph indent, run into the text, bold caps and lowercase).

19.5.2 ***Italics.***—Use italics as follows:

- For level 4 heads (second-level sideheads)
- When terms are given as terms and letters as letters (see also 6.6.7, Punctuation, Coined Words, Slang):

In his handwriting the *n*'s look like *u*'s.

No punctuation is needed after the word *handwriting* in the sentence above.

- When indicating the first use of a technical term, especially when accompanied by a definition (see also 6.6.7, Punctuation, Coined Words, Slang):

The page number is called the *folio.*

- For titles of books and journals, proceedings, symposia, plays, paintings, long poems, musical compositions, space vehicles, planes, and ships (see also 8.4, Capitalization, Titles and Headings):

USS *Constitution*

Verdi's *Requiem*

JAMA

- For some non-English words and phrases (see also 10.1, Non-English Words and Phrases; Accent Marks [Diacritics]) that are not shown in the current edition of *Merriam-Webster's Collegiate Dictionary* or in accepted medical dictionaries. Italics are not used if words or phrases are considered to have become part of the English language, eg, café au lait, in vivo, in vitro, en bloc.
- For lowercase letters used in alphabetic enumerations of items or topics (the parentheses are set roman): (*a*), (*b*), (*c*), etc
- For genus and species names of some microorganisms, plants, and animals when used in the singular and the names of a variety or subspecies. Plurals or adjectival forms and class, order, family, or tribe names are not italicized (see also 12.12, Nomenclature, Organisms):

  Chlamydia trachomatis (*But:* chlamydia, not italic, when referring to any species or to the genus broadly)

  Streptococcus (*But:* streptococcus organisms, streptococcal, streptococci)

- For restriction enzyme abbreviations (see also 12.6.1, Nomenclature, Nucleic Acids and Amino Acids)
- For gene, genotype, and locus symbols (see also 12.6.2, Nomenclature, Human Gene Nomenclature) and animal genetic terms (see also 12.6.5, Nomenclature, Animal Genetic Terms)
- For chemical prefixes (*N*-, *cis*-, *trans*-, *p*-, etc) (see also 12.4.4, Nomenclature, Chemical Names)
- For mathematical expressions such as lines, variables, unknown quantities, and constants (see also 18.0, Mathematical Composition). Numerals or abbreviations as for trigonometric functions and differentials are not italicized:

  $\sin x = a/b$

- For some statistical terms (see also 17.5, Statistics, Statistical Symbols and Abbreviations):

  P r df U z R^2

- For the abbreviation for acceleration due to gravity, *g*, to distinguish it from g for gram (see also 11.11, Abbreviations, Clinical and Technical Terms)
- For legal cases (see also 2.12.50, Manuscript Preparation, Legal References), eg, *Roe v Wade*
- For the term *sic* (see also 6.5.2, Punctuation, Brackets, Insertions in Quotations)
- In formal resolutions, for *Resolved*
- Sparingly, for emphasis

19.5.3 ***Small Caps.***—Use small capital letters as follows:

- AM and PM in time (see also 15.6.5, Units of Measure, Time)
- BC, BCE, CE, and AD (see also 11.3, Abbreviations, Days of the Week, Months, Eras)
- Some prefixes in chemical formulas (L for levo-, D for dextro-) (see also 12.4.4, Nomenclature, Chemical Names)

ACKNOWLEDGMENT

Principal author: Jane C. Lantz, ELS

ADDITIONAL READINGS AND GENERAL REFERENCES

Bruno M, ed. *Pocket Pal: A Graphic Arts Production Handbook.* 15th ed. Memphis, Tenn: International Paper Co; 1992.

The Chicago Manual of Style. 14th ed. Chicago, Ill: University of Chicago Press; 1993:767-772.

Craig J. *Designing With Type.* New York, NY: Watson-Guptill Publishers; 1992.

Korger H. *Handbook of Type and Lettering.* New York, NY: Design Press; 1992.

Tufte ER. *Envisioning Information.* Cheshire, Conn: Graphics Press; 1990.

CHAPTER 20

20.0 COPYEDITING AND PROOFREADING MARKS

20.1 ■ **COPYEDITING MARKS.**—Use the following examples as a guide to copy marking. See 20.2.1, Editing on Hard Copy, for a demonstration of their use.

bullet	• (indicate point size)
set in italics	published in JAMA
set in boldface	Comment
set in roman	*terms such as provision and delivery* (set roman)
delete underlining (italics)	in vivo, in vivo
capitals	National institutes of Health
small capitals	406 BC, 4 PM, PCO_2, Case
italic capitals	usa
lowercase a capital letter	She was President of the committee. (lc)
lowercase a capital series	TABLE 5. FACILITIES AND ORGANIZATIONS OF 47 DIVISIONS OF SURGICAL ONCOLOGY
superscript	Studies by Savrin et al 8 show results similar to those reported by Barrorso. 9
subscript	H_2O
en dash	basement membrane-like
em dash	CASE 1.--
apostrophe	'
period	That is all
comma	Groups 1, 2, and 3 all received 10 mL of bacterial suspension.

semicolon	He was generous; he had the fault.
colon	The briefest commandment is this: Don't.
insert parentheses	Her pulse rate was normal (72 beats per minute).
hyphen	symptom = free interval
insert a hyphen	followup period
close up	follow ing
plus sign	The mean change in systolic blood pressure was +4.2 mm Hg. (plus)
minus sign	The value could not exceed -1. (minus)
insert word(s)	A group has been assembled. (of volunteers)
change word(s)	Doors which close usually open. (that)
transpose elements	will answer only to his name (tr) will only to his name answer (tr)
correct a typographic error	The complicatex xeptic ulcer (d p)
delete elements	computed axial tomography
delete and close up	computerized tomography
insert space	underway (#)
mark Greek letter	µg/dL (Gk lc mu)
indent 1 em space	1 Symptoms
indent 2 em spaces	2 Fever
flush left	[Table stub
flush right	Signature]
center element	]Centerhead[
set as 2 lines, centered	]Gross and Microscopic Examination [
paragraph	¶ Cholecystectomy is one of the most common elective surgical procedures and a major source of hospitalization.

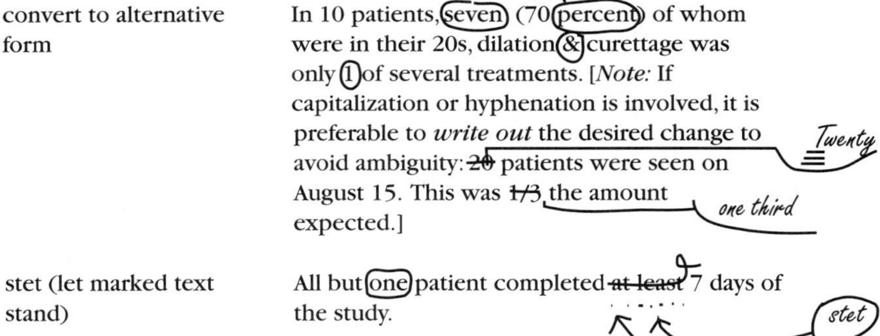

convert to alternative form	In 10 patients, seven (70 percent) of whom were in their 20s, dilation & curettage was only 1 of several treatments. [*Note:* If capitalization or hyphenation is involved, it is preferable to ***write out*** the desired change to avoid ambiguity: 20 patients were seen on August 15. This was 1/3 the amount expected.]
stet (let marked text stand)	All but one patient completed at least 7 days of the study.

20.2 ■ **COPYEDITING SAMPLES.**—The following examples have been copyedited, first in the traditional way with pen or pencil on paper, and second in an electronic format, showing 1 form of electronic editing, sometimes called redlining or revision marking. When using the redline function, the copy editor should consider the readability of the changes. For example, deletion of a hyphen in the redline function is not legible because the strikethrough line merely overstrikes the hyphen. Retyping the word unhyphenated is plainer to the reader. Likewise, retyping whole words in which parts are changed may make review of the document easier.

20.2.1 *Editing on Hard Copy.*

REPORT OF A CASE

Case 1.--A nineteen-year-old woman was seen for the 1st time in may of 1992 with complaints of stabbing pain of one years duration in the posterior aspect of the left calf from the knee downwards, throbbing sensations on the dorsum of the left foot and ankle and edema of the foot and leg.

Her history revealed that the patient had "fleshy tumors" of the left leg since she was 1-1/2 years old. Since then she'd undergone nine or ten operations for removal of these tumors, the last 1 having been performed in 1991. There was no known family hisotry or congenital vascular malformations. The patient was not known to have any allergies was atking no medication.

20.2.2 ***Electronic Text Editing.***—Insertions are underlined and deletions are struck through. When copyediting is done electronically, the copy editor also serves as the typesetter by inserting codes into the electronic manuscript file that tell the compositor how the type should appear. These codes do not ordinarily print out on the edited typescript. In the example below, codes for small caps and a mixed fraction have been inserted into the electronic file so that these typographic characteristics appear correctly on the made-up page. Other types of codes the copy editor inserts may be for font type and weight, column width, heading styles, and superscripts and subscripts.

~~REPORT OF A CASE~~ **REPORT OF A CASE**

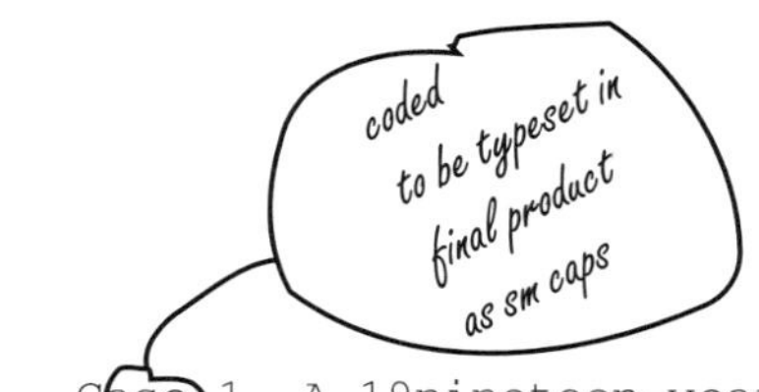

_______Case 1. A 19~~nineteen~~-year-~~-~~old woman was seen
for the first~~1st~~ time in M~~m~~ay ~~of~~ 1992 with complaints
of stabbing pain of 1~~one~~ year's duration in the
posterior aspect of the left calf from the knee
downward~~s~~, throbbing sensations on the dorsum of the
left foot and ankle, and edema of the foot and leg.

Her history revealed that she had~~the patient~~ had
“fleshy tumors” of the left leg since she was 1-1/2
years old. Since then she had~~'d~~ undergone 9~~nine~~ or
10~~ten~~ operations for removal of these tumors, the last
one~~1~~ ~~having been performed~~ in 1991. There was no known
family histo~~t~~ry of~~r~~ congenital vascular malformations.
The patient was not known to have any allergies and was
ta~~at~~king no medication.

coded
to be typeset
in final
product
as
mixed
fraction

20.3 ■ **PROOFREADING MARKS.**—The following marks are made in the margins of the proof. See 20.4, Proofreading Sample, for examples of their use.

- delete
- delete and close up
- close up entirely; take out space

(#)	add space; insert a space
∧	caret; insert addition
(eq #)	equalize space where indicated
(stet)	let marked text stand as set
[1]	indent 1 em space
[2]	indent 2 em spaces
¶	begin a new paragraph
⌒	no paragraph; run in
⊙	period
∧,	comma
∧;	semicolon
∧:	colon
∨' ∨' ∨'	apostrophe or single quotation marks
∨" ∨"	double quotation marks
(prime) → ′	prime sign
=	hyphen
(equals) → =	equals sign
1/N	en dash
1/M	em dash
(/)	parentheses
[/]	brackets
{/}	braces
(wf)	wrong font
(lc)	lowercase
(c+lc)	lowercase with initial capitals
(c+sc)	small capitals with initial capitals
(caps)	set in large capitals

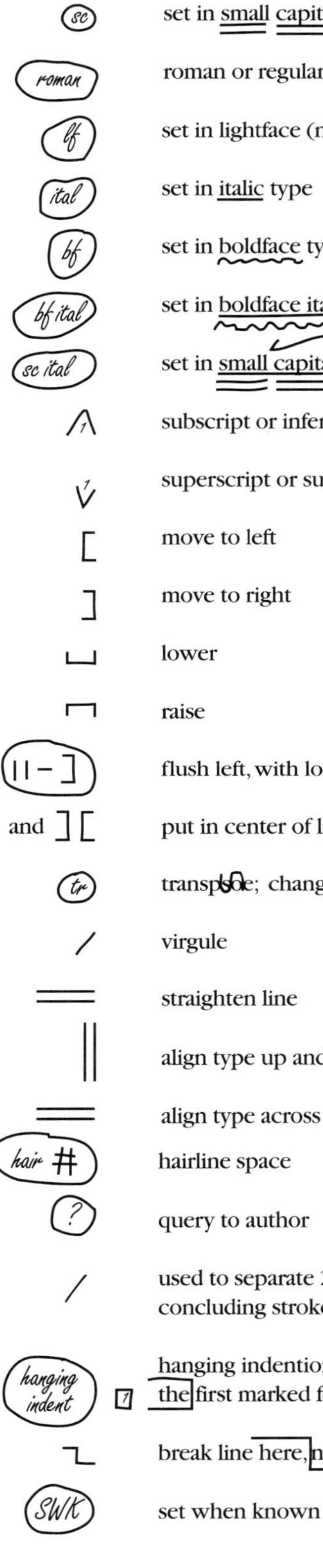

set in small capitals

roman or regular type (lightface)

set in lightface (not italic or boldface) type

set in italic type

set in boldface type

set in boldface italic type

set in small capital italic type

subscript or inferior letter or figure

superscript or superior letter or figure

move to left

move to right

lower

raise

flush left, with longest line flush right

put in center of line or page

transpose; change order the

virgule

straighten line

align type up and down

align type across

hairline space

query to author

used to separate 2 or more marks and often used as a concluding stroke at the end of an insertion

hanging indention—this style should have all lines after the first marked for the desired indention

break line here, not elsewhere

set when known

20.4 ■ **PROOFREADING SAMPLE.**—The following example shows how a proof is marked by the proofreader or copy editor and how these corrections then appear in the revised proof.

Proofread version:

Report of a Case

CASE 1.—A 19-year-old woman was seen for the first time in May 1992 with complints of stabbing pain of 1 year's duration in the posterior aspect of the right calf from the knee downward throbbing sensations on the dorsum of the left foot and ankle and oedema of the foot and leg.

Her history revealed that she had had "fleshy tumors" of the leg since she was 1 1/2 years old. Since then, she had undergone 9 10 oeprations for revmoal of these tumore, the last one in 1991. There was no known family history of congenital vascular malformations. The patient was not known to have any allergies and was taking no medication.

Corrected version:

REPORT OF A CASE

CASE 1.—A 19-year-old woman was seen for the first time in May 1992 with complaints of stabbing pain of 1 year's duration in the posterior aspect of the left calf from the knee downward, throbbing sensations on the dorsum of the left foot and ankle, and edema of the foot and leg.

Her history revealed that she had had "fleshy tumors" of the left leg since she was 1 1/2 years old. Since then, she had undergone 9 or 10 operations for removal of these tumors, the last one in 1991. There was no known family history of congenital vascular malformations. The patient was not known to have any allergies and was taking no medication.

ACKNOWLEDGMENT

Principal author: Jane C. Lantz, ELS

Chapter 21

21.0 Glossary of Publishing Terms

This glossary is intended to define terms commonly encountered during editing and publishing as well as those industry terms that also have a more common vernacular meaning. The glossary is not all-inclusive. New terms and new usage of existing terms will emerge with time and advances in technology. Definitions for the terms herein were compiled from the eighth edition of this manual and the sources listed at the end of the chapter.

AA—Author's alteration; a change or correction made by an author; used in correcting proofs (compare **EA** and **PE**).

access—The ability to locate specific information in a body of stored data. Data stored on magnetic tape are accessed sequentially; data stored on disks may be randomly accessed.

acid-free paper—Paper made from alkaline sizing, a treatment that improves the paper's resistance to liquid and vapor and improves the paper's permanence (see also **sizing**).

advertorial—Promotional or advertising content that has the appearance of editorial content (see 3.12.3, Ethical and Legal Considerations, Advertorials).

against the grain —See **grain direction.**

align—To place text or graphic material to line up horizontally or vertically with related elements.

alphanumeric—Letters, numbers, and symbols used as a code, eg, for a computer command.

ANSI—Acronym for American National Standards Institute, Inc.

art repair, art rebuilding—Replacing text, symbols, arrows, and lines on line art to produce illustrations that are consistent in format, type, and size.

artwork—Illustrative material, such as photographs, drawings, and graphs, intended for reproduction (see 2.14, Manuscript Preparation, Figures).

ascender—The part of lowercase letters, such as *d*, *f*, *h*, and *k*, that extends above the midportion or x-height of the letter (see **x-height,** compare **descender**).

ASCII—Acronym for American Standard Code for Information Interchange; a code representing an alphanumeric group of characters recognized by most computers and computer programs (pronounced *askey*).

ASCII file—A computer file containing only ASCII-coded text.

asterisk—A character (*) used as a reference mark.

ASTM—Abbreviation for American Society for Testing and Materials.

author's editor—An editor who substantially edits an author's manuscript and prepares it to meet the requirements for publication in a particular journal (see also **editor**).

backstrip—A strip of paper affixed to the bound edges of paper that form a journal's spine.

backup—Saving copies of digital files on disk, tape, or other medium.

bad break—A poorly arranged or potentially confusing arrangement of type occurring at the end of a line or the bottom or top of a page or column. Examples include a paragraph ending with 1 or 2 words at the top of a page or column (see **widow**) or at the bottom of a page or column (see **orphan**), a subheading falling on the last line of a page or column, an improperly hyphenated word or acronym, or the second part of a properly hyphenated word starting a page.

bandwidth—The capacity of a communication system to transfer data.

basis weight—The weight of paper determined by the weight in pounds of a ream (500 sheets) of paper cut to a standard size for a specific grade. For example, 500 sheets, 25×38 in, of 80-lb coated paper will weigh 80 lb.

baud rate—The speed at which data are transmitted through a communications line (eg, telephone line); 1 baud is equal to 1 bit per second.

BBS—Abbreviation for bulletin board system.

binary system—A system of numbers using only the digits 1 and 0 for all values; it is the basis for digital computers.

binding—The process by which printed units or pages are attached to form a book, journal, or pamphlet, including operations such as folding, collating, stitching, or gluing (see also **loose-leaf binding, perfect binding, saddle-stitch binding,** and **selective binding**).

bit—A binary digit, either 0 or 1; the smallest unit of digital information.

bit map—The digital image of a page or unit to be printed that indicates every bit (or spot) to be printed (see also **tag, tagged,** and **TIFF**).

bit-map fonts—Low-resolution fonts designed for computer screens only (eg, Chicago, Geneva, New York); any font with the name of a major city.

black—One of the 4 process printing colors (see **CMYK**).

blanket—A fabric coated with rubber or other material that is clamped around a printing cylinder to transfer ink from the press plate to the paper (see also **offset printing**).

bleed—A printed image that runs off any edge of a printed page. A partial bleed extends above, below, or to the side of the established print area but does not continue off the page (see also **live area**).

blind folio—A page number counted but not printed on the page (see **folio**).

blind image—An image that fails to print because of ink receptivity error.

blueprint, blackprint—A photoprint made from film that is used to check position and relative arrangement of text and image elements.

body type—The type characteristics used for the main body text of a work.

boilerplate—A section of text that can be reused without changes.

boldface (bf)—A typeface that is heavier and darker than the text face used (see 19.0, Typography).

bouncing reject—A rejected manuscript that is returned to the editorial office with request for reconsideration (see 3.11.2, Ethical and Legal Considerations, Editorial Responsibility for Rejection).

bps—Abbreviation for bits per second. A measurement of the speed with which data travel from one place to another.

broadside—Printed text or illustrations positioned on the length rather than the width of the page, requiring the reader to turn the publication on its side to read it; usually used for tables and figures that are wider than the normal width of a publication.

browser—See **Web browser.**

bug—Something that causes an error in computer software or hardware (see **virus**).

bullet—An aligned dot of a heavy weight (•) used to highlight individual elements in a list (see **centered dot**).

byline—A line of text at the beginning of an article listing the authors' names (compare **signature**) (see 2.2, Manuscript Preparation, Bylines and End-of-Text Signatures, and 3.1.1, Ethical and Legal Considerations, Authorship: Definition and Criteria).

byte—A unit of digital information that can code for a single alphanumeric symbol; 1 byte equals 8 to 32 bits.

CAD—Abbreviation for computer-assisted design.

caliper—Thickness of paper or film measured in terms of thousandths of an inch (mils or points); also the tool used to measure the thickness of paper.

call-outs—Quotes of text reprinted in typeface, usually bolder and larger than that of the original text, to place emphasis, improve design, or fill white space.

camera-ready—Copy, including artwork and text, that is ready to be photographed for reproduction without further composition or alteration.

CAP—Abbreviation for computer-assisted publishing.

CAR—Abbreviation for computer-assisted reading.

caret—A symbol (/\) indicating where to insert a correction or additional material.

case—The cover of a hardbound book (see also **lowercase** and **uppercase**).

CD—Abbreviation for compact (or computer) disc containing data.

CDI—Abbreviation for interactive compact disc containing data.

CD-ROM—Abbreviation for compact (or computer) disc read-only memory; a compact disc containing data that can be read by a computer. Many CD-ROMs are interactive and have sound, graphic images, and video.

cell—In tables or spreadsheets, a unit in an array formed by the intersection of a column and a row; in computer terminology, a basic subdivision of a memory that can hold 1 unit of a computer's basic operating data unit (see also 2.13.4, Manuscript Preparation, Table Components).

centered dot—A heavy dot (●) used to highlight individual elements in a list (see **bullet**). Also, a lighter centered dot (·) is used in mathematical composition to signify multiplication and in chemical formulas to indicate hydration.

central processing unit (CPU)—The part of a computer that performs all the main functions of the system.

CEPS—Acronym for color electronic prepress systems; electronic color equipment used to perform electronic retouching, cloning, and pagination.

character—A letter, numeral, symbol, or punctuation mark.

character count—The process of estimating the amount of space that typed or computer-printed copy will occupy on a published page. A character count is made by counting the number of characters and spaces in an average line of the manuscript, multiplying that number by the number of lines on the manuscript page, and multiplying that number by the total number of manuscript pages. Most word-processing programs will provide an exact character count and word count.

Chromalin—The trade name for a proof made from color separations that shows all colors as a single composite. This is used by publishers to approve color separations and by printers to match colors at press time.

circulation—The total number of copies of a publication sold and distributed (see also **controlled circulation**).

citation analysis—An analysis of the number of times a published article is cited in the reference list of subsequently published articles (see also **impact factor**).

close up—To eliminate the space between 2 characters or the space left between 2 characters after deleting another character.

CMYK—Abbreviation for the 4 process printing colors: cyan, magenta, yellow, and black.

codes—Combinations of letters, numbers, and symbols entered through a keyboard that instruct a computer how to format and compose a document or file (see also **tag** and **tagged**).

colophon—A summary of information about the publication or the publication's production methods or specifications; also the publisher's emblem or trademark (see also **masthead**).

color breaks—Separating elements of a piece of artwork that will print in more than 1 color. A second or third color proof may be attached to a black proof to show the color screen on artwork.

color proofs—Photomechanical or digital representations of color.

color separation—The result of the process of separating original color images, from transparencies or reflective art, into the 4 process printing colors (cyan, magenta, yellow, and black).

compatible—A term describing an environment in which one computer will accept and process data from another computer without conversion of code modifications; also a term describing the ability to use hardware and software together on one computer platform.

composite figure—A figure that is composed of more than one type of element (eg, halftone, line art, 4 colors).

composition—The arrangement of type and typographic characteristics for printing.

compression—A computer technique of eliminating redundant information, such as blank lines from a document or white space from an image, to reduce the file size for faster transmission or more compact storage of data.

computer-assisted composition—A process in which text in digital form is recorded on a magnetic medium (magnetic tape, hard disk, diskette, optical drive) and processed through a set of typesetting parameters stored in a computer that dictate the type size and font, hyphenation and justification, character and word spacing, and all typographical requirements needed to typeset the text. The data stream created from this process is used to drive an image setter for typesetting and printing a page of text.

condensed type—Characters set narrower than normal, fitting more text in one line than in another line of the same width (see 19.0, Typography).

context-sensitive editor—A software program that uses document structure to determine which elements are appropriate to insert in a particular context within a document (eg, SGML editor).

continuous tone—An image that has gradations of tone from dark to light, in contrast to an image formed of pure blacks and whites, such as a pen-and-ink drawing or a page of type (see also **halftone** and **duotone**).

controlled circulation—Copies of a publication distributed to a select list of recipients without charge (see also **circulation**).

copy—Any matter, including a manuscript in handwritten, typescript, or digital format, artwork, photographs, tables, and figures, to be set or reproduced for printing (see also **hard copy**).

copy editor—An editor who prepares a document or other copy for publication, making alterations and corrections to ensure accuracy, consistency, and uniformity (see also **editor**).

copy fitting—Estimating the space required to print a given amount of copy in a specific type size, typeface, and format. The number of characters in the manuscript is estimated and divided by the number of characters per pica for the typeface and type size to be used in the published version; this number is divided by the number of picas of the typeset line, and then by the number of lines of type per page. The result is an estimate of the number of published pages the manuscript will occupy (see also **character count**).

copyright—The law protecting an author's rights to published and unpublished works created by that author (see 3.6.2, Ethical and Legal Considerations, Copyright: Definition, History, and Current Law).

cover—The front and back pages of a publication. The 4 pages making up the covers in a publication are often designated covers 1, 2, 3, and 4. Covers 1 and 4 are outside pages, and covers 2 and 3 are inside pages.

cover stock—Paper used for the cover, usually heavier than the paper used for the body of the publication.

CPI—Abbreviation for characters per inch.

CPU—See **central processing unit.**

crop—To reduce the size of an image by removing extraneous areas, usually along 1 or more edges.

crop marks—Lines placed on the sides, top, and bottom of a photograph or illustration indicating the size or area of the image to be reproduced.

cursor—In computer terminology, an on-screen indicator, such as a blinking line, arrow, hollow square, or other image (usually mouse or keystroke driven), that marks a designated place on the screen and indicates current point of data entry or modification, menu selection, or program function.

cyan—One of the 4 process printing colors (cyan, magenta, yellow, and black); a shade of blue (see **CMYK**).

dagger—A character (†) used as a reference mark or to indicate a death (see also **double dagger** and 2.13, Manuscript Preparation, Tables).

data—Factual information (eg, measurements) used in calculation, analysis, and discussion; information in digital form that can be organized, manipulated, stored, and transmitted.

data bank—A compilation of information stored in a computer for retrieval and use.

database—A collection of stored data from which information can be extracted and organized in various forms and formats, usually for rapid search and retrieval.

debug—To trace and correct errors in a computer program.

demand printing—A part of the publishing industry that creates short-run, customized print publications quickly and on individual request.

demographic versions—Different versions of an issue of a publication containing specific inserts targeted for specific readers; the inserts are usually advertisements.

descender—The part of such letters as *p*, *q*, and *y* that extends below the main body of the letter or baseline (compare **ascender** and **x-height**).

desktop color separation—A computer file format that separates an encapsulated PostScript (EPS) color file into the 4 color elements: cyan, magenta, yellow, and black (see **encapsulated PostScript**).

desktop publishing (DTP)—A microcomputer-based publishing system consisting of a computer, pagination software, scanner, and output device.

digitize—To transform a printed character or image into bits or binary digits, so that it can be entered into and manipulated in a computer.

DIRFT—In quality terminology, abbreviation for do it right the first time.

disk—A circular plate coated with a magnetic substance and used for the storage and retrieval of data.

diskette—A disk coated with magnetically sensitive material used for storage of information, usually in personal computers.

display type—Type that differs from the body type of the text of a printed work. Display faces are used in titles, headings, and subheadings and are usually larger than the body type.

document—Organized coherent information in written, printed, or digital format.

document delivery— A type of service that allows users to search online databases of indexes and tables of contents to identify articles and request copies of those articles to be delivered by mail, by fax, or online.

DOS—Abbreviation for disk operating system (pronounced *doss*); operating system used by most PC-compatible computers and workstations.

dot—In a halftone, an individual printing element or spot (see also **dot grain, dots per inch,** and **halftone**).

dot grain—A printing defect that causes 2 dots to print larger than they should, resulting in darker tone and color than intended.

dot matrix printer—A device that produced hard copy from a series of wires (pins) that strike against an ink source. The dots created form characters. Quality varies; manuscripts printed on dot matrix printers may not be easily read by some optical scanners for typesetting because the spaces between the dots create an uneven structure (see also **ink-jet printer, laser printer,** and **line printer**).

dots per inch (DPI)—A measure of the resolution of a printed image (see **spots per inch**).

double dagger—A character (‡) used as a reference mark (see also **dagger** and 2.13, Manuscript Preparation, Tables).

double spread—Printed material (text, tables, illustrations) that extends across 2 pages (left- and right-hand pages); also called a 2-page spread.

download—The process of transferring digital files from a remote computer to a local computer.

DPI—See **dots per inch.**

drive—The computer hardware, consisting of the motor, read/write heads, and electronics, that is used with a disk.

drop folio—A page number printed at the bottom of the page (see **folio**).

dropped cap—A production term indicating that the initial letter of a word (usually beginning a paragraph) will be set in boldface, larger than the body text (see also **initial**).

DSSSL—Abbreviation for document style semantics and specification language; an output specification standard used with SGML-coded documents and a DTD to drive a typesetter or printer (see also **specifications, SGML,** and **DTD**).

DTD—Abbreviation for document type definition; in an SGML (coded) digital document, the DTD is the ASCII file that is separate from the text document and that defines the elements and structure of that document. Without a DTD, the SGML tags are meaningless (see also **ASCII** and **SGML**).

dummy—A layout of a page to represent the size and appearance after printing.

duotone—A 2-color halftone reproduction from a black-and-white photograph (see also **halftone**); usually reproduced in black and one other color.

EA—Abbreviation for editor's alteration or correction (compare **AA** and **PE**).

editor—(1) By occupation, someone who directs a publication or heads an editorial staff and/or decides on the acceptability of a document for publication (eg, editor, editor-in-chief); manages a publication (eg, managing editor); prepares a document for publication by altering, adapting, and refining it (eg, copy editor, author's editor). (2) In computer terminology, a program used to create text files or make changes to an existing file. Text or full-screen editors allow users to move through a document with direction keys, keystrokes, and a mouse- or command-driven cursor. Line editors allow the user to view the document as a series of numbered lines (see also **context-sensitive editor** and **SGML editor**).

editorial—(1) Of or relating to an editor or editing. (2) A written expression of opinion that may reflect the official position of the publication. (3) Published material that is not promotional in nature (eg, not an advertisement).

editorial assistant—One who assists in the editorial procedures and processes of editing and publishing.

e-journal—Electronic journal; a journal published in digital format (ie, online, CD-ROM) that is accessed via a computer.

elite type—Typewriter type that equals 12 characters to the inch (see also **pica type**).

ellipses—A series of 3 periods (. . .) used to indicate an omission or that data are not available.

em—A measurement used to specify to the typesetter the amount of space desired for indention, usually equal to the square body of the type size (eg, a 6-point em is 6 points wide).

e-mail—Electronic mail; an online system that allows people to send messages to each other through their computers.

em dash—A punctuation mark used to indicate an interruption or break in thought in a sentence; also used after introductory clauses and before closing clauses or designations (compare **en dash** and see 6.3, Punctuation, Hyphens and Dashes).

emulsification—A condition in offset printing that results from a mixing of the water-based fountain solution and oil-based ink on the press (see also **fountain**).

emulsion side—The side of a photographic film to which a chemical coating is applied and on which the image is developed.

en—Half an em (see also **em**).

enamel—The surface of shiny coated paper.

encapsulated PostScript (EPS)—A file format that stores images in a trademarked page description language (PostScript and an optional bit-map equivalent for screen display). Used best for high-resolution black-and-white line art and image interchange on a Macintosh computer.

en dash—A punctuation mark (longer than a hyphen and half the length of an em dash) used in hyphenated or compound modifiers (compare **em dash** and see 6.3, Punctuation, Hyphens and Dashes).

end mark—A symbol, such as a dash (—) or an open square (□), to indicate the end of an article; often used in news stories.

e-publication— Electronic publication; a work published in digital format (eg, online, CD-ROM) that is accessed via a computer.

expanded type—Type in which the characters are wider than normal (see 19.0, Typography).

face—The open side of a publication.

F & G—Abbreviation for folded and gathered signatures of a publication for final review before publication (see also **signature**).

FAQs—Acronym for frequently asked questions; often used by Web site and home page designers to help users access and search for information and resolve common problems.

fax—Short for facsimile; transmission of printed or digitized material through telephone lines.

figure—An illustration, eg, photograph, drawing, graph (see 2.14, Manuscript Preparation, Figures).

file—A collection of related, digitally stored information that is recognized as a unit by a computer.

filler—(1) Editorial content used to fill white space created by articles or advertisements not filling an entire page. (2) Chemicals used to fill the spaces between fibers in paper to improve the paper's opacity.

finish—The surface of paper.

firewall—In computer terminology, a security software program or device that blocks or restricts entry into a local area network from the Internet.

floppy disk—A flexible disk coated with magnetically sensitive material used for temporary storage of information, usually used with personal computers (see also **diskette**).

flush—Lines of type aligned vertically along the left margin (flush left) or the right margin (flush right).

flush and hang—To set the first line flush left on the margin and indent the remaining lines.

flyleaf—Any blank page at the front or back of a book.

folio—A page number placed at the bottom or top of a printed page (see also **dropped folio** and **blind folio**).

font—A complete assortment of characters in one face and size of type (see 19.0, Typography).

foot—The bottom of a page (compare **head**; see also **running foot**).

form, press form—A group of assembled pages (usually 8, 12, 16, or 32 pages), printed at the same time, then folded into consecutively numbered pages (see also **signature**).

format—The shape, size, style, margins, type, and design of a publication.

FOSI—Abbreviation for formatting output specification instance; an output specification standard used with an SGML-coded digital document and a DTD to drive a typesetter or printer (see also **specifications, SGML,** and **DTD**).

fountain—In offset (lithographic) printing, the part of the press that contains the dampening device and solution (usually water, buffered acid, gum, and alcohol); in nonoffset printing, the part of the press that contains the ink.

FPO—Abbreviation meaning for position only; refers to low-resolution graphics used in place of high-resolution graphics to show placement of artwork and photographs before printing.

FPS—Abbreviation for frames per second.

FTP—Abbreviation for file transfer protocol. A method for moving files between 2 Internet sites.

function key—A key on a computer keyboard that gives an instruction to the machine or computer, as opposed to the keys that indicate letters, numbers, and punctuation marks; often labeled F (eg, F1, F2).

galley proof—A proof of typeset text copy run 1 column wide before being made into a page.

gatefold—A foldout page.

GB—Gigabyte; a unit of computer storage, approximately equal to 1 billion bytes.

ghost author—An author who meets all criteria for authorship but is not named in the byline of a publication (see 3.1.2, Ethical and Legal Considerations, Guest and Ghost Authors).

ghosting—Shadows produced by uneven ink coverage (variations are caused by wide contrasts in the colors or tones being printed).

GIF—Abbreviation for graphics interchange format.

glossy—A photograph or line art printed on smooth shiny paper that traditionally has been required by some publishers for print reproduction.

gopher—An online browser that allows a user to locate online addresses and topics in text-only format (no graphics).

grain direction—The direction of the fibers in a sheet of paper created when the paper is made. When the fibers of the paper are parallel to the forward motion of the paper machine, the resulting paper will have a quality called "with the grain." Paper made with the fibers passing perpendicular to the forward motion of the paper machine will have a quality called "against the grain."

granularity—The level of specificity with which parts of a digital document are identified by a context-sensitive editor.

graphical user interface (GUI)—Pronounced *gooey;* a computer display format that allows the user to select commands, run programs, and view lists of files and other options by pointing a cursor to icons or menus (text lists) of items on the screen.

gutter—The 2 inner margins of facing pages of a publication, from printed area to binding.

hairline—The thinnest stroke of a character.

hairline rule—A thin rule, usually measuring one-half point.

halftone—A black-and-white continuous tone artwork, such as a photograph, that has shades of gray (see also **duotone** and 2.14, Manuscript Preparation, Figures).

halftone screen—A grid used in the halftone process to break the image into dots. The fineness of the screen is denoted in terms of lines per inch (eg, 120, 133, 150).

H & J—Abbreviation for hyphenation and justification; the determination of line breaks and the division of words into lines of prescribed measurement.

hard copy—Printed copy in contrast to copy stored in digital format.

hardware—Machinery, circuitry, and other physical entities (compare **software**).

head—The top of a page (compare **foot**; see also **running head**).

head margin—Top margin of a page.

home page—The first screen a user views when connecting to a specific site on the World Wide Web.

HTML—Abbreviation for hypertext markup language; codes (tags) used to prepare a file containing both text and graphics for placement on the Internet via the World Wide Web (see also **tag**).

http—Abbreviation for hypertext transfer protocol; a computer connection used at the beginning of a World Wide Web address to connect with and transfer information and graphics across the Web.

hyperlinks—The nonlinear relating of information, images, and sounds that allows a computer user to jump quickly from one topic, item, or representation to another by clicking a mouse-driven cursor on a word or icon.

icon—A small graphic image, usually a visual mnemonic, displayed on a computer screen, easily manipulated by the user, that represents common computer commands (eg, a trash can may represent a command for deleting unwanted text or files).

image setter—A device that plots an array of dots or pixels onto photosensitive material (film) line by line, until an entire page is created (including text, graphics, and color). The film can be output as a negative or positive with resolutions from 300 to 3000 dots per inch (see also **dots per inch**).

impact factor—A measure of the frequency with which the average article in a journal has been cited in a particular year. It helps to evaluate a journal's relative importance when compared with others in the same field. The impact factor is calculated by dividing the number of current citations to articles published in the 2 previous years by the total number of articles published in those 2 years. It tends to discount the advantage of journals that produce large, citable bodies of literature due to thickness of issue, frequency of issuance, or years in print. See also **citation analysis.**

imposition—The process of arranging pages or press forms of a publication so that the pages will be in sequential order when printed, folded, and bound into a publication; a guide or list showing the sequential order of pages.

impression—The transfer of an ink image by pressure from type, plate, or blanket to paper. The speed of a sheet-fed printing press is measured by the number of impressions printed per hour.

indent—To set a line of type or paragraph in from the margin or margins (see 19.0, Typography).

inferior—See **subscript.**

initial—A large letter, the first letter of a word used to begin a paragraph, chapter, or section. A "sunken or dropped initial" cuts 2 or 3 lines down into the text; a "stickup initial" aligns at the bottom with the first line of text and sticks up into the white space above (see also **dropped cap**).

ink fountain—Device on the press that supplies the ink to the inking rollers.

ink-jet printer—A device by which ink is forced through a series of nozzles; this method of printing is usually used to produce the mailing address or a short message to the subscriber (see also **laser printer, line printer,** and **dot matrix printer**).

input—To enter information, instructions, and text into a computer system; or that which is entered.

in register—See **register.**

insert—Printed material (a piece of paper or multiple pages) that is positioned between the normal pages of a publication during the binding process. The insert is usually printed on different paper than that used in the publication; it is often an advertisement.

interface—The ability of individual computers to interact; also, the actual hardware that performs the function.

Internet—A large international computer network that provides access to a variety of information and databases.

Internet Service Provider—A commercial entity that provides access to the Internet.

intranet—A private network with restricted access to specific users (eg, employees of a company or members of an organization).

ISBN—Abbreviation for International Standard Book Number (eg, the ISBN for this manual is 0-683-40206-4).

ISO—Abbreviation for International Organization for Standards.

ISSN—Abbreviation for International Standard Serial Number (eg, the ISSN for *JAMA* is 0098-7484).

IT—Abbreviation for Information Technology.

italic—A typestyle with the top portion of characters slanting upward and to the right (*italic*) as opposed to roman type (see 19.0, Typography).

JPEG—A file interchange format.

justify—To add or delete space between words or letters to make copy align at the left and right margins (see also **margin** and **unjustified** and 19.0, Typography).

kerning—To modify spacing between characters, usually to bring letters closer together.

keyboard—Input device of a computer or typesetter, with keys representing letters, numbers, punctuation marks, and functions that give instructions to the computer.

keyline—Tissue or acetate overlay separating or defining elements and color for line art or halftone artwork.

ladder—Four or more hyphens appearing at the end of consecutive lines; a typographic pattern to be avoided.

LAN—Acronym for local area network. A computer network restricted to an immediate area (eg, a building, floor of a building, or a department).

laptop—A portable computer.

laser printer—A high-quality, moderate-speed printer (see also **dot matrix printer, ink-jet printer,** and **line printer**).

layout—A drawing showing a conception of the finished product; includes sizing and positioning of the elements.

leaders—A row of dots or dashes designed to guide the reader's eye across space or a page.

leading—Pronounced *ledding;* the spacing between lines of type (also called *line spacing*); a carryover term from hot metal composition. For example, 9-point type on 11 points of line space allows 2 points of leading below the type (see 19.0, Typography).

legend—A caption or description accompanying a figure, photograph, or illustration (see 2.14, Manuscript Preparation, Figures).

ligature—Two or more connected letters, such as œ, set as connected (see 19.0, Typography).

line art—Illustration composed of lines and/or lettering, eg, charts, graphs (see 2.14, Manuscript Preparation, Figures).

line printer—A machine, driven by a computer, that prints out stored data one line at a time (see also **dot matrix printer, ink-jet printer,** and **laser printer**).

line spacing—See **leading.**

lines per inch (LPI)—A unit of measurement for halftone screens.

listserv—A digital mailing list program that manages e-mail addresses of an online discussion group. The listserv program duplicates the messages sent by individual users and automatically sends them to every user in the group.

lithographic printing—Formal term for *offset printing*.

live area—The area of a page within the margins (see also **margin**).

login—The name used to gain access to a computer system or network.

logo—One or more words or other combinations of letters or designs often used for easy recognition and promotion of company names, trademarks, etc.

long page—A page that runs longer than the live area or margins of the page (see also **live area**; compare **short page**).

loose-leaf binding—Binding that permits pages to be readily removed and inserted (compare **perfect binding, saddle-stitch binding,** and **spiral binding**).

lowercase—Letters that are not capitalized.

macro—A series of automatically executed computer commands activated by a few programmed keystrokes; useful for repetitive tasks.

magenta—One of the 4 process printing colors (cyan, magenta, yellow, and black); a shade of red (see **CMYK**).

mainframe—A large, powerful, central processing computer.

makeready—The part of the printing process that immediately preceded the actual press run, in which colors, ink coverage, and register are adjusted to produce the desired quality; may also apply to the binding process (see also **register**).

makeup—The arranging of type lines and illustrations into pages or press forms for review or printing (see also **imposition**; compare **live area**).

margin—The section of white space surrounding typed, composed, or printed copy (see also **white space**).

markup—The process of marking manuscript copy with directions for style and composition (see also **imposition**).

master proof—The set of galley or page proofs that carries all corrections and alterations.

masthead—A boilerplate listing of editorial, production, and publishing staff; editorial boards; contact information; subscription and advertising information; important disclaimers (see also **boilerplate** and **colophon**).

matte finish—The surface of dull-coated paper.

MB—Megabyte; a unit of computer storage, equal to approximately 1 million bytes.

measure—The length of the line (width of the column) in which type is composed or set.

memory—The part of a computer in which digital information is permanently stored (see also **RAM**).

menu—A series of options in a software program, usually presented on the computer screen as a list of text options.

MHz—Megahertz; a unit that measures a computer system's cycle speed; 1 MHz equals 1 million cycles per second.

modem—Modulator-demodulator; an electronic telecommunication device that converts computer-generated data (digital signals) into analog signals that can be carried over telephone lines.

moiré pattern—An undesirable wavy pattern caused by incorrect screen angles, overprinting halftones, or superimposing 2 geometrical patterns.

monitor—A video output device for the display of computer-generated text and graphics (see also **screen**).

mouse—A hand-operated device that controls the movement of a cursor on a computer screen.

MSL—Abbreviation for must start left. See also **MSR**.

MSR—Abbreviation for must start right. See also **MSL**.

multimedia—Interactive electronic products created from digitized data reformatted to include text, images, and sound that allow the user to interact with the information on a computer screen.

multitasking—Performing simultaneous functions or manipulations on one computer or workstation, or performing simultaneous data manipulations in one computer program.

network—Two or more computers connected to share resources (see also **Internet** and **intranet**).

newsgroup—The common nomenclature for Usenet News, a tool for group discussion on the Internet. Newsgroups function as group e-mail by providing a posting site for discussion on a particular topic. One can participate by posting a query or by reading answers to queries that have already been posted.

oblique—Type that is slightly slanted but not italic (see also **italic**).

OCR—Abbreviation for optical character reader (or recognition); in digital composition and typesetting, an OCR input device is capable of scanning a typescript and replicating the typed characters. An OCR device creates a digital document that can be edited, as opposed to a scanner, which simply transfers images from paper to a digital file.

offset, offset printing—Commonly used term for offset lithographic printing; a printing method in which an image is transferred from an inked plate cylinder to a blanket made of rubber or other synthetic material and then onto a sheet of paper.

on-demand printing—See **demand printing**.

opaque—To paint out on the negative those areas that are not to be printed.

operating system—A program that controls the overall operations of a computer system, intermediating between the application software programs and the hardware, such as MS-DOS, UNIX, or OS/2.

optical character recognition/reader—See **OCR**.

orphan—One or 2 short words at the end of a paragraph that fall on a separate line (compare **widow,** see also **bad break**).

outline halftone—A portion taken from a halftone that is the shape or modified shape of a subject (see **halftone**).

out of register—See **register**.

overlay—A hinged flap of paper or transparent plastic covering for a piece of artwork. It may protect the work and/or allow for instructions or corrections to be marked for the printer or camera operator.

overprinting—Printing over an area or page that has already been printed.

overrun—Production of more copies than the number ordered (see also **press run** and **print order**).

page proof—A proof set or printed in the form of the finished page (see also **proof**).

paginate—To number, mark, or arrange the pages of a document, manuscript, article, or book.

Pantone Matching System colors—See **PMS**.

paragraph—(1) A unit of text set off by indentation, horizontal space, bullets, or other typographical device. (2) A character (¶) used as a reference mark (see 2.13, Tables).

parallel— A character (‖) used as a reference mark (see 2.13, Manuscript Preparation, Tables).

paste-up—A mock assembly of the elements of type and artwork as a guide to the printer for makeup.

PC—Personal computer, usually self-contained (keyboard, monitor, printer, central processing unit, and memory devices), as opposed to a terminal or networked computer; often used to refer to IBM-compatible computers.

PDF—Abbreviation for page description format.

PDL—Abbreviation for page description language.

PE—Printer's error or publisher's error; used in correcting proofs to indicate an error attributable to the printer or publisher (see also **AA** and **EA**).

peer review—The process by which editors ask experts to read, criticize, and comment on the suitability of a manuscript for publication (see 4.0, Editorial Assessment and Processing, and 3.11.6, Ethical and Legal Considerations, Editorial Responsibility for Peer Review).

peer-reviewed journal—A journal containing editorial content that is peer reviewed.

penalty copy—Copy that is difficult to typeset (heavily corrected, difficult to read, heavy with tabular material, etc) for which the typesetter charges more than the regular rate.

perfect binding—Process in which signatures are collated, the gutter edge is cut and ground, adhesive is applied to the signatures, and the cover is applied (compare **loose-leaf binding, saddle-stitch binding,** and **spiral binding**).

perforate—To punch lines of small holes or slits in a sheet so that it can be torn off with ease.

photostat—A camera process that duplicates graphic matter; also the graphic matter thus produced.

pica—A unit of measure; 1 pica equals approximately $\frac{1}{6}$ in or 12 points (see also **point**).

pica type—Typewriter type that equals 10 characters to the inch (see also **elite type**).

pixel—A unit in a digital image; the smallest point of a bit-mapped screen that can be assigned independent color and intensity.

plate—(1) A sheet of metal, plastic, rubber, paperboard, or other material used as a printing surface; the means by which an image area is separated from a nonimage area. (2) A full-page, color book illustration, often printed on paper different from that used for the text matter.

PMS (Pantone Matching System) colors—A color identification system matching specific shades of approximately 500 colors with numbers and formulas for the corresponding inks, developed by Pantone Inc.

pockets—Sections on a binder in which individual signatures are placed and then selected as required for each copy to be bound (see also **signature**).

point—The printer's basic unit of measurement, often used to determine type size; 1 point equals approximately $\frac{1}{72}$ in); 12 points equal 1 pica (see also **pica**).

preprint—An article or part of a book printed and distributed or transmitted digitally before publication and/or review.

press form—See **form.**

press plates—The plates used to print multiple copies on the press (see also **plate**).

press run—The total number of copies of journals, books, or other materials printed.

print order—The number of copies of printed material ordered.

printout—Paper output of a printer or other device that produces normal-reading copy from computer-stored data.

process printing colors—Cyan, magenta, yellow, and black (CMYK); used to produce color illustrations in print publications.

program—A set of instructions for a computer. To program is to create such a set of instructions.

programmable key—A key on a computer's keyboard that, when pressed alone or in combination with other keys, produces a computer command (see also **macro** and **function key**).

proof—A hard copy of the text and graphic material of a document used to check accuracy of text, composition, positioning, and/or typesetting (see also **hard copy**).

proofreader—One who reads or reviews proofs for errors.

publisher—A person or entity that directs the production, dissemination, and sale of information.

pullout quotes—See **call-outs.**

ragged right—Type set with the right-hand margin unjustified (or ragged).

RAM—Acronym for random access memory; temporary computer memory used by a computer to hold data currently being processed or created that are lost when the computer is shut down.

raster image processor (RIP)—A device that produces a digital bit map to show an image's position on a page before printing (see also **bit map**).

RC (resin-coated) paper—Paper used in composition to produce a type proof of the quality needed for photographic reproduction.

ream—500 sheets of paper (see also **basis weight**).

recto—A right-hand page (compare **verso**).

redlining—A software program that shows changes made in a document to be seen on screen and on a printed typescript for review by the editor and author. Also called revision marking, strikethrough.

register—To print an impression on a sheet in correct relationship to other impressions already printed on the same sheet, eg, to superimpose exactly the various color impressions. When all parts or inks match exactly, they are *in register.* When such impressions are not exactly aligned, they are said to be *out of register.*

remake—To alter the makeup of a page or series of pages.

reprint—A reproduction of an original printing in paper or digital format.

reproduction proof—A high-quality proof for use in photoengraving or offset lithography.

resolution—A measurement of the visual quality of an image according to discrimination between distinct elements; the fineness of detail that can be distinguished in an image (see also **dots per inch**).

reverse-out, reverse text, or **reverse image**—Text or image that appears in white surrounded by a solid block of color or black.

RGB—Abbreviation for red, green, blue, the primary additive colors used in color computer monitors.

right-reading—Produced to read as original copy from right to left, as in right-reading film (compare **wrong-reading**).

RIP—See **raster image processor**.

river—A streak of white space running down through lines of type, breaking up the even appearance of the page; to be avoided.

roman—A typestyle with upright characters, as opposed to *italic* (see **italic** and 19.0, Typography).

RTF—Abbreviation for rich text format; a generic word-processing format that uses ASCII codes to preserve the formatting of a file (see also **ASCII**).

runaround—Type composed or set to fit around an illustration, box, or other design element.

run in—To merge a paragraph with the preceding paragraph.

running foot—A line of copy, usually giving publication name, subject, title, date, volume number, and/or authors' names, appearing at the bottom of consecutive pages.

running head—A line of copy, usually giving publication name, subject, title, date, volume number, and/or authors' names, appearing at the top of consecutive pages.

runover—Material not fitting in the space allowed (see also **live area** and **long page**).

saddle-stitch binding—Process by which signatures, or pages, and covers are assembled by inserting staples into the centerfold (see also **loose-leaf binding, perfect binding,** and **spiral binding**).

sans serif—An unadorned typeface; a letter without a short line projecting from the top or bottom of the main stroke of the letter, such as sans serif (compare **serif** and see 19.0, Typography).

scaling—Determining the appropriate size of an image and the amount of reduction or enlargement needed for the image to fit in a specific area.

scanner—A device that produces color-separated film or images; or a device that uses an electronic reader (eye) to transform type, characters, and images from a printed page into a digital form (see also **OCR**).

score—To indent or mark paper or cards slightly so they can be folded exactly at certain points.

screen—(1) The dot pattern produced to show tint or shade of color (see also **halftone screen**). (2) The face of a computer monitor.

scribe—Thin strips of nonprinting areas, such as those between figure parts.

selective binding—A method of binding in which specific contents of each copy produced are determined by instructions transmitted electronically from a computer. Signatures, or specific groups of pages, are selected to produce a copy for a specific recipient or recipient group (see also **binding** and **signature**).

self-cover—A cover for a publication that is made of the same paper used for the text and printed as part of a larger press form.

serif—An adorned typeface; a short, light line projecting from the top or bottom of a main stroke of a letter (compare **sans serif** and see 19.0, Typography).

server—A computer software package or hardware that provides specific services to other computers.

SGML—Abbreviation for standard generalized markup language; an international system of codes that determine the structural elements and hierarchy of those elements in a digital document. The content of the document is defined by its structure rather than its printed or composed appearance. The text is stored in ASCII and the codes (or tags) of the elements are recorded in a document type definition (DTD). An SGML editor (software program) uses the DTD to validate the coding. The SGML-coded text and the DTD make a digital document more portable and readable by a variety of platforms (see also **ASCII** and **DTD**).

SGML editor—A context-sensitive editor based on SGML (see also **context-specific editor**).

short page—In makeup, a page that runs shorter than the established live area (see also **makeup** and **live area**; compare **long page**).

show through—Inking that can be seen on the opposite side of the paper, because of either the heaviness of the ink or the thinness of the paper.

sidebar—Text or graphics placed in a box and printed on the right or left side of a page.

signature—(1) A printed sheet comprising several pages that have been folded, so that the pages are in consecutive order according to pagination. (2) A line of text appearing at the bottom of an article that lists the author(s).

sink—Starting type below the top line of the live area, which leaves an area of white space (see also **live area** and **white space**).

sizing—A process of adding material to a paper to make it more resistant to moisture.

slug—A line or lines of copy inserted to draw the attention of the reader, often set between rules in enlarged, bold type.

small caps—Capital letters that are smaller than the typical capital letters of a specific typeface, usually the size of the x-height of the font (see also **x-height** and 19.0, Typography).

software—Computer programs (compare **hardware**).

solid—Style of type set with no space between lines.

solidus—A forward slanted line (/) (see also **virgule** and 6.4, Punctuation, Virgule [Solidus]).

spacing—Lateral spaces between words, sentences, or columns; also paragraph indentions (see also **line spacing** and **leading**).

specifications—Often called "specs" for short; instructions given to the printer that include numbers of copies (print run); paper stock, coating, and size; color, typography, and design.

spine—The backbone of a perfect-bound journal or book. The width of the spine depends on the number and thickness of pages in the publication (see also **perfect binding**).

spiral binding—A process of binding a publication with wires or plastic in a spiral form inserted through holes along the binding side (see also **loose-leaf binding, perfect binding, saddle-stitch binding,** and **selective binding**).

spot color—One or more extra colors on a page.

spots per inch—A measure of the resolution of a printed image (see **dots per inch**).

standard generalized markup language—See **SGML**.

stet—Instruction that marked or crossed-out copy or type is to be retained as it originally appeared.

stock—Type of paper for printing.

storing data—Placing data in computer storage by recording the data in digital form on a magnetic, optical, or other medium, such as disks and tapes, either inside or outside the computer.

straight copy—Material that can be set in type with no handwork or special programming (copy that contains no mathematical equations, tables, etc).

strikethrough—To mark a character or amount of text for deletion by superimposing a line through the main body of the character(s).

strip—To join film in a unit according to a press imposition before platemaking.

style—A set of uniform rules to guide the application of grammar, spelling, typography, composition, and design.

subhead—A subordinate heading (see 19.0, Typography).

subscript—A number or symbol that prints partly below the baseline, eg, A_2 (inferior).

subscription—The price for a publication; usually set in annual terms.

superior—See **superscript.**

superscript—A number or symbol that prints partly above the baseline, eg, A^2 (superior).

SWK—Abbreviation for set when known.

SWOP—Abbreviation for specifications for web offset publications; a color proofing system used to check color consistency.

tag—To insert a style or composition code in a computer file or document.

tagged—Coded.

TCP/IP—Abbreviation for Transmission Control Protocol/Internet Protocol; the language governing communication between computers on the Internet.

tear sheet—A page cut or torn from a book or periodical.

text—The main body of type in a page, manuscript, article, or book.

TIFF—Acronym for tagged image file format; a file format that allows bit-mapped images to be exchanged between different computer applications; the preferred format for halftones (see also **bit map** and **halftones**).

tints—Various even tone areas of a solid color, usually expressed in percentages.

tip-in, tip-on—A sheet of paper or a signature glued to another signature before binding (see also **signature**).

TOC—Abbreviation for table of contents.

toner—Imaging material or ink used in photocopiers, computer printers, and some off-press proofing systems.

trademark—A legally registered word, name, symbol, slogan, or any combination of these, used to identify and distinguish products and services and to indicate the source and marketer of those products and services (see 3.6.14, Ethical and Legal Considerations, Trademark).

transpose (tr)—A proofreading and editing term meaning to switch the positions of 2 elements (eg, characters, words, sentences, or paragraphs).

trapping—The process of printing 1 ink on top of another to produce a third color.

trim—The edges that are cut off 3 sides—the top (head), bottom (foot), and right (face)—of a publication after binding.

trim line, trim marks—The line or marks indicated on copy to show where the page ends or needs to be cut.

trim size—The final size of the publication.

TTP—Abbreviation for text transfer protocol; a method for moving text from one place to another on the Internet (see also **FTP** and **Internet**).

turnaround time—The period of time between any 2 events in publishing (eg, between manuscript submission and acceptance, between manuscript scanning and telecommunication to the printer).

typeface—A named type design, such as Baskerville, Helvetica, or Times Roman, produced as a complete font (see 19.0, Typography).

type gauge—A type-measurement tool calibrated in picas and points.

typescript—A manuscript output by a computer printer or in typewritten form.

typesetter—A person, firm, or machine that sets type.

typestyle—The general characteristics of a typeface (eg, roman, bold, italic, and condensed) (see also **typeface** and 19.0, Typography).

underrun—Production of fewer printed copies than was ordered (see also **press run, print order,** and **overrun**).

UNIX—Not an abbreviation or acronym; a powerful operating system.

unjustified—A ragged or uneven margin (compare **justify** and see 19.0, Typography).

upload—To transfer a digital file or data from a local computer to a remote computer.

uppercase—A capital letter.

URL—Abbreviation for uniform resource locator; an address for a document or information available via the Internet or World Wide Web (eg, http://www.ama-assn.org).

verso—A left-hand page (compare **recto**).

virgule—A forward slanted line (/) used to separate numbers, letters, or other characters (see also **solidus**).

virus—A computer program, usually hidden in another program, that replicates and inserts itself into other programs without the user's knowledge and frequently causes harm to the programs or destroys data.

VR—Abbreviation for virtual reality.

WAIS—Abbreviation for wide-area information server (see **server**).

WAN—Abbreviation for wide-area network (see **network**).

watermark—An image or set of characters produced by thinning a specific area of paper that is visible when the paper is held up to light; often used to show a company logo.

web, Web—(1) Short for offset lithographic printing press. (2) Short for online text and graphical information accessed via a computer browser (see also **World Wide Web**). (3) A continuous roll of paper.

Web browser—A program for quickly searching and accessing information on the World Wide Web.

web press—A lithographic press that prints on a continuous roll (web) of paper.

well—A part of a journal, usually the middle pages, in which advertising is not allowed; usually reserved for important scientific and clinical articles in biomedical journals. Regular features, such as news articles, essays, letters, and book reviews, are typically run outside the editorial well, where ad interspersion may be allowed.

white space—The area of a page that is free of any text or graphics (compare **live area**).

widow—A short line ending a paragraph and positioned at the top of a page or column, to be avoided (compare **orphan**; see also **bad break**).

word processor—A general term for a computer program with which text consisting of words and figures can be input, edited, recorded, stored, and printed.

World Wide Web (WWW)—Online text and graphical information accessed via a Web browser (see also **Web**).

wrong font (wf)—Incorrect or inconsistent type size or typeface (see also **font**).

wrong-reading—Produced to read as a mirror image (from left to right) of the original copy, usually refers to film (compare **right-reading**).

WWW—See **World Wide Web.**

WYSIWYG—(Pronounced *wizzy wig*); acronym for what you see is what you get; meaning that which is displayed on the computer screen is essentially how the final product will appear after printing.

x-height—A vertical measurement of a letter, usually equal to the height of a lowercase letter without ascenders or descenders (ie, x) (see also **ascenders** and **descenders**).

yellow—One of the 4 process printing colors (cyan, magenta, yellow, and black) (see **CMYK**).

ACKNOWLEDGMENTS

Principal author: Annette Flanagin, RN, MA

The following reviewed this section and offered suggestions for revision: Charl Richey, Mary Steermann.

DEFINITIONS FOR THIS GLOSSARY WERE COMPILED FROM THE FOLLOWING SOURCES

A Glossary of Printing and Publishing Terms. Dayton, Ohio: Mead Corp; 1995.

Glossary of Common Internet Terms. Lawrence, Kan: Allen Press Inc; July/August 1995:7. Allen Press Inc Journal Promotion Series.

Glossary of technical terms. In: *The Chicago Manual of Style.* 14th ed. Chicago, Ill: University of Chicago Press; 1993:831-859.

Graphic arts terms. In: Bruno MH, ed. *Pocket Pal: A Graphic Arts Production Handbook.* 15th ed. Memphis, Tenn: International Paper Co; 1992:185-214.

Internet Literacy Consultants. ILC Glossary of Internet Terms. Available at: http://www.matise.net/files/glossary.html. Accessed October 16, 1996.

Lawson AE, Agner D. *Printing Types.* Boston, Mass: Beacon Press; 1990.

Merriam-Webster's Collegiate Dictionary. 10th ed. Springfield, Mass: Merriam-Webster Inc; 1993.

Merriam-Webster's WWWebster Dictionary. Available at: http://www.m-w.com. Accessed November 12, 1996.

Microsoft Encarta [book on CD-ROM]. Funk & Wagnalls Corp; 1994.

The Allen Press Guide to Electronic Publishing. Lawrence, Kan: Allen Press Inc. Allen Press Inc Journal Promotion Series.

The American Heritage Dictionary of the English Language. 3rd ed. Boston, Mass: Houghlin Mifflin Co; 1992.

CHAPTER 22

22.0 RESOURCES

Works consulted in the preparation of this manual are cited in and listed at the end of each chapter.

22.1 ■ READINGS.

22.1.1 *Dictionaries*

The American Heritage Dictionary of the English Language. 3rd ed. Boston, Mass: Houghton Mifflin Co; 1992.

Dorland's Illustrated Medical Dictionary. 28th ed. Philadelphia, Pa: WB Saunders Co; 1994.

Merriam-Webster's Collegiate Dictionary. 10th ed. Springfield, Mass: Merriam-Webster Inc; 1993. Also available at: http://www.m-w.com.

Flexner SB, ed in chief; Hauck LC, managing ed. *The Random House Dictionary of the English Language.* 2nd ed, unabridged. New York, NY: Random House; 1993.

Stedman's Medical Dictionary. 26th ed. Baltimore, Md: Williams & Wilkins; 1995.

22.1.2 *Guides to General, Scientific, and Technical Usage*

American Psychological Association. *Publication Manual of the American Psychological Association.* 4th ed. Washington, DC: American Psychological Association; 1994.

ASM Style Manual for Journals and Books. Washington, DC: American Society of Microbiology; 1991.

Bernstein TM. *The Careful Writer: A Modern Guide to English Usage.* New York, NY: Atheneum; 1984.

Bernstein TM. *Dos, Don'ts & Maybes of English Usage.* New York, NY: Times Book; 1977.

Bernstein TM. *Miss Thistlebottom's Hobgoblins: The Careful Writer's Guide to the Taboos, Bugbears and Outmoded Rules of English Usage.* New York, NY: Simon & Schuster; 1971.

Bishop CT. *How to Edit a Scientific Journal.* Philadelphia, Pa: ISI Press; 1984.

Brooks BS, Pinson JL. *Working With Words: A Concise Handbook for Media Writers and Editors.* 2nd ed. New York, NY: St Martins Press; 1993.

The Chicago Manual of Style. 14th ed. Chicago, Ill: University of Chicago Press; 1993.

Day RA. *How to Write & Publish a Scientific Paper.* 4th ed. Phoenix, Ariz: Oryx Press; 1994.

Day RA. *Scientific English: A Guide for Scientists and Other Professionals.* 2nd ed. Phoenix, Ariz: Oryx Press; 1996.

Dodd JS, ed. *The ACS Style Guide: A Manual for Authors and Editors.* Washington, DC: American Chemical Society; 1985.

Fishbein M. *Medical Writing: The Technic and the Art.* 4th ed. Springfield, Ill: Charles C Thomas Publisher; 1978.

Follett W; Barzun J, ed. *Modern American Usage: A Guide.* New York, NY: Hill & Wang; 1966.

Fowler HW; Gowers E, ed. *A Dictionary of Modern English Usage.* 2nd ed. New York, NY: Oxford University Press; 1965.

Fowler HW. *The New Fowler's Modern English Usage.* 3rd ed. New York, NY: Oxford University Press; 1997.

Gordon KE. *The Transitive Vampire: A Handbook of Grammar for the Innocent, the Eager, and the Doomed.* New York, NY: Times Books; 1984.

Gordon KE. *The Well-Tempered Sentence: A Punctuation Handbook for the Innocent, the Eager, and the Doomed.* New Haven, Conn: Ticknor & Fields; 1983.

Huth EJ. *How to Write and Publish Papers in the Medical Sciences.* 2nd ed. Baltimore, Md: Williams & Wilkins; 1990.

Jablonski S. *Dictionary of Medical Acronyms & Abbreviations.* 2nd ed. Philadelphia, Pa: Hanley & Belfus Inc; 1993.

King LS. *Why Not Say It Clearly: A Guide to Expository Writing.* 2nd ed. Boston, Mass: Little Brown & Co Inc; 1991.

Logan CM, Rice MK. *Logan's Medical and Scientific Abbreviations.* Philadelphia, Pa: JB Lippincott Co; 1987.

Longman's Language Activator. White Plains, NY: Addison Wesley; 1993.

Maggio R. *The Dictionary of Bias-Free Usage: A Guide to Nondiscriminatory Language.* Phoenix, Ariz: Oryx Press; 1991.

Marriott FHC. *A Dictionary of Statistical Terms.* 5th ed. Essex, England: Longman Scientific & Technical; 1990.

Miller C, Swift K. *The Handbook of Nonsexist Writing.* New York, NY: Lippincott & Crowell; 1980.

Moxley JM. *Publish, Don't Perish: The Scholar's Guide to Academic Writing and Publishing.* Westport, Conn: Praeger Publishers; 1992.

Rubens P, ed. *Science and Technical Writing: A Manual of Style.* New York, NY: Henry Holt & Co; 1992.

Schwartz M, and the Task Force on Bias-Free Language of the Association of American University Presses. *Guidelines for Bias-Free Writing.* Bloomington: Indiana University Press; 1995.

Strunk W Jr, White EB. *The Elements of Style.* 3rd ed. New York, NY: Macmillan Publishing Co Inc; 1994.

Council of Biology Editors Style Manual Committee. *Scientific Style and Format: The CBE Manual for Authors, Editors, and Publishers.* 6th ed. New York, NY: Cambridge University Press; 1994.

Sutcliffe AJ, ed. *The New York Public Library Writer's Guide to Style and Usage.* New York, NY: HarperCollins Publishers; 1994.

Warriner JE. *English Grammar and Composition: Complete Course.* Franklin ed. New York, NY: Harcourt Brace Jovanovich Publishers; 1982.

Webster's Dictionary of English Usage. Springfield, Mass: Merriam-Webster Inc; 1989.

Zinsser W. *On Writing Well: An Informal Guide to Writing Nonfiction.* 2nd ed. New York, NY: Harper & Row Publishers Inc; 1980.

22.1.3 *Guides to Illustration Design and Format*

Briscoe MH. *Preparing Scientific Illustrations: A Guide to Better Posters, Presentations, and Publications.* 2nd ed. New York, NY: Springer-Verlag; 1996.

Cleveland WS. *The Elements of Graphing Data.* Summit, NJ: Hobart Press; 1994.

Council of Biology Editors Scientific Illustration Committee. *Illustrating Science: Standards for Publication.* Bethesda, Md: Council of Biology Editors Inc; 1988.

Tufte ER. *Envisioning Information.* Cheshire, Conn: Graphics Press; 1990.

Tufte ER. *The Visual Display of Quantitative Information.* Cheshire, Conn: Graphics Press; 1983.

Tufte ER. *Visual Explanations: Images and Quantities, Evidence and Narrative.* Cheshire, Conn: Graphics Press; 1997.

22.2 ■ PROFESSIONAL WRITING, EDITING, AND COMMUNICATIONS ORGANIZATIONS AND GROUPS.

American Medical Writers Association
9650 Rockville Pike
Bethesda, MD 20814
Telephone: (301) 493-0003
Fax: (301) 493-6384
E-mail: amwa@amwa.org
Newsletter: *AMWA News*
Journal: *AMWA Journal*

Association of Earth Science Editors
781 Northwest Dr
Morgantown, WV 26505
Telephone: (304) 599-2865
(304) 285-4679
Newsletter: *The Blueline*

Board of Editors in the Life Sciences
PO Box 824
Highlands, NC 28741-0824
Telephone: (202) 334-2230
Fax: (704) 526-9138
Newsletter: *BELS Letter*

Council of Biology Editors, Inc
60 Revere Dr
Suite 500
Northbrook, IL 60062
Telephone: (847) 480-6349
Fax: (847) 480-9282
E-mail: cbehdqts@aol.com
Journal: *CBE Views*

European Association of Science Editors
c/o Maeve O'Connor
49 Rossendale Way
London NW1 OXB, England
Telephone: 171-3889668
Fax: 171-3833092
E-mail: secretary@ease.org.uk
Newsletter: *EASE Bulletin*

International Committee of Medical Journal Editors
c/o Secretariat Office
Annals of Internal Medicine
Independence Mall West
Sixth Street at Race
Philadelphia, PA 19106-1572
Telephone: (800) 523-1546, extension 2631

Society for Scholarly Publishing
10200 W 44th Ave
Suite 304
Wheat Ridge, CO 80033
Telephone: (303) 422-3914
Newsletter: *Scholarly Publishing Today*
Journal: *Journal of Scholarly Publishing*

Society for Technical Communication
901 N Stuart St
Suite 904
Arlington, VA 22203-1854
Telephone: (703) 522-4114
E-mail: stc@stc-va.org
Newsletter: *Intercom*
Journal: *Technical Communication*

22.3 ■ **ONLINE RESOURCES.**—Biomedicine is well represented by a wide variety of online resources, including large bibliographic databases, full-text databases, cataloging databases, and online journals. Timeliness and flexibility make these online resources particularly attractive to health professionals and researchers as an aid to biomedical investigation. Online searching has revolutionized the ease and efficiency with which biomedical and scientific research is performed. These databases provide organized and easy access to vast caches of information and are invaluable when used properly, but frustrating and potentially expensive when not. For the uninitiated, access and retrieval can be daunting. Without proper technique, a search can easily be too broad or too narrow, or so far afield as to retrieve virtually useless information. Many commercial services offer software interfaces that make it easier for a novice, although some rudimentary training is still required. Training or the assistance of a well-trained online researcher, such as a research librarian, can help ensure that information obtained from a search is appropriately sensitive and specific—that is, that the search is broad enough to capture all relevant articles but not so broad that it retrieves unrelated or irrelevant information.

To present an organized approach to the vast number of online services and access methods available for biomedical bibliographic databases, at this time, this section first provides a description of selected databases, followed by descriptions of the common access methods. Larger and more established databases that provide coverage for a significant number of years and reference a broad base of journals for the particular area of interest have been included.

Many online services began as counterparts to print index services, but the scope of the online services has expanded greatly. Some online services have become new entities unto themselves with resources and features far exceeding those of the original product. The online format has allowed for enhancement of the different index services and the inclusion of increasingly larger tracts of information. Most bibliographic services now include abstracts, comments, corrections, and even proceedings from applicable meetings and conferences.

Another valuable feature of some online databases and services is the built-in thesaurus or subject-heading trees. The thesaurus or index tree provides subject-heading vocabulary arranged hierarchically for precise retrieval of indexed literature. This allows the researcher to broaden or narrow the search parameters within a given subject area by simply scrolling up or down the hierarchically arranged subject index. The subject-heading tree also furnishes a visual representation of the subject-heading index logic. These thesauruses are usually part of the database or else an enhancement provided as part of a commercial software interface.

22.3.1 *Databases.*

BIOSIS: BIOSIS began as the online counterpart to *Biological Abstracts,* the BioSciences Information Services' print index service. BIOSIS is used for biological and biochemical research. The span of coverage is 1969 to the present. BIOSIS references approximately 6500 peer-reviewed journals.

CA Search: CA Search began as the online counterpart to *Chemical Abstracts,* the American Chemical Society's print index service. The focus of CA Search is on chemistry, toxicology, and chemical engineering literature. The span of coverage is 1967 to the present.

CINAHL (Cumulative Index to Nursing and Allied Health): The CINAHL database began as the online counterpart to the *Cumulative Index to Nursing and Allied Health Literature*, and is now the print index of the Glendale Adventist Hospital of Loma Linda, Calif. The focus of the database is nursing and the allied health professions literature. The span of coverage is 1983 to the present. The CINAHL references approximately 550 peer-reviewed journals.

EMBASE: EMBASE began as the online counterpart to *Excerpta Medica* and *Drug Literature Index,* Elsevier Publishing's print index services. EMBASE is used for biomedical and drug research. It focuses more on European sources of biomedical literature, which can be helpful when searching clinical applications and pharmacologic techniques not in common practice in North America. The span of coverage is 1974 to the present. EMBASE references approximately 3500 peer-reviewed journals.

HEALTHSTAR (Health Planning and Administration/Health Services, Technology, Administration and Research): HEALTHSTAR is an online bibliographic database that provides access to published literature covering health services technology, administration, and research. It is produced cooperatively by the National Library of Medicine and the American Hospital Association. HEALTHSTAR is the merger of HEALTH (Health Planning and Administration), produced in cooperation with the American Hospital Association, and HSTAR (Health Services/ Technology Assessment Research), initiated by the National Library of Medicine's National Information Center on Health Services Research and Health Care Technology. HEALTHSTAR incorporates the subject scopes of both HEALTH and HSTAR by citing literature on health care administration, economics, planning, and policy, as well as health services research, clinical practice guidelines, and health care technology assessment. It includes relevant MEDLINE records from 1975 forward, CATLINE records from 1985 forward, and unique records from 3 other sources. There is some overlap between the HEALTHSTAR database and MEDLINE, but duplicate retrieval can be avoided by using a specific search technique that can exclude MEDLINE references.

MEDLINE: MEDLINE began as the online counterpart to *Index Medicus*, the US National Library of Medicine's general medicine print index service, the *Index to Dental Literature*, and the *International Nursing Index*. Its sources include the biomedical, dental, health care administration, and nursing literature. The span of coverage is 1966 to the present. MEDLINE references approximately 3900 peer-reviewed journals. MEDLINE is the best known and most widely used of the online biomedical bibliographic databases. It includes abstracts, comments, and corrections where applicable. MEDLINE is one of a family of databases, designated MEDLARS, produced by the US National Library of Medicine.

PsychINFO: PsychINFO began as the online counterpart to *Psychological Abstracts*, the American Psychological Association's print index service. The focus of the database is psychology and related fields, such as sociology and psychiatry. The span of coverage is 1967 to the present.

Other US National Library of Medicine (NLM) Databases: Medical Literature Analysis and Retrieval System (MEDLARS) is the computerized database system of the NLM. MEDLARS consists of nearly 40 online databases, of which MEDLINE is the most renowned. Following are some of the other NLM online databases.

AIDSDRUGS. The companion database to AIDSTRIALS. This database contains descriptive information about the agents being tested in clinical trials.

AIDSLINE. The focus of the database is acquired immunodeficiency syndrome (AIDS) and related topics. AIDSLINE provides bibliographic citations to journal articles, government reports, technical reports, meeting proceedings, monographs, special publications, theses, books, and information on audiovisual materials. AIDSLINE provides AIDS literature and information from MEDLINE, CANCERLIT, HEALTHSTAR, CATLINE, AVLINE, and BIOETHICSLINE databases. AIDSLINE references more than 3000 peer-reviewed journals.

AIDSTRIALS. The database provides information on clinical trials related to AIDS, AIDS-related opportunistic diseases, and human immunodeficiency virus infection.

Avline. This focus of the database is biomedical audiovisual materials and computer software information from the NLM since 1975.

Bioethicsline. This database provides bibliographic citations to literature on ethics and public policy issues in health care and biomedical research and is maintained by NLM and the Kennedy Institute of Ethics at Georgetown University, Washington, DC. It also provides citation of newspaper articles, court decisions, bills, laws, and information on audiovisual material. The span of coverage is 1973 to the present.

Cancerlit. This database is produced by the US National Cancer Institute in cooperation with NLM. The focus of the database is major cancer topics. The span of comprehensive coverage is 1976 to the present (some citations are as early as 1963).

Catline. This database contains bibliographic records of virtually all of the cataloged titles in the NLM collection. This includes monographs, monograph series, serials, audiovisual series, and manuscripts. The span is the 15th century to the present.

Chemline. This database is an online dictionary of chemical substances. Each record is for a particular substance and provides information on the structure and nomenclature, synonyms, and Chemical Abstract Service registry numbers.

Histline. This database began as the online counterpart to *Bibliography of the History of Medicine*. It now offers bibliographic citations on the history of medicine and other related subjects. The span of coverage is 1964 to the present and includes citations to monographs, journal articles, and publications from congresses and symposia. References are primarily derived from MEDLINE and CATLINE.

Pdq. This is a menu-driven database maintained by the US National Cancer Institute for recent advances in cancer treatment, cancer treatment protocols, clinical trials, and a directory of physicians, institutes, and organizations involved in cancer treatment and research.

Toxline. This database is a collection of bibliographic citations in the area of pharmacologic, biochemical, and toxicologic effects of drugs and other chemicals. The citations are provided by a variety of subfile producers, including NLM, the Hazardous Materials Technical Center, and the Toxicology Research Projects.

Bibliographic vs Full-Text Searches: Searching a particular topic by means of bibliographic indexing terms will be most effective when that topic has been assigned a subject heading within a given database. The precise and defined organization of subject headings and, where available, the logical outline of a subject-heading index tree or thesaurus allow for narrow or broad searching depending on the researcher's needs.

By contrast, a successful full-text search depends on correctly anticipating the exact words used in the text. Different modes of expression and a desire to capture all pertinent references in a full-text database can make a search so broad it becomes useless. Even correctly anticipating the author's phrasing can occasionally be foiled, on rare occasions, by typographical errors or technical mishaps when the text is electronically transferred into a full-text database. Full-text searching can become difficult and time-consuming. However, a full-text search can be the best way to locate an article that references the brand name of a drug or a particular service, a jargon phrase, or cutting-edge technology not yet provided a subject heading. Many of the bibliographic databases allow for full-text searching of their abstracts simultaneously with a subject-heading search, which can be quite useful. A full-text article correctly identified also provides more information than an abstract in a bibliographically organized database and allows for downloading of the entire article when no hard copy is available. Most full-text databases are provided by commercial online services. Some are also available on CD-ROM services.

22.3.2 *Access.*

CD-ROM Systems: CD-ROM refers to read-only access to a database that is contained on a compact disc (CD). Read-only means that information cannot be saved to the disc, but information can be downloaded from the CD. CD-ROM access to bibliographic and full-text database services can be valuable to those who lack online access or to someone who uses a particular database frequently. The information provided by CD-ROM access is not as timely as a direct online connection, since the discs must be updated periodically. Most services send either monthly or quarterly updates for their discs. Thus, when a disc is newly updated, the quality and outcome of the search are similar to those of an online search of the same database. A CD-ROM search can also be time-consuming when a number of discs must be searched (such as searching a sizable database over a large span of years). This necessitates the loading and reloading of the CDs, which is easily overcome on a network service that has downloaded the discs en masse.

The CD-ROM format offers many advantages. One CD can hold full text records of an entire monograph series or a several years of a complete journal. A CD-ROM service can also offer rapid access to full-color graphics and tables. Many CD-ROM services offer enhanced versions of databases by combining a number of pertinent databases or a database with monographs and other reference sources that can be researched by a single search technique. There are also CD-ROM services that have interface software that links to the Internet. This interface updates and enhances the information contained on the CD-ROM, making it as current as its online counterpart.

The Internet: The Internet can provide direct access to online interfaces for many databases and the World Wide Web. Many commercial services provide access to the Internet and also provide software that offers assistance in navigating the Internet's many sites and access points. The Internet also allows for the exchange of information and full-text files.

One helpful way to access information is through the World Wide Web (WWW). Many organizations, government agencies, and publishers, such as the American Medical Association, US National Institutes of Health, and US National Library of Medicine, have organized "home pages" or "Web sites." From a WWW home page, the user can connect to other Internet sites by means of the "links" provided. The home page is usually organized by subject matter or specialty and, when well organized, leads one in a logical fashion to links with other related information sources.

Another useful aspect of the Internet is the potential for dialogue with authors and fellow researchers. Newsgroups allow for just such a connection and provide a forum for collecting information, leads, and opinions. A user "subscribes" to a group where news, information, and questions are posted to be answered by anyone accessing the newsgroup by adding the group to his or her newsgroup address book. The posted query is ideally answered by someone who has the knowledge and expertise required, or who can refer one to a colleague who does. A list of medically related newsgroups is maintained by The Johns Hopkins University (http://world-health.net/newsgroup.html). Newsgroups run the gamut from diabetes discussion groups (misc.health.diabetes) to telemedicine groups (sci.med.telemedicine) and even politics (talk.politics.medicine).

22.3.3 ***Resources***.—The aforementioned list of databases and access methods and services is by no means comprehensive. For more detailed information, contact a research librarian. One good resource for general information on particular databases and for locating the services that provide access to each database is the *Gale Directory of Databases*.

The following is a sample of World Wide Web addresses and home pages (the addresses are subject to change):

AltaVista*	http://altavista.digital.com/
American Medical Association (access to *JAMA* and the AMA *Archives* Journals)	http://www.ama-assn.org/
Annals of Internal Medicine	http://www.acponline.org/journals/annals/annaltoc.htm/
British Medical Journal	http://www.bmj.com/bmj/
Centers for Disease Control and Prevention	http://www.cdc.gov/
Human Genome Database	http://gdbwww.gdb.org/
Infoseek*	http://guide.infoseek.com/
Institute of Medicine	http://www.nas.edu/iom/
The Lancet	http://www.thelancet.com/
National Academy of Science	http://www.nas.edu/
National Institutes of Health	http://www.nih.gov/
National Library of Medicine	http://www.nlm.nih.gov/
Nature	http://www.nature.com/
New England Journal of Medicine	http://www.nejm.org/
Oncolink	http://cancer.med.upenn.edu/
Physician's Guide to the Internet	http://www.webcom.com/pgil/
PubMed	http://www.ncbi.nlm.nih.gov/PubMed
Science	http://science-mag.org/
Virtual Hospital	http://vh.radiology.uiowa.edu/
Web Crawler*	http://webcrawler.com/
World Health Organization	http://www.who.ch/
Yahoo*	http://www.yahoo.com/

*World Wide Web search engines.

22.4 ■ OTHER SERVICES.

Copy Editor (newsletter)
Editorial Office
149 Fifth Ave
Suite 1207
New York, NY 10010-6801
Telephone: (212) 757-2645
Fax: (212) 995-2147
E-mail: maryproto@delphi.com
World Wide Web: http://www.copyeditor.com (on which a comprehensive guide called Workshops for Copy Editors is also available)

The Editorial Eye (newsletter)
EEI
66 Canal Center Plaza
Suite 200
Alexandria, VA 22314-5507
Telephone: (703) 683-0683
Fax: (703) 683-4915
E-mail: info@eei-alex.com
World Wide Web: http://www.eei-alex.com/eye/

Grammar Hotline Directory
Writing Center
Tidewater Community College
1700 College Crescent
Virginia Beach, VA 23456
(Updated annually in January; send a self-addressed stamped envelope.)

Language Research Service
PO Box 281
Springfield, MA 01102
(Questions answered about entries in *Merriam-Webster's Collegiate Dictionary*; send a self-addressed stamped envelope.)

Purdue University On-Line Writing Lab (OWL)
E-mail: owl@sage.cc.purdue.edu
World Wide Web: http://owl.trx.purdue.edu

ACKNOWLEDGMENTS

Principal authors: Roxanne K. Young, ELS, for sections 22.0 through 22.2 and 22.4; Brian P. Pace, MA, Assistant Editor, *JAMA*, for section 22.3.

INDEX

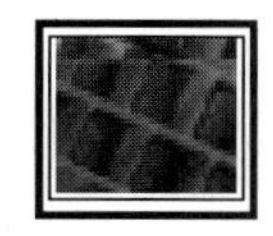

ACKNOWLEDGMENT

Principal author: Jane C. Lantz, ELS